Behavioral Endocrinology

Behavioral Endocrinology

edited by Jill B. Becker, S. Marc Breedlove, and David Crews

A Bradford Book
The MIT Press
Cambridge, Massachusetts
London, England

Second printing, 1992
© 1992 Massachusetts Institute of Technology

This book was set in Trump and Helvetica by Asco Trade Typesetting Ltd., Hong Kong and was printed and bound in the United States of America.

Library of Congress Cataloging-in-Publication Data

Behavioral endocrinology/Jill B. Becker, S. Marc Breedlove, and
  David Crews, editors.
  p. cm.
 "A Bradford book."
 Includes bibliographical references and index.
 ISBN 0-262-02342-3. —ISBN 0-262-52171-7 (pbk.)
 1. Psychoneuroendocrinology. 2. Hormones—Physiological effects.
3. Physiology, Comparative. I. Becker, Jill B. II. Breedlove, S.
Marc. III. Crews, David.
 [DNLM: 1. Behavior—drug effects. 2. Hormones—metabolism.
3. Psychophysiology. WK 102 B419]
QP356.45.B444 1992
152—dc20
DNLM/DLC
for Library of Congress   91-29932
                CIP

Contents in Brief

Contents in Detail

Preface

What is behavioral endocrinology, and why study it? All of us understand the importance of behavior—it is the fabric of society. Endocrinology is the study of hormones, the chemical messengers that travel through the bloodstream to transmit information from one part of the body to another. The brain is often a source or a target of these messengers, and behaviors originate from brain activity, so hormones sometimes have a powerful effect on behavior. During the past fifty years or so, the field of behavioral endocrinology has arisen to study how hormones alter behavior and also how behavior affects hormone release.

Why should anyone offer or take a course in behavioral endocrinology? Many people in our society believe that hormones can affect our moods and behavior. It is widely accepted that some athletes taking anabolic steroids can become dangerously aggressive, that some women experience intense mood shifts during parts of their menstrual cycle, and that men and women are biologically destined to differ in mathematical and other intellectual abilities. There are also strongly held but quite divergent opinions about whether people are "born with" a homosexual orientation, whether hormones force men to be promiscuous, and whether the mental abilities of women are affected by their menstrual cycle, as well as about the extent to which males and females differ and are similar. Although many of our social policies and attitudes are built upon these opinions, remarkably little solid information is available to evaluate the ideas. However, we do have some information, some hints of what is going on, and a scientific point of view reveals the important issues and complications inherent in all of these questions. Thus, we can use this information to temper our judgments and decisions. We are not suggesting that instruction in behavioral endocrinology should be required of all students, just that the questions addressed in such a course are relevant to all of our lives.

Psychologists and neuroscientists have long been interested in how thoughts, memories, and behavior patterns are physically represented in the nervous system. These are very challenging questions that will not be fully answered for a long time. The only practical approach to the study of these questions is to compare individuals who display a particular behavior to individuals who do not display that behavior. If the nervous system of one group has a different structure or physiological response than the nervous system of the other group, then that difference may be responsible for the differences in their behavior. Hormones are excellent candidates as causes of such differences: If animals treated with a hormone act differently from animals not treated with that hormone, then we can examine where the hormone goes in the animals' body and what the hormone does there, keeping a special lookout for effects on the nervous system. If we track down these two questions with enough ingenuity and caution, we will eventually discover the changes in the structure or function of the nervous system that caused the change in behavior. As we will see, scientists have made considerable progress in answering these questions for simple behaviors in animals and, by building upon such knowledge, we should one day understand the factors affecting more complicated human behaviors.

Biologists have long recognized that hormones can have profound influences on the physiology of animals. What is sometimes overlooked is the effect these same hormones can have on behavior and how the behavioral experience of the animals can in turn affect hormone release. Also, because males and females produce different hormones, it is important for biologists to be aware of how these different hormones may affect their anatomical or physiological measures. Furthermore, many stressful experiences, including some found in the laboratory, can cause the release of hormones that will affect most physiological processes. Even nonstressful experiences, such as exposure to an animal of the opposite sex, can affect hormone release. Finally, because hormones are released in particular patterns across the day, a drug or manipulation that has one effect on an animal in the morning may have no effect (or an opposite effect) in the late afternoon! Only by learning about how hormones affect behavior and how behavior affects hormones can biologists remain alert for such complications.

What does this textbook offer? Because we believe these issues are important and interesting, we have tried to produce a textbook on behavioral endocrinology for undergraduates who have had little previous exposure to physiology. Our aim is to reach students who have taken an introductory survey course in biology or physiological psychology. This book will allow those with such preparation to learn in some detail what hormones are, how they affect cells, and how such effects can alter the behavior of animals. We assume that the reader may need a refresher course and have therefore written an introductory chapter to cover this basic material. Therefore the first chapter is longer than is traditional for textbooks these days. However, much of the chapter will be familiar to all students, although most students will find some material that is new to them. Furthermore, nearly all of the topics in chapter 1 will resurface later and will be dealt with in more detail in subsequent chapters.

Every textbook reflects the strengths and interests of its authors. First of all, we felt it was important to address the question of whether hormones also alter the behavior of that most fascinating and troublesome animal species, humans. Although the data for humans are, in almost all respects, less conclusive and more conflicting than those for other animals, we believe it is important to review human data with an open yet critical mind. Some students will be uncomfortable with the ambiguity inherent in such a careful discussion, but we believe it is important that our conclusions be thorough and cautious. More research is needed to determine how different hormones affect behavior in humans. However, only by accurately and objectively representing what is currently known can we hope to ask the important questions in future research.

Second, we wanted to produce a text that considered more than just rats, mice, and humans, despite the fact that the vast majority of studies focus on these three species. As Frank Beach, one of the founders of behavioral endocrinology, stated, an appreciation of the variety of ways different species solve life's problems (mate selection, copulation, and food gathering, among others) has importance for understanding both the general and special ways in which hormones and behavior are interrelated. Thus, we will discuss the effects of hormones on the behavior of frogs, snakes, lizards, birds, hyenas, and insects. Because rats are far and away the most studied species, we will talk about them a great deal, but we hope to stir interest in other organisms as well.

Finally, we consciously decided to present a broad continuum of levels of analysis, from the molecular to the evolutionary. We will discuss in some detail the ways genes work, the structure of cells, the interactions of endocrine organs, the behavior of individuals, the structure of social hierarchies, and the evolution of mating systems, all in one book! There are very few fields of study in which one could even attempt such an integration.

For some of us, the range of approach in this field of study is another attraction of behavioral endocrinology. Because of the diversity of expertise involved, we chose to ask experts in each field of research to write chapters for this book. We know that there are style differences among chapters, and we hope that this is not too distracting. We hope readers agree that each author's enthusiasm for his or her subfield comes through and gives the student a feeling for the excitement of research in behavioral endocrinology. So get started, have fun, and let us know what you think about the book and this field.

Contributors

Michael J. Baum

Department of Biology
Boston University

Jill B. Becker

Department of Psychology
The University of Michigan

S. Marc Breedlove

Department of Psychology
University of California, Berkeley

Eliot Brenowitz

Department of Psychology
University of Washington

C. Sue Carter

Department of Zoology
University of Maryland

David Crews

Departments of Zoology and Psychology
The University of Texas, Austin

John Dark

Department of Psychology
University of California, Berkeley

Stephen E. Glickman

Department of Psychology
University of California, Berkeley

Elizabeth Hampson

Department of Psychology
University of Western Ontario

Darcy B. Kelley

Department of Biological Sciences
Columbia University

Doreen Kimura

Department of Psychology
University of Western Ontario

Edward P. Monaghan

Department of Psychology
University of California, Berkeley

Lawrence P. Morin — Department of Psychiatry
State University of New York, Stony Brook

Jay S. Rosenblatt — Institute of Animal Behavior
Rutgers University

Robert M. Sapolsky — Department of Biological Sciences
Stanford University

Rae Silver — Department of Psychology
Barnard College

Edward M. Stricker — Department of Behavioral Neuroscience
University of Pittsburgh

James W. Truman — Department of Zoology
University of Washington

Joseph G. Verbalis — Department of Medicine
University of Pittsburgh School of Medicine

Behavioral Endocrinology

I Introduction

1 Introduction to Behavioral Endocrinology

Jill B. Becker and S. Marc Breedlove

In this first chapter we review the basic principles of how hormones and the nervous system work. That means that this information will be packed rather densely. But students should have been exposed to most of the information before, and virtually all of these topics will be dealt with in specific examples in later chapters. This chapter is intended to be used as a reminder and a reference source for the basic concepts needed to appreciate the information given in the chapters that follow.

Some of the questions you should focus on while reading this chapter include: What are hormones, what are the different kinds of hormones, and how do they change biological processes? How does the brain control hormones, and how do hormones affect the brain? How does one measure behavior and hormones?

The Study of Behavioral Endocrinology

Behavioral endocrinology is the study of how hormones influence an animal's behavior. The Swedish scientist A. A. Berthold is credited with conducting the first formal experiments in behavioral endocrinology in 1849. We have learned a great deal since Berthold's time, but the basic logic and experimental design used for demonstrating a causal relationship between hormones and behavior is the same now as it was then.

Berthold removed the testes of a rooster and observed the animal's behavior. He found that the rooster no longer crowed nor engaged in sexual or aggressive behavior. When Berthold reimplanted one testis in the body cavity, the castrated rooster once again began crowing and also exhibited normal sexual behavior and aggression. The reimplanted testis did not reestablish nerve connections, so Berthold concluded that some chemical, produced by the testes and released into the general circulatory system, influenced the rooster's behavior.

We now know that the effect produced by the grafted testis can be mimicked by administering the hormone **testosterone** to a castrated rooster. Testosterone is the main hormone synthesized and released by the testes of male vertebrates. A causal relationship between the presence of a certain hormone (testosterone) in the circulatory system and behavior (crowing, sexual behavior, aggressive behavior) is established by conducting experiments to show that when the hormone is present, certain behaviors are more likely to occur.

The same kinds of experiments are conducted in behavioral endocrinology today. In order to show that a particular behavior is influenced by a particular hormone, the scientist must demonstrate that the frequency of the behavior changes when the endocrine gland producing the hormone is removed and that the frequency of the behavior can be returned to normal by providing the animal with the missing hormone(s).

Berthold's experiment also illustrates that the study of behavioral endocrinology is the study of two related systems. First, we must learn about the endocrine system, represented by the testes in this case. Of course, neither the testes nor the testosterone these glands released into the bloodstream completely determined the rooster's behavior. Other factors such as the time of day, the presence of a hen or a rival rooster, and so on, also made a difference. But the testosterone released from the testes reached the brain. There the hormone acted on nerve cells (neurons) in various brain regions and changed the likelihood that those behaviors would appear under the appropriate circumstances. Therefore, to understand how the hormone influenced behavior, we must study a second system, the nervous system.

Inherent in our discussion of how hormones can influence an animal's behavior is the idea that if hormones produce a change in an animal's behavior, there has been some sort of change in the animal, probably in its brain. We can try to find out which parts of the brain have been changed, how they have been changed, and how those modifications have caused an alteration in behavior. Conversely, if hormones cause alterations in the brain, there should be a corresponding change in the behavior or the physiology of the animal that we may be clever enough to detect.

Behavioral Methods: Field versus Laboratory Studies

Obviously, experiments in behavioral endocrinology require the assessment and measurement of behavior. Most people assume that this is the easy part: Sit and watch. However, there are many ways to measure behavior, including ways that may not be valuable. To discuss the issues involved in methodology, we must first consider two very different types of research: laboratory versus field research. Surely the best way to understand behavioral endocrinology is to observe the creatures of interest in their normal habitat: deer in the woods, mice in the fields, and monkeys in the jungle. But research in the field is a great challenge. Conditions are not necessarily conducive to humans. Many important variables are beyond inspection or control, and unexpected turns of events are common. Therefore, it is difficult to observe the exact same phenomena twice. Consequently, two researchers trying to study the same things may observe and report very different field results. The difficult task of field researchers is to try to achieve consistent, repeatable results. Only then can they feel confident that they understand the phenomena.

The consistency field researchers strive for is in fact the great advantage of laboratory research because the investigator in the laboratory can control and keep constant so many variables. Temperature, humidity, food and water

Table 1.1 Behavioral Assessment of Neurological Function in Animals: Summary of Features of Behavior and Appearance That Can Be Examined

MEASURE	SPECIFIC FEATURE
Appearance	Body weight, core body temperature, eyes, feces, fur condition, genitals, muscle tone, pupils, responsiveness, saliva, teeth, toenails, vocalizations
Sensory and sensorimotor behavior	Response to auditory, olfactory, somatosensory, taste, vestibular, and visual stimuli presented both in the home cage and in an open field
Posture and immobility	Behavior when spontaneously immobile, posture and muscle tone when immobile; tonic immobility or animal hypnosis; environmental influences on immobility
Movement	General activity, movement initiation, turning, climbing, walking, swimming, righting responses, limb movements, mouth and tongue movements
Species-typical behaviors	All species-typical behaviors including grooming, food hoarding, foraging, taste aversion, sleep, maternal behavior, sexual behavior, play, nest building, and burying
Learning	Classical conditioning, instrumental conditioning, and learning sets, especially including measures of spatial learning, avoidance learning, and conditioned taste aversion

Adapted from Whishaw et al., 1983.[1099a]

availability, even, in some cases, the genetic make-up of the subjects, can all be controlled. If laboratory rats of strain X are kept in conditions Y and given hormone Z, then they should display the same behaviors each time, and to a great extent they do. As will become obvious at various places in this book, however, there are plenty of individual differences even in the laboratory setting. But as more and more conditions are standardized to achieve consistency from laboratory results, you run a risk that what you are learning is applicable only to the laboratory! So the strength of field research becomes more evident: validity. If you do learn something in the laboratory and then can repeat this observation in the field, you know it is valid for the world-as-it-is. Ideally, laboratory workers read the field reports to help them judge which phenomena may be relevant outside the laboratory and therefore valid. In turn, if field researchers suspect, for example, that hormones are affecting a particular behavior, they may try to test that notion under the more controlled conditions of the laboratory.

To obtain results in the laboratory that approximate conditions in the field, the scientist must approach the experimental question from the perspective of the animal. If your subject is a rat, you need to "think like a rat." In other words, you should design your behavioral tests to take advantage of the normal behavior of the animal in the wild. Whishaw and colleagues[1099a] have described in exacting detail methods that can be used to analyze the behavior of the laboratory rat. Some of these ideas are summarized in table 1.1. This approach can be applied to the study of other species in the laboratory. The exact details of the behavioral tests will vary with the species, but the methods used to observe, analyze, and challenge the neurological functions of an animal can be generalized to any species. These authors argue that with the careful observation and description of an animal's appearance and behavior, "meaningful generalizations about the organization of the nervous system [can] later be made"[1099a] This is also true for the behavioral endocrinologist who wants to make meaningful generalizations about the influence of hormones on the nervous system.

Experimental Design

The challenge of obtaining meaningful behavioral results in the laboratory can also be addressed by careful construction of the experimental procedures, i.e., experimental design. There are a number of important things to consider here. For example, let's say that you have decided to investigate the effect of estrogen on sexual behavior in female rats. What groups will you compare? In order to control circulating estrogens in your animals, you may want to begin with animals that have had their own source of estrogen (the ovaries) removed (i.e., **ovariectomized** animals). One way to test the effect of estrogen on sexual behavior in these ovariectomized rats would be to test all the animals first in the absence of estrogen. Then you could give the animals estrogen and repeat the behavioral test (this is known as a sequential design, repeated measures, or a within-animal comparison). One thing you need to be aware of, however, is that sometimes experimental procedures themselves can change an animal's behavior. For example, perhaps the experience of the first test would affect performance in the second test regardless of hormone treatment. So it is important to run a control group that is tested a second time without receiving the hormone. Another way to conduct the experiment would be to use a simultaneous design (between-animal comparison). With this experimental design, each ovariectomized rat would be tested only once. One group would receive the hormone treatment—say, estrogen dissolved in sesame oil—while the control group would receive injections of the sesame oil vehicle without the estrogen. The behavior of the two groups of animals during the test would then be compared to see if the hormone has affected the behavior.

The advantage of the sequential design is that usually fewer animals are needed. The behavior of each animal during the two tests can be compared, and this tends to reduce variability in the data. On the other hand, if your procedures are causing changes in the animals' behavior for reasons other than the hormone treatment, a simultaneous design may be the best way to test your hypothesis. There are more complex experimental designs, but they are essentially variations and combinations of these two basic protocols.

Behavioral Observations

Next, you must decide how you will define and quantify the behavior. You must also choose your testing environment and procedures. Most behavioral

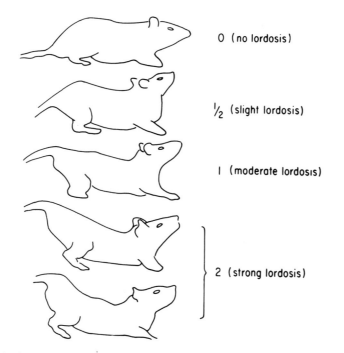

0 (no lordosis)

½ (slight lordosis)

1 (moderate lordosis)

2 (strong lordosis)

Figure 1.1 Lordosis in the female rat. These drawing were traced from single frames of films of rat mating encounters. Note the arching of the back with elevation of the head and rump. (From Brink et al., 1978.[151a])

experiments involve procedures that require an observer to make decisions about the animals' behavior. For example, a female rat exhibits a number of behaviors before she is mounted by a male that have been termed "proceptive" behaviors: She will hop and dart, and display ear wiggling in response to a male. You must decide if you are going to record these behaviors; if so, you must define them so that they are always scored in the same way. When a male rat mounts a receptive female rat, she will arch her back (head and rump are elevated) and deflect her tail to one side. This is a reflexive behavior known as **lordosis**, and it permits the male to achieve intromission (i.e., place his penis in her vagina). You must decide how to quantify this behavior. You could count the number of times the rat displays lordosis in proportion to the number of mounts, measure the amount of time the rat is in lordosis, judge the completeness of the lordosis (figure 1.1), or make-up some combination of these.

Because behavioral observation often requires making subtle judgments, it is also important that the observer be unaware of the specific treatment that an animal has received (this is known as being "blind" to the experimental conditions). This is usually achieved by coding the animals or treatments to hide their identity from the observer, thereby preventing any expectations the observer may have from coloring his judgment. It is also a good idea to have more than one observer score the behavior and to test the reliability of the data across observers. In other words, do both observers score the behavior the same way? This knowledge is important for several reasons. First, you want to be sure that the data have internal consistency, i.e., that all animals were scored the same way. Second, you want to be sure that your definitions are precise enough to allow two observers using these definitions to obtain the same results. If so, then other investigators will be able to repeat your methods and replicate your results.

Other Considerations

Other things that need to be considered include when to make your behavioral observations and what dose or treatment regimen to use for the hormone administration. When in doubt, it is best to be guided by endogenous, physiological concentrations of the hormone (if they are known) and what is already known about the temporal relations between the endogenous hormone fluctuations and the behavior under consideration.

When considering dose, some investigators might be tempted to begin with high doses of a hormone just to be sure that they see an effect. Results from high doses, however, can be very misleading. A bell-shaped curve showing the relationship between a hormone and a behavior is frequently found in behavioral endocrinology. This means that within a particular range of doses, the higher the dose, the more effective the hormone at producing a change in a behavior. But even higher doses of the hormone might have no effect or even an opposite effect on the behavior.

Alternatively, when a behavior is altered *only* by a large dose, it is possible that the extremely high dose has made the animal sick or disoriented and thereby has had a crude effect on behavior that is unrelated to the normal actions of the hormone. This latter concern is especially important when a large dose of a drug or hormone *decreases* a behavior because the animal may display the behavior only when it is feeling comfortable and relaxed. Similarly, you must always be concerned when a treatment alters behavior in the same way that general stress might alter it; perhaps the treatment distressed the animal and thereby changed the behavior, but this reflects nothing about any normal influence of that hormone on that behavior.

There are many ways to administer hormones. Steroid hormones are not very soluble in water, so they are usually dissolved in oil and injected just under the skin (subcutaneously [SC]). Another way to administer hormones is to pack solid hormone into a piece of silicone rubber (the brand name is Silastic) tubing and seal the ends. This Silastic implant is placed under the animal's skin. The hormone will slowly diffuse through and out of the tubing. By varying the thickness and length of the tubing, the amount and duration of hormone to be delivered can be adjusted. This method has the advantage that hormone can be delivered for long periods of time without the repeated stress of frequent injections. The disadvantages are that you do not always know how much hormone you are delivering, and, as we will learn, endogenous hormones are not released in such a constant fashion.

It may be desirable in some experiments to deliver hormone directly to specific areas of the brain in order to localize the brain area mediating a particular behavior. In order to do this, a small cannula (a hollow piece of stainless steel tubing) is tamped full of hormone at one end. The end of the cannula containing the hormone is then introduced into an animal's brain in a specific location. If the behavior is changed by this local application of hormone, the question to be asked is whether you can be sure that the effect is specific to the hormone and that it acted in that particular area of the brain. Maybe the cannula damaged the brain, causing the observed effect, or perhaps the hormone diffused to another area of the brain a few millimeters away. Therefore, cannulae containing control hormones (i.e., biologically inactive versions of the same hormone) and cannulae containing the active hormone placed in other brain regions should not produce the same effect.

Thus, the study of hormones and behavior in the laboratory requires a design that will accurately measure and evaluate the effect of experimental manipulation on the behavior. In order to produce results that can be generalized to animals outside the laboratory, it is a good idea to use behavioral tests that reflect naturally occurring behaviors and hormone treatments that closely approximate endogenous hormone secretions.

Relating Behavior to Brain: Highlights of Chapters to Follow

Using procedures such as these and others, scientists have investigated how hormones affect behavior, and that is the topic of this book. Investigators have studied the way hormones affect neuronal function as well as how the brain is organized. For example, we know that there are specific areas of the brain that are responsible for sexual behavior and that the areas of the brain important for sexual behavior are different for males and females. In chapter 2 you will learn how the hormones produced by the fetus are responsible for the sexual differentiation of the brain. In fact, some hormones determine whether certain neurons live or die (chapters 2, 11). You will learn how this exciting field of research has demonstrated that sex differences in both reproductive behavior and brain morphology are determined by the hormonal milieu in which neurons develop.

In the second section of the book, the consequences of hormonal influences on brain development for sexual behavior and courtship will be explored in greater detail. You will learn about the intricate hormonal cycle that coordinates the simultaneous production of eggs with the onset of sexually receptive behavior in many female mammals in chapter 3. You will also learn that more than one strategy has evolved to maximize the possibility that fertilization of the egg will take place. In chapter 4 you will learn, among other things, how scientists have been able to determine that different areas of the brain are important for sexual arousal and sexual motivation in males. Then we will consider how the data from nonhuman animals relates to what we know about hormonal influences on sexual behavior in humans (chapter 5).

In chapter 6 we will learn more about the diversity of hormone-behavior relations that have evolved in various species. We will see that even though the hormone-behavior relations may appear to be very different, the same neuroendocrine systems are involved in controlling reproductive behaviors. Part II concludes with a discussion of courtship behavior. Frogs, birds, and fish have evolved different mechanisms to convey to members of their own species information about their reproductive status and fitness. Hormonal influences on sensory receptors, muscle development, and the electrical activity and morphology of neurons in the brain all play a role in ensuring that males and females of a species find and select their mates. But there is a rich diversity among species in where and when hormones produce their effects.

In the third part of the book we learn how hormones are also important for nonsexual behaviors. The hormones of pregnancy, for example, facilitate the initiation of parental behavior (chapter 8). Hormones can influence aggressive behavior both by their effects on the brain and by their effects on the pheromones secreted by an animal that affect the aggressive behavior of others (chapter 9). Chronic stress has a profound impact on the secretion of hormones by the adrenal gland, and these hormones can have dire consequences for an animal, affecting energy availability, growth, reproduction, and the immune system (chapter 10). You will also learn that hormones can act on specific areas of the brain to affect sensorimotor and cognitive function. Basic studies have investigated some of the possible underlying neural processes involved in these functions for nonhuman animals (chapter 11), and correlative experiments have suggested the presence of similar effects of hormones on cognitive function in humans (chapter 12).

In the fourth part of the book we learn that hormone-behavior relations are reciprocally related. We will have seen many examples of the ways in which secreted hormones alter behavior, but conversely, exposure to stimuli and even the execution of behavior itself can affect hormonal secretions in turn. Chapter 13 describes many of the various ways in which behavior and experience can affect hormones. Chapter 14 describes the research on invertebrate systems that has demonstrated the ways in which various behaviors triggered by different hormones interact to ensure successful metamorphosis. For ingestive behavior, we learn that hormones can affect eating and drinking and that these behaviors affect the secretion of many hormones (chapter 15). Finally, we learn how endogenous biological rhythms coordinate the many endocrine systems, serving as one of the major organizing forces for hormone-behavior relations (chapter 16). Each chapter describes what is known about how hormones affect behavior and the underlying neural mechanisms mediating these hormone-behavior relations. This means that in addition to understanding how behavior is studied, we must also have a basic understanding of both the nervous system and the endocrine system.

Basic Concepts in Cell Biology

Experiments similar to those performed by Berthold are still conducted today to establish hormone-behavior relations. Of course, today's behavioral endocrinologist can investigate the underlying neural mechanisms mediating hormone-behavior relations, the subcellular events that occur in response to hormones, and even the molecular biology of those subcellular responses. Therefore, today's student of behavioral endocrinology must become familiar with the basic mechanisms of neural and cellular function to understand hormone-brain interactions.

Before we discuss how and where hormones act in the brain to influence various components of an animal's behavior, we will first review some basic facts and principles of biology, endocrinology, and biopsychology. As mentioned earlier, these ideas will be important for an understanding of the topics to be discussed later in the book. This discussion is not intended to be a comprehensive review or "everything you ever wanted to know" about the brain and endocrine systems. Instead, it is a brief introduction (or review) of some basic ideas that can also be referred to when reading the rest of the book if questions arise. For more details and further explanations of the subject material, additional readings are suggested at the end of this chapter.

The Biology of Eucaryotic Cells

All complex biological organisms are made up of individual eucaryotic cells that contain a spherical-shaped nucleus, in which the genetic material for the organism is stored, and the surrounding cytoplasm, which contains many subcellular organelles that perform diverse functions. While the number of cells in an organism and the complexity of relations between cells varies considerably across species, most of the cellular processes that eucaryotic cells carry out are found in all species. In particular, the ways in which genes store or encode the information needed to produce an organism is a fascinating story that seems to change little across species from worms and flies to people. The genetic code and its regulation are important for two reasons. First, the modern behavioral endocrinologist takes advantage of these principles and methods when asking questions about hormones and behavior. Second, in this book we will discuss the effects of many hormones that *produce their effects by activating specific genes.* Therefore, a brief overview of how the instructions contained in the genome are carried out has become important for the understanding of how hormones produce their effects.

THE GENETIC CODE
The genetic information for each cell is stored in fiber-like structures called chromosomes. The chromosomes are actually long, twisted molecules of **deoxyribonucleic acid** (or **DNA**) that remain in the cell's nucleus. DNA is composed of four different molecules called **nucleotides** (so called because they were originally isolated from cell nuclei). The nucleotides form a long chain with a sugar (deoxyribose) linking them together. Two of these DNA chains wind around each other in the famous double helix. DNA codes for the sequence of amino acids that go into individual proteins. Some of these pro-

1. DOUBLE STRANDED DNA

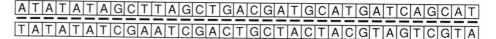

2. TRANSCRIPTION: single strand DNA to single strand RNA

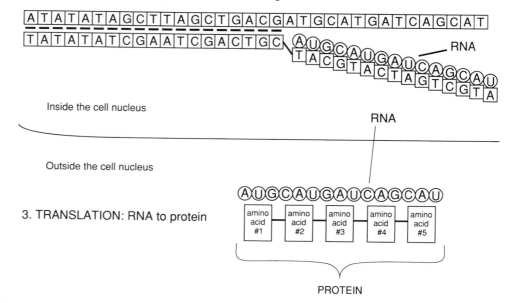

Inside the cell nucleus

Outside the cell nucleus

3. TRANSLATION: RNA to protein

PROTEIN

Figure 1.2 The four nucleotides that make up each DNA molecule (adenine, thymine, guanine, and cytosine) are represented schematically in this figure by boxes with the letters A, T, G, and C, respectively. The four nucleotides in RNA (adenine, uracil, guanine, and cytosine) are represented by circles with the four letters A, U, G, and C. (1) In forming the double-stranded DNA molecule, each nucleotide is always paired with only one of the other base pairs: C with G, T with A. Normally, the two strands are tightly twisted around each other in a "double helix." (2) For transcription to occur, the two strands of the DNA molecule must first unwind. The single strands of DNA can then serve as templates for synthesis of single strands of RNA. Each of the four DNA nucleotides always codes for only one of the four RNA nucleotides (C for G, G for C, T for A, and A for U). The newly synthesized RNA can then leave the nucleus. (3) Translation of the sequence of amino acids to make up a protein occurs outside the nucleus. Each series of three RNA nucleotides is the code for one particular amino acid to be added to the chain. A short series of amino acids is called a peptide; a long series of amino acids is a protein.

teins are packaged by the cell for export, others are enzymes that allow the cell to make other molecules or perform certain functions. Amazing as it may seem, all genetic instructions come down to which particular proteins are to be made in different cells at different times.

A particular piece of DNA that contains the instructions for making a protein is known as a gene. In order for DNA to produce a protein, the gene must first be **transcribed** (figure 1.2). During this process of transcription, a single strand of DNA serves as a template for the assembly of a string of nucleotides forming **ribonucleic acid (RNA)**. Each of the four different DNA nucleotides has a tendency to pair with only one particular RNA nucleotide. There are, therefore, four

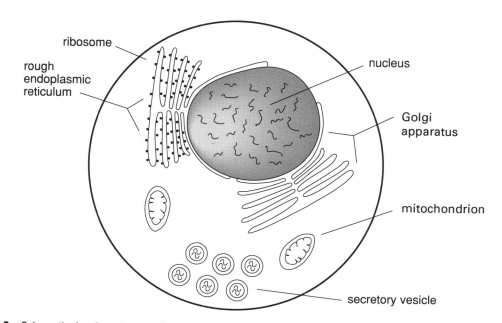

Figure 1.3 Schematic drawing of some of the subcellular organelles found in eucaryotic cells. The genetic material (large strands of DNA coiled into chromosomes) is sequestered within the nucleus of the cell (depicted as fibers within the nucleus). Protein synthesis occurs on the ribosomes in the rough endoplasmic reticulum. Additional processing takes place in the Golgi apparatus, where proteins that were synthesized for export are sequestered in secretory vesicles. Mitochondria provide energy for cellular metabolism.

different RNA nucleotides, each complementary to a DNA nucleotide. The newly transcribed string of RNA nucleotides forms a molecule known variously as the "message," the "transcript," or messenger RNA (**mRNA**).

Since each DNA nucleotide is transcribed as a specific RNA nucleotide, the code for an amino acid sequence is now contained within the series of RNA nucleotides. The mRNA leaves the nucleus for the cytoplasm, where protein synthesis occurs when the genetic instructions encoded in the mRNA transcript are **translated** into a chain of amino acids. A series of three nucleotides constitutes the name (also referred to as the **codon**, or code) for which of the 20 or so different amino acids will be added to the chain. A long series of such triplets codes for a long series of amino acids, and that is what constitutes a protein. This flow of information from the gene to a protein is the foundation upon which modern molecular biology is built (figure 1.3).

SUBCELLULAR ORGANELLES

Outside the nucleus but within the cytoplasm of the cell are a number of subcellular organelles that serve different specific functions. For example, **mitochondria** provide energy to the cell. **Ribosomes** (themselves made up of special, ribosomal, RNA) are the site of protein synthesis, i.e., translation. The **endoplasmic reticulum** (literally, a network of membranes) and **Golgi apparatus** assist with protein synthesis and transport within the cell. Proteins that

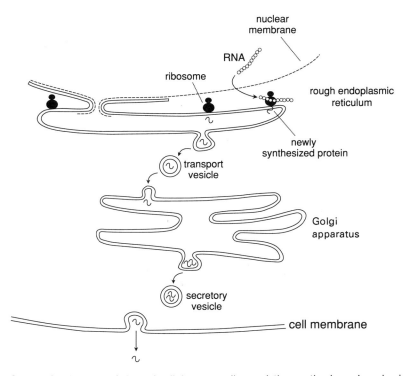

Figure 1.4 Schematic close-up of the subcellular organelles and the synthesis and packaging of protein into secretory vesicles for release by exocytosis. mRNA leaves the nucleus, and protein synthesis occurs on the ribosomes in the rough endoplasmic reticulum. Newly synthesized proteins undergo additional processing in the rough endoplasmic reticulum and are then transported to the Golgi apparatus, where they are packaged into secretory vesicles for release by exocytosis. The movement of the protein from synthesis, packaging, and release by exocytosis is indicated by the arrows. (Adapted from Shepherd, 1988.[939a])

are destined for secretion from the cell or insertion into the cell's own membrane are synthesized on ribosomes found within the endoplasmic reticulum. Together, the ribosomes and endoplasmic reticulum are referred to as the **rough endoplasmic reticulum** because in electron micrographs the ribosomes appear as bumps on the membranes of the endoplasmic reticulum. This is illustrated schematically in figure 1.4.

The Secretory Process

All cells in an organism engage in protein synthesis. However, some cells use proteins or other chemicals produced by enzymes (which are themselves protein) for communication between cells. We will be interested in three different types of these intercellular chemical messengers: (1) **hormones**, produced by endocrine cells and released into the circulatory system, (2) **neurotransmitters**, produced by neurons and released at the synapse, and (3) **neurohormones**, produced by specialized neurons known as neurosecretory cells. The three types of chemical messengers differ in where they are produced, where they are released, and the distance the chemical has to travel to produce an effect. These methods of communication differ, therefore, in the speed of the message and the type of information they convey. Nevertheless, cells using these different methods produce, package, and secrete their different chemical messengers in much the same way. With this idea in mind, we shall examine the mechanisms involved in a generic model of the secretory process in all cells.

The general model for the secretory process is based on the now classic work of George Palade (for a review see Palade and Farquar.[794a]) Palade was investigating the synthesis and secretion of proteins by the pancreas using what has become known as the pulse-chase method. First, in order to detect newly synthesized proteins, Palade labeled an amino acid with radioactivity. That is, one or more of the nonradioactive atoms in the molecule was replaced by a radioactive isotope (e.g., an ordinary hydrogen [^{1}H] atom was replaced with a tritium [^{3}H] atom, or an ordinary carbon [^{12}C] atom was replaced with a ^{14}C atom). The radioactive amino acid was initially injected into a rat all at once to make the pulse. This was followed by administration of more *nonradioactive* amino acid, so that the amount of amino acid available would be constant throughout the experiment. As a result of ongoing protein synthesis, the radioactive amino acid was incorporated into protein for a brief period of time before it was diluted (chased) by the nonradioactive amino acid.

Palade followed the fate of the radioactively labeled amino acids as they were incorporated into newly synthesized proteins by locating radioactivity within pancreatic cells at different times after the pulse. He found radioactivity first in newly translated proteins as they were produced by the ribosomes of the rough endoplasmic reticulum. The radioactive protein was later found packaged into transport **vesicles** (sphere-shaped sacks). Still later, these radioactivity-filled vesicles were found in the Golgi complex.

In the Golgi complex, the protein was packaged into **secretory vesicles** and was released from the pancreas by a process known as **exocytosis** (figure 1.5). Exocytosis is the fusion of a secretory vesicle with the extracellular membrane and the subsequent discharge of the vesicle contents outside the cell. Exocytosis is an active process that requires both energy and the presence of free calcium ions. Endocrine cells, neurons, and neuroendocrine cells all use exocytosis to release secretory products.

In some hormones and neurotransmitters the synthesis of the secretory product and its packaging into vesicles differ from this model. In fact, steroid hormones are probably not packaged into vesicles at all. But in all other cases, the Golgi apparatus (or an analogous structure) is involved in the formation of the secretory vesicles, the secretory product is packaged into secretory vesicles, and release occurs by exocytosis.

These are the general processes mediating protein synthesis and secretion. In order to understand the ideas discussed in the following chapters, you need to be familiar with these basic relations between DNA, RNA, and proteins. A more detailed look at these processes is the concern of molecular biologists. For now, we are ready to consider the details of the nervous and endocrine systems.

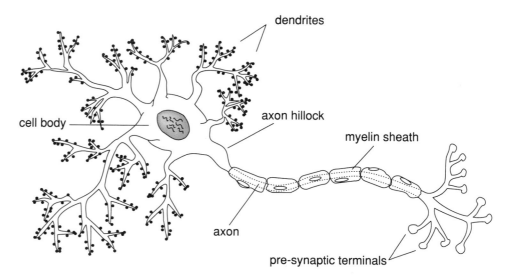

Figure 1.5 In neurons, as for other eucaryotic cells, the nucleus is sequestered in the cell body or soma. Dendrites project in tree-like formation from the soma and receive information from other neurons. A single axon projects from the cell body, through which information is transmitted to other neurons. When the membrane potential at the axon hillock reaches a certain threshold, an action potential is generated and is transmitted down the axon to the presynaptic terminal, where the neurotransmitter is released by exocytosis.

Basic Concepts in Neurobiology

The adult human brain contains from 30 to 100 billion neurons, whereas in the tobacco hornworm moth (*Manduca sexta*) it is estimated that there are 30 to 100 thousand neurons. But in both moths and humans neurons behave very much alike—they share characteristics that allow them to receive, process, and transmit information.

Parts of the Neuron

Most neurons have three structural components: the **cell body**, the **dendrites**, and the **axon** (figure 1.5). Neurons have an outer membrane made of a double layer of fat-like molecules (lipids) with proteins that float within the lipid membrane. As in almost all other cells, the neuronal cell body (or soma) has a nucleus as well as the various subcellular organelles typical of eucaryotic cells.

Extending from the cell body are two different types of projections, axons and dendrites (figure 1.5). Dendrites are usually widely branching fibers that receive information from other neurons. Axons are single fibers that extend from the cell body and transmit information to other neurons. The site where the axon leaves the cell body appears to be slightly swollen and is therefore called the **axon hillock**. The axon usually branches many times at its terminal end, so that multiple contacts can be made with many different target neurons. At the end of each axon branch is a swelling known as the **presynaptic termin-**

al. The site where the presynaptic terminal contacts another neuron is known as a **synapse**.

The Membrane Potential and Action Potentials

Neurons can receive and transmit information because, unlike most other types of cells, their membranes are electrically excitable. Because there are more negatively charged ions inside neurons than outside, the cells have a **polarization** or electrical charge across the membrane called the **resting potential**. All cells have a resting potential that they actively defend, but it is a change in the membrane potential that is the result and cause of the transmission of information between neurons.

If an electrical stimulus is applied to the neuronal membrane to make the potential across the membrane *less* negative (i.e., the inside becomes less negative than the outside), then we say that the membrane has become **depolarized**. If an electrical stimulus makes the potential across the membrane *more* negative (i.e., the inside becomes even more negative than the outside), then the membrane is said to be **hyperpolarized**. Such changes in membrane polarization can be caused by an experimenter using electrical stimulation, but in the normally functioning nervous system changes in membrane polarization are brought about by different means, as we shall soon see.

However the membrane polarization is altered, and whether the alteration is a depolarization or a hyperpolarization, the membrane will **passively conduct** this change in potential along the membrane away from the site that was stimulated. This type of conduction is called **decremental conduction** because the change in membrane potential is smaller farther from the site of stimulation. The analogy frequently used is that of a ripple created by dropping a pebble into a calm pool of water. The wave created by the pebble becomes smaller as the distance from the site of impact increases. The change in membrane potential created is also referred to as a **graded potential**. This is because the size of the change in membrane potential is proportional to the size of the stimulus. Going back to our analogy, if you drop a large rock into the pool of calm water, you will produce bigger waves than you would with a pebble.

The events that normally produce changes in neuronal membrane potential occur at the synapse. A **presynaptic** neuron releases its **neurotransmitter**, and this produces changes in the membrane potential of the **postsynaptic** neuron. The postsynaptic response in the next neuron is passively conducted by decremental conduction. The response is also a graded potential, so it is proportional to the amount of neurotransmitter released at a synapse. Throughout the dendrites and cell body, any stimulation of the neuron results in a graded potential and decremental conduction of that potential away from the many sites of stimulation. Because it is literally covered with synapses, each neuron receives input from thousands of other neurons. The neuron integrates the many depolarizations and hyperpolarizations received by the dendrites and cell body. But it is at the axon hillock that the *net* polarization determines whether this neuron has become sufficiently depolarized to pass on the information to other neurons.

If the net depolarization of the membrane potential at the axon hillock reaches a certain threshold, the axon becomes depolarized, an **action potential** is generated, and the neuron is said to "fire." This action potential is an all-or-none phenomenon; once an action potential has been generated in the axon hillock, it cannot be stopped, and the strength of the signal does not diminish as it travels down the axon at some 10 to 100 miles per hour (mph). If, as is usually the case, the axon branches, the action potential travels down each branch, and available neurotransmitter is released at each synapse. Action potentials are relatively easy to measure by a variety of electrophysiological techniques.

Synaptic Transmission

The process of communication between two neurons relies on the release of a chemical messenger, the **neurotransmitter**. When the action potential arrives at the presynaptic terminal, the terminal releases neurotransmitter. The released neurotransmitter crosses the synapse and is detected by postsynaptic receptors. Release of a neurotransmitter and its reception by the postsynaptic neuron is a process known as **synaptic transmission**. This term reflects two important aspects of this process: synaptic, because it only occurs at a synapse; transmission, because information is communicated or transmitted between two cells. Synaptic transmission relies on (1) the availability of neurotransmitter, (2) the release of neurotransmitter by exocytosis, (3) the binding of the postsynaptic receptor by the neurotransmitter, (4) the response of the postsynaptic cell, and (5) the subsequent removal or deactivation of the neurotransmitter.

AVAILABILITY OF NEUROTRANSMITTER: SYNTHESIS AND
PACKAGING INTO VESICLES

Most neurotransmitters are small molecules, about the size of a single amino acid, but neurotransmitters can also be larger proteins or peptides. Some of the substances that are currently thought to be neurotransmitters are listed in table 1.2. The synthesis of a neurotransmitter varies according to the size of the molecule. Protein and peptide neurotransmitters are synthesized as described above, in the cell body, and then packaged into secretory vesicles (which in neurons are called **synaptic vesicles**). Once the proteins or peptides have been manufactured and packaged into vesicles in the cell body, they are transported down the axon to the presynaptic terminal for release. If the neurotransmitter is a small molecule, synthesis does not occur only in the cell body. The enzymes for neurotransmitter synthesis are assembled in the cell body and transported to the presynaptic terminal. The neurotransmitter is then synthesized and packaged into synaptic vesicles in the presynaptic terminal, close to where it will be needed.

Table 1.2   Partial List of Putative Neurotransmitters and Releasing Factors

---

Acetylcholine

Monoamines
   Catecholamines
      Dopamine (DA)
      Norepinephrine (NE)
      Epinephrine (EPI)
   Indoleamines
      Serotonin (5-hydroxytryptamine, 5-HT)
      Histamine

Amino acids
   Glutamate
   Gamma-aminobutyric acid (GABA)
   Glycine
   Aspartate

Purines
   Adenosine

Peptides
   Dynorphin
   Enkephalin
   Substance P
   Neurotensin
   Bombesin
   Somatostatin
   β-Endorphin
   Neuropeptide Y
   Cholecystokinin (CCK)
   Oxytocin
   Vasopressin
   Angiotensin II
   Vasoactive intestinal polypeptide (VIP)
   Corticotropin-releasing hormone (CRH)
   Growth hormone-releasing factor (GRF)
   Thyrotropin-releasing hormone (TRH)
   Gonadotropin-releasing hormone (GnRH)

EXOCYTOSIS

When a neuron fires, the arrival of the action potential at the presynaptic terminal causes calcium influx into the terminal. The availability of free calcium results in release of the neurotransmitter from the presynaptic terminal by exocytosis. The neurotransmitter diffuses across the synaptic cleft, where it contacts postsynaptic receptors—large protein molecules or multiprotein complexes that recognize and bind to the neurotransmitter (figure 1.6).

RECEPTOR BINDING

When the neurotransmitter contacts the postsynaptic receptor, the two molecules are thought to fit together in such a way that for a short time they are bound to each other. Because a particular neurotransmitter will fit into only some receptors, such **receptor binding** is usually conceptualized as a "lock and

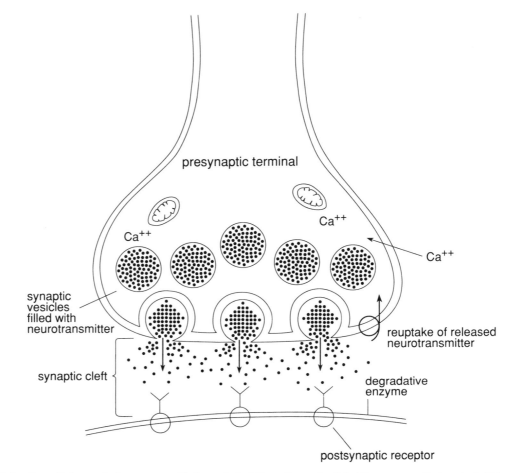

Figure 1.6 Synaptic transmission occurs with the arrival of the action potential at the presynaptic terminal. This causes an increase in calcium (Ca2+) influx and results in movement of the synaptic vesicles filled with neurotransmitter to the presynaptic terminal membrane, where the membranes fuse and neuro-transmitter is released by exocytosis. The neurotransmitter diffuses across the synaptic cleft to bind to the postsynaptic receptors, where a graded potential is generated in the postsynaptic cell. (The synaptic vesicles are depicted with only one membrane, but their membranes are also lipid bilayers as depicted for the extracellular membrane.)

key" association between the two molecules. But the binding is also reminiscent of the way Velcro works. When two complementary strips of Velcro come in contact, they stick together, but they can also be pulled apart with no change in the shape or usefulness of either. Thus, when the two are attached, they are bound to each other, but this is not a permanent attachment. Similarly, a neurotransmitter has an affinity for its receptor, so it sticks to the receptor for a brief time and then is released.

The binding of the neurotransmitter at the postsynaptic receptor induces changes in the electrical potential of the postsynaptic neuronal membrane. The change in membrane potential is proportional to the amount of neurotransmitter released. A neurotransmitter can produce either inhibition (by hyperpolarization) or excitation (by depolarization) of the membrane of the postsynaptic cell. The particular neurotransmitter and the particular post-synaptic receptor determine the direction of the response. If the postsynaptic response is hyperpolarization, the chance of depolarization occurring at the axon hillock is ultimately reduced, and therefore the cell is inhibited from firing. Conversely, if the postsynaptic response is depolarization, the cell is excited. In either case, the information from this synapse is summated with all of the other information arriving at this postsynaptic neuron, and when the **threshold** is reached at the axon hillock this neuron will fire.

DEACTIVATION OF THE NEUROTRANSMITTER
A neurotransmitter is available only briefly to bind to the postsynaptic re-ceptors and then is rapidly deactivated. Deactivation occurs through either degradative enzymes present in the synaptic cleft or removal of the neuro-transmitter by reuptake into the presynaptic terminal. Nevertheless, a brief exposure of the receptor to the neurotransmitter is quite effective at pro-ducing a postsynaptic response.

Some Simple Pharmacology

To investigate how specific neural systems interact with the endocrine sys-tem, it is often helpful to be able to manipulate neuronal activity. Because pharmacological manipulations are frequently used, it is a good idea to become familiar with the general principles and terminology used to describe the ways in which drugs can influence neuronal activity.

Drugs that act on the brain to influence an animal's behavior usually do so by altering neurotransmitter activity, and there are a number of different ways that drugs can produce their effects. Many drugs are thought to act on specific neurotransmitter systems and therefore alter activity in specific populations of neurons. For example, **neurotransmitter synthesis** can be prevented or de-creased by drugs that affect the *synthetic enzyme for a neurotransmitter.* When neurotransmitter synthesis is blocked, the amount of neurotransmitter available for release is decreased, so there is decreased neurotransmitter activ-ity. Alternatively, **storage** in synaptic vesicles can be prevented with drugs that make *synaptic vesicle membranes leaky.* This results in depletion of neuro-transmitter stores and again decreases neurotransmitter activity.

Other drugs block or stimulate the **release** of specific neurotransmitters. Still other drugs act by **blocking receptors**, so that the real neurotransmitter cannot bind to the receptors. Drugs that *prevent a neurotransmitter from binding* to its receptor are called receptor **antagonists**. For example, drugs used to treat patients with schizophrenia such as haloperidol, chlorpromazine, and clozapine (i.e., neuroleptics or antipsychotic drugs), are antagonists at recep-tors in the brain for the neurotransmitter dopamine. Other drugs act by bind-ing to a receptor and *mimicking the normal neurotransmitter.* Such drugs are called receptor **agonists**. An example of a receptor agonist is Valium, a benzo-

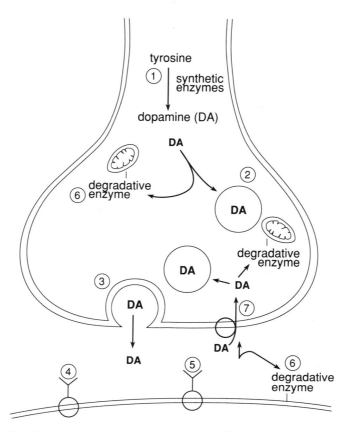

Figure 1.7 Possible sites of drug action in a dopamine (DA) neuron. These same sites can be affected by drugs in neurons that use other neurotransmitters. Drugs can also influence the endocrine system by acting at analogous sites. 1, Synthesis; 2, storage; 3, release; 4, receptor-agonist; 5, receptor-antagonist; 6, degradative enzymes; 7, reuptake. (Adapted from Cooper et al., 1991.[221a])

diazepine that mimics the effect of the endogenous neurotransmitter gamma-aminobutyric acid (GABA) to decrease anxiety. Other drugs interfere with the **deactivation** of a neurotransmitter after it has been released, thereby prolonging the action of a neurotransmitter. This can be done by blocking reuptake (as cocaine does for catecholamines) or inhibiting degradative enzymes. Finally, drugs that **prevent an action potential** from occurring can *block neuronal activity* throughout the brain and the peripheral nervous system. Drugs such as tetrodotoxin (pufferfish poison) and others that block neural activity are quite lethal. The various ways in which drugs can affect neuronal activity are illustrated schematically in figure 1.7 for a neuron that uses dopamine (DA) as its neurotransmitter.

Basic Concepts in Neuroendocrinology

In vertebrates, the central nervous system develops from a long hollow tube of cells called the neural tube. As the brain develops, the neural tube forms three outpouchings. The adult brain is divided into subdivisions based on these

Table 1.3 Major Subdivisions of the Vertebrate Brain

Forebrain	Telencephalon	Olfactory bulbs Cerebral hemispheres Basal ganglia
	Diencephalon	Epithalamus Thalamus Hypothalamus
Midbrain	Mesencephalon	Tectum Tegmentum
Hindbrain	Metencephalon	Cerebellum Pons
	Myelencephalon	Medulla oblongata

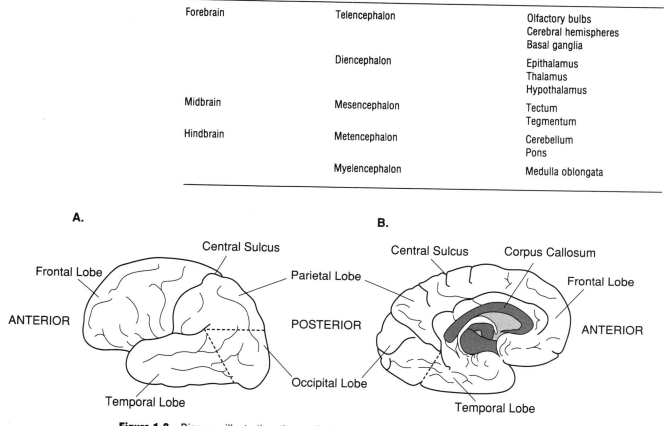

Figure 1.8 Diagram illustrating the cortical regions in the human brain. *A*, View of the lateral surface of the cerebral hemispheres. *B*, View of the medial surface of the cerebral hemispheres. The cerebral cortex is divided into four main lobes: the frontal lobe, the parietal lobe, the temporal lobe, and the occipital lobe. (Adapted from Shepherd, 1988.[939a])

embryological formations of forebrain, midbrain, and hindbrain (table 1.3). In mammals, the cerebral hemispheres of the forebrain comprise the largest portion of the brain. These include the cerebral cortex, the basal ganglia, and the limbic system. The cortex can be subdivided into four lobes: frontal, parietal, occipital, and temporal (figure 1.8; see also chapter 12). However, for behavioral endocrinologists, most interest focuses upon a relatively small region at the base of the forebrain, a part of the diencephalon called the hypothalamus. As we will see, the hypothalamus warrants this attention because it exerts a profound influence on the secretion of nearly every known hormone (figure 1.9)

Hypothalamic-Pituitary Relations in Vertebrates

By definiton, hormones are substances produced by a gland that are carried by the circulatory system to a distant target organ to cause an effect. The brain is a

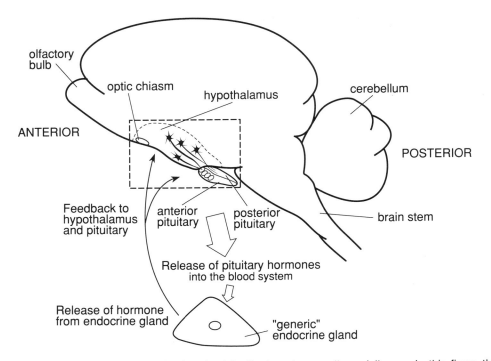

Figure 1.9   The hypothalamic-pituitary-endocrine gland feedback system—a "generic" case. In this figure the brain is viewed from the side. There are two different classes of neurosecretory cells in the hypothalamus, as illustrated schematically in this figure. The first class of hypothalamic neurosecretory cells send their axons to the median eminence (see figure 1.10). There the cells deliver releasing factors onto blood vessels in the hypophyseal portal system. The releasing factors travel to the anterior pituitary to stimulate or inhibit the release of anterior pituitary hormones. The second class send their axons down the pituitary stalk and terminate near blood vessels in the posterior pituitary. When these neurons fire, they release neurohormones (either oxytocin or vasopressin) directly into the circulatory system. Hormones from the anterior pituitary or neurohormones from the posterior pituitary reach their target glands and induce hormone release. Hormones released from the endocrine gland feed back to both the hypothalamus and pituitary. Stippled box indicates region of close-up in figure 1.10.

target organ for many of these hormones and in turn regulates their secretion. Although the relations between the brain and the endocrine system in vertebrates are conceptually simple, as with most biological systems the details can be quite complex.

In vertebrates, the hypothalamus is the neural control center for all endocrine systems. Although it is relatively small, there are a number of specialized nuclei (i.e., functional groups of neurons) within the hypothalamus (figure 1.10). These nuclei are involved in the regulation and integration of endocrine and physiological functions and behaviors. For example, the suprachiasmatic nucleus (so called because of its location above the optic chiasm) is involved in the maintenance and coordination of biological rhythms, and the medial preoptic area and ventromedial hypothalamus are involved in sexual behavior (among other functions). You will learn much more about the various hypothalamic nuclei and their many functions in the chapters that follow.

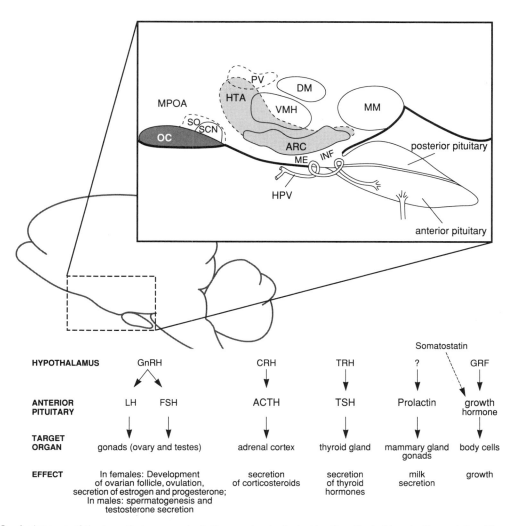

HYPOTHALAMUS	GnRH		CRH	TRH	?	Somatostatin GRF
ANTERIOR PITUITARY	LH	FSH	ACTH	TSH	Prolactin	growth hormone
TARGET ORGAN	gonads (ovary and testes)		adrenal cortex	thyroid gland	mammary gland gonads	body cells
EFFECT	In females: Development of ovarian follicle, ovulation, secretion of estrogen and progesterone; In males: spermatogenesis and testosterone secretion		secretion of corticosteroids	secretion of thyroid hormones	milk secretion	growth

Figure 1.10 A close-up of the hypothalamus and pituitary region indicated by the stippled box in figure 1.9, with a schematic representation of the relations between hypothalamic-releasing factors, pituitary hormones, and their target glands. A solid arrow indicates a stimulatory effect, a dashed arrow indicates an inhibitory effect. The releasing factors are released by neurons in the hypothalamus and diffuse through the hypophyseal portal blood vessels (HPV) to the anterior pituitary. 1. Gonadotropin-releasing hormone (GnRH) stimulates the pituitary to release luteinizing hormone (LH) and follicle-stimulating hormone (FSH). LH and FSH in turn stimulate their primary target organs, the gonads, to promote spermatogenesis in the testes or development of eggs in the ovary. 2. Corticotropic hormone (CRH) stimulates the pituitary to release adrenocorticotropin (ACTH), which acts primarily on the adrenal cortex to induce the release of corticosteroids. 3. Thyrotropic-releasing hormone (TRH) stimulates the release of thyroid-stimulating hormone (TSH) from the pituitary, which acts primarily on the thyroid gland to stimulate the release of thyroid hormones. 4. Scientists are still uncertain about the hypothalamic-releasing factor that induces prolactin release. At high concentrations, dopamine will inhibit prolactin release. Prolactin has a wide range of actions in the body and the brain. Prolactin gets its name from its effect on the mammary gland promoting milk secretion. In conjunction with LH, prolactin also act to promote gonadal function. 5. Somatostatin inhibits, while growth hormone-releasing factor (GRF) stimulates, the release of growth hormone (GH) from the anterior pituitary. GH stimulates growth of cells, this including bone growth as well as growth of other cells in the body. Neuroanatomical abbreviation: ARC, arcuate nucleus; DM, dorsomedial nucleus; HPV, hypophyseal portal vessels; HTA, hypophysiotropic area; INF, infundibular stalk; ME, median eminence; MM, mammillary nucleus, MPOA, medial preoptic area; OC, optic chiasm; PV, paraventricular nucleus; SCN, suprachiasmatic nucleus; SO, supraoptic nucleus; VMH: ventromedial hypothalamic nucleus. (Adapted from Shepherd, 1988.[939a])

Specialized types of neurons in the hypothalamus have evolved that allow the brain to influence the secretions of the endocrine system. These neurons communicate directly with endocrine systems and are called **neurosecretory cells** because they release their products not into a synapse but into blood vessels that carry the neurotransmitter to other organs to produce its effect. Such neurotransmitters can be thought of, therefore, as **neurohormones**.

The hypothalamus is directly above a very important endocrine gland, the **pituitary**. The pituitary gland (sometimes called the **hypophysis**) is sandwiched between the roof of the mouth and the hypothalamus. Cradled in a small nook of the cranium, the pituitary is actually attached to the hypothalamus by a slender stalk. As we will see, the hypothalamus receives information about external conditions from other brain regions and, using this information, controls secretions from the pituitary. The hypothalamic neurosecretory cells exert their control over the pituitary in two quite different ways.

As illustrated schematically in figure 1.9, neurosecretory cells in the hypothalamus are associated with the both the anterior and posterior lobes of the pituitary gland (there is also a slim intermediate zone in the pituitary, but it will not concern us). One type of neurosecretory cell releases its neurohormones onto specialized blood vessels that supply the *anterior* pituitary to stimulate the release of hormones. These neurohormones are also called **releasing factors** because they stimulate or inhibit the release of hormones by cells in the anterior pituitary gland. The other type of hypothalamic neurosecretory cell sends axons into the *posterior* pituitary to release its neurohormones directly into the general circulatory system.

HYPOTHALAMIC CONTROL OF THE ANTERIOR PITUITARY
It was widely accepted for some time that the hypothalamus produced releasing factors that acted on the anterior pituitary to stimulate or inhibit pituitary hormone secretion. However, isolation of a releasing factor did not occur until the early 1970s. The convention now is to call a substance a releasing factor until it has been chemically isolated and characterized. Once its chemical structure is known, it is called a **releasing hormone**. We will use the term releasing factor as a generic term to refer to both.

Releasing factors are secreted into a specialized system of blood vessels that runs between the base of the hypothalamus and the anterior pituitary lobe (or **adenohypophysis**) as opposed to the posterior pituitary lobe (or **neurohypophysis**). The hypothalamic-pituitary portal system is actually a profuse tangle of small blood vessels (i.e., capillaries) that use blood flow to deliver the hypothalamic-releasing factors to the pituitary. There are many different types of cells in the anterior pituitary: Some release growth hormone (GH) and are called somatotrophs; other cells (lactotrophs) release prolactin (Prl), and so on (see table 1.4). Each of these specialized pituitary cells is controlled by specialized hypothalamic releasing factors. The pituitary cells respond to the releasing factors by either increasing or decreasing their production and release of pituitary hormones (see figure 1.10).

Table 1.4 Vertebrate Endocrine Glands and Some of the Hormones They Are Known to Secrete

ENDOCRINE GLAND	HORMONES SECRETED
Anterior pituitary	Growth hormone (GH) Prolactin (Prl) Melanophore-stimulating hormone (MSH) Adrenocorticotropin (ACTH) Luteinizing hormone (LH) Follicle-stimulating hormone (FSH) Thyroid-stimulating hormone (TSH)
Posterior pituitary	Arginine vasopressin (AVP; also known as antidiuretic hormone [ADH]) Oxytocin
Thyroid gland	Thyroxin Calcitonin

Adrenal cortex	Glucocorticoids
	    Corticosterone
	    Cortisol
	Mineralocorticoids
	    Aldosterone

Adrenal medulla	Epinephrine Norepinephrine Enkephalins Endorphins
Kidney	Renin
Liver	Preangiotensin
Pancreas	Insulin Glucagon
Stomach and intestines	Gastrin Secretin Cholecystokinin (CCK) Vasoactive intestinal peptide (VIP) Bombesin Somatostatin
Pineal gland	Melatonin

Gonads: Ovary	Estrogens
	    Estradiol (E2)
	    Estriol
	    Estrone
	Progesterone

Gonads: Testis	Androgens
	    Testosterone (T)
	    Dihydrotestosterone (DHT)
	    Androstenedione

The pituitary hormones are released into the bloodstream and subsequently act on peripheral endocrine glands to stimulate or inhibit *their* function and hormone release. The hormones produced by the various endocrine target glands then feed back to both the hypothalamus and the pituitary. In this way, the hormonal production of the endocrine glands can be continuously monitored and regulated by the brain (see figures 1.9 and 1.10).

For example, the hypothalamus manufactures and releases corticotropic-releasing hormone (CRH) into the portal blood system. CRH reaches the pituitary and stimulates corticotrophs there to release adrenocorticotropin (ACTH) into the general circulation. ACTH travels to the adrenal glands (just above the kidneys), which in turn release various corticosteroid hormones (such as cortisol) into the bloodstream. This pattern of control holds for all the anterior pituitary hormones: Neurosecretory cells in the hypothalamus release their releasing factors into the portal system. The releasing factors act on specific pituitary cells to stimulate or inhibit the release of their particular hormone. The anterior pituitary hormone travels through the general circulation to affect the hormonal secretions of the target organ(s).

We can use this same example to illustrate another basic feature of hypothalamic-pituitary interactions: negative feedback. The adrenal steroids, released in response to pituitary ACTH (itself released in response to hypothalamic CRH), travel through the bloodstream to reach the entire body, including the brain and pituitary. At these two sites, the adrenal hormones act to stem the flow of CRH from the hypothalamus and inhibit the responsiveness of pituitary adrenotrophs. Both actions result in decreased ACTH release. Lowered ACTH levels then result in a decrease in any additional release of adrenal hormones. The negative feedback loop of information means that the release of adrenal cortex hormones is (normally) self-limiting. The adrenal cortex hormones turn off the stimulus that caused them to be secreted in the first place. In turn, as the blood concentration of adrenal cortex hormones falls, CRH and ACTH levels are released from inhibition, and adrenal cortex hormone levels rise again. Thus, the negative feedback aspect of this loop helps to maintain relatively constant levels of adrenal hormones. If they get too high, CRH and ACTH levels are inhibited. If blood concentrations of adrenal cortex hormones fall too low, CRH and ACTH levels rise to bring them up again.

This negative feedback effect is a general phenomenon characteristic of the regulation of the hypothalamus and anterior pituitary. To cite another example, the hypothalamus also makes and releases thyrotropin-releasing hormone (TRH). TRH stimulates the pituitary to release thyroid-stimulating hormone (TSH). TSH stimulates the thyroid gland to release thyroxine and other thyroid hormones. These thyroid hormones then have a negative feedback effect, reducing hypothalamic release of TRH and pituitary release of TSH. When thyroid hormone levels fall below a certain level, TRH and TSH are released again to restore them.

While the negative feedback loop *tends* to keep hormone concentrations in blood relatively constant, there are also conditions under which the feedback system results in regular cycles of varying hormone concentrations. This occurs during the reproductive cycle in females (chapter 3), during pregnancy (chapter 8), and with endogenous rhythms (chapter 16). For example, during the female's reproductive cycle, estrogen exerts both negative and positive feedback effects on the hypothalamus. During initial development of an egg (or oocyte), a small amount of estrogen is produced and released by the ovary (see figure 3.1 in chapter 3). This inhibits hypothalamic release of gonadotropins-releasing hormone (GnRH) and pituitary release of luteinizing hormone (LH) as a negative feedback effect. Then, as the oocyte becomes mature, there is a rapid increase in estrogen release from the ovary. Instead of inhibiting GnRH and LH release, however, this rapid increase in estrogen has the opposite effect. It *stimulates* a pulse of GnRH release from the hypothalamus. This GnRH pulse induces a pulse of LH release from the pituitary, which is crucial for the final maturation and release of the mature egg (see chapters 2 and 3).

HYPOTHALAMIC NEUROSECRETORY CELLS AND THE POSTERIOR PITUITARY

Oxytocin and vasopressin are hormones made by neurosecretory cells in the hypothalamus. Oxytocin and vasopressin are both neurohormones and neurotransmitters. Some of these cells send their axons down to the median eminence and into the posterior pituitary. When these neurons fire, oxytocin or vasopressin is released from the posterior pituitary directly into the bloodstream. You can think of oxytocin and vasopressin as hypothalamic neurohormones that affect target organs directly, without using pituitary cells or their hormones as intermediaries. However, not all neurons that make oxytocin or vasopressin project to the posterior pituitary. Some of the hypothalamic cells that make these hormones project to the brain and spinal cord, synaptically releasing their products upon neurons.

Oxytocin release into the bloodstream triggers milk ejection during nursing and uterine contractions for childbirth. In fact, hospitals often administer a synthetic version of oxytocin, called pitocin, to induce or speed delivery. Vasopressin is vital for fluid conservation. Additional functions of oxytocin and vasopressin will be discussed in chapters 3, 8, and 15. Oxytocin and vasopressin are "sister" hormones—their chemical structures are very similar. This structural similarity probably reflects a common evolutionary origin of these hormones. Amphibians, for example, have one such hormone, called vasotocin, which has actions reminiscent of both oxytocin and vasopressin.

Most vertebrates produce these hormones, but there are species variations in the molecular structure of the actual hormones produced and in the functions of these hormones. Table 1.4 lists some of the endocrine glands and the hormones that they produce in most vertebrate animals (mammals, reptiles, amphibians, fishes, and birds). The relations among the hypothalamic-releasing factors, anterior pituitary hormones, and their target endocrine glands are illustrated schematically in figure 1.10. Each releasing factor stimulates the release of a specific hormone (or, in the case of GnRH, release of two hormones). These hormones are released by the pituitary into the bloodstream and are then carried to their target organs, where they produce their specific effects, usually stimulating the target organs to release hormones of their own.

Mechanisms of Hormone Action

OVERVIEW: STEROIDS VERSUS PEPTIDE HORMONES

Hormones fall into two general classes based on their molecular structures. The first class comprises steroid hormones produced by the gonads and adrenal cortex and the steroid-like hormones produced by the thyroid gland. The steroid hormones are all synthesized from the common precursor cholesterol (see figure 2.2 in chapter 2). The thyroid hormones have a steroid-like three-dimensional structure that influences their chemical properties, making them behave like steroids. Because these hormones share many common properties they are usually discussed together. The second class of hormones comprises the glycoprotein hormones (LH, follicle-stimulating hormone [FSH]) and protein or peptide hormones. We hinted earlier that these different hormones are synthesized and packaged for secretion in different ways.

The protein and peptide hormones are chains of amino acids and are processed as described earlier for proteins generally. The glycoprotein hormones undergo additional processing in the Golgi apparatus, where a sugar group (glycogen is the basic building block in sugars, hence the "glyco" prefix) is added to the protein prior to packaging into vesicles. Steroid hormones, on the other hand, are synthesized from precursors in the smooth endoplasmic reticulum, processed further in the mitochondria, and then returned to the smooth endoplasmic reticulum for final processing. The thyroid hormones are synthesized from amino acids that form a complex steroid-like structure. It is currently believed that, unlike protein hormones, steroid and steroid-like hormones are not stored in vesicles. It is thought that they simply diffuse out of cells after synthesis. Release of these hormones is, therefore, governed primarily by the rate at which they are synthesized.

The molecular structure of a hormone is also important because of the way it can act upon other cells. Protein, peptide, and glycoprotein hormones do not readily pass through cell membranes, so they usually act upon receptors found in the outer membrane of responsive cells. Only cells containing the appropriate receptor can respond to a particular hormone. The hormone and receptor have complementary shapes (as we discussed for a neurotransmitter and its receptor) that result in the binding of the hormone to the receptor. Protein, glycoprotein, and peptide hormones bind to specific receptor molecules that span the cell membrane and trigger intracellular chemical reactions that can have a wide range of effects, as we will see.

In contrast, because steroid hormones are lipid soluble they are thought to pass through the extracellular membrane. Inside the cell, steroid hormones bind to specific receptor proteins, and this steroid-receptor complex then binds to DNA. The binding of the hormone to DNA results in an increase or decrease in synthesis of specific proteins that also can begin a wide range of effects.

PROTEIN HORMONES

Among the vertebrates, protein hormones include the hypothalamic-releasing factors as well as the pituitary hormones (table 1.4). The posterior pituitary hormones oxytocin and vasopressin are each peptides composed of only nine amino acids. Insulin, another vital protein hormone, consists of about 100 amino acids and is released from the pancreas. Like other proteins, the molecular structure of these hormones is coded for by genes in DNA.

The binding of a protein hormone to its receptor sets into motion a chain of chemical events inside the cell. One of the first events is the activation of a second messenger system that results in a cascading series of reactions within the cell. The exact second messenger varies among the protein hormones, but all are thought to employ second messenger systems to induce a response in target cells. The initial response of the target cell is much like that of a neuron responding to a neurotransmitter, i.e., a change in membrane potential. The particular chain of subsequent events depends upon the type of receptor that was activated and the state of intracellular events that existed before the hormone arrived. Figure 1.11 is a diagram of the rather complicated cascade of chemical reactions triggered by the arrival of a glucagon molecule at a target cell.

The regulation of receptors for protein hormones is thought to be mediated by negative feedback mechanisms similar to those operating at neurotransmitter receptors. In general, the number and activity of these receptors are inversely regulated by the amount of hormone or neurotransmitter available. When neurotransmitter release or protein hormone release is high, a "downregulation" of receptors occurs, so that even more hormone is needed to induce a biological response. In contrast, when hormone release is low, the receptors' response can become supersensitive to stimulation by protein hormones, i.e., less hormone is required to produce the same biological response. This negative feedback system serves to maintain a relatively constant biological response even when the endocrine system may be damaged or altered. For each hormone and receptor, however, there are also other factors that are important in the regulation of receptor activty, including the regulation of receptors by steroid hormones.

One example of the operation of the negative feedback mechanism carried to an extreme occurs in people with adult onset diabetes (also known as type II, or insulin-independent diabetes mellitus). This form of diabetes, as suggested by its name, develops late in life and is usually associated with obesity. Unlike type I diabetes (in which individuals do not produce enough insulin), in type II diabetes insulin secretion is elevated, and peripheral insulin receptors are decreased in number and insensitive to insulin. It is as though the elevated insulin secretion has desensitized the insulin receptors. Alternatively, it may be that the decreased receptor response has resulted in increased insulin secretion. Frequently, after weight loss, these individuals regain normal insulin secretion and sensitivity.[778a] Why some individuals develop this abnormality in the negative feedback response to insulin is not known.

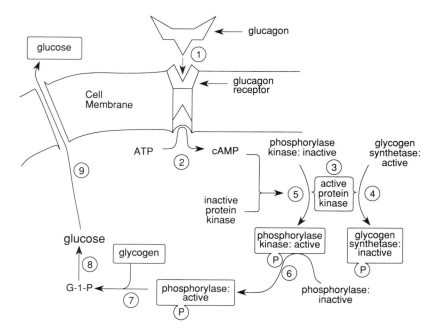

Figure 1.11   Cascade of events triggered by the arrival of a glucagon molecule at a target cell. Glucagon binds to its cell membrane receptor (1). This stimulates the activity of an effector enzyme that promotes the formation of cyclic adenosine monophosphate (cAMP) from adenosine triphosphate (ATP) inside the cell (2). cAMP, known as the second messenger, activates one of a class of enzymes known as protein kinases (3). This particular protein kinase catalyzes the phosphorylation (i.e., the addition of phosphate groups [P]) of other specific enzymes (4, 5, and 6), which in turn catalyze the metabolism of glycogen to glucose-1-phosphate (G-1-P) (7) and then the generation of glucose (8), which is released from the cell (9). (Adapted from Norman and Litwack, 1987.[778a])

STEROID HORMONES

In vertebrates, steroid hormones are often referred to by the organ of their origin. For example, the hormones produced by the ovaries and testes (or gonads) are referred to as the gonadal steroids. The principal products of the testes are the androgens, testosterone and dihydrotestosterone. The ovaries primarily make two types of steroid hormones, estrogens and progestins. Examples of estrogens include estradiol, estriol, and estrone. Progesterone is the principal example of a progestin, so-named because it promotes gestation or pregnancy. It should be noted, however, that testosterone is a precursor to estrogen, so the ovaries also make testosterone. Conversely, estrogen is a metabolite of testosterone, so the testes also produce some estrogen.

The hormones secreted by the cortex of the adrenal gland are known as the adrenal steroids or corticosteroids. The corticosteroids include two classes of steroid hormones. These are the glucocorticoids and the mineralocorticoids. The glucocorticoids, in general, increase circulating glucose. Cortisol and corticosterone are examples of glucocorticoids. Cortisone is a synthetic version of cortisol that is used medicinally. Androgens (testosterone, dehydroepiandrosterone, and so on) are also produced by the adrenal cortex and are released in response to ACTH, as are the mineralocorticoids that regulate water balance (e.g., aldosterone). In fact, over 50 adrenal steroid hormones can be released in response to ACTH from the pituitary. As we will learn in chapter 10, scientists suspect that there are other hormones determining which steroids the adrenals will produce.

One word of caution may be needed here. Although the principal secretion of the testes in most male vertebrates is testosterone, the testes also secrete small amounts of estrogens, as noted earlier. Similarly, ovaries and adrenals also produce androgens. Thus, the idea that androgens are "male" hormones while estrogens are "female" hormones is overly simplistic; both sexes make both classes of hormone albeit in quite different proportions (see chapter 2). The proportions and specific androgens or estrogens that are produced also vary with the species. For example, the stallion has exceptionally high concentrations of estradiol.

The third organ to release steroid-like hormones is the thyroid gland. As noted before, the thyroid hormones look and behave very much like steroids in that they are lipid soluble and not released by exocytosis. The principal thyroid hormones are triiodothyronine, abbreviated T3, and thyroxine (also known as tetra-iodothyronine, abbreviated T4).

Steroid hormones (and thyroid hormones) act quite differently from protein hormones. They are lipophilic and therefore readily cross the lipid cell membrane. Target cells are those that contain protein receptor molecules that recognize and bind to a particular steroid. Once the steroid binds to its receptor, the steroid-receptor complex binds to DNA and thereby manages to either increase or decrease transcription of specific genes (probably by triggering the winding or unwinding of DNA coils), changing the production of a wide variety of proteins. Thus, steroid hormones can **regulate gene transcription** (or expression) and can therefore exert powerful influences upon the development and differentiation of cells.

Another difference between steroids and protein hormones occurs in the regulation of their receptors. Steroid hormone receptors are sometimes regulated by a positive feedback system. In other words, in the absence of testosterone, for example, the number of testosterone receptors decreases. Therefore, it is sometimes necessary to treat an animal repeatedly with a steroid hormone to induce sufficient numbers of receptors to get a biological response. The number of receptors that can be induced by this mechanism is finite, however, so that if excess hormone is present for a prolonged period of time, eventually no receptors will be available to bind hormone.

Selective gene activation or regulation is an important concept. Even though all of the cells in an animal contain the same genetic material (about 100,000 genes in the human), the genes used, or **expressed**, by individual cells vary. Genes that are expressed in a cell are those genes that are transcribed to produce proteins. Most cells express the genes that contain the information needed to produce the synthetic and housekeeping organelles, so some genes are expressed in most cells. Then there are some genes that are expressed in only a particular cell type. For example, it has been estimated that liver cells express about 30,000 genes and various neurons express about 50,000 genes, and that about 20,000 of these genes are common to both liver cells and neurons. It is also important for a cell to be able to adapt to the changing needs of an organism. So the expression of genes is regulated by information obtained from within the cell and by information from external sources. One way that the expression of genes can be regulated is through hormonal input.

Endocrine Methods

BIOASSAY
In the old days, the only way to measure the concentration of a hormone in blood or in an organ was to reconstruct in the laboratory some physiological system that normally responds to the hormone. For example, what if you wanted to measure the testosterone concentration in a sample of blood plasma from a bull? You could castrate adult male rats, thereby depriving them of their own gonadal steroid hormones; you would then notice that the prostate glands surrounding the urethra become smaller afterward and that injections of testosterone make them bigger again. The weight of these glands can serve as a biological assay, or **bioassay**, of androgen concentrations. If you now inject the rat with a solution containing hormones extracted from the plasma of a steer (i.e., a castrated bull), kill the rat and then weigh its prostate, you would see little or no growth, whereas injecting a solution of hormones extracted from the plasma of a bull should induce considerable growth of the rat's prostate. Such bioassays are effective but not very convenient or sensitive. Furthermore, minor differences in the way the rats are treated or the glands dissected can dramatically affect the bioassay results. This makes it difficult sometimes to compare results of bioassays from different investigators because not all laboratories measure a substance in the same way.

RADIOIMMUNOASSAY
These days the most common method for measuring hormone concentrations in blood is the **radioimmunoassay**, or RIA. (The RIA was invented by Rosalyn Yalow and Seymour Berson, for which they won the Nobel prize.) To measure the testosterone concentrations in bull plasma with an RIA, you need three things: (1) testosterone (T) of known purity that was either expressly manufactured (known as "synthetic" hormone because it was synthesized by humans in either a chemistry laboratory or by the enslavement of bacteria) or was "purified" from some animal product (testes perhaps) by the use of biochemical methods; (2) testosterone that has been radioactively labeled (T*). By detecting the radioactive particles given off by the radioactive isotopes, it is possible to quantify the total radioactivity and therefore the total number of so-called "hot" T* molecules. Nonradioactive T molecules may be referred to as "cold" T; (3) an **antibody** that recognizes and attaches itself to testosterone. Antibodies are large, complex proteins made by an organism to attach to invaders

and mark them for destruction (see chapter 10). We can inject a rabbit with the substance of interest and later withdraw some of the rabbit's plasma to harvest the antibodies it made to the substance of interest, in this case, testosterone.

With these three reagents (each of which can be purchased commercially for most hormones) it is possible to assay the concentrations of testosterone in the sample of bull plasma. We refer to the bull's own testosterone as "endogenous testosterone" because it was made inside the bull and contrasts with "exogenous" testosterone that we introduce in either the bull or the plasma sample. If we were to add the antibodies that recognize testosterone to the sample, they would bind the testosterone more or less irreversibly. Unfortunately, there are no simple ways to count the antibodies. On the other hand, if we added the antibodies to our exogenously supplied "hot" T^*, then separated the leftover free T^* from the T^* bound by antibodies, we could use Geiger counter-like machines to detect the antibody-T^* complexes by measuring the radioactive T^*.

So what would happen if we added a known amount of hot T^* to our plasma sample and then added the antibodies? After waiting awhile for the antibodies to bind to both T and T^*, we would separate out the leftover, unbound T^*. If there were no endogenous testosterone in the sample, we would get just as many antibody-T^* complexes (measured by the amount of radioactivity) as we would get if we added antibody and T^* to water instead of plasma. But if there were some endogenous testosterone in the plasma sample, some of the antibodies would stick to that testosterone (which of course would not be "hot"), and therefore fewer antibody-T^* complexes would be made. In fact, the more endogenous testosterone that is present, the more hot molecules would be displaced and therefore fewer antibody-T^* complexes would be detected when we measure the radioactivity. We can find out how much hot T^* will be displaced by a given amount of testosterone by measuring out different amounts of "cold" T of known purity (say 50, 100, 250, and 500 micrograms [μg] worth) and seeing exactly how much T^* is displaced by each. From this information we could generate a standard curve that would allow us to determine exactly how much testosterone exists in each of our biological samples.

Summary

Behavioral endocrinology joins together the fields of neuroscience, endocrinology, and psychology to ask important and exciting questions about how changes in the endocrine system can influence the brain and behavior. In this chapter we have reviewed some of the basic concepts important to the study of the nervous and endocrine systems. Some of the most important concepts are summarized below.

1. The methods used to measure and evaluate behavior must be just as precise and exacting as the methods used to quantify hormones. In many ways, the behavioral component of these experiments is much more difficult than the biochemical methods discussed. This is because the methods to quantify

behavior frequently depend on visual observation. Thus, a great deal of time is needed to conduct precise and accurate measures of behavior.

2. We will study three different types of intercellular messengers: neurotransmitters, neurohormones, and hormones. Most of these intercellular messengers are packaged into secretory vesicles for release by exocytosis. Differences among these messengers lie in where they are produced, where they are released, and the distance that must be traveled to produce an effect. Neurotransmitters are produced by neurons in the brain, released at the synaptic terminal, and diffuse across the synaptic cleft to produce a response at the postsynaptic membrane. Neurohormones are produced by neurons in the brain, released from synaptic terminals into the bloodstream, and produce their effects at target organs. Hormones are produced by endocrine cells, released into the bloodstream, and produce their effect at distant target organs.

3. Communication between neurons occurs through the release by exocytosis of chemical messengers known as neurotransmitters. The neurotransmitter is released at the synapse and binds to a postsynaptic receptor. This process is known as synaptic transmission. The binding of the neurotransmitter to the receptor results in a change in the membrane polarization of the postsynaptic cell. This influences whether or not the postsynaptic cell will fire an action potential. Drugs that produce changes in neuronal activity usually do so by influencing one or more components of synaptic transmission.

4. Neurohormones known as releasing factors are released by neurosecretory cells in the hypothalamus. These releasing factors travel through a specialized system of blood vessels to reach the anterior pituitary to control the release of pituitary hormones. The pituitary hormones enter the bloodstream to regulate the release of hormones from the peripheral endocrine glands. Negative and positive feedback from the endocrine glands to the brain and pituitary results in coordination of the neuroendocrine systems.

5. Hormones are classified according to their molecular structure as either steroid or protein hormones. Both kinds of hormones produce their effects on target tissues by binding to specific receptors. The process induced by the binding of a hormone to the receptor is very different depending on whether the hormone is a protein or a steroid. Protein hormones induce their effects by binding to membrane-associated receptors and causing intracellular changes by activation of a second messenger system. Steroid hormones bind to intracellular receptors, and the steroid-receptor complex alters gene expression.

6. Genetic information is coded by the DNA found in the nuclei of eucaryotic cells. Particular lengths of DNA known as genes are transcribed into a string of specific RNA nucleotides that leave the nucleus. In the cytoplasm of the cell, RNA is translated into a specific sequence of amino acids. A short sequence of amino acids is called a peptide; a long sequence is called a protein. The genetic code is important for our understanding of information in later chapters for two reasons. First, steroid hormones produce their effects by altering gene expression, and this can be shown to be related to the behavioral effects of steroid hormones. Second, releasing factors, neurotransmitters, and

some hormones are proteins or are synthesized from proteins. One way to measure changes in production of these molecules is to quantify the production of the mRNA that codes for these proteins.

Sources of Additional Information

Textbooks

Rosenzweig, M. R., and Leiman, A. L. (1989) Physiological Psychology (2nd ed.). Random House, New York.

Cooper, J. R., Bloom, F. E., and Roth, R. H. (1991) The Biochemical Basis of Neuropharmacology (6th ed.). Oxford University Press, New York.

Norman, A. W. and Litwack, G. (1987) Hormones. Academic Press, San Diego.

Shepherd, G. M. (1988) Neurobiology (2nd ed.). Oxford University Press, New York.

Review Articles

On the secretory process in eucaryotic cells: Palade, G. E. and Farquar, M. G. (1981) Cell biology. In L. H. Smith and S. O. Thier (Eds.), Pathophysiology: The Biological Principles of Disease. W. B. Saunders, Philadelphia, pp. 1–56.

On behavioral techniques in the laboratory: Whishaw, I. Q., Kolb, B., and Sutherland, R. J. (1983) The analysis of behavior in the laboratory rat. In T. E. Robinson (Ed.), Behavioral Approaches to Brain Research. Oxford University Press, New York, pp. 141–202.

2 Sexual Differentiation of the Brain and Behavior

S. Marc Breedlove

This next introductory chapter is made necessary by a quite fundamental fact of life on this planet: sex. Almost all of the more complex animals on this planet are either male or female, and this difference has remarkably wide-ranging consequences for both physiology and behavior. The processes that lead to external and internal differences between the sexes are fairly well understood, and, as you will see, hormones play a pivotal role in these differences. We even know something about how the brains of males and females came to be different, but deciding how those differences affect behavior remains a challenge.

How do males and females develop differently, what controls those differences, and when do they arise? What biological factors influence sex differences in behavior, and are such factors at work in humans? How might environmental and biological influences interact during the development of sex differences?

Introduction

Every toddler quickly learns that humans come in two basic anatomical packages. (To quote one such source, "boys stick out and girls are neatly tucked in.") Thereafter, the tendency to classify animals, people, their accessories (e.g., boats, cars), and their behavior as either feminine or masculine becomes, for most of us, deeply ingrained and virtually reflexive. We are used to thinking that the ultimate criterion for gender is based upon external genitalia: Is there a penis or a vagina? But many other parts of the body, including the brain, are also different in male and female mammals, and, as we shall see, it is possible for an individual to be masculine in some body regions and feminine in others.

We are going to explore what is known about how males and females develop different bodies, brains, and behaviors—a process known as **sexual differentiation**. The principles of development of physical sex differences in humans have already proved to be very similar to those in other mammals. However, when we consider sex differences in behavior and the structure of the nervous system, it has been more difficult to decide whether the processes at work in other animals also apply to humans. Our strategy will be to gain a firm understanding of sexual differentiation in animal models and then to see which mechanisms apply to humans. Chapter 7 will discuss ways in which sexual differentiation in some nonmammalian vertebrates (frogs, electric fish, and songbirds) is similar and ways in which it is different from that in mammals.

Sexual Reproduction in Vertebrates

Keep in mind that mammals are the minority and that for most animal species on this planet (i.e., most of the invertebrates) there is only one sex. Some animals can reproduce by **parthenogenesis** (literally "virgin birth"). These parthenogenetic females give rise to daughters that are genetically identical to the mother. You will learn more about a parthenogenetic vertebrate in chapter 6. Many invertebrate species (e.g., slugs, worms, jellyfish) are **monoecious**, meaning that all individuals are alike and are hermaphroditic. Each individual has both male and female reproductive organs and can reproduce as either or both. Note that, unless the hermaphrodite self-fertilizes, it is still reproducing sexually.

On the other hand, almost all vertebrates and many invertebrate species are **dioecious**, meaning that there are two distinct sexes. Another term with a similar meaning is **gonochorism**, the specialization of gonads (i.e., ovaries or testes) in the two sexes to produce different **gametes** (i.e., eggs or sperm).

Sexual reproduction, by combining chromosomes from different individuals, clearly helps to bring together in a single individual all the advantageous mutations that have arisen in many separate individuals. However, evolutionary theorists have yet to reach a consensus on why almost all vertebrates reproduce sexually.

Sex Determination

You may already know that sex chromosomes normally determine whether we develop as boys or girls. The mother's egg always contains one X chromosome, and if it is fertilized by a sperm carrying another X chromosome, the baby will be a female, but if the father contributes a Y chromosome, the baby will be a male. These rules of sex determination hold for mammals and will be discussed later.

First, however, you should be warned that the mechanisms of sex determination vary dramatically in other vertebrates. In birds the female has two different sex chromosomes (known as W and Z), while the male has two Z chromosomes. Consequently, it is the mother's contribution that determines the sex of the offspring, depending on which sex chromosome was carried by the egg before it was fertilized. Some reptiles have sex chromosomes, but in other reptile and amphibian species it is the temperature at which the eggs are incubated that determines the sex![167]

Among the invertebrates, many species have no sex determination at all because, as mentioned above, each individual has both sets of reproductive organs. Other invertebrates, such as the fruit fly, *Drosophila melanogaster*, have two distinct sexes and, like mammals, use sex-determining chromosomes. Finally, some invertebrate species have some individuals that are hermaphroditic, whereas other individuals are one sex or the other.

Sexual Differentiation in Mammals

The Process of Sexual Differentiation

How does the presence of the Y chromosome cause male development and the absence of a Y chromosome result in female development? The chain of events during sexual differentiation is well understood in placental mammals such as ourselves and was largely worked out by Alfred Jost in the 1950s and 1960s.[542] A simplified summary is that genetic sex determines gonadal sex, and gonadal sex determines phenotypic sex. Recall that an individual's phenotype is the sum total of all the physical characteristics she or he possesses. Clearly, our phenotype changes with time, and we call those changes with time development or ontogeny or aging. In contrast, our genotype, i.e., the sum total of all genetic information contained in one's DNA, is fixed at fertilization. Except for rare mistakes in duplication, our genotype does not change. So what do we mean by saying genetic sex determines gonadal sex, which determines phenotypic sex?

The Y chromosome does not seem to do very much (as many people have guessed). Early in development, both XX and XY individuals have gonads that do not yet resemble either testes or ovaries and are therefore called "indifferent" (figure 2.1*A*). The one crucial task performed by at least one gene on the Y chromosome is the transformation of this originally indifferent gonad into a testis. This gene on the Y chromosome has been found, and the structure of the protein it encodes, the testis determination factor (TDF), was recently determined.[117] If the cells of the indifferent gonad contain a Y chromosome with the TDF gene, they begin to develop as a testis. In the absence of a TDF gene, the gonad develops as an ovary. Thus, genetic sex (whether the individual is XX or XY) determines gonadal sex (whether there are ovaries or testes). Thereafter, the rest of sexual differentiation is driven not by the sex chromosomes directly but by the hormones secreted by the gonads.

THE ROLE OF GONADAL HORMONES IN SEXUAL DIFFERENTIATION
OF THE BODY
If the indifferent gonad develops as an ovary, it appears to secrete very little hormone prenatally, and the fetus develops into a female. But if the gonad develops into a testis, several hormones are secreted, and these hormones instruct the rest of the body to develop in a masculine fashion. Thus, genetic sex, via the presence or absence of TDF, determines gonadal sex, which, through hormonal secretions, determines phenotypic sex. In other words, differences between males and females arise indirectly as a function of the hormones secreted by the gonads, not as a direct influence of sex chromosomes.

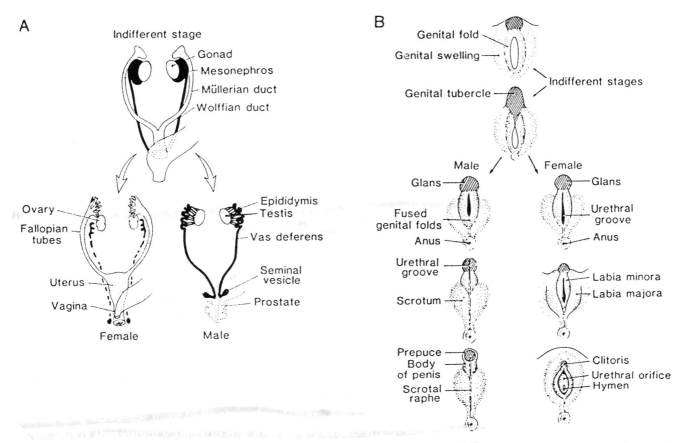

Figure 2.1 Fetal development of male and female reproductive tracts. *A*, Early in development (top) internal organs are "indifferent" because they appear identical in the two sexes. There are two duct systems, the müllerian and Wolffian ducts, connecting the indifferent gonads to the body wall. In females (lower left), the müllerian ducts grow and differentiate to form fallopian tubes, uterus, and the inner portion of the vagina. In males (lower right) it is the Wolffian ducts that develop, forming the epididymis, vas deferens, and seminal vesicle. The prostate arises from nearby tissues. *B*, External genitalia also begin as indifferent (top). In males (left), the genital tubercle grows to form a penis, and genital folds fuse, forming the scrotum and enclosing the urethral groove to form the urethra. In females (right), the genital tubercle develops into the clitoris, and genital folds form the labia and outer vagina. Hormones drive this sexual differentiation of the urogenital system. (From Wilson et al., 1980.[1103a])

TESTICULAR SECRETIONS DRIVING MASCULINE DEVELOPMENT

The testicular secretions that drive masculine development are the peptide hormone known as the müllerian regression factor (MRF) and the steroid hormone testosterone. At first, both XX and XY individuals have two sets of "ducts" connecting the indifferent gonad to the exterior: the müllerian ducts and the Wolffian ducts (figure 2.1A). MRF is secreted only by testes and, true to its name, causes the müllerian ducts to regress. Ovaries do not secrete MRF, and consequently the müllerian ducts develop into the fallopian tubes, uterus, and inner vagina. In adult females, these structures form the pathway through which the ripened egg will be fertilized, the embryo will be nurtured, and the fetus brought to the outside world.

   The second testicular secretion directing masculine development is the steroid hormone testosterone. Testosterone has masculinizing effects on many parts of the developing body including, as we will see later, the brain. One effect of testosterone is the acceleration of development of the Wolffian ducts, a process known as virilization. In the absence of testosterone, the Wolffian ducts remain only as tiny remnants. Only with testosterone stimulation do the Wolffian ducts form the epididymis, vas deferens, and seminal vesicles. In the adult male, these structures lead from the testis to the penis and deliver sperm for reproduction. Testosterone also directs the masculine development of the genital skin into the penis and scrotum (the pouch of skin that holds the testes). In the absence of testosterone, these genital regions form a clitoris, the outer vagina and the labia surrounding the vagina (figure 2.1B). The masculinizing influence of testosterone on the external genitalia is aided by an enzyme called 5α-reductase that is present in the genital skin and converts testosterone to dihydrotestosterone (DHT; figure 2.2). DHT binds the androgen receptors more effectively than does testosterone, and thus the reductase enzyme serves to amplify the effects of androgen locally. We know that the virilization of the Wolffian ducts does not require this amplification because little or no reductase is found there during that period.

Anomalies in Sexual Differentiation

Occasionally individuals are born with an abnormal complement of sex chromosomes. Turner's syndrome results when only a single sex chromosome is present (denoted as XO). Such individuals develop abnormal but recognizable ovaries and, in the absence of testicular secretions, a feminine body. Unfortunately, they also usually suffer from mental retardation and other defects resulting from the poorly understood consequences of having only one X chromosome. No individuals have been found without any X chromosome— i.e., there are no known cases of YO, which indicates that such a condition is lethal during early development. In XXY (Klinefelter's syndrome) or XYY individuals, the gonads develop as testes and result in a masculine phenotype, again with occasional mental retardation and sterility. These chromosomal

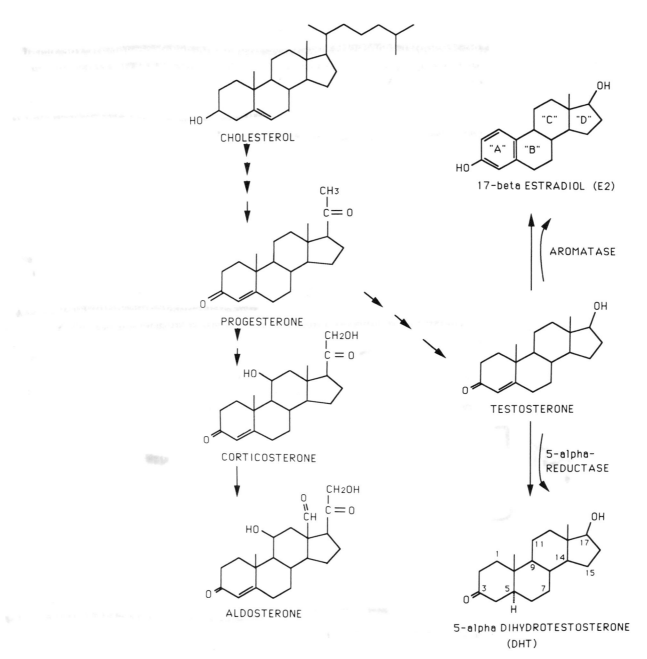

Figure 2.2 Steroids are synthesized from cholesterol that is either eaten or manufactured from simpler compounds. Cholesterol (top left) consists of four connected rings of carbon atoms. In chemical convention, each line represents a bond between carbon atoms; double lines represent double bonds, but most of the Cs are omitted here for clarity. Cholesterol can be converted to progesterone through four chemical reactions (represented by four arrows), each catalyzed by a specific enzyme. Progesterone in turn can be converted to the glucocorticoid called corticosterone, which in turn can be converted to the mineralocorticoid aldosterone (bottom left). Alternatively, a series of enzymes can transform progesterone to testosterone (middle right). The various carbon atoms of steroids are numbered by convention (lower right). The enzyme 5α-reductase acts to reduce the number 5 carbon atom by

abnormalities underscore the simple rule that when a Y chromosome is present, the indifferent gonads will develop as testes.

On the one hand, sexual differentiation appears rather simple because testicular secretions drive masculinization. However, to produce the male phenotype, TDF, two hormones (MRF and testosterone), many enzymes (including 5α-reductase and the enzymes needed for steroid manufacture), and several receptors (those for androgen and those for MRF) must all be expressed by the individual's genes. Thus, there are many steps in which a missing or defective gene can cause things to go awry. Because such mistakes are not lethal, each has been found in humans.

One interesting anomaly in sexual differentiation is the testicular feminization mutation (TFM), also known as androgen insensitivity. These animals have a defective structural gene for the androgen receptor and therefore fail to respond to androgen. The TFM mutation is on the X chromosome and is transmitted by female carriers who, of course, have a second X chromosome with a normal androgen receptor gene. Half of the eggs produced by such a carrier will receive the X chromosome with the TFM gene. If such an egg is fertilized by an X-bearing sperm, another female carrier will result. But when an egg with the TFM gene is fertilized by a Y-carrying sperm, problems arise. The resulting offspring will develop testes (due to normal TDF activity from the Y), and the testes will secrete MRF, which will cause the müllerian ducts to regress. Furthermore, the testes will also secrete testosterone, but, because the individual lacks functional androgen receptors, the genital epithelium fails to respond to the androgen and therefore develops in a feminine fashion, i.e., with a clitoris, labia, and a shallow vagina. Thus, the individual will be born looking like a normal female, and in humans the condition may not be detected until puberty, when the absence of menstruation brings the attention of a doctor.

Androgen-insensitive humans look, act, and think of themselves as females despite their XY genotype, testes, and sterility. TFM defects have also been found in mice, rats, cats, and goats.[984] One aspect of sexual differentiation unique to humans that is illustrated by androgen insensitivity is the development of breasts. The extent of breast development seems to depend on the ratio of estrogens to androgens—the higher the ratio the greater the development. These steroids have their greatest effect upon breast development during

---

adding a hydrogen atom to it. This hydrogen is added in the alpha position, meaning that it projects slightly below the plane of the figure (indicated by a broken line). A hydrogen atom is also added to the number 4 carbon (not shown), and hence the result is known as dihydrotestosterone (DHT). 5α-DHT is an important androgen. If the hydrogen is added to the number 5 carbon in the beta direction (catalyzed by 5β-reductase), the resulting 5β-DHT has no biological activity. An enzyme called aromatase (because it aromatizes the A ring of carbon atoms) converts testosterone to 17β-estradiol (upper right). The hydroxy group (OH) attached to the number 17 carbon atom is in the beta position, meaning that it projects slightly above the plane of the figure. 17α-Estradiol has no biological activity. The conversion of testosterone to either estrogen or DHT is a one-way process, i.e., neither estradiol nor DHT is converted back to testosterone.

Table 2.1 Possible Genetic Defects Resulting in Abnormal Sexual Phenotype

Predict, for each of the cases below, the sexual phenotype of the following structures: gonads, müllerian duct features, Wolffian duct features, external genitalia. Later, after we have discussed sex differences in neural structure, you may want to deduce whether they would appear feminine or masculine in these instances. We provide an answer for the first two cases.

1. An XY individual in which both testes fail to develop (or are removed).

   Here you would predict that there would be no gonads; in the absence of MRF the müllerian duct structures would develop in the feminine fashion, and, due to the absence of androgen, Wolffian ducts and external genital features would be phenotypically female.

2. An XY individual in which one testis fails to develop (or is removed).

   The single testis should produce enough androgen to at least partially masculinize the external genitalia and Wolffian duct structures. It turns out that müllerian regression factor (MRF) must act locally because when this experiment is performed, the müllerian duct structures partially develop on the side where the testis is removed.

3. An XX individual in which both ovaries fail to develop.

4. An XY individual in which androgen receptors are absent (i.e., testicular feminization mutation [TFM]).

5. An XY individual in which the enzyme 5 α-reductase is absent.

6. An XO individual (Turner's syndrome).

7. An XY individual in which MRF is defective or absent.

8. An XY individual in which MRF receptors are defective or absent.

9. An XY individual with an additional X chromosome (47 XXY; Klinefelter's syndrome).

10. An XY individual with an additional Y chromosome (47 XYY).

puberty, exerting only subtle effects thereafter. Human TFM individuals typically develop phenotypically female breasts because their testes and adrenals secrete small amounts of estrogen. This does not amount to much estrogen but, because of the inadequate androgen receptors, the functional ratio of estrogens to androgens is high. There are also instances of incomplete androgen insensitivity, which results in an intermediate sexual phenotype that may be obvious at birth.

Sexual differentiation of genetic females can also be disturbed by early exposure to androgen. The most common such syndrome is **congenital adrenal hyperplasia** (CAH), so called because these individuals are born with enlarged adrenal glands. These individuals lack an enzyme that converts androstenedione to cortisol in the adrenal cortex. Because there is little cortisol to provide negative feedback, the hypothalamus and pituitary release more corticotropic-releasing hormone (CRH). This causes the pituitary to release more adrenocorticotropic hormone (ACTH). Consequently, the adrenal gland grows larger (hence the term hyperplasia, meaning an excessive number of cells) and releases more steroid hormone in response to ACTH. However, some of the androstenedione that would normally be converted to cortisol is instead made into androgen as a "spillover" product. Because the adrenal cortex is unable to make cortisol to bring CRH and ACTH levels back down, this high androgen secretion will continue unless the individual is treated. When this prenatal condition occurs in females, their bodies are exposed to androgen and therefore are partially masculinized, i.e., the clitoris is enlarged and the labia may resemble a scrotum. Such individuals are usually identified at birth, and with present-day treatment the phallus is surgically reduced to resemble a more normal clitoris and exogenous cortisol is administered to reduce ACTH release, thereby halting excess androgen production. Such individuals are sometimes referred to as hermaphrodites. This term is not quite correct because they do not possess testes and, unlike true hermaphrodites, cannot reproduce as males. Thus, CAH individuals are more properly "pseudo-hermaphrodites." Not long ago, they were often untreated, and they and their families experienced a good deal of confusion about their actual gender.

Some XY individuals either lack MRF or the receptors to respond to MRF. Such individuals look like men but during surgery are found to have a moderately developed uterus and remnants of fallopian tubes!

An especially intriguing human example of abnormal sexual differentiation is the person in whom inadequate 5α-reductase (which is required to convert testosterone to DHT in the external genitalia) is produced by an XY fetus. The child is born with slightly ambiguous genitalia—labia (with testes inside) and an enlarged clitoris. This partial masculinization is presumed to be the result of testicular testosterone acting without the amplification provided by reductase in the external genitalia.[519] These individuals are usually raised as females, but at puberty the rise in testicular androgen secretion causes the phallus and scrotum to grow and the body to develop in a male fashion, i.e., narrow hips, male-like breasts, muscular build, and, eventually, slight beard growth. This genetically transmitted condition is fairly common in one area of the Dominican Republic, where such individuals are known as "guevedoces"—a name that means literally: testes at 12 years old. At this age the individuals start wearing male clothes, assuming male tasks, and having girlfriends.

It has been suggested that these cases prove that early testosterone masculinizes the human brain in terms of gender identity and sexual preference and that social influences contribute little to these characteristics. This view contends that the guevedoces grow up to be men despite having been raised as girls. However, it is hard to rule out the possibility that the villagers treat these children differently from normal girls. Certainly the existence of a nickname for the condition means that they are aware of the possibility. Furthermore, there are considerable advantages to be gained from being a male in that society. Thus, an alternative explanation is that early hormones have *no* influence on human gender identity, that humans are quite malleable, and that when confronted with an altered body and residing in a society that permits it, they can change sexual identities at puberty.

In summary, in placental mammals sex chromosomes guide the development of the gonads, and then gonadal secretions coordinate the sexual differentiation of the body. Both males and females have the capacity to respond to the masculinizing influence of testicular secretions, and both male and female bodies can develop in a feminine fashion in the absence of those hormones.

Masculinization of the Ability to Ovulate by Testicular Hormones

The first demonstration that early steroids could permanently masculinize the nervous system took place in 1933, but it was not originally recognized as such. It was known that the pituitary was crucial for ovulation (i.e., the production and expulsion of a mature egg) because when the pituitary was removed, ovulation ceased. Furthermore, when bits of ovary were implanted in the eyes of female rats, the ovarian fragments still ovulated. This finding demonstrated that hormones alone could control ovulation, even when the nerves innervating the ovary were cut. But when Pfeiffer[815] implanted bits of ovary in the eyes of male rats, the fragments did not ovulate. Pfeiffer very reasonably concluded that it was the male rats' pituitary that could not support ovulation. We will discuss ovulatory cycles, including the menstrual cycle, in chapter 3.

Pfeiffer then went on to show that testicular secretions in the first few days of life determined whether a rat would later, as an adult, be competent to induce ovulation. When male rats were castrated shortly after birth, they could support ovulation (in surgically implanted ovaries, of course) as adults. When newborn female rats were given subcutaneous grafts of testicular tissue, they could not support ovulation as adults in either their own or surgically provided ovaries. (Later experimenters showed that a single injection of testosterone during the first week of life had the same effect as a testicular graft: The rat became permanently incompetent to support ovulation.) Pfeiffer concluded that exposure to androgen early in life somehow masculinized the pituitary and that ovulatory incompetence was an indication of the masculinization that took place.

CONTROL OF OVULATORY COMPETENCE BY THE BRAIN

In the meantime, Geoffrey Harris was championing the idea that, while the pituitary was the "master gland" regulating hormone secretion, it was in turn controlled by the brain. The idea that the brain plays a role in triggering ovulation was supported by the existence of "induced ovulators" (such as rabbits and cats; see chapter 3). In these animals, ovulation is triggered by the stimulation of copulation itself. Rabbits could be induced to ovulate by gently stimulating the vagina and cervix with a blunt glass rod. These findings indicated that the nervous system must be somehow involved in the control of ovulation. Because there were no nerve fibers from the brain to the anterior pituitary, Harris proposed that the sensory stimulation of copulation eventually reached a part of the brain called the hypothalamus and that the hypothalamus in turn released some chemical factor to stimulate the pituitary. Harris and others had previously noted that the hypothalamus was close enough to the pituitary to allow such chemical control. In fact, electrical stimulation of the hypothalamus could itself induce ovulation. Harris' vision of hypothalamic domination of the pituitary was amply confirmed[465] (see chapter 1).

So, did Pfeiffer's hormone manipulations of rats masculinize the pituitary or the hypothalamus? Harris proved that the pituitary of male rats could in fact support ovulation. He removed the pituitary of female rats and, in a very demanding surgical procedure, implanted a male rat's pituitary in its place. If the surgeon succeeded in connecting the blood supply (that is, the hypothalamic-pituitary portal system) to the pituitary, the rat could support ovulation.[466] This demonstration proved that the male's pituitary was competent to support ovulation.

Pfeiffer's experiments therefore had to be reinterpreted. By elimination, one might conclude that the brain, probably the hypothalamus, had been permanently altered and made incompetent for ovulation by early androgen exposure. This idea was eventually proved to be correct. Specifically, for ovulation to take place the female rat hypothalamus must release a surge of gonadotropin-releasing hormone (GnRH) in response to estrogen stimulation. This "positive feedback" effect of estrogen on GnRH differs from the more usual situation in which steroids inhibit further GnRH release (the negative feedback described in chapter 1). The pulse of GnRH causes the pituitary to release a pulse of luteinizing hormone (LH), which causes the ovary to expel the egg. We now know that the hypothalamus of male rats does not show the positive feedback effect and therefore does not release the pulse of GnRH needed for ovulation.

Interestingly, primates differ from rodents in this regard. Males can show a positive feedback response to estrogen. In fact, male monkeys receiving an ovarian implant can support ovulation.[779] No one knows why primates differ from rodents in this way. But in rodents the same testicular signals that instruct the body to develop a male phenotype also masculinize (or, more properly, defeminize[1099]) the brain to prevent ovulatory capacity.

MASCULINIZATION OF BEHAVIOR BY TESTICULAR HORMONES EARLY IN LIFE

Phoenix and associates[817] studied copulation in rodents, especially the receptive behavior of female guinea pigs. For copulation to take place among rodents, the female must arch her back to elevate the rump and head and, in species that have a tail, move the tail to one side (see figure 1.1). This posture is called lordosis, and it can serve as a measure of the female's receptivity to mating. Normally, female rodents exhibit this lordosis reflex in response to mounting from a male only during a particular part of the ovulatory cycle. When the ovaries are removed, the animal becomes behaviorally unreceptive (i.e., she fails to exhibit lordosis). A female rat can be made receptive again by being given injections of estrogen for 1 to 2 days and then a single injection of progesterone. This regimen simulates the sequence of steroids normally produced during the ovulatory cycle. Approximately 6 hours after the progesterone injection, the female becomes receptive—i.e., for a few hours she will display the lordosis posture in response to the mounting of a male. We say that the estrogen and progesterone "activated" the lordosis behavior.

When the same hormonal regimen that activates behavioral receptivity in ovariectomized females is given to a castrated male, the male shows almost no lordosis in response to another male's mounting. (Normal male rats readily mount and thrust their pelvis against the backside of just about any other rat they bump into, especially if that rat is smaller. If the mounted rat is a male and, as in the case just mentioned, fails to show a lordosis response, the first male will eventually stop mounting him.) The fact that males are not induced to show lordosis after being given the same hormones that activate lordosis in females indicates that male and female rats must be different. Because the central nervous system (CNS) mediates behavior, it is likely that the nervous system holds the difference. In other words, the male and female nervous systems are not alike in their behavioral responsiveness to hormones.

Phoenix and colleagues asked whether the same factor that masculinized the bodies and ovulatory competence of rodents also masculinized their ability to show a lordosis response to adult steroids. They found that female guinea pigs that had been exposed to testosterone prenatally showed little or no lordosis behavior when given estrogen and progesterone in adulthood. This result inspired the "organizational hypothesis": that early androgens permanently alter the developing brain, causing it to function in a masculine manner in adulthood. In other words, sexual differentiation of the nervous system, and consequently behavior, is guided by the same steroid cues that drive sexual differentiation of the body.

Testicular steroids normally exert a masculinizing influence on the body early in development, during the first trimester of pregnancy in humans. After that time, androgens come to be increasingly less effective, so that by adulthood steroids can exert only modest effects on these structures. Little is understood about why the body stops responding to steroids, but restricted "sensitive periods" such as this are common in development. The organizational hypothesis proposed that the nervous system also was sensitive to the masculinizing influence of steroids for only a brief period in development. In rats, for example, injections of testosterone on the day of birth or up to the tenth day of life can render a female anovulatory and unlikely to display lordosis. However, by the twelfth day of life, even large doses of steroids have little effect on these measures.

The organizational hypothesis had an immediate and profound effect upon the field of behavioral endocrinology. Many researchers tried to see whether other sex differences in adult behavior were determined by early androgen exposure. In each case, the prediction was clear—exposure of young animals to androgen should make their behavior more masculine in adulthood, and the absence or removal of androgen should result in more feminine adult behavior. Furthermore, particular behaviors could be affected by steroid treatment only during a sensitive period, which varied from species to species and for different behaviors. Although there were some interesting exceptions,[37] these predictions were often borne out for many other behaviors as well (e.g., taste preferences, aggression, rough and tumble play, masculine copulatory behavior).

The organizational hypothesis presented a nice clear picture: The same hormonal signals that guide the sexual differentiation of the genitalia also guide the sexual differentiation of the brain. Individuals with penises need not bother with the neural circuitry that supports ovulation or display lordosis behavior, whereas individuals with vaginas develop lordosis "circuits" and therefore show the sex-appropriate behavior. In the case of both the genitalia and the nervous system, androgen secretions from the fetal testes drive masculine development. If a newborn female rat is exposed to androgen, it may be too late to cause a penis to develop, but the adult rat will be unable to support ovulation and much less likely to display lordosis than an untreated female. If a newborn male rodent is deprived of his testes, he will still have a penis in adulthood (because the testes did their prenatal work), but he will act like a female: Given the right hormones in adulthood, he will show lordosis behavior.

PARADOXICAL EFFECT OF EARLY ESTROGEN TREATMENT ON THE CENTRAL NERVOUS SYSTEM

Not only will a single injection of testosterone permanently masculinize the behavior of a newborn female, so will a single injection of estrogen! Such early estrogen treatment has little or no effect on the genitalia but drastically masculinizes ovulatory competence and lordosis behavior.[133, 344] In fact, microgram for microgram, estrogen is more effective than testosterone for masculinizing ovulation and lordosis behavior. These findings at first challenged the organizational hypothesis. Why should an ovarian steroid cause masculinization? Why don't estrogens from the newborn females's ovaries (or prenatal estrogen from the mother's ovaries) masculinize them normally? The organizational hypothesis was rescued from these vexing questions by a very helpful offspring—the aromatization hypothesis.

The chemical structure of testosterone and estrogen are very similar. In fact, testosterone can be converted to estrogen by a single chemical reaction, the substitution of a hydroxy group for a double-bonded oxygen and simultaneous losses of a hydrogen atom and a methyl group. These substitutions make the A ring resemble benzene, a process that chemists refer to as aromatization (figure 2.2). Originally, this term referred to the fact that benzene-like compounds were literally aromatic (i.e., fragrant). The aromatization of testosterone to estrogen is greatly facilitated by the enzyme aromatase. Importantly, the reverse reaction, the conversion of estrogens back to testosterone, is energetically very expensive, very rare, and functionally insignificant. These biochemical facts of life mean that tissues containing aromatase can convert testosterone to estrogen and thereby make use of estrogen receptors.

It was soon demonstrated, in adult[771] and newborn[841] rats, that the hypothalamus contained aromatase. Furthermore, when rats were injected with radiolabeled testosterone, a small but significant amount of radiolabeled

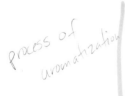
Process of aromatization

estrogen appeared in the brain,[690] and some of that estrogen was bound to estrogen receptors. Thus, systemic testosterone could wind up stimulating estrogen receptors in the hypothalamus. The aromatization hypothesis proposed that it was in fact the aromatized estrogenic metabolites of testosterone that masculinized the developing rodent brain. That was why injections of estrogen to newborn females could permanently render them anovulatory and less likely to display lordosis. If it seems paradoxical that a "feminine" hormone like estrogen could be responsible for masculinization, remember that both sexes normally secrete the same steroids, albeit in different proportions. Also, remember that testosterone is a normal precursor for the synthesis of estrogen. It seems that natural selection shows no concern for our labels of what is feminine or masculine.

There was a problem with this theory, of course—how do females normally escape masculinization? Although the ovaries of fetuses and newborns secrete very little steroid, all fetuses are exposed to rather high levels of estrogens produced by the mother's ovaries during pregnancy. (Steroids readily pass through the placental barrier.) What prevents these maternal estrogens from masculinizing female offspring? A protein called α-fetoprotein (AFP) was found in the plasma of perinatal rodents. AFP binds estrogen but not testosterone. It is now generally accepted that AFP works in rat fetuses of both sexes to bind maternal (or fetal) estrogen and limit its entry to the developing brain (see figure 2.2). Male fetuses circumvent this barrier by secreting testosterone, which bypasses AFP. The testosterone enters brain cells, where it is locally aromatized to estrogen, beyond the reach of AFP, and triggers (through estrogen receptors) some cascade of events that prevents the normal expression of ovulation and lordosis. Injections of exogenous estrogens swamp the AFP molecules, allowing some estrogen to reach the brain. Interestingly, although a clear homologue of rodent AFP is found in primates, it does not bind estrogen. As we will see, this and other findings cast doubt on the role of aromatization in the masculinization of the human CNS.

There are several situations in which hormones passed between mother and fetus or between fetuses can affect sexual differentiation. For example, farmers have known for centuries that a female calf born with a male twin may be sterile as an adult. The likelihood that such cows, known as freemartins, will be sterile correlates with the amount of overlap between the twins' placentas.[634] In rats there is a similar but more subtle effect on the receptivity of females developing near males in utero.[213] For both cows and rats, fetal testicular hormones appear to be able to cross from one fetus to the other and thereby influence sexual differentiation. It also appears that the male fetuses of pregnant rats exposed to stress have slightly lower than normal levels of fetal androgen and adult masculine copulatory behavior, due perhaps to maternally secreted opiates that damp fetal GnRH release (see chapter 4) and therefore testosterone secretion.

Finally, from this discussion you might think that the sexual differentiation of the brain and sexual behavior are passive in females. But recent research suggests that the presence of a small amount of estrogen (from the mother prenatally or from the developing ovary postnatally) may be necessary for the full expression of feminine sexual behavior and other sex-related behaviors in female rats and mice.[299, 1038] Thus AFP may serve to regulate, not completely prevent, estrogen's access to the brain.

Detailed Mechanisms of Sexual Differentiation

Discovery of Sex Differences in Neural Structure

Until the 1970s, almost all researchers agreed that early steroid administration could indeed permanently alter the structure of the brain and thereby permanently alter behavior. However, this belief rested on indirect evidence. Just as particle physicists spoke of atoms and electrons without ever actually seeing them, behavioral endocrinologists spoke of the androgenic organization of neural structure without actually seeing any changes in the brain. They inferred the organization of the brain by the changes in behavior. Since the nervous system controls behavior (barring the existence of spirits or demons), the existence of sex differences in behavior implies that there are sex differences in neural structure. Although there were those who worried that sex differences outside the nervous system, most obviously in the structure of the genitalia, might be responsible for differences in behavior,[90] later studies amply vindicated the notion that male and female brains are built differently.

Darwin coined the term sexual dimorphism to refer to the tendency in many species for the two sexes to have very different body shapes or sizes. For example, lions, peacocks, and gorillas exhibit moderate to great sexual dimorphism, but seagulls, hyenas, and many snakes and fish show little or none. One of the first reports of sexual dimorphism in neural structure that generated a great deal of interest was from Raisman and Field,[835] who examined the preoptic area (POA) of the hypothalamus in rats. Using electron microscopy, they carefully classified and counted synapses in this area and found that females had more of a particular synapse type than males. Furthermore, in complete accord with the organizational hypothesis, early androgen manipulations could reverse the sex difference seen in adulthood. Because earlier work had shown that lesions or stimulations of the POA could alter reproductive behavior and ovulation, and because synapses were known to play a crucial role in neural function, this finding generated a great deal of enthusiasm and, because the work involved was very tedious and time consuming, admiration. This was also the exact sort of sexual dimorphism researchers were prepared for—subtle and requiring great technological skill to detect.

MACROSCOPIC SEXUAL DIMORPHISM IN THE BRAIN

In 1976 the assumption that neural sexual dimorphisms would be subtle was blown apart. Nottebohm and Arnold[783] reported that the brain nuclei of songbirds displayed sex differences that were so large one could detect them without a microscope at all! Each of these nuclei (remember that a cluster of neurons found within the CNS is known as a nucleus and is different from an individual cell's spherical repository of chromosomes, also known as a nucleus) had been shown by lesion and electrical stimulation experiments to be involved in birdsong production. Nottebohm and Arnold, studying canaries and zebra finches, in which males do almost all of the singing, found song control nuclei that were five to six times larger in males than in females (figure 2.3).

Soon thereafter, a deluge of sex dimorphisms in neural structure were reported, some subtle, some large, some involving the number or shape of synapses, the length of dendrites, the number of neurons, the amount of neurotransmitter available, and so on (for reviews, see Arnold and Gorski[38]; Fishman and Breedlove[354]; DeVries et al.[281]). By now the list of articles describing sex differences in neural structure is too long to be reviewed comprehensively. Instead, we will concentrate in this chapter on a few of the well-studied systems, and the ontogeny of several other interesting systems will be discussed in chapter 7.

PROMINENT SEXUAL DIMORPHISM IN THE RAT HYPOTHALAMUS

We have already mentioned the preoptic area (POA); lesions of the POA stop male copulatory behavior in a striking variety of species. Thus, Roger Gorski and his colleagues carefully examined the POA and found a nucleus in this region that was five to six times larger in males than in females, a difference so prominent that one could distinguish brain slices from the two sexes with the naked eye (figure 2.4). They named this region the sexually dimorphic nucleus of the POA (SDN-POA).[424] The sex dimorphism of the SDN-POA obeyed beautifully the rules of the organizational hypothesis: castration of males on the day of birth caused their SDN-POAs to be smaller (i.e., less masculine) in adulthood, while androgen treatment of newborn females caused their SDN-POAs to be larger in adulthood. In fact, if females were exposed to androgens both before and just after birth, their SDN-POAs were as big as those of normal males. In other words, early androgen exposure determined the size of the SDN-POA in adulthood. The longer the early androgen exposure, the larger the SDN-POA (figure 2.4). Furthermore, manipulations of androgens in adulthood had no effect on the volume of the SDN-POA. There was great hope, therefore, that the SDN-POA might provide an anatomical signature of androgen's masculine organizing influence upon the rat nervous system.[423]

How do early androgens orchestrate the masculine development of the SDN-POA? First, one can look at the ontogeny of the SDN-POA: When does it first become detectable and when does the sex difference in size first arise? Jacobson and Gorski found that the SDN portion of the POA was visible as early as the twentieth day of gestation, but volume did not differ between the sexes until the day of birth (the twenty-third day of gestation) and became most prominent on the tenth day of life.[529] Of course, just because the sex difference in SDN-POA volume is not visible before birth does not mean that androgen is

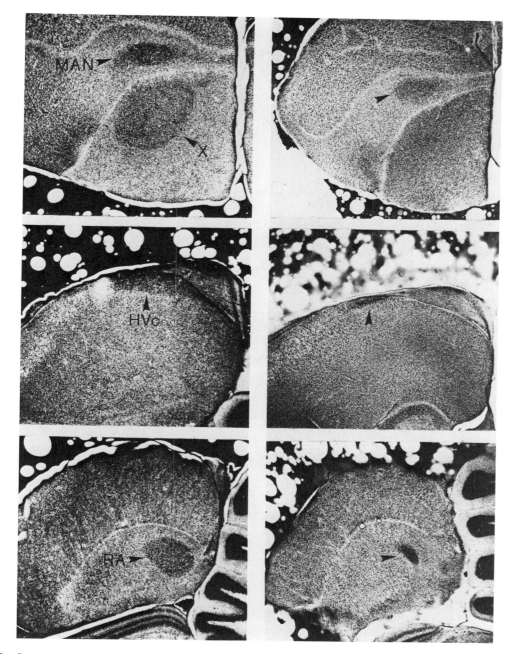

Figure 2.3   Sexually dimorphic neural regions of the songbird brain. In these frontal sections of Nissl-stained material you can compare the sizes of nuclei MAN and area X (top) in males (left) and females (right). Middle panels depict nucleus HVc, bottom panels depict nucleus RA. All of these nuclei are involved in song learning or production, which is primarily performed by males in both canaries and zebra finches. The volume of these nuclei is greater in males than in females because of the early actions of steroids (see chapter 7). For a schematic representation of the connections between these nuclei, see figure 7.9. (Courtesy of Arthur Arnold.)

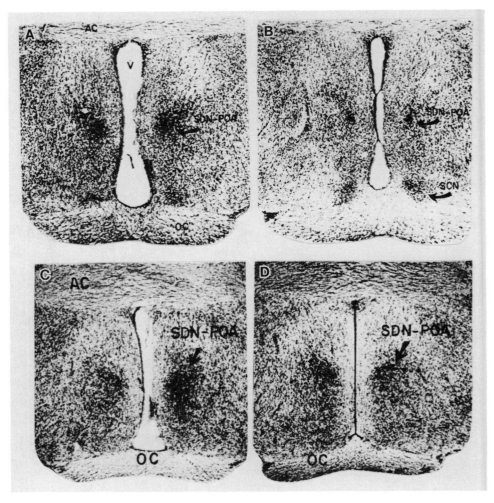

Figure 2.4   The sexually dimorphic nucleus of the preoptic area (SDN-POA) of rats. This region is three to five times larger in volume in male rats (A) than in female rats (B). Perinatal treatment of females with either testosterone (C) or the synthetic estrogen diethylstilbestrol (D) masculinizes, i.e., enlarges the SDN-POA. AC, anterior commissure; OC, optic chiasm; SCN, suprachiasmatic nucleus; V, ventricle. (Courtesy of Roger Gorski.)

not driving processes before birth that will cause the later dimorphism. In fact, it appears that there are sex differences in the production of neurons in the SDN before birth. When a cell duplicates its DNA (to provide a full set to each daughter cell), it must use thymidine and other nucleotides to synthesize a new set of chromosomes (see box 2.1). Jacobson and colleagues injected pregnant rats with radiolabeled thymidine. If the fetuses were killed a few hours later, all the radioactivity was found along the rim of the brain's ventricles, in the so-called ventricular zone, indicating that the dividing cells were found there. Several days after injecting the thymidine, some neurons were found to have radioactivity in their nuclei, indicating that a cellular "ancestor" of that

Box 2.1 Thymidine Autoradiography to Detect the Time of Neurogenesis

Even we multicellular organisms begin as a single cell. The zygote duplicates the DNA and divides, leaving both daughter cells with a complete genetic blueprint. Cycles of mitosis continue to form an embryo, fetus, juvenile, and adult. Even in adulthood, some cells such as blood cells and glia, continue to divide. But the cells that give rise to neurons generally stop dividing early in life, shortly after birth in humans. The time of the final division that gives rise to a neuron is known as the "birthdate" of that cell. The timetable of divisions that give rise to different neuronal populations is relatively fixed—motoneurons are born well before birth, interneurons later, and glia continue to be born in the adult CNS. Outer cortical neurons are born later than neurons of the inner cortex, and so on. The birthdate of particular cells can be determined by labeling the DNA that is copied before division. If we inject a radiolabeled precursor to DNA called thymidine, it will be used to provide the thymine (see chapter 1) in new DNA being produced at that time. Once the animal grows up, we can examine cells to see whether they have radioactivity in their nuclei. If so, one of their "ancestors" was preparing to divide back at the time we injected the thymidine. If injections of thymidine before day 14.5 of development result in labeled motoneurons in adulthood but injections after 14.5 days never label them, we can conclude that those cells are all born by 14.5 days. In rats, neurons of the POA generally are born between 14 and 16 days postconception. However, neurons in the SDN portion of the POA are born a little later, at 16 to 18 days of gestation. This later birthdate coincides with a time during which males have elevated systemic levels of androgen. Furthermore, male rats appear to be producing more neurons during this later period than are females, so it may be that androgen somehow augments neurogenesis in the SDN-POA, thereby making the nucleus larger.

neuron was about to divide on the day the thymidine was injected. In the parlance of the trade, one refers to the "birthdate" of cells, i.e., the day of the final division that produced that cell and its sister cell. It turns out that all of the neurons of the SDN-POA are born by the eighteenth day of gestation. What's more, on the seventeenth day of gestation, more SDN-POA neurons are being born in males than in females.[528] It is important to note that a consequence of this early sex difference in SDN-POA neurogenesis will not become manifest as a sex difference in volume for another five to six days.

The next obvious question about the SDN-POA is, when during development can steroids exert their effects, and which steroids are effective? We mentioned briefly earlier that testosterone could affect the volume of the SDN-POA only when it was administered perinatally. More specifically, it was found that either prenatal or neonatal injections of testosterone could masculinize the SDN-POA of females. However, prenatal injections were more effective than postnatal ones, and androgen had to be given during both periods to bring about complete sex reversal of SDN-POA volume (i.e., make it as big as that found in normal males). As to which hormone does the work, perinatal estrogen is more effective than testosterone in masculinizing SDN-POA volume, and the other major active metabolite of testosterone, DHT, has no measurable effect upon the SDN-POA. It appears then, that in normal males testicular testosterone is aromatized to estrogen (possibly within the developing SDN-POA itself) and that estrogen is actually guiding the masculine development of the nucleus. This inference is supported by examination of TFM rats. Although these XY individuals produce testes and testosterone, they lack the androgen receptors to respond and therefore develop a feminine exterior phenotype. However, the TFM animals possess estrogen receptors[41] and aromatase[876] and, in accord with the aromatization hypothesis of brain sexual differentiation and in contrast to their feminine bodies, TFM animals have a large, masculine SDN-POA. Thus, androgen receptors per se do not appear to cause the masculinization of the SDN-POA of rats. Rather, it is the aromatized metabolites of testosterone that direct the masculine development of this nucleus. The SDN-POA follows the rules not only of the organizational hypothesis but of the aromatization hypothesis as well.

The excitement about the SDN-POA was slightly diminished for a time when Gorski's group reported that no deficit in masculine sexual behavior was caused by lesions of the SDN-POA,[33] even though similar sized lesions of the dorsal POA outside the SDN region significantly decreased the likelihood of ejaculation. However, another group found that lesions of the SDN portion of the POA decreased male sexual behavior in rats who were sexually naive.[268] Specifically, lesioned animals were less likely to reach ejaculation and took longer to mount, achieve intromission, and ejaculate than normal males. The deficit caused by the lesion was relatively subtle, disappearing with additional sexual experience. But, since Gorski's laboratory had used sexually experienced male rats, perhaps the subtle effect of SDN-POA lesions was masked.

Spinal Nucleus of the Bulbocavernosus

One way to overcome the problem of understanding the functional significance of a sex difference in the nervous system is to deliberately choose a system so simple that its function is relatively obvious. Such a simple sexual dimorphism is found in the spinal cord. The muscles that attach to the penis (figure 2.5) are quite likely to play a role in sexual behavior, and so too are the spinal motoneurons that innervate and control those muscles. Thus the striated muscles bulbocavernosus (BC), levator ani (LA), and ischiocavernosus, all of which attach to the base of the penis, became an object of study of neural sexual differentiation. The BC and IC are present in human males (the BC is under voluntary control and is used to eject the last drops of urine) and in females (except that in females they attach to the base of the clitoris, the BC, under voluntary control in women, constricts the opening of the vagina). The BC and IC are smaller in women than in men, but in rats the sexual dimorphism of these muscles is much more drastic. Adult female rats lack them altogether.

Given the sexual dimorphism of the muscles of the perineum (the so-called pelvic floor region including the genitalia), it is not surprising that the spinal motoneurons controlling these muscles also display a dimorphism. The motoneurons innervating the BC and LA are found in a distinctive position and

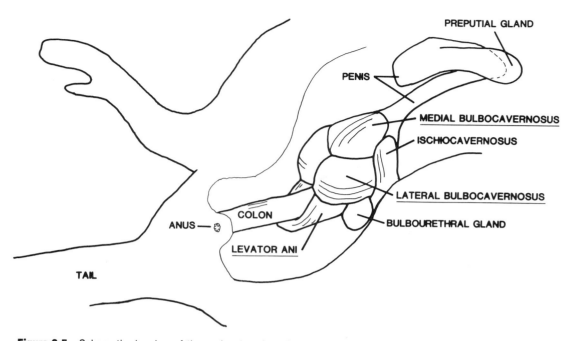

Figure 2.5 Schematic drawing of the perineal region of a male rat. The striated muscles bulbocavernosus and levator ani are innervated by the spinal nucleus of the bulbocavernosus (SNB). The levator ani, which attaches to the base of the penis and wraps around the colon, is sometimes called the dorsal bulbocavernosus. The bulbocavernosus looks similar in males of many species, including humans, but the levator ani may be restricted to rodents. (From Breedlove, 1984.[142a])

collectively are called the spinal nucleus of the bulbocavernosus (SNB). There are more SNB cells in male rats than in females, and they are larger in males (figure 2.6). The motoneurons innervating the external anal sphincter are also located in the SNB region, and it is these cells that occupy that nucleus in female rats.

Female rats begin life with BC, LA, and IC muscles attached to the base of the clitoris,[209] and SNB motoneurons have made functional synapses with these muscles.[838] Despite all this effort, the SNB cells and perineal muscles die in the first weeks of life in female rats. This degeneration is averted in males by the intervention of androgen, and the SNB system can be permanently saved in females with a single injection of androgen early in life[144, 145] (figure 2.7). Aromatized metabolites of testosterone do not seem to affect the survival of SNB cells or their targets. For example, TFM rats (which possess normal levels of testosterone, aromatase, and estrogen receptors) develop a completely feminine SNB system, apparently because they lack the androgen receptors to prevent the death of these cells. Once the SNB cells and their target muscles have died, androgen cannot resurrect them. Thus, the basis of the sensitive period during which steroids can organize the SNB system is determined by how far the degeneration has proceeded. If the organizational actions of steroids in

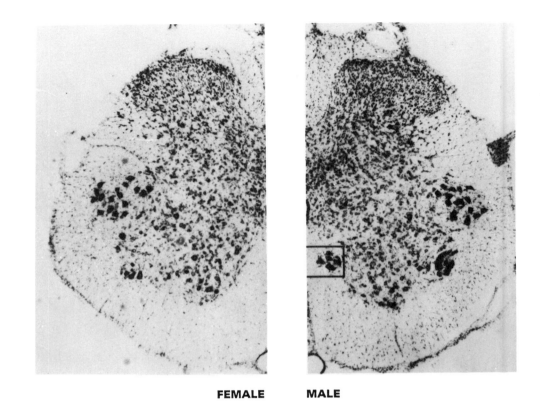

FEMALE   **MALE**

Figure 2.6 Photomicrographs of cross-sections of the lumbar spinal cord of an adult female (left) and an adult male rat (dorsal is up). The spinal nucleus of the bulbocavernosus (SNB) is a readily recognized, discrete nucleus of motoneurons in males (within the 3-sided box on the right). Most of these motoneurons innervate either the bulbocavernosus or the levator ani, but some innervate the external anal sphincter, and it is these scattered motoneurons that occupy this area in female rats. The human homologue of the SNB occupies a more ventral position and is known as Onuf's nucleus.

other systems involve the prevention of cell death, a similar mechanism may be behind other sensitive periods.[599]

How does early androgen prevent the death of BC and LA muscles and their SNB motoneurons? It appears that androgen directly prevents the degeneration of the muscles and that the survival of the SNB motoneurons is a secondary response to the sparing of their muscle targets. Several lines of evidence support this idea. First, androgen can maintain the muscles in newborn females even after the motoneurons have been removed.[352] Second, androgen receptor blockers interfere with testosterone's effects better when they are injected directly into the muscle rather than into the general circulation.[352] Finally, while the BC muscles of newborn rats can bind androgen, neither SNB cells or other spinal motoneurons can accumulate steroid until after the sensitive period for sparing the system.[355] Thus, androgens affect the *target* of SNB

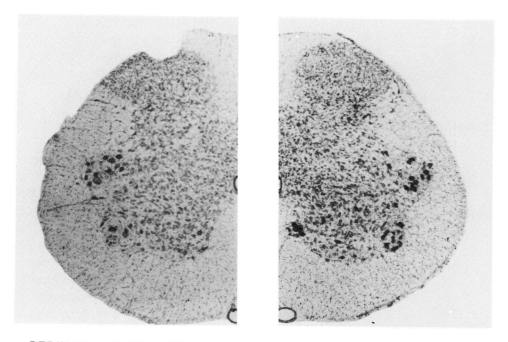

PERINATALLY TREATED MALE   NEONATALLY TREATED FEMALE

Figure 2.7 Photomicrographs of spinal cord sections from an adult male rat that was treated with antiandrogen before birth and castrated at birth (left). This treatment causes the bulbocavernosus and SNB motoneurons to die. Conversely, perinatal androgen treatment, in this case with DHT, preserves the muscles and SNB cells in a female rat (right).

motoneurons, thereby sparing them from cell death and leading to the sexual differentiation of the spinal cord. Future research must address which genes are being turned on or off in these muscles when androgen prevents their degeneration.

Features that Differ Between the Sexes

Notice that this diversity of sex differences makes it very difficult to refer to someone as being simply "male" or "female" because it is possible for an individual to be masculine in some body or brain regions and feminine in others. With our more informed view of sexual differentiation, we need to specify which character we are interested in before deciding whether it is masculine or feminine. We can also refine our use of the terms feminization and masculinization. When a normally masculine characteristic develops, we can describe that process as masculinization and a treatment that prevents that structure from forming as demasculinizing. Similarly, the development of a feminine characteristic is feminization, whereas the prevention of the appearance of a female characteristic is defeminization. Normally, of course, males are both masculinized (in terms of genital structure, copulatory behavior, SDN-POA,

SNB, and so on) and defeminized (in terms of müllerian duct structures, ovulatory competence, lordosis responsiveness, and so on). Females are normally both feminized and demasculinized. In most discussions, one refers to any move in the female direction as feminization and any move in the male direction as masculinization.

Sexual Differentiation of the Human Central Nervous System

There is no doubt that men and women look and act differently. Sex differences in behavior are more prominent in some cultures than others but are never quite absent. What is controversial is the question of how boys and girls grow up to be so different—is it the result of their biological differences or the result of their different experiences while growing up? This question is a subset of the ongoing "nature versus nurture" debate—to what extent is our behavior affected by our genome (nature) or our experience (nurture)? This is a complex and sometimes emotional debate that is of interest to almost everyone. Several different disciplines, including behavioral genetics,[822] animal behavior,[15] and developmental neurobiology[832] attempt to address this question, each from a slightly different approach.

In the field of behavioral endocrinology, the nature–nurture debate is so confined that it may one day be resolved. Because so much is known about sexual differentiation of the body, the question of sexual differentiation of the brain and behavior can be boiled down to this: If there is a biological influence on the sexual differentiation of human behavior, then steroid hormones mediate that influence. So we can ask, Do differences in early steroid hormone secretions alter the human nervous system or behavior? It is a great intellectual advantage to be able to pare down a question to a readily comprehensible form that can be tested. Nonetheless, the complexity of behavior and the nervous system, coupled with the difficulties and limitations of working with human subjects, have so far given us only a partial answer.

Remember that the principles by which testicular secretions direct masculine development of the body are much the same in all mammals, including humans. Do the sex differences in prenatal steroid exposure also cause sex differences in the development of the human nervous system and therefore sex differences in behavior? To address that question, we can first ask whether there is sexual dimorphism in the human nervous system.

Sexual Dimorphism in the Human Central Nervous System

Nineteenth century researchers noted that men have heavier brains than women, and some of these (male) workers viewed this finding as the natural result of the intellectual superiority of men (for reviews, see Gould[429] and Swaab and Hofman[1015]). But of course men also have larger bodies than women, and if you measure brain weight relative to body weight or height, the sex difference disappears, or favors women. There is a tendency to dismiss the obvious sex difference in brain weight because of the sex difference in body size, but it is worthwhile to examine this tendency. How does brain size come to mirror body size? There are three general ways it could come about: (1) The nervous system might monitor body size and adapt itself to follow suit, (2) the nervous system might instruct the body how much to grow, or (3) some other signal (e.g., growth or thyroid hormone) might independently control body and brain growth. Which of these three mechanisms cause men to have heavier brains than women? We don't know. Whichever mechanism is at work, it seems likely that the sex difference in body and brain size is the result of biological influences, specifically, prenatal hormones. This idea is supported by the fact that a small (2–3%) but reliable sex difference in human brain size, corrected for height, arises by 2 years of age,[794, 1015] presumably (but not necessarily) before parents' treatment of infants could have much effect. By the way, it is not clear that this sexual dimorphism leads to sex differences in intelligence.

THE SEXUALLY DIMORPHIC NUCLEUS OF THE PREOPTIC AREA
The two prominent sex differences in the rat CNS that were discussed earlier, the SDN-POA and the SNB, have both been examined in human tissues. Two different research teams have examined the human POA, and while the two teams have some minor disagreements about nomenclature, they both agree that there is at least one nucleus in the human POA that is larger in men than in women. The human nuclei have a somewhat different shape than the rat SDN-POA, and the degree of sexual dimorphism is much less pronounced than in rats. Is this nucleus in the human POA really the equivalent of the rat SDN-POA, or is the human nucleus really a different nucleus that just happens to be dimorphic? This difficult question will be addressed by future research comparing the developmental origins of the nuclei in the two species; if they arise in a similar way by similar mechanisms, then the nuclei were probably present in the ancestral species common to rat and man and may even have been sexually dimorphic since then! Even if the human POA nucleus turns out to be unrelated to the rat SDN-POA (i.e., the result of evolutionary "convergence"), it seems unlikely that anyone would have noticed the sexual dimorphism in humans without the impetus provided by the animal research.

THE SPINAL NUCLEUS OF THE BULBOCAVERNOSUS
The SNB is more easily defined in humans—it is the group of motoneurons that innervates the BC and IC muscles found in both men and women and looks very much the same in male rats and humans. The nucleus of motoneurons innervating these perineal muscles is called Onuf's nucleus.[789] Onuf's nucleus looks much the same in humans, monkeys, cats, and dogs but is found in a slightly different location in the human spinal cord than in the rat SNB. Since women have smaller BC and IC muscles than men, one might expect a sex difference in the number of Onuf's nucleus motoneurons, and men do, in fact, have more cells there.[368] Also as one might expect, the sex difference is more subtle in humans than in rats, since female rats lose the

BC altogether after birth. Furthermore, dogs also have a sex difference in the number of Onuf's motoneurons (again favoring males), and prenatal androgen treatment of females leaves them with a masculine number of cells in Onuf's nucleus. Thus, it seems likely that the sexual dimorphism in human Onuf's nucleus is in fact biologically determined by sex differences in prenatal steroid secretion, just as occurs with its rat homologue, the SNB.

Sexual Orientation

Many people would like to know whether these biological influences upon the developing nervous systems of animals are also at work in humans. More specifically, some have wondered whether early, prenatal steroid exposure influences sexual orientation. Do heterosexual men and homosexual women prefer female sexual partners because androgen organized their developing brains in a "masculine" fashion? Or, conversely, is the sexual orientation of homosexual men and heterosexual women (i.e., a preference for male partners) the result of low prenatal androgen levels? It's easy to pose these questions conversationally, but exceedingly difficult to answer them scientifically. It is impossible to monitor prenatal steroid levels without incurring substantial risk to the fetus. Also, it would be unethical to manipulate the prenatal steroid environment of humans to try to determine sexual orientation. Thus, the only way to answer this question is to make use of correlational data, and those data, as you might have guessed, give equivocal answers at best (see also chapter 4).

First, there have been many studies that have failed to find any difference between heterosexual and homosexual men (or women) in terms of adult plasma androgen or estrogen levels.[712] Of course, animal models might suggest that any androgenic effect on sexual orientation should occur early in life, perhaps even prenatally. However, there is no technically feasible way to monitor fetal steroid levels in a large number of individuals. There have been reports that homosexual and heterosexual men differ in their response to injections of estrogen.[304, 406] Specifically, it is said that homosexual men show a greater positive feedback response of LH levels when given an injection of estrogen. The rat models of sexual differentiation suggest that this positive feedback response is feminine. The reasoning continues that a prenatal androgen shortage might result in only a partial masculinization of brain circuits concerned with sexual orientation or gender identity and ovulatory competence.

However, you may remember that primates are not very sexually dimorphic in terms of ovulatory capacity, so it is not clear whether this is indeed an exclusively feminine trait in humans. Furthermore, there have been several failures to replicate these observations.[483] Finally, rather than prenatal androgen altering both sexual orientation and gonadotropin regulation, it is always possible that something about the homosexual experience causes the subtle changes in gonadotropin regulation. In that case, sexuality might be unrelated to prenatal steroids. Similarly, although there is a report that a region of the POA (which may or may not be homologous to the rat SDN-POA) is larger in heterosexual men than homosexual men,[623] it is not yet known whether the difference in the brain is the *cause* or a *result* of the development of sexual orientation. Thus, there is no irrefutable evidence that prenatal hormones affect sexual orientation in humans. The subjective experience of the majority of homosexuals and heterosexuals is that, from their very earliest remembrance, the object of their sexual interest has been unchanged. Although of course this experience is consistent with a prenatal determination, it proves nothing. One's earliest memories of language may be of English, but of course that is strictly because of experiences that predate those memories.

Sex Differences in the Lateralization of Cognitive Functions in Humans

Another area of research into human sexual dimorphism revolves around the issue of cerebral asymmetry or lateralization. As you may know, some higher cognitive functions seem to be primarily controlled in one cerebral hemisphere or the other. For example, speech seems to be controlled by the left cerebral hemisphere in most of us (including most left-handed people). This conclusion was first reached in the nineteenth century by neurologists examining the postmortem brains of stroke and accident victims who were left aphasic (i.e., unable to speak or understand speech). Later it became possible to inject a fast-acting anesthetic into the carotid artery supplying one hemisphere and observe a short-lasting speech deficit when the drug was given on the left. Spatial reasoning, on the other hand, is usually carried out by the right hemisphere. The extent to which a function is carried out by one hemisphere rather than another is referred to as lateralization.[982] There have been several reports of a sex difference in the degree of lateralization of cognitive functions.[695] When such a sex difference is seen at all, it is very subtle, and many studies have failed to find a difference.[346]

An exciting finding of the 1970s was that of Wada and colleagues, who reported that the planum temporale, a flat region of the human temporal lobe thought to be involved in speech, was usually larger on the left than on the right.[1083] This anatomical asymmetry fitted well with what was known about the functional lateralization of speech. What's more, these scientists reported that the asymmetry of the planum temporale, while present in both sexes, was more prominent in men. That is, while most women had a larger planum temporale on the left, the right side was occasionally equal to or larger than the left, and women were more likely than men to show this unusual pattern.

What made the report from Wada and colleagues exciting was the possibility that the sex difference in structural asymmetry might be a reflection of sex differences in functional asymmetry. There were several reports indicating that various functions were more evenly distributed on the left and right brain halves of women than of men. For example, most of us can pick words out of noise better with our right ear (and hence the left side of our brain) than with our left ear. But, in general, women show less discrepancy in the performance of the two ears than do men. It makes sense that the left side of the brain, which performs most language processing, would have a larger planum temporale. Furthermore, because women are less lateralized in auditory processing than men, the more symmetrical planum of women may be responsible. Similarly, men are more likely to detect written words briefly flashed to their right visual field than the left visual field. While women also perform better with right visual field presentation, they are more likely than men to do about as well on either side. However, no one has found a sex difference in asymmetries in visual processing brain regions.

There is a report that prenatal steroids can masculinize females in terms of cerebral lateralization.[489] Women who were prenatally exposed to the synthetic estrogen diethylstilbestrol (DES; a drug that was used to prevent miscarriages in the 1950s and early 1960s) were compared to their unexposed sisters. Whether presented with visual or auditory stimuli, DES-treated women were more strongly lateralized than their sisters at word detection. Thus, in keeping with the aromatization hypothesis, prenatal estrogens may masculinize cognitive function. These ideas about lateralization of cognitive function will be discussed further in chapter 12.

Sexual Dimorphism in the Pathway Communicating Between the Two Hemispheres

The major pathway that transmits information from one half of the brain to the other is the corpus callosum. The corpus callosum consists of the axons from millions of neurons that carry information from each hemisphere to the other. Seen in midline cross-section, the corpus callosum resembles a leech. At the caudal end (i.e., the end nearest the back of the head), the corpus callosum is shaped something like a bulb, and this bulbous region is called the splenium. It was reported that the splenium of the corpus callosum was more bulbous in females than in males[272] (figure 2.8). Since this portion of the corpus callosum consists of axons connecting the two cortical areas that process vision, i.e., the occipital cortex, the report of a more bulbous splenium in women could be related to less lateralized visual processing in females. In other words, perhaps the two hemispheres share information more readily in women than in men because of a greater number of callosal axons.

There have been several problems with the tale of sexual dimorphism in the human corpus callosum. First, there may not be a sex difference in the number of axons because there is no sex difference in the overall cross-sectional area of the corpus callosum, only in the shape of the caudal end. Perhaps this means that in women a greater proportion of the corpus callosum axons is invested in one task rather than another, but no one has found a way to demonstrate that. A second problem is the number of failures of other researchers to replicate the original finding.[1107] To see the sex difference in shape, one must adhere very strictly to a remarkably complicated series of steps to define the splenium. If deviation from these steps occurs in measuring the splenium, no sex difference is apparent. The very particular steps one must go through to see a sex differ-

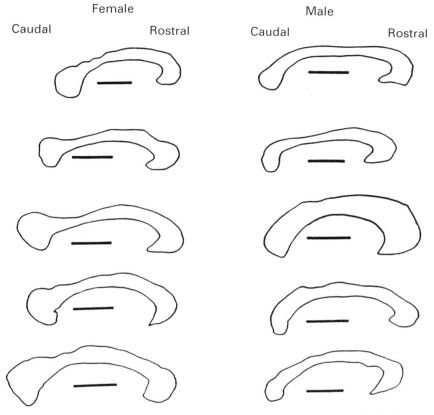

Female   Male

Caudal   Rostral   Caudal   Rostral

Scale: 2 cm

Figure 2.8   Drawings of midline cross-sections illustrating the sexual dimorphism of the corpus callosum of humans. The splenium, which forms the caudal corpus callosum, is more bulbous in females than in males. The sex difference appears to be due to a difference in shape rather than a difference in total area of the cross-sections. (Reprinted from DeLacost and Holloway, 1982.[272])

ence illustrate how subtle the difference is and how difficult it is to understand just what the difference really means. On the other hand, some other laboratories have been able to replicate the originally described sex difference in splenial "bulbosity" of the corpus callosum and have also reported the necessity of following the very detailed method of measuring the splenium. If one accepts that there is a sexual dimorphism in the corpus callosum, it is possible that sex differences in the cognitive or social experiences of young children are responsible for the sex difference in the corpus callosum. However, there is one report that the sex difference in the corpus callosum is present in fetal human material,[269] which would suggest that prenatal factors such as hormones are responsible for the dimorphism in the corpus callosum. Unfortunately, this report, too, is contested.[105] We are left with the impression that there is a sexual dimorphism in the human corpus callosum, but it is subtle. Whether this sexual dimorphism in corpus callosum structure is the cause or the result of sex differences in the lateralization of cognitive function or is completely unrelated to lateralization, is even less clear.

Summary and Conclusions

During sexual differentiation the presence of a Y chromosome transforms the indifferent gonad into a testis. In the absence of the Y chromosome the gonad becomes an ovary. Thereafter, the sexual differentiation of the male relies on the fetal testes production of MRF and testosterone. This means that both primary sex characteristics (penis, scrotum, and so on) and secondary sex characteristics (e.g., facial and axillary hair, muscle) depend on hormonal secretions for phenotypic expression. The absence of testicular secretions results in the development of feminine primary and secondary sex characteristics.

The brain is also "organized" by the presence or absence of testicular secretions during perinatal development. In rodents, testosterone masculinizes the brain to prevent ovulatory capacity and establish male-typical sexual behavior. Estrogen is equally capable of masculinizing the brain. In the male this is thought to reflect the conversion of testosterone to estrogen (aromatization) within the brain. Female rodents are protected from their own and their mother's estrogen by the presence of AFP in the blood. This protein binds to estrogen and limits its entry into the brain. However, a small amount of estrogen gains access to the brain in females, and this may be important for the expression of feminine sexual behavior in the adult.

Primates may be very different from rodents in the mechanism(s) mediating sexual differentiation of the hypothalamus. Two points are important here. First, it does not seem likely that the aromatization of testosterone to estrogen is important for sexual differentiation of the hypothalamus in primates. Second, the hypothalamus of the male in primates retains the capability of supporting ovulation. This characteristic is lost during sexual differentiation of the hypothalamus of male rodents.

The number of brain regions that have been found to be sexually dimorphic in rodents is substantial, and this number will undoubtedly continue to increase as more brain regions are investigated. Processes mediating the expression of sex-related differences vary with the brain region. The gonadal steroid hormones can exert effects both directly on neurons and by exerting a tropic effect on the target muscles of motoneurons. In both cases, there are apparently gonadal hormone effects both on neuron survival and on the morphology of the surviving neurons.

While considerable effort has been expended over the years to document sexual dimorphism in the brains of humans, the confirmatory evidence is surprisingly meager. Evidence in support of sex-related differences in the hypothalamus and spinal cord is most compelling. Other sex-related differences tend to be more subtle. Whether there is any evidence to support a role for sexual differentiation of the human brain in the establishment of sexual behavior or sexual preference is still controversial.

For the next five chapters we will be considering the mysterious and fascinating world of sexual behavior. It is in this arena that most people already consider hormones to have a great deal of influence. Indeed, rats are very unlikely to display sexual behavior without the appropriate hormones (either from their internal supplies or administered by an experimenter). This close correlation between hormones and sexual behavior is the reason we devote five chapters (nearly a third of the book) to courtship and copulatory behavior; few behaviors are so reliably altered by hormone treatment in so many species. In later chapters we will find that the effects of hormones on some other behaviors are more subtle and more likely to vary from one species to another. Therefore, you should appreciate how reliably and robustly hormones affect reproductive behaviors.

But as you will see, not even rats are hormone-driven automatons. When we give animals hormones we change the probability that they will show male- or female-like behaviors, but there are still individual differences in response. For example, some male rats refuse to copulate even though they have plenty of the apparently appropriate hormones (i.e., androgens), and some male mice strains continue to copulate even after castration! Furthermore, even when females are in "heat," they can still be rather selective about which males they will allow to mount if they are given the opportunity to choose.

By the time you read about human sexual behavior in chapter 5, you should certainly be prepared for some ambiguity in the relations between hormones and sexual behavior. Natural selection has also produced species in which hormones have, of necessity, become uncoupled from reproductive behavior, as chapter 6 attests. Hormones also affect many of the courtship behaviors attending copulation, and chapter 7 gives you a glimpse of the remarkable species diversity of such behaviors and the diverse ways in which hormones influence them.

These chapters should teach you that hormones are not "love potions" that force animals to copulate willy-nilly but coordinators of reproduction. The same hormones that prepare the production of eggs, sperm, and other physiological processes *directly* involved in reproduction also prepare the nervous system to display courtship and copulatory behaviors that are also required for reproduction. As hormonal influence upon reproductive organs evolves, so too do the hormonal effects upon the nervous system. The nervous system is a very complex organ that processes a great deal of information at a rapid clip, and hormones are just one source, albeit an important one, of information about reproduction. The animal's previous experiences, level of arousal, and even general health are all integrated by the nervous system and affect the behavior displayed.

3 Neuroendocrinology of Sexual Behavior in the Female

C. Sue Carter

We begin our study of sexual behavior with females. In many species females display cycles of reproductive function, and behavior is an integral part of that cycle. For example, female rats ovulate about every 4 days and will, for a period of a few hours during that time, allow males to copulate with them. This receptivity on the part of the female occurs at a particular point in the ovulatory cycle that favors fertilization and pregnancy. The receptive behavior is coordinated by the same gonadal hormones that guide ovulation. The close correlation between female receptivity and gonadal hormones has made it possible to discover a good deal about how hormones affect this and other feminine sexual behaviors.

What sexual behaviors do females display, which hormones affect these behaviors, and where do the hormones act to exert these effects? When during the ovulatory cycle will females of various species, including humans, mate, and how do pregnancies affect the probability of mating?

Introduction

As described in chapter 2, steroid hormones may affect behavior either through organizational effects on the developing nervous system or through activational effects in adults. Organizational and activational effects of hormones are not mutually exclusive phenomena. In fact, as will be discussed in this chapter, organizational effects of gonadal hormones on sexual differentiation of the brain may not be manifest in sexually dimorphic behavior in the adult without the additional activational stimulus of specific gonadal hormones.

This chapter will focus on the activational effects of hormones that influence adult female sexual behavior. However, these behavioral actions are dependent upon the previous hormonal experiences of the individual. Early hormone exposure can alter the birth, survival, or death of neurons. In addition, the capacity of a given cell to produce chemicals or respond to subsequent neuroendocrine changes within the body can be regulated during development. Thus, the organizational effects of hormones are thought to produce sex differences in the patterns of neural connections and functions within the brain. By comparison, activational effects of hormones are transient and tend to coordinate behavior with an internal event, such as ovulation or sperm production, or an external event, such as the presence of a sexual partner.

In addition to sex differences, there also are significant species differences in reproductive behaviors. In spite of interspecific variation in the patterns of sexual behavior, it has been possible to compare the behavioral effects of a variety of hormones across species. Most of the available research examining the mechanisms underlying female sexual behavior has been conducted in rodents, such as rats, mice, and hamsters. References to a variety of other species are included here to illustrate other principles relating to behavioral endocrinology.

Definitions Important for Studies of Female Sexual Behavior

For simplicity, feminine sexual behavior can be divided into two components. Precopulatory behaviors, leading to copulation, may be described as courtship behaviors. Copulatory behaviors, usually defined by reflexive postures, are often considered separately from courtship. The reflexive sexual posture, called **lordosis**, is similar across many species (see figure 1.1 in chapter 1 for an illustration of the lordosis posture in the rat). Both courtship and copulatory behaviors may be influenced by hormones. However, courtship behaviors vary across species, and researchers have tended to focus on the more stereotyped components of sexual behavior, such as lordosis.

COURTSHIP BEHAVIORS
Under natural conditions, courtship interactions prior to or associated with sexual behavior function to permit mate selection.[683] Both sexes usually participate in mate selection. However, sex differences in gamete (i.e., egg and sperm) production are associated with sex differences in reproductive strategies. For example, females may ovulate on a periodic or cyclic basis. In contrast, at least during breeding seasons, males maintain a relatively constant supply of sperm. Consequently, females have fewer potential opportunities than do males to produce offspring. It was assumed for many years that females would be more likely to select a single sexual partner, whereas males would be more likely to have several sexual partners. Parentage can be determined by comparing the profile or fingerprint of DNA contained in every cell of an individual. Recent studies using DNA fingerprinting suggest that absolute sexual exclusivity may be rare in both sexes. These studies have indicated that in species in which the female simultaneously rears multiple young it is not uncommon to find litters that are sired by more than one male. This has been found to be true even in species that have been considered to be socially monogamous.[191] Additional discussions of the adaptive significance of courtship behaviors can be found in chapters 6 and 7.

For the female, the hormonal events associated with ovulation promote social affiliation, courtship, and subsequent copulation.[282] Under laboratory conditions in rats, estrogen increases a female's willingness to approach a male and induces sexual solicitations, known as **proceptive behavior**. In the rat there are three components to proceptive behavior: **approach**, **orientation**, and **run-**

away. In the rat, proceptive behaviors include an approach to the male followed by sniffing and grooming (orienting) as well as ear wiggling and hopping and darting. Ear wiggling is an extremely rapid vibration of the head that makes it appear as though the ears are wiggling and usually occurs in response to an approach and contact by the male. Hopping and darting consist of a rapid hop with almost rigid legs combined with fast "darting" movements away from the male (runaway). This sequence of behaviors frequently induces the male rat to chase after the female rat.

McClintock argues that these behaviors are not necessarily always solicitatious behaviors and that they also can serve to pace the rate of mating. Repeated intromissions (insertions of the penis into the vagina) are necessary for ejaculation. During copulation in rats, the male's intromissions trigger progesterone secretion (and other hormonal changes) in the female; this production of progesterone is necessary for successful implantation of fertilized eggs. The optimal number of intromissions and the interval between intromissions necessary to induce the progestational state needed for pregnancy is species specific. In many species pregnancy cannot occur in the absence of an appropriate pattern of vaginal-cervical stimulation. The female can pace the timing of copulations with solicitations of the male.[683]

If the female is permitted to set the pace of intromissions, she will choose a pace that optimizes pregnancy induction. This has been demonstrated in experiments that permit the female to control interactions with a male. If a test apparatus is designed so that the female pushes a lever to open a partition that allows a male to enter or that allows the female to escape from the male, the female will slow the pace of mating. As a result, the female requires fewer intromissions to trigger the progestational state.[683] When animals mate in a large group environment, or when a pair of familiar male and female rats mate, it is the female that initiates copulatory sequences by engaging in solicitatious behavior. Under these circumstances, the female normally sets the pace for mating. Thus, these precopulatory behaviors and the pacing of copulatory events can regulate the female's reproductive success.

In addition to facilitating proceptive behaviors, estrogen can also enhance the attractivity of the female (i.e., her value as a stimulus capable of evoking sexual responses from a male rat).[91] For example, estrogen priming can induce the production of stimuli such as odors, sounds, or physical changes in the female that make her more attractive to the male; concurrently, estrogen promotes proceptive behaviors that are associated with positive responses to a male's physical advances. Prolonged exposure to progesterone, which normally occurs in pregnancy, may inhibit subsequent proceptivity, sexual attractivity, and ovulation.

Thus, for the female, courtship involves behaviors that typically occur when a female is sexually receptive and the concurrent production of specific odors, sounds, and other physical stimuli that signal the female's estrous condition. Specific courtship behaviors vary with the species. Examples of the role of organizational and activational effects of hormones in the development of courtship are discussed in chapter 7.

COPULATION

Studies of the physiological mechanisms responsible for female sexual behavior have focused most often on the analysis of copulatory reflexes.[282] Sexual receptivity in rodents and a variety of other mammals has been operationally defined by the occurrence of lordosis. Lordosis is usually characterized by immobility on the part of the female and an arching of the back, which in conjunction with hindleg extension elevates the rump and head. In species with a long tail, the female may also deviate the tail to one side. In some cases, lordosis is seen prior to male contact, but most commonly this posture is elicited by male mounting or manual stimulation of the female's flank and hindquarters. In rats it is common to calculate a **lordosis quotient** (LQ). The LQ is the ratio of the number of lordosis postures shown in response to a fixed number of mounts (usually 10) $\times$ 100. Thus, if a female shows five lordosis responses to ten mounts she is said to have an LQ of 50 and would be assumed to be moderately receptive.[91] In a number of species, such as voles and hamsters, it is difficult for a male to mount a "nonreceptive" female, preventing the calculation of an LQ. In the latter cases, the sexual receptivity of the female may be indexed by the frequency of lordosis or the duration of the lordosis posture during a fixed test period with a sexually active male.

ESTRUS AND THE ESTROUS CYCLE

The time during a female's reproductive cycle when she is sexually receptive, or willing to mate, is known as estrus. Behavioral estrus is sometimes called heat. The cyclic ovarian events that determine when an animal comes into estrus is known as the estrous cycle. The specific events of the estrous cycle will be described in detail later. In primates, the ovarian cycle is referred to as a menstrual cycle. The menstrual cycle is characterized by uterine bleeding, known as menstruation. Although there is some cyclicity in sexual behavior during the menstrual cycle[1086] (see chapter 5), female primates will mate throughout the menstrual cycle, and a true estrus is not seen in primates. In the estrous cycle of rodents and other nonprimates, menstrual bleeding does not occur, although in a few species, such as dogs, bleeding is associated with ovulation.

Basic Neuroendocrine Functions in the Female

Ovarian Function and Behavioral Receptivity

The gonads have two important functions. They produce ova or sperm (i.e., **gametogenesis**), and they synthesize gonadal steroid hormones (i.e., **steroidogenesis**). Gonadal steroids in turn coordinate neuroendocrine aspects of reproduction, including sexual behavior.

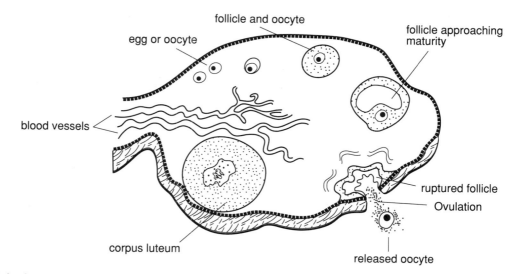

Figure 3.1 Schematic representation of the cycle of follicular development, ovulation, and corpus luteum development in the mammalian ovary. The developing oocyte is nurtured by the follicle, and this is referred to as the follicular phase of the ovarian cycle (depicted as follicle and oocyte; the follicle is approaching maturity). The period around the time when the follicle ruptures, releasing the oocyte (ovulation) is referred to as the periovulatory period. The follicle that remains in the ovary after ovulation becomes the corpus luteum. The phase of the ovarian cycle during which the hormone secretions of the corpus luteum prepare the uterus for implantation of a fertilized egg is called the luteal phase (in species that have an active corpus luteum). See text for additional details.

The primary functional components of the mammalian female gonad (ovary) are the eggs, follicles, and corpus luteum (figure 3.1). Each egg is surrounded by a follicle, which nurtures the developing egg or oocyte, a process called **oogenesis**. The major hormonal function of the follicle is the production of estrogens, including estradiol, estriol, and estrone. When an egg ovulates (is physically expelled) from a follicle, the follicle may be converted into a new structure called a corpus luteum. The corpus luteum is a source of progesterone and other hormones that prepare the uterus for implantation of the fertilized egg.

Mammalian ovarian function involves cycles of follicle development, ovulation (of a small number of follicles), and subsequent corpus luteum formation. In many species, the hypothalamic-pituitary axis regulates ovarian activity, and one or more eggs are produced at regular intervals. However, as described later, not all animals ovulate "spontaneously." There are a number of different patterns of hormone secretion. These patterns in a variety of mammals are reviewed in detail by Feder[342, 343] and Morali and Beyer.[746]

PHASES OF THE OVARIAN CYCLE

In animals that ovulate spontaneously, the duration of an ovarian cycle can vary from approximately 4 days (in mice, rats, and hamsters), to approximately 16 days (in guinea pigs) or longer (in primates). Each phase of the ovarian cycle is usually referred to by the events that are occurring in the ovary during that phase (figure 3.1).

Follicular Phase The cycle begins with the development of the egg. During this phase, luteinizing hormone (LH) and follicle-stimulating hormone (FSH) are released by the pituitary to induce the ovary to begin gametogenesis. The follicle nurtures the egg and also produces estrogen. This phase is referred to as the follicular phase. The follicular phase lasts from 3 days in rodents to 10 to 14 days in humans.

Periovulatory Period As the egg matures, the rate of estrogen secretion increases. A surge of estrogen precedes ovulation and induces the release of a pulse of gonadotropin-releasing hormone (GnRH) from the hypothalamus, which in turn induces a pulse of LH release by the pituitary. The pulse of LH causes the follicle to rupture, resulting in ovulation. This is referred to as the periovulatory period because it describes the sequence of events surrounding ovulation. LH also induces a preovulatory surge of progesterone release from the ovaries. In some animals (e.g., rats and hamsters) the preovulatory surge of progesterone triggers the onset of sexually receptive behavior. The periovulatory period takes about 12 hours in most rodents; in humans it occurs over a period of 1 to 2 days. In rodents, behavioral estrus occurs in association with the periovulatory period.

Luteal Phase The follicle, once it has ruptured and expelled its egg, is transformed into a new endocrine organ known as the corpus luteum (named for the fact that it appears as a "yellow body"). In some animals (e.g., rats and mice) the corpus luteum is not spontaneously retained (i.e., is not "functional"). In such species the corpus luteum is retained only in the event of a pregnancy, signaled by vaginal-cervical stimulation. In turn, progesterone secreted by the corpus luteum plays a major role in the implantation of the egg in the uterine wall and the maintenance of pregnancy. In other species, including primates, the corpus luteum is spontaneously functional. In humans, progesterone and estrogen are secreted by the corpus luteum for a period of about 10 days. This postovulatory period is referred to as the luteal phase. In a nonpregnant female the duration of the luteal phase is determined by the life of the corpus luteum. If an egg is fertilized, implantation in the uterus is facilitated by the luteal phase hormones. The controversial drug RU-486 (the abortion pill) produces its effect by blocking the action of progesterone, thus preventing implantation.

Menstrual Phase In primates, menstruation occurs after the fall in progesterone and estrogen secretion, associated with regression of the corpus luteum. The long (menstrual) cycle of primates results in a build-up of the uterine wall (endometrium), and sloughing of the endometrium results in uterine bleeding. In species such as rodents, which have shorter (estrous) cycles, the endometrial wall is thinner and does not bleed, and there is no event analogous to menstruation.

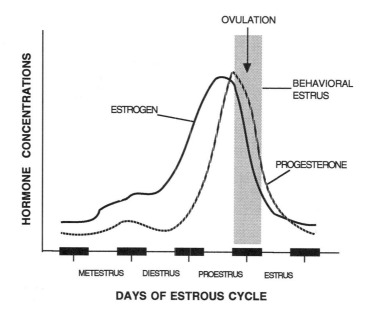

Figure 3.2 Relative concentrations of estradiol and progesterone in serum during the estrous cycle of a female rat. The days of the 4-day estrous cycle (metestrus, diestrus, proestrus, and estrus) are determined from examination of the vaginal epitheleum (slides containing cells from the walls of the vagina are examined under a microscope). Nights are represented by the dark bars on the X axis. Behavioral estrus (dark hatched column) usually begins on the night of proestrus. In the absence of mating, behavioral estrus can persist for 12 hours or more.

ASSOCIATION BETWEEN THE OVARIAN CYCLE, REPRODUCTIVE BEHAVIOR, AND OTHER NEURAL AND PERIPHERAL SYSTEMS IN RODENTS

Ovarian hormones coordinate sexual receptivity, mating, and sperm availability with ovulation. In many species female copulatory behaviors are tightly regulated by ovarian hormones. The 4-day estrous cycle of the rat is an example of the tight regulation that exists between hormones and behavior.

In rats the 4 days of the cycle are usually described relative to the day of ovulation (figure 3.2). **Metestrus** is a day of reduced hormonal and behavioral activity and is the day following ovulation. **Diestrus** is the day associated with the onset of follicular activity and estrogen secretion. **Proestrus** is the day before estrus and includes the major hormonal events that induce behavioral estrus. The GnRH and LH surges that trigger eventual ovulation usually occur on the evening of proestrus. Behavioral estrus and copulatory behavior are first seen on proestrus. **Estrus** describes the day of the estrous cycle on which ovulation actually occurs.

The ovary (possibly with assistance from the adrenal) produces pulses of estrogens, some androgens (testosterone or others), and a surge of progesterone and other progestins on proestrus. These hormones enter the general circulation and act sequentially throughout the body to prime the nervous system, pituitary, uterus, vagina, mammary glands, and other tissues for behavioral estrus and subsequent ovulation, pregnancy, and lactation.

The lordosis posture results from a cascade of spinal reflexes that are modulated by specific brain regions and neurochemicals that will be described below. Lordosis can be elicited at the level of the spinal cord by strong somatosensory (i.e., tactile) stimuli. However, in tests with males, lordosis is infrequent in prepubertal females or in adult females following removal of the ovary (ovariectomy or spaying). Thus, in many mammals,[309, 1086] ovarian secretions acting on the nervous system are essential for the normal expression of female sexual behavior.

OTHER CONSIDERATIONS

Sexual behavior in females is clearly influenced by ovarian function. However, it is also important to remember that many aspects of reproduction are regulated by environmental stimuli such as photoperiod, food, and water. Environmental regulators produce seasonal variations in sexual activity in many species. In addition, reproductive old age or senescence can limit reproduction. In small rodents, spontaneous ovulation may occur under optimal environmental conditions to permit frequent pregnancies. In large mammals such as some primates and ungulates, spontaneous ovulation is regulated by seasonal factors to ensure the birth of young during a period of resource availability (such as spring in the northern hemisphere). Thus, sheep have an 8-month gestational period, and their breeding season begins during times of decreasing day length (fall in the northern hemisphere), so that the young are born in spring, when food is available. The importance of biological rhythms in the regulation of endocrine systems and cycles will be discussed in greater detail in chapter 16.

Variation in Mechanisms Mediating Ovulation

Ovulation may either be timed by endogenous stimuli, as described above, or *induced* by exogenous stimuli. In some animals sexual receptivity occurs in spontaneous cycles, but ovulation does not occur without copulation (**induced ovulation**). In other species both behavioral estrus and ovulation are induced by specific stimuli (**induced estrus and ovulation**).

INDUCED OVULATION

Induced ovulation usually relies on the presence of copulatory stimuli from the male to provide the surge of hypothalamic-pituitary hormones required to trigger egg release. This is considered an opportunistic reproductive strategy. In induced ovulators (such as rabbits, cats, and ferrets) the ovary may produce waves of follicles during the reproductive season and remain quiescent at other times. These animals come into a period of behavioral estrus, during which follicles are activated to produce mature eggs. The follicle does not rupture and ovulation does not occur, however, unless the animal mates during this period.

In cats, ferrets, and rabbits, as the waves of ovarian follicles mature, the ovary secretes estrogen. Estrogen in turn induces, within a day or more, behavioral estrus leading to mating. In these species, copulatory stimuli from the male (usually vaginal-cervical stimuli) are essential for the induction of ovulation. Copulation activates a neural response that results in hypothalamic release of GnRH, which in turn induces pituitary release of LH to induce rupture of the follicle and ovulation. Progesterone is probably not essential to trigger female receptivity in induced ovulators, but it may play a role in the termination of estrus.[190, 343]

INDUCED ESTRUS AND OVULATION

In some animals (such as prairie voles) both estrus and ovulation are induced. These animals may remain reproductively inactive until stimuli from a male are present. Thus, the stimuli from the male can regulate the reproductive condition of the female, guaranteeing that a male partner will be present when the female becomes sexually active.

This pattern of induced reproductive condition is typical of highly social mammals, including prairie voles. These animals are thought to rely on chemical signals, biologically active odors or pheromones, from the male to activate ovarian estrogen secretion. Prairie voles show no indication of cyclic ovarian activity, and, in the absence of male-related stimuli, female prairie voles do not show behavioral estrus. After an initial exposure to a male or male pheromones, estrogen is secreted, which primes the female. After a day or more of male exposure, sexual receptivity is usually observed, and ovulation is induced by about 10 to 12 hours following coitus. Progesterone secretion follows ovulation by a day or more in this species. In this case, progesterone probably functions primarily to inhibit receptivity in prairie voles.[190]

The musk shrew also relies on social stimuli for the induction of lordosis. Virgin female musk shrews are not receptive but begin to show sexual behavior within 1 hour of male exposure.[857] It was originally believed that this species was capable of steroid-independent sexual receptivity.[309] Female musk shrews will mate while the ovary is hormonally quiescent. In addition, ovarian estrogen or exogenous estrogen at doses that mimic those found in intact females are not effective in inducing sexual receptivity. However, recent studies by Rissman and her associates[857] have revealed that the ovary is involved in sexual receptivity, apparently through the use of androgens.

Doses of androgens near the physiological range are capable of inducing receptivity in the musk shrew. Thus, like males of many species, female shrews may utilize androgens to regulate sexual activity. It appears that these androgens are behaviorally most effective following conversion (aromatization) into estrogens.[857] Enzymes capable of aromatizing androgens to estrogens exist within the brain, suggesting the possibility that androgens enter the brain in that form and are converted within brain tissue to estrogens. The musk shrew is a tropical species and is found in breeding condition throughout the year. Rissman and associates[857] suggest that this mechanism would allow year-round breeding while minimizing the systemic exposure of the female to estrogen, which is potentially toxic.

Socially induced estrus and ovulation are primary modes of reproductive activation in some species and also may be alternative modes of reproduction in animals that are usually characterized as having spontaneous or cyclic ovulation. Under suboptimal environmental conditions, such as irregular light cycles or limited availability of food or water, even species that usually show cyclic patterns of spontaneous estrus and ovulation can revert to socially induced reproductive activation. Such flexibility in patterns of reproduction is especially characteristic of rodents, such as mice and rats, that inhabit highly variable environments.

SYNCHRONY OF OVARIAN CYCLES

Another consequence of the influence of social stimuli on ovarian cycles is the phenomenon of estrous synchrony. When female rats or mice are housed together, "cycles change in length until estrus is synchronized within the social group; as a consequence, females tend to come into heat and ovulate on the same day."[683]

McClintock[683] has demonstrated that this coordination of estrous cycles in rats is modulated by airborne chemicals. If rats are housed in separate cages but have a common air supply, estrous synchrony develops. The synchrony of cycles involves the coordination of at least two different chemosignals or pheromones. These two pheromones have opposing effects, one shortening the estrous cycle and enhancing the probability of the female coming into estrus and ovulating and the other lengthening the cycle while suppressing estrus and ovulation.

A similar phenomenon has been reported in human females. Female coeds living together in a residential women's college have been reported to show menstrual cycle synchrony after a period of 4 to 7 months.[682] A second study investigating menstrual synchrony in college-age women found that the amount of time women spent together, not just the sharing of common living quarters, determined whether two women would become synchronous. Over a 4-month period, women who identified each other as close friends became synchronous for the onset of menstruation.[435] The mechanisms mediating this effect in humans are unknown.

Pregnancy and the Ovarian Cycle

Pregnancy inhibits ovarian cycles. However, on the day of birth (parturition) or shortly thereafter, females of some species come into estrus. This is referred to as postpartum estrus. In addition, in some instances reproductive cycles are suspended during lactation. Thus, there is a complex interaction between pregnancy, lactation, and the ovarian cycle.

POSTPARTUM ESTRUS

Once a female rodent has successfully mated, the physiology of pregnancy suspends the ovarian cycle. However, in many species, females show behavioral receptivity in the period just prior to or following parturition, and ovulation also follows birth. Postpartum estrus is similar but not identical to a cyclic estrus. The duration of mating during the postpartum period is typically less extended than that in cyclic estrus.[683] Postpartum estrus seems to maximize the reproductive potential of a female; litters conceived in postpartum estrus are born at approximately the time that the older litter is weaned (21 to 23 days after the birth of the older litter).

In addition, in monogamous or pair-bonding species such as prairie voles, females in postpartum estrus may be very selective in their choice of a sexual partner. Monogamous females usually mate preferentially with their familiar partner and often will attack unfamiliar males.[191] Thus, in species with a monogamous mating system, partner familiarity can play a particularly important role in the expression of sexual activity in the postpartum period.

The endocrinology of postpartum estrus is not well documented. However, it is likely that female rodents come into estrus as a result of exposure to estrogen that is secreted during pregnancy or during the peripartum. Even in species like rats that rely on sequential exposure to estrogen and progesterone for cyclic estrus induction, females can respond to estrogen alone if the hormone is present over an extended period of days. In most mammals the progesterone level is elevated throughout pregnancy and falls rapidly just before parturition. Progesterone relaxes the smooth muscle of the uterus, and a decline in progesterone may be necessary for the uterine contractions associated with delivery. There also may be a surge of progesterone during the postpartum period in some species.

In rats there is evidence that oxytocin, which promotes parturition, also can facilitate female sexual behavior in estrogen-primed females.[179] Thus, prolonged exposure to estrogen and progesterone during pregnancy and the subsequent decline in progesterone would set the stage for postpartum estrus. In some cases a second surge of progesterone and a parturitional surge of oxytocin also may be components of the timing mechanisms that link postpartum estrus and parturition.

LACTATIONAL INHIBITION OF FEMALE SEXUAL BEHAVIOR

After a brief period of postpartum estrus, females that nurse their young may experience an inhibition of ovarian cycles and female sexual receptivity. Follicular maturation and ovarian steroid production often are inhibited during lactation. The absence of appropriate steroid hormone priming presumably results in the absence of female sexual behavior. However, lactational acyclity is not absolute, and, especially when food is plentiful, females may resume cycling and ovulate before lactation ceases. Prolonged exposure to the two major hormones of lactation, prolactin and oxytocin[1109] or the endogenous opiates[976] also may inhibit sexual behavior.

Reproductive Inhibition

Both spontaneous and induced ovulators can fail to cycle or show sexual behavior in the presence of other females. This reproductive inhibition may
occur in young females, resulting in a delay in the onset of ovarian activity
(puberty).[1062] In addition, reproductive inhibition has been described in adult,
cycling, or postpartum estrous females.[158, 308] In highly social species, including monogamous mammals such as prairie voles,[190] small social primates
known as marmosets, and even female-only parthenogenic lizards (see chapter
6), it is common for only the oldest or dominant female within a group or
family to reproduce. A particularly extreme case of reproductive inhibition
occurs in the naked mole rat, in which only one female within a colony of
hundreds is cycling or capable of reproduction.[940]

Reproductive inhibition or delay can be adaptive. Inhibited females may
assume other functions within the family or gain benefits by waiting to
reproduce.[1090] In addition, although they delay their own reproduction, such
females may indirectly enhance their reproductive fitness by increasing
the probability that a larger portion of the family (carrying at least some of
their own genes) will survive. Group living may be generally stressful, and
stress can inhibit reproduction[22] (see also chapter 10). However, it also has
been shown in a variety of mammals that females can emit chemical signals
or pheromones that inhibit or delay the reproduction of other members of
their group.[158, 308, 683, 1062]

Expression of Feminine Sexual Behavior in Adulthood

Physiological Mechanisms Regulating Female Sexual Behavior in Rodents

In ovary-intact female rodents, lordosis is rare during the metestrous and di-
estrous phases of the female's estrous cycle. Female rats with a 4-day cycle
usually show lordosis during the evening of proestrus and, if unmated, remain
sexually receptive through the day of estrus. These effects can be shown
to be hormone dependent.

ESTROGEN
The actions of various endocrine factors in sexual behavior are species specific.
However, the most consistent element regulating female reproductive behavior is the steroid hormone estrogen. Estrogen plays the major coordinating
role in female reproduction through its ability to stimulate or regulate various
target organs including the nervous system.

The presence or absence of a given receptor can allow or prevent the cellular
actions of a given hormone.[644, 812] Estrogen receptors are distributed in particular regions of the brain and spinal cord (figure 3.3) and show remarkable consistency in their location across a variety of vertebrate species. Regulation of
receptors can occur through changes in the number of receptors or through

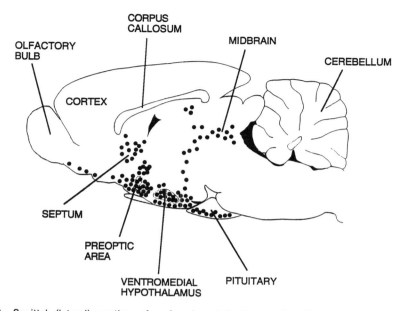

Figure 3.3 Sagittal (lateral) section of a female rat brain showing the relative distribution of estradiol-concentrating cells. Areas of highest concentration are represented by dots. Highest concentrations are found in the preoptic area, hypothalamus (especially the ventromedial hypothalamus), amygdala (not shown), septum, and midbrain central gray (Pfaff and Schwartz-Giblin, 1988). These distributions were determined by examining autoradiograms of brain slices. Radioactively labeled estradiol is injected into an ovariectomized rat. After the radioactively labeled estradiol has circulated throughout the body for a few hours, it will be selectively retained by cells that contain estrogen receptors. The brain can then be sliced and the location of the estrogen receptors determined.

changes in the affinity of a receptor for the hormone. A molecule that binds to a receptor is called a ligand, and when a ligand has a weak affinity for a receptor, it does not bind very tightly to the receptor. Very high concentrations may therefore be required to elicit a biological response.

During periods of hormone deprivation the sensitivity to estrogen decreases. This is thought to be primarily due to a decrease in the number of estrogen receptors. If hormone treatment is initiated, estrogen receptors are self-nduced over a period of hours or days. It is generally assumed that the induction of estrogen receptors is essential for centrally mediated female sexual receptivity.

A number of other hormones may influence behavior through their interactions with estrogen and its receptors. In general, receptors may respond to a variety of molecules with similar structures; however, the binding affinity may be weaker for some structures than others. Therefore, other hormones or neurotransmitters can influence the effect of estrogen by competing with estrogen for the receptor.

The behavioral effects of estrogen usually require at least 24 hours to be expressed, and the hormone is most effective if given in discontinuous pulses.[210, 812] Endogenous hormone secretion is often pulsatile, and these pulses may be necessary for normal hormonal action. Uninterrupted, prolonged exposure to estrogen can result in a relative insensitivity to its behavioral effects, probably caused by a decrease in the number of receptors.

Pulsatile estrogen treatment produces rapid (within minutes) and long-lasting effects that eventually result in polypeptide or protein synthesis in neurons containing estrogen receptors.[812] Injection of protein synthesis inhibitors disrupts the ability of steroids to facilitate female sexual behavior. Various neurochemicals or receptors also may be synthesized under the influence of estrogen or progesterone. Of importance to female sexual behavior in the rat is the estrogen-dependent induction of receptors for progesterone.[931] Progestin receptors are probably essential to permit a normal behavioral response to the endogenous preovulatory surge of progesterone that triggers the onset of lordosis.

PROGESTERONE

In estrogen-primed female rats progesterone clearly enhances lordosis behavior.[88] However, progesterone is not effective in inducing lordosis in ovariectomized females that have not received estrogen. Because progestin receptors are induced by estrogen, estrogen indirectly regulates the behavioral effects of progesterone. In addition, under conditions in which estrogen, without progesterone, induces lordosis it is possible that estrogen acts in part through stimulation of progestin receptors.[931] Species that do not depend on progesterone for the induction of estrus such as prairie voles[190, 216] and ferrets[80] nonetheless have progestin receptors in their brains; the function of these receptors is unknown at present.

ANDROGENS

In female rats androgens released during mating may pace patterns of female sexual behavior by inhibiting receptivity.[330] Mating-timed inhibitions of receptivity are probably adaptive in reducing risks, such as predation, associated with sexual behavior. From the male's perspective, turning off the female's receptivity would help to protect his copulatory "investment" in the female.

Androgens also have been implicated in the induction of female sexual behavior in a variety of species (reviewed in Rissman[857]).[941] However, at least in rodents, androgens are probably not normally essential for estrus induction. As discussed earlier, the female musk shrew may rely on androgens as a prohormone from which brain tissues can produce estrogens. Androgens may be important for the motivational components of female sexual behavior in humans and other primates.[942, 1086] The latter hypothesis will be discussed in chapter 5.

Interactions Between Sexual Behavior and Gonadal Steroid Hormones

The onset of sexual receptivity and lordosis usually follows within 1 to 4 hours after the preovulatory surge of progesterone. By this time, the female also has been exposed to increasing concentrations of follicular estrogen. Without estrogen priming progesterone does not induce the onset of sexual receptivity. The onset of lordosis precedes ovulation by about 10 to 12 hours, and this timing provides an opportunity for mating to occur and sperm to reach the ovary prior to or immediately following ovulation.[19, 20, 683]

The priming of progesterone receptors by estrogen is functionally important, at least in female rats. As discussed in chapter 1, steroid hormones characteristically induce the production of their own receptors. In addition, estrogen also induces the production of progesterone receptors. Thus, estrogen priming results in the induction of progesterone receptors, reducing the amount of progesterone required to induce sexually receptive behavior. Through this mechanism, estrogen acts to regulate directly the effect of progesterone on female sexual receptivity.

The duration and termination of sexual receptivity also may be regulated in part by the same hormones that induce estrus. If estrogen is withdrawn, receptivity is lost within a matter of hours. In addition, prolonged exposure to progesterone inhibits subsequent sexual receptivity, even in species that rely on progesterone for estrus induction.[343] The ability of progesterone to initially facilitate and later inhibit receptivity is termed the biphasic effect of progesterone. Within a given estrous cycle, the duration of behavioral estrus is probably regulated by declining concentrations of estrogen and long-term exposure to progesterone. Furthermore, once the hypothalamus has been exposed to progesterone, there is a down-regulation of progesterone receptors and therefore a refractory period. Thus, unlike the initial effect of estrogen described earlier, progesterone does *not* induce an increase in the number of its receptors but actually *causes a decrease* in receptor availability. A period of a relatively low hormone level followed by reexposure to estrogen to induce progesterone receptors and then to progesterone to activate the receptor response is usually necessary to reinstate sexually receptive behavior.

Copulatory stimuli play a major role in inhibiting subsequent female sexual receptivity and thus in inducing sexual satiety. Copulatory stimulation releases progesterone and other neurochemicals, which may combine with prolonged exposure to progesterone to terminate the sexual receptivity of a recently mated female.[20, 187]

Species vary in the amount of time spent in copulatory activities. Female guinea pigs may become unreceptive after experiencing a single ejaculation, whereas rats may mate for several hours,[20, 683] and female prairie voles remain behaviorally receptive for a day or longer.[190] Different patterns of postcopulatory progesterone release[191] or species differences in sensitivity to progesterone's inhibitory effects may contribute to species differences in patterns of sexual behavior.

Neural Regulation of Feminine Sexual Behavior

Pfaff and Schwartz-Giblin[812] offer a schematic description of the nervous system based in part on the embryology of neural development. Using this model, they have divided the nervous system into functional modules or subdivisions that include the forebrain, hypothalamus, midbrain, lower brainstem, and spinal cord.

FOREBRAIN

As far as we know, no part of the forebrain is essential for the appearance of lordosis, and, in fact, the forebrain may inhibit the lordosis reflex. Within the forebrain, lesions in adult animals of the cerebral cortex, septum, preoptic area, and olfactory bulb do not eliminate female sexual receptivity. When tested in confined cages with highly motivated males, lesioned females have high lordosis quotients and may even respond more easily or show lordosis postures of a longer duration than those seen in nonlesioned females.[812] These findings are complicated by the disruption of various sensory systems that occur with such lesions and may indicate that females have less fear of the males or are interpreting differently other sensory experiences such as genital stimulation. In addition, female rats that have been decorticated as infants do not show an enhanced lordosis response and are less responsive to males when tested under conditions of low estrogen.[192] In general, the presence or absence of a particular neural tissue may affect behavior in more than one way, depending on the age at which the lesion occurs and the conditions of behavioral testing.

HYPOTHALAMUS

The hypothalamus has long been viewed as a critical component of the circuitry needed for female sexual behavior. Of particular importance within the hypothalamus is the ventromedial hypothalamic (VMH) nucleus (see figure 3.3 and chapter 1). This small concentration of cells plays a critical role in lordosis behavior. Lesions of the VMH usually disrupt lordosis behavior, particularly if the female is tested under conditions in which she cannot escape male mounting. However, smaller VMH lesions are less effective than large lesions, and small lesions may not inhibit lordosis under test conditions in which the female regulates the copulatory interactions. Under the latter conditions, females with small VMH lesions exhibit lordosis behavior but spend more time than normal females in areas of the test cage that cannot be reached by the males. Thus, it has been suggested that, following the lesion, stimuli from the male have become more aversive. Conversely, it can be argued that under normal conditions hypothalamic neurons regulate the interpretation of somatosensory input as either aversive or not.[931]

Estrogen, progesterone, and other neurochemicals may interact within the VMH to facilitate or inhibit the expression of female sexual behavior. One of the brain areas that concentrates steroid hormones is the basal hypothalamus. Facilitative effects on lordosis in ovariectomized female rats can be measured following small implants of estrogen and progesterone,[886] and these effects are selectively localized in the VMH. Hormonal effects within the VMH may be mediated by modulation of the intensity or interpretation of sensory inputs such as tactile stimuli. Such modulation could then alter the probability that the female would remain in the presence of the male or would show lordosis if mounted.

MIDBRAIN

Estrogen receptors also are localized within the midbrain central gray. Neurons from the ventromedial hypothalamus send axons to the midbrain central gray, as do neurons in the spinal cord receiving information from sensory systems that are important for lordosis. This connection may be important, therefore, in the activation of lordosis behavior.[866] Destruction of this area reduces lordosis in female rats, while electrical stimulation in the midbrain can facilitate lordosis.

LOWER BRAINSTEM AND SPINAL CORD

Fibers from the brainstem descend to the spinal cord through the vestibulospinal and reticulospinal tracts.[812] Reticulospinal pathways in particular are believed to be hormone dependent. Postural adjustments associated with lordosis are presumably integrated in these areas. Complete spinal transections eliminate lordosis, but relatively large lesions may have little effect on this behavior as long as the lateral funiculus, containing the above mentioned tracts, is intact.

The Neural Circuit Mediating the Lordosis Reflex

Using the units of the brain described earlier, Pfaff and Schwartz-Giblin[812] have proposed a model for the neural circuits regulating the lordosis reflex in the rat (figure 3.4). The lordosis reflex in the rat begins in response to sensory stimuli applied by the male during mounting. Sensory input is relayed from the sensory receptors into the spinal cord, where input converges on interneurons. Activation of these interneurons can trigger lordosis. If the spinal cord is isolated from the brain, however, females do not exhibit lordosis. It is concluded, therefore, that additional neural circuitry is normally necessary for initiation of lordosis.

Stimuli received from mounting are relayed from the spinal interneurons to ascending fibers that project to the reticular formation in the medulla and the midbrain central gray. This circuit is activated whenever a female is mounted by a male, even if she is not behaviorally receptive. It is the activation of hypothalamic neural centers by estrogen and, in some cases, progesterone that determines whether this sensory input will trigger lordosis. These hormones also influence the attractiveness of the rat, so a female that is not receptive is also not as attractive to a male rat and is less likely to be mounted in the first place.

Estrogen and progesterone act in the VMH to promote lordosis. This has been demonstrated in a number of ways. First, as discussed earlier, the VMH contains neurons that accumulate estrogen and progesterone, indicating that the appropriate receptors are found in the area. Local implants of estrogen into

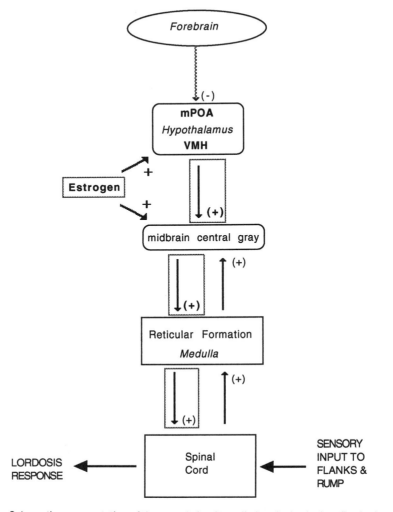

Figure 3.4 Schematic representation of the neural circuit mediating the lordosis reflex in the rat. Sensory input on the rump and flanks from the male mounting the female is received at the spinal cord. This sensory information is relayed to ascending fibers that project to the medullary reticular formation and the midbrain central gray. This circuit is activated by sensory input whenever it is received. The lordosis reflex is triggered, however, only if the female rat has been previously exposed to estrogen (indicated by the hatched boxes around the descending arrows). strogen acts in the medial preoptic area (mPOA) and the ventromedial hypothalamus (VMH) regions of the hypothalamus and in the midbrain central gray (indicated by the arrows with +) to enhance the excitability of midbrain target neurons, so that the lordosis reflex is triggered in response to mounting by a male rat. The forebrain can inhibit the lordosis reflex when conditions are not favorable for mating. Large arrows at bottom indicate sensory input and motor output. Smaller vertical arrows indicate the direction of information flow and whether the stimulus is excitatory (solid arrows with [+]) or inhibitory (stippled arrow with [−]). (Adapted from Pfaff and Schwartz-Giblin, 1988.[812])

the VMH will facilitate lordosis, whereas estrogen implants elsewhere have little effect. Implants of antiestrogens in the VMH inhibit behavior. Other experiments have demonstrated specific effects of estrogen on electrical activity and gene expression in neurons located within or near the VMH.

Axons from neurons in the VMH project to the midbrain central gray. Activation of VMH neurons by estrogen results in an increase in the electrical excitability of midbrain target neurons. This in turn activates descending projections that control the motor neurons involved in the lordosis reflex. According to this model, when a female is mounted by a male, if estrogen has potentiated neural activity in the VMH, the output circuitry is excited, and the lordosis reflex is initiated.

This is, of course, a highly simplified summary of the lordosis reflex. Other input to neurons in this circuit (e.g., from the forebrain) can also modulate neuronal activity, thus affecting the probability of lordosis. In addition, there are hormonal effects on neurons in the midbrain central gray as well as on sensory receptors that also affect responsiveness within the circuit. For additional details, the reader is referred again to the review of Pfaff and Schwartz-Giblin.[812]

Neurohormone and Neurotransmitter Regulation of Feminine Sexual Behavior

Neurohormones and neurotransmitters capable of influencing other aspects of reproduction such as ovulation, maternal behavior [573](see also chapter 8), and lactation[473] can also influence female sexual behavior. Knowledge of a species' reproductive strategy and mating system may provide powerful clues about those agents that will be most likely to influence behavior within that species.

A given neurotransmitter or neurohormone may have different actions when present at different sites in the brain. It is also possible and in fact common for a neurohormone or neurotransmitter to facilitate a behavior at one time and inhibit it at another time. These phenomena may be due to differences in receptor physiology or to changes in the circulating hormonal milieu that can alter the neural substrate(s) upon which the neurohormone or neurotransmitter must act. The following is an attempt to synthesize and simplify the roles of a number of neuroactive agents thought to play a role in female sexual behavior.

GnRH
GnRH neurons have their cell bodies in the preoptic area of the hypothalamus with axons that project primarily to the median eminence. Terminals in the median eminence release GnRH into hypophyseal portal vessels. A surge of GnRH carried from the hypothalamus to the pituitary triggers the release of FSH and LH from the pituitary gland. FSH and LH in turn circulate to the ovary and induce ovulation.

Of potential importance to behavior is the fact that GnRH axons also project to the midbrain central gray. Thus, GnRH may also be released in the brain to influence the probability that lordosis will occur. GnRH administered locally to the midbrain central gray potentiates lordosis behavior. Conversely, antisera to GnRH in the central gray can block lordosis. In spontaneous ovulators, such as rats, GnRH that is endogenously released into the central gray prior to ovulation may help to ensure that female sexual receptivity is synchronized with ovulation.[812]

OXYTOCIN

Oxytocin has traditionally been studied as a posterior pituitary hormone with peripheral actions in birth and lactation. However, it is now known that oxytocinergic neurons (in the paraventricular nucleus of the hypothalamus) release oxytocin into the brain as well as into the bloodstream. Receptors for oxytocin are widespread in the nervous system as well as in the breasts and uterus. The possible role for oxytocin in sexual behavior is particularly interesting because of the unique neuroanatomy of the cells that manufacture this hormone.[473] Oxytocinergic cells are usually separated by glia, but these glia can be retracted within a matter of minutes. This leaves the oxytocin neurons electrically coupled to each other with the potential for synchronous, pulsatile release of hormone.

Peripheral stimuli, such as touch or cervical stimulation, during copulation can trigger the release of oxytocin. Injections of oxytocin stimulate sexual behavior in female rats that are primed with subthreshold doses of estrogen and/or progesterone.[34, 179, 801] In fact, estrogen induces an increase in oxytocin receptors in the VMH. Thus, during estrus, copulatory stimulation that triggers the release of oxytocin could provide a cascade of events that eventually leads to a surge of oxytocin and an enhanced receptor response (reviewed by Carter[188]).

Implantation of oxytocin within the VMH in estrous female rats did not affect lordosis quotients, but females showed reduced aggression and increased physical contact with the male. Since oxytocin is normally released as a result of copulation and not prior to coitus, the normal role of oxytocin may be important for sexual satiety and pair-bonding.[188, 1109]

Centrally released oxytocin also may play a role in the autonomic events (e.g., changes in heart rate) that accompany sexual behavior. Synchronous release of oxytocin into the peripheral circulation could enhance uterine contractility and thus sperm transport. Finally, exposure to long-term or high concentrations of oxytocin may contribute to the sexual satiety that follows extended mating and to the lactational inhibition characteristics of female sexual behavior.[188, 1109]

PROLACTIN

A second lactational hormone, prolactin, also may play a role in female sexual behavior. Prolactin-containing cells are found primarily in the anterior pituitary but also have been identified in the arcuate nucleus of the hypothalamus (near but not within the VMH). Axons from these neurons project throughout the brain. In particular, there is a projection to the midbrain central gray. Infusions of prolactin into the midbrain central gray can facilitate lordosis in female rats pretreated with low doses of estrogen.[812] The functional significance of prolactin in female sexual behavior is not well understood. However, like oxytocin, prolactin is released in the postpartum period and might synergize with estrogen to time the onset or duration of postpartum estrus.

CATECHOLAMINES

Two catecholamines, dopamine and norepinephrine, also have been implicated in female sexual behavior. The neurochemical events that precede the release of GnRH and oxytocin may also facilitate female sexual receptivity. For example, norepinephrine turnover in the hypothalamus has been correlated with GnRH and oxytocin release, which in turn can facilitate lordosis.

A direct facilitative effect of norepinephrine on lordosis is thought to be due to the activation of a specific class of norepinephrine receptors called α_1-adrenergic receptors found within the VMH. Infusion of norepinephrine into the medial preoptic area or VMH can activate lordosis in animals treated with estrogen. Drugs that block α_1-adrenergic receptors (α_1-antagonists) reduce lordosis. If the axons from the norepinephrine cell bodies in the locus coeruleus that project to the hypothalamus are severed, lordosis is blocked.[812]

Norepinephrine may in part induce these effects on lordosis by modulating progestin binding. Treatment with α_1-adrenergic antagonists can prevent the estrogen-induced increase in progesterone receptors.[744] Norepinephrine, therefore, could facilitate lordosis directly through its effects on adrenergic receptors in the VMH or preoptic area, or indirectly by regulating the release of oxytocin and GnRH.

The catecholamine dopamine may be important for promoting proceptive motor behaviors, including general movement as well as ear wiggling, hopping, and darting. The ascending dopamine projection from the midbrain to the basal ganglia is typically associated with the execution of stereotyped movements (movements that are always done in the same way) and increased sensorimotor responsiveness. Gonadal hormone-induced activation of dopamine activity, therefore, may promote responsiveness of the female to stimulation by the male as well as the exhibition of proceptive behaviors. Some of these ideas will be discussed in chapter 11. This dopamine system, therefore, may participate in the fine-tuning of motor patterns in female sexual behavior, but it is probably not directly involved in the lordosis reflex. There are also dopaminergic neurons contained within the hypothalamus (the incertohypothalamic dopamine neurons). These dopaminergic neurons are implicated in male sexual behavior (see chapter 4), but their role in female sexual behavior has not been demonstrated.

ACETYLCHOLINE

Acetylcholine is a neurotransmitter with widespread neural activity. Acetylcholine cell bodies in the basal forebrain project to the medial basal hypothalamus. Estrogen can increase the activity of choline acetyltransferase, an enzyme necessary for acetylcholine synthesis, and increase the number of acetylcholine receptors in the VMH. These effects were found in female rats but not male rats. The estrogen-induced increase in acetylcholine receptors in the VMH increases the number of cells that respond electrophysiologically to acetylcholine. Clemens and associates[212, 214] have shown that drugs that stimulate acetylcholine receptors can facilitate lordosis in female rats, and drugs that specifically inhibit acetylcholine receptors inhibit lordosis. By applying cholinergic agonists and antagonists locally at specific sites in the brain, they have found that acetylcholine facilitates lordosis when applied to the medial preoptic area, VMH, or midbrain central gray but not when applied to the reticular formation or frontal cortex. Maximum cholinergic facilitation required estrogen pretreatment of animals. Thus, acetylcholine terminals in the hypothalamus are thought to participate in the estrogen-induced facilitation of lordosis behavior.

SEROTONIN
Among the other neurotransmitters that are implicated in female (and male) sexual behavior is serotonin (5-hydroxytryptamine, 5-HT). Drugs that inhibit serotonin facilitate lordosis in several species including rats[600, 715] and hamsters.[189] Excess serotonin is associated with hyperreactivity to stimuli such as touch; thus, reduced serotoninergic activity might synergize with specific opiates (see later discussion) to modulate the reactivity of the estrous female to painful or aversive stimuli. In addition, serotonin receptors are regulated by estrogen. We can speculate that serotonin, if released during mating, could also play a role in inhibiting further sexual behavior and thus inducing sexual satiety.

GAMMA-AMINOBUTYRIC ACID (GABA)
GABA is generally viewed as an inhibitory neurotransmitter and may also regulate lordosis. Drugs that block GABA can facilitate lordosis, and drugs that stimulate GABA receptors usually inhibit sexual behavior. Schwartz-Giblin and colleagues[931] postulate that estrogen-dependent inhibitions of GABA may act to increase synaptic efficiency (possibly in the spinal cord). Blocking GABA is thought to increase sensitivity to light somatosensory stimuli and thus regulate lordosis behavior at the spinal cord level. GABA neurons are widespread throughout the nervous system and play an important role in the regulation of other processes, including the release of oxytocin.[573] Thus, GABA could have indirect effects on sexual behavior through its actions on other systems.

ENDOGENOUS OPIATES: β-ENDORPHINS AND ENKEPHALINS
In addition to modulating her behavioral arousal, the estrous female must be selectively sensitive or insensitive to contact behaviors, including copulatory stimuli, that might otherwise be aversive.[809] The endogenous opiates, including the β-endorphins and enkephalins, are generally associated with reducing

pain perception but probably also have a role in the modulation of female sexual and social behavior.[22, 976, 1101]

In general, high concentrations of opiates have been associated with the inhibition of sexual behavior and other aspects of reproduction.[813] Opiate treatment reduces GnRH release, and opiate antagonists such as naloxone increase GnRH release. Opiate antagonists facilitate some components of female sexual behavior, possibly through secondary actions on the release of GnRH.[22, 961] High concentrations of opiates, including β-endorphins released during stress, may serve to prevent sexual activity at times when the environment is inappropriate. Opiate release during mating also could inhibit subsequent sexual behavior and thus may be part of the mechanism responsible for sexual satiety. Other possible functions of endogenous opiates in reproduction have been extensively reviewed elsewhere.[22, 813, 976, 1101]

Injections of naloxone or other β-endorphin antagonists into the midbrain central gray facilitate lordosis. This raises the possibility that somatosensory inputs, pain inhibition, autonomic functions, and other fundamental behavioral components of sexual behavior are regulated in the midbrain.[812]

Another class of endogenous opiates, the enkephalins, may have effects that are opposite to those of β-endorphins and thus facilitate female sexual behavior. Enkephalins act on different receptors and in different brain regions than the β-endorphins. Enkephalins are thought to modulate the effects of more arousing hormones and to induce a level of analgesia. Analgesia, especially of the peripheral tissues, is thought to be necessary to allow the female to cope with aversive or painful stimuli encountered during sexual behavior.[809, 931] In spite of its length, the above list of neurohormones and neurotransmitters capable of influencing female sexual behavior is not exhaustive. As new biologically active substances are discovered within the nervous system, they are usually tested for their effects on lordosis, and many prove to be behaviorally active. New neurochemicals remain to be discovered, and many behavioral functions of the well established hormones and neurotransmitters remain to be explored.

Summary

1. In general, at least in rodents, estrogen-priming must occur first if other hormones or neurotransmitters are to facilitate female sexual behavior.

2. In spontaneous ovulators with short estrous cycles, progesterone is the major ovarian hormone that times the onset of female sexual receptivity as measured by lordosis. However, other neurochemicals can "substitute" for or synergize with progesterone in estrus induction. Substances that are released prior to ovulation, including norepinephrine, GnRH, oxytocin, prolactin, enkephalins, and acetylcholine, are all capable of inducing or facilitating female sexual behavior.

3. Chemicals that are released during or as a consequence of mating are most likely to inhibit or abbreviate behavioral estrus. Progesterone, dopamine,

oxytocin, prolactin, serotonin, GABA, and β-endorphins, under certain conditions, inhibit female sexual receptivity. Inhibitory processes are needed to produce cyclic patterns of reproduction. At least some of the neurochemicals that inhibit female sexual behavior also may be involved in postcopulatory sexual satiety.

General Summary and Conclusions

1. Feminine sexual behavior consists of proceptive or courtship behaviors and sexual receptivity or copulatory behaviors. Both of these components are influenced by estrogen and progesterone in most mammals, with the exception of primates. In addition to bringing a male and female together, proceptive behaviors may serve to optimize the pace of the mating sequence for promotion of pregnancy. Copulation requires that a female exhibit a characteristic posture known as lordosis in response to mounting by a male. Females exhibit this reflex when they are sexually receptive during estrus.

2. The phases of the ovarian cycle in spontaneous ovulators are the follicular phase, periovulatory phase, and luteal phase. Not all animals have a luteal phase because, in the absence of copulation, the corpus luteum may not be functional (e.g., in rats, hamsters, and mice). Primates additionally have a menstrual phase. The follicle develops during the follicular phase. The egg is released and animals become sexually receptive during the periovulatory phase. The remaining follicle becomes the corpus luteum in animals with a luteal phase, releasing progesterone and estrogen to prepare the uterus for implantation. In animals with a menstrual phase, the demise of the corpus luteum results in the sloughing off of the uterine lining.

3. In induced ovulators, the ovary produces follicles, and the animals become sexually receptive, but ovulation occurs only if the animal copulates. In other animals, the presence of a male is required to induce both behavioral estrus and ovulation.

4. Estrogen primes progesterone receptors. Therefore, without pretreatment with estrogen, progesterone does not induce sexual receptivity. These hormones also mediate the termination of sexual receptivity. When estrogen is withdrawn, receptivity is lost within hours. Progesterone has a biphasic effect. In the initial phase, progesterone stimulates sexually receptive behavior. However, if progesterone is continuously present for a period of time (as happens as a result of copulation, during the luteal phase, or during pregnancy), receptivity is inhibited.

5. The lordosis reflex is initiated in the rat when, following exposure to estrogen and progesterone, mounting by a male triggers specific sensory input to the midbrain central gray. When converging input from the hypothalamus (and in particular the VMH) and other forebrain structures facilitates neural activity in the midbrain neurons, the sensory input triggers the lordosis reflex.

6. Our understanding of how the lordosis response is modulated by other neural systems is still quite rudimentary compared with our understanding of the basic neural circuit. However, we know that estrogen influences neuro-

transmitter and neurohormone activity in a number of systems that project to the VMH or the midbrain. These systems are, therefore, implicated in modulation of lordosis behavior. Such systems include the norepinephrine and acetylcholine systems as well as GABA, enkephalin, GnRH, oxytocin, and prolactin-releasing neurons. Studies of neuroendocrine correlates of female sexual behavior have focused on the analysis of relatively simple behaviors like lordosis in laboratory rodents. This approach has been productive. However, there is increasing awareness that sexual behaviors occur within social and ecological constraints.[158] More modern approaches to the analysis of female sexual behaviors include this broader perspective and take advantage of species diversity to understand the physiology of female behavior.

Acknowledgments

The animal research described here as the work of the author was conducted under the sponsorship of the National Science Foundation and the National Institutes of Health.

4 Neuroendocrinology of Sexual Behavior in the Male

Michael J. Baum

The sexual behaviors of both females and males are complex, but in males the role of peripheral structures (e.g., the penis) is more obvious. As we will see, hormones may affect male sexual behavior by acting upon such peripheral structures. However, pharmacological and anatomical studies indicate that hormones also have two distinct effects on the brain, influencing male sexual motivation and performance independently. Normally, there is a coordinated effort involving different metabolites of a single hormone, to prepare both central and peripheral structures for copulation. Once again, hormones, by virtue of their widespread influence throughout the body, provide this coordination.

What are the components of male sexual behavior? Which hormones affect these components? Where do the hormones act? What are the neural mechanisms controlling male sexual behavior and which neurotransmitter systems are involved? How can we measure sexual motivation and sexual performance separately?

Introduction

As described in chapter 1, one of the first experiments conducted in behavioral endocrinology demonstrated that castrating a rooster inhibited its ability to mate with a hen, and this coincided with a reduction in the size of the rooster's comb. Like the rooster's comb, the nervous system is a target for androgenic hormones secreted by the testes. These early observations laid the groundwork for numerous later experiments investigating the actions of androgens on both the nervous system and other androgen-sensitive target tissues. Androgens can act directly upon the brain to affect an animal's behavior. Through its action on other androgen-sensitive tissues, including the accessory sex organs (e.g., prostate gland, seminal vesicles) androgen may also affect behavior indirectly. This chapter will concentrate on the actions of androgens in the adult and fetal brain that contribute to masculine sexual motivation and the control of mating behavior in the male.

We will consider the neuroendocrine mechanism controlling the secretion of the primary androgen secreted by the testes, testosterone. Then we will discuss the contribution of two neural metabolites of testosterone, estrogen and 5α-dihydrotestosterone (DHT), to the control of sexual motivation and mating in adult males. Next, we will consider some of the underlying neural mechanisms that mediate the actions of androgens on masculine sexual performance. This includes inputs from the olfactory system, basolateral amygdala, and medial preoptic area to the motor systems that control the pelvic movements necessary for mating in male vertebrates. The role of particular neurotransmitter systems as well as neuropeptides that modulate aspects of masculine coital function will be discussed. Finally, we will examine the role of estrogen and testosterone in regulating the perinatal development of neural systems that control masculine sexual motivation and performance in adulthood. The male rat and ferret serve as model systems for addressing these issues.

Definitions Important for Studies of Male Sexual Behavior

A distinction between **sexual motivation** and **coital performance** will be emphasized throughout this chapter. This distinction is especially striking when one considers mating in male vertebrates. A poignant example is the diabetic man, whose penile erectile capacity is compromised due to disease-induced damage to the innervation of the erectile tissues of the penis. Unfortunately, the diabetic man's motivation to engage in sexual activity remains at normal levels. Such a mismatch in motivation and performance capacity is a major source of discontent and psychological suffering in such patients. Considerable research using animal models has concentrated on the different neuroendocrine mechanisms controlling penile erection and sexual motivation. For example, studies using the male rat have analyzed penile erectile function by recording the latency (i.e., time to first occurrence) of erection as well as the number of discrete erections shown by a rat when restrained on its back with the penile sheath retracted by the experimenter.

Other studies have assessed erectile function and mating performance in male rats during direct interactions with an estrous female. In this situation a receptive female is placed in a chamber with the male being tested, and the observer records the occurrence of mounts, intromissions, and ejaculations over time. In rats, as in many rodent species, the male displays a series of discrete mounts of the female partner that are accompanied by penile erection and intromission into the vagina. The male dismounts after each intromission. After 5 to 15 such mounts with intromission, the male ejaculates a copulatory "plug" composed of secretions of the prostate, seminal vesicle, and coagulating gland plus sperm from the testes. Deposition of this copulatory plug against the female's cervix ensures that sperm will pass into the uterus, thereby heightening the likelihood that fertilization of ova will occur in the female's fallopian tubes. Following ejaculation, a period of sexual quiescence ensues for several minutes (the postejaculatory interval or refractory period), whereupon the male resumes mating.

Great species variations exist in the behavioral patterns displayed by male vertebrates during mating. For example, many species of fish perform stereotyped courtship movements that entice the female to deposit eggs in a nest, whereupon the male positions himself over these eggs and deposits his sperm. In avian species the male exhibits a wide variety of courtship displays, including vocalization (crowing or singing), strutting, mounting, and deposition of sperm through direct cloacal contact with the female. The pattern of mating displayed by the male rhesus monkey resembles that shown by the male rat described earlier. By contrast, the male ferret mates by grasping the female's neck, mounting, and exhibiting episodes of pelvic thrusting (accompanied by penile erection). Once the erect penis is inserted into the female's vagina, thrusting ceases, and the intromission is maintained for many minutes, even after the ejaculation of sperm. Specific patterns of masculine courtship and coital behavior have evolved in different species to maximize the chances of reproductive success. These behaviors develop within the constraints of that species' physiology, social organization, and environmental ecological setting. Additional discussion of social, environmental and evolutionary constraints on behavior is found in chapter 6.

Counting the incidence or timing the duration of neck grip, mounting, intromission, and ejaculation serves as a useful index of masculine coital performance. However, these parameters of sexual activity provide only partial insight into an animal's level of sexual motivation. Sexual motivation is a conceptual term that refers to the inclination of an individual to seek out and approach a female for the purpose of mating. Masculine sexual motivation has been measured experimentally in several different ways. In some studies the male is given the opportunity to obtain access to an estrous female by performing an operant response, such as moving over a fixed distance in a maze or pressing a lever. Another approach has been to assess the reinforcing value of access to an estrous female by seeing whether a male rat will develop a preference for a site in which he has previously had the opportunity to mate with a female (i.e., will he develop a conditioned place preference for the estrous female). Examples of each of these different methods of measuring males' sexual motivation will be given as we consider the action of sex steroids (androgens versus estrogen), different brain regions (basolateral amygdala versus the medial preoptic area [POA], and various neurotransmitters in controlling motivational versus performance aspects of masculine sexual activity.

Basic Neuroendocrine Relations in the Male

Feminine gonadal function is generally cyclic and synchronized to ensure the periodic release of ova from ovarian follicles (see chapter 3). Two steroid hormones, estrogen and progesterone, are secreted sequentially. By contrast, in males the production of both sperm and steroid hormones by the testes occurs tonically for considerable periods of time. Germ cells in the seminiferous tubules divide and differentiate into sperm. Testosterone is produced by Leydig cells located in the interstitial space between these tubules. Testosterone is produced by the Leydig cells in response to the stimulatory action of the pituitary gonadotropin, luteinizing hormone (LH).

The secretion of LH is ultimately controlled by the neuropeptide gonadotropin-releasing hormone (GnRH), which is released in a pulsatile fashion (depending on the species, one to two pulses/hour) from nerve terminals in the median eminence at the base of the brain. GnRH passes into portal blood vessels that traverse the pituitary stalk and then enter the anterior pituitary gland. Here GnRH interacts with membrane receptors in gonadotrophs, thereby stimulating the release of LH as well as follicle-stimulating hormone (FSH). Pulses of LH are detected by membrane receptors in the Leydig cells of the testes, and a pulsatile pattern of testosterone secretion results. Testosterone released from the testes influences both the expression of masculine sexual behavior in adulthood and the perinatal differentiation of brain mechanisms destined to control masculine sexual motivation and performance.

There is considerable variation among vertebrate species in the seasonal pattern of testosterone secretion and in the sensitivity of the brain to the actions of testosterone. In many instances, the entire hypothalamic-pituitary-testis axis undergoes a yearly regression. In such seasonal breeders the output of GnRH and LH, and consequently of testosterone, is dramatically reduced as the animal passes out of breeding condition. The testicular production of mature sperm also ceases as a consequence of hormonal deprivation. In most vertebrates the reproductive axis resumes its function as the next breeding season approaches. However, there are some interesting exceptions to this rule, as discussed in chapter 6. The timing of these periods of testicular regression and regrowth in some species is often linked to changes in the prevailing photoperiod—i.e., the relative duration of day and night (see chapter 16). For example, in male sheep, peak testicular secretion of testosterone, spermatogenesis, and maximal breeding activity occur in the fall, in response to shortening day length. Gestation in this species lasts 5 months, and therefore lambs are born in the spring, when conditions are optimal for survival of the newborn.

In male ferrets, breeding occurs in the spring, when the days are growing longer. In this species, gestation lasts only 41 days, and thus conditions are again optimal for the survival of the newborn offspring. In addition to governing the seasonal cycle of testosterone secretion, differences in photoperiod may also affect responsiveness of the nervous system to circulating hormones. For example, castrated hamsters kept under short-day photoperiods exhibit masculine sexual behavior in response to exogenous testosterone less readily than do castrates kept under long-days.[722] In the adult male rat, however, the testicular secretion of testosterone occurs throughout the year, with pulsatile variations in output occurring on an hourly basis. Seasonal variations in male laboratory rats' behavioral responsiveness to testosterone have not been reported.

Before the onset of puberty and the establishment of adult reproductive function, testosterone secretion by the testes in male vertebrates is more episodic or pulsatile in nature. Episodes of testosterone secretion occur at the same time as the occurrence of sexual differentiation of the external and internal genital structures and the brain. The exact timing of perinatal testosterone secretion differs widely among species, depending on the length of gestation and the speed of neural and somatic development. In all species a period exists after birth when the reproductive neuroendocrine axis is relatively quiescent. At some point, however, this system is reactivated, whereupon puberty occurs, and adult levels of testicular steroidogenesis coupled with spermatogenesis are established.

Expression of Masculine Sexual Behavior in Adulthood

You will recall from chapter 2 that testosterone itself may induce its effects by acting both directly on the nervous system and on peripheral non-neural tissue (i.e., muscles, sensory receptors, accessory sex organs). Alternatively, testosterone may be converted either in brain or peripheral tissue to a metabolite that has specific effects on the target tissue. There are two questions, therefore, that must be considered regarding the role of testosterone in masculine sexual behavior in adults. First, what is the site of action of testosterone and its metabolites to promote expression of male sexual behavior (i.e., the central nervous system, peripheral tissues, or both)? Second, what hormone(s) are necessary for expression of masculine sexual behavior? It is possible that there may be more than one active hormone and that multiple hormones acting at multiple sites may be needed to produce the full expression of masculine sexual behavior. As we shall see, this latter scenario appears to be the case. It took a while, however, for scientists to reach this conclusion.

Role of Testosterone and its Neural Metabolites

As stated at the outset, castration of a male chicken reduces the expression of masculine sexual behavior. Similar results have been seen in species representing all vertebrate classes. Likewise, in men, hypogonadism (i.e., lack of testes or testicular secretions), which result from a congenital failure of GnRH neurons to develop, blocks the normal occurrence of puberty and the associated increments in sexual motivation and the capacity for penile erection.[260] Soon after testosterone was first synthesized in the 1930s, Stone[994] showed conclusively that administration of this hormone to castrated rats reliably restored all aspects of mating.

These findings, together with later demonstrations that testosterone is the primary steroid secreted by the testes in almost all male vertebrates, provided strong evidence that testosterone activates mating behavior in adult male vertebrates. Studies carried out on male rats and dogs by Hart[469] also showed that castration eliminated penile erections, whereas testosterone replacement restored them. Thus, both erection and mating rely on the actions of testosterone.

Experiments conducted with guinea pigs[446] and rats[251] suggested that only a threshold concentration of circulating testosterone is required to activate masculine sexual behavior and erectile function. Typically, the concentration of androgen in plasma in males of these species greatly exceeds the minimal amount sufficient to sustain males' sexual performance. By contrast, in some other species (ferret,[84] rhesus monkey[719]) males' mating performance varies dramatically as a function of the circulating testosterone concentrations.

Although testosterone is clearly required for penile erection and the expression of sexual behavior, for many years it was not clear whether these effects of testosterone resulted from the action of the steroid in the central nervous system or, alternatively, in non-neural tissues. Indeed, sensory receptors on the surface of the glans penis, whose size and number are stimulated by testosterone, have been identified in several species.[816] It seemed possible that testosterone activated erection and mating by enhancing the sensory responsiveness of these receptors. Nevertheless, such effects of testosterone could not explain its activational effects on measures of sexual motivation in the absence of genital contact with a female.

In the late 1960s Baulieu and associates[71] showed that the stimulatory action of testosterone on cells of the prostate gland as well as on those of the genital skin actually depends on its conversion by 5α-reductase into DHT. It is DHT that promotes the growth and secretory activity of target cells after interacting with specific androgen receptor proteins. Subsequently, 5α-reductase and androgen receptors were found in those neural sites (preoptic and hypothalamic areas) that are thought to participate in the control of mating behavior (details later). In light of these findings, it was surprising to discover that administration of DHT to castrated rats failed to activate mating. This was true regardless of whether DHT was given systemically[684] or implanted directly into the POA.[536] Interestingly, however, administration of DHT to castrated rats did activate penile erections displayed when rats are restrained on their backs.[438] This may occur through an action of androgen receptors in the lumbar spinal cord.[143] Systemic treatment with DHT, therefore, duplicated all of the effects of testosterone on the putative sensory receptors of the glans penis and activated penile erections, yet these rats failed to mate.

In contrast, Davidson[257] found that testosterone, implanted directly into the POA, facilitated sexual behavior. This suggests that testosterone, not DHT, activates mating through a direct effect on the male rat's nervous system. However, at about the same time that the experiments on the behavioral effects of DHT were being conducted, it was found that administration of estrogen strongly facilitated mounting and intromissive behavior in castrated male rats.[258] This was surprising, in that estrogen had been thought to be exclusively a "female" steroid. It soon became apparent, however, that the aromatizing enzymes that convert androgen to estrogen (discussed in chapter 2) are present in the hypothalamic and limbic forebrain structures of adult males and females of essentially all vertebrate species.[771] Furthermore, specific receptors for estrogen are present in these same brain regions in both sexes.[1082]

A comparison of the effects of testosterone, DHT, and estrogen on the mating behavior and erectile function of castrated adult male rats is shown in

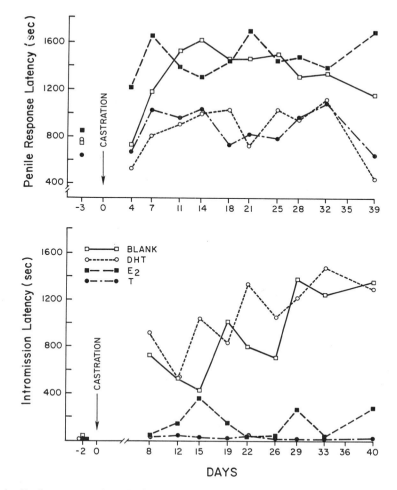

Figure 4.1 Penile response (erection) latencies of male rats (top) tested while restrained on their backs and intromission latencies (bottom) of the same rats when tested with an estrous female. Groups of male rats were tested repeatedly after castration and SC insertion of Silastic capsules containing nothing (blank), 5α-dihydrotestosterone (DHT), estradiol (E$_2$), or testosterone (T). The data illustrate that E$_2$ has little restorative effect upon the reflexive erections but does facilitate actual mating. DHT, on the other hand, facilitates erections but not mating. T, which can be metabolized to either E$_2$ or DHT, maintains both types of behavior. (From Meisel, O'Hanlon, and Sachs, 1984.[705])

figure 4.1.[705] Prior to castration, males showed equivalent short latencies (i.e., little delay) to first intromission (in tests with estrous females) and to first penile erection (in tests while restrained on their backs). Following castration, males receiving subcutaneous implants of Silastic capsules containing testosterone continued to show similar first intromission and erection latencies. Castrated males given blank capsules showed lengthened response latencies; in other words, it took longer before they showed the behaviors. Males given estrogen showed intromission latencies that closely resembled those of testosterone-treated males, whereas their erection latencies resembled those of males given blank capsules. Conversely, males treated with DHT showed first intromission latencies resembling those of males with blank capsules, but their erection latencies resembled those of males treated with testosterone.

It is important to note that castrated males given estrogen in this experiment managed to achieve erections that were sufficient to allow penile intromission in tests with estrous females. Thus, estrogen by itself, presumably acting through the nervous system, activates both mounting and intromission in the male rat. Meisel and colleagues[705] suggest, however, that an androgenic stimulus may normally be required for full erectile function. In the rat this function is mediated in part by the spinal nucleus of the bulbocavernosus (SNB) system, which is sensitive to testosterone and DHT (see chapter 2). The SNB system is critical to the deposition of copulatory plugs containing sperm in the female's vagina and the resultant occurrence of pregnancy.[895] It seems likely that an androgen (perhaps DHT) is also required for full penile erection in other species, including the male ferret (see later).

Much evidence suggests that both estrogen and androgen (either testosterone itself or DHT) contribute to the activation of masculine sexual activity, including penile erection, in the male rat and in males of numerous other vertebrate species.[81] In the ferret, for example, sc injections of either testosterone or estrogen to castrated males facilitated neck gripping, mounting, and pelvic thrusting behavior to equivalent degrees (figure 4.2[72]). Interestingly, ovariectomized females given these same steroids showed no pelvic thrusting or mounting and less neck gripping than did males. This was presumably because the neural mechanisms governing masculine coital function are less developed in females due to the lack of perinatal steroidal exposure (see later section in this chapter and chapter 2). At first glance, it appears that estrogen duplicated all of the behavioral effects of testosterone, suggesting that an estrogen, formed directly in the brain, may normally mediate all of the behavioral actions of circulating androgen. Other data suggest, however, that estrogens only partially duplicate the behavioral effects of testosterone.

A striking difference between the actions of estrogen and testosterone was obtained when ferrets' masculine sexual motivation was assessed by allowing subjects to choose between approaching and interacting with either estrous or anestrous females in the opposite goal boxes of a T-maze[77] (figure 4.3). Gonadectomized male and female ferrets were tested in this situation repeatedly while receiving daily injections of oil vehicle, testosterone, or estrogen. When treated with oil vehicle, males and females both showed equivalent preferences for estrous and anestrous females. Nor did either sex display a preference during extinction trials when no stimulus animals were placed in the respective goal boxes of the T-maze. When treated with testosterone, males showed a distinct preference for the estrous female, whereas females did not. Again, preferences of both sexes for the two (now empty) goal boxes returned to chance levels during extinction trials. Finally, when given estrogen, neither males nor females displayed a preference for estrous or anestrous females. These results suggest that estrogen is unable to duplicate the activational effect of testosterone on male ferrets' motivation to approach and interact with

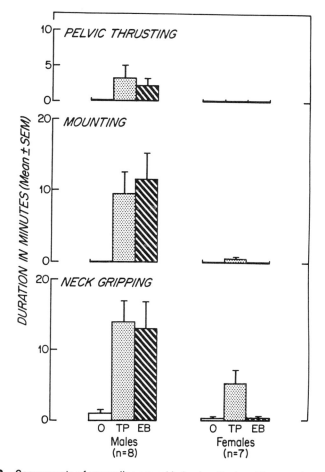

Figure 4.2 Components of masculine sexual behavior displayed by gonadectomized male and female ferrets 10 to 14 days after the onset of daily SC injections of oil vehicle (O), testosterone propionate (TP; 5 mg/kg), or estradiol benzoate (EB; 10 μg/kg). Note the similar behavioral effects of TP and EB in males and the relative ineffectiveness of either hormone in females. Data are expressed as mean ± SEM; (Data adapted from Baum, 1976.[72])

an estrous female, even though once confronted directly with such a female, the estrogen-treated male readily neck grips, mounts, and exhibits pelvic thrusting behavior towards the female (see figure 4.2). Although estrogen activates these latter behaviors in castrated male ferrets as readily as testosterone, it is considerably less effective than testosterone in promoting intromission. Perhaps androgen is required for full erection in the ferret as in the male rat.

In addition to rat and ferret, estrogen activates aspects of masculine sexual behavior in several other mammalian species including hamster, pig, deer, sheep, and cow (reviewed in Baum et al.[81]), in two avian species, quail and ring dove (reviewed in Balthazart et al.[47]), and in one reptilian species, the lizard.[236] Thus, the ability of estrogen to duplicate the activational effect of testosterone on masculine sexual behavior is widely represented among vertebrates. In-

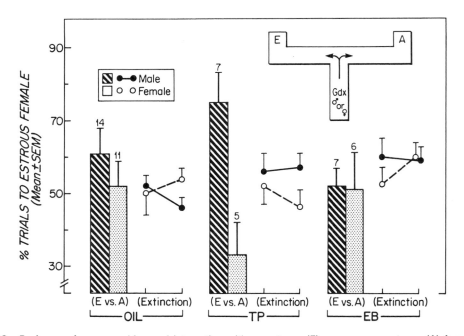

Figure 4.3 Preference for approaching and interacting with an estrous (E) versus an anestrous (A) female in a T-maze displayed by gonadectomized (Gdx) male and female ferrets tested 7 to 14 days after the onset of daily injections of oil vehicle, testosterone propionate (TP; 5 mg/kg), or estradiol benzoate (EB; 12 μg/kg). Stimulus females were absent from the goal boxes during the 2 days of extinction tests given under each hormone condition. TP caused males to approach an estrous female more effectively than did EB. Neither hormone caused female subjects to approach an estrous female. Data are expressed as mean ± SEM. (From Baum et al., 1990.[75])

terestingly, no one has been able to demonstrate any activational effects of estrogen in male primates, including man.

Species differences also exist in the ability of DHT to activate masculine sexual behavior. DHT exerts only minimal activational effects on mating in castrated male rats and hamsters, whereas in the lizard, mouse, guinea pig, and rhesus monkey DHT has been shown to stimulate rather high levels of this behavior. In avian species, such as the dove and quail, the evidence strongly supports the obligatory role of estrogen in the activation of this behavior. In mammalian species, however, the case is less clear cut. In primates, neither estrogen nor DHT nor their combination can duplicate the activational effects of testosterone on masculine sexual performance.[719] By contrast, in male rats and hamsters the combination of estrogen and DHT can duplicate all of the effects of testosterone on mating behavior and erectile function.[86, 266]

Either systemic administration or direct intracranial infusion of drugs that inhibit the aromatization of androgen to estrogen effectively reduces mounting and intromissive performance in testosterone-treated castrated rats.[206] Thus, it seems that the neural formation of estrogen from circulating testosterone is normally required for the activation of these behaviors. In other work,[139] systemic administration of a drug that blocks the 5α-reduction of testosterone reduced the ability of testosterone treatment to activate penile erection in castrated rats that were tested while restrained on their backs. This result suggests that DHT normally is required for the activation of erectile function in this species.

McGinnis and Dreifuss[692] measured nuclear androgen and estrogen receptor levels in the hypothalamus, preoptic area, amygdala, and septal region in gonadally intact male rats and in castrated rats treated with estrogen, DHT, or a combination of these metabolites of testosterone. They found that estrogen plus DHT elevated nuclear estrogen and androgen receptor levels in these neural tissues as readily as did testosterone treatment. Yet, at the low doses of estrogen and DHT administered, castrated males displayed little sexual behavior. In contrast, gonadally intact animals and testosterone-treated castrates mated readily. Based on these observations, the authors argue that testosterone itself, not estrogen or DHT, is normally responsible for the full activation of mating in adult male rats. However, these experiments do not rule out the possibility that all three hormones normally contribute to the expression of male sexual behavior.

To summarize, there is evidence of central activation of male sexual behavior both by neural estrogenic metabolites of testosterone and by androgens (perhaps testosterone itself). Although it is well established that either testosterone or estrogen will activate masculine sexual behavior when implanted into the medial POA/anterior hypothalamic region of castrated rats, there is no agreement about the precise localization of hormone action within the POA anterior hypothalamus continuum. Numerous other types of experiments, including demonstrations of the antagonistic effects of aromatase inhibitors on mating in males of several species, point to a role for estrogen in controlling this behavior. More work is needed to resolve the relative contributions of testosterone, DHT, and estrogen to the activation of masculine sexual motivation, the coordination of the motoric behaviors (mounts or pelvic thrusts with or without intromission) involved in mating, and the occurrence of penile erection.

There is also clear evidence of androgenic effects on peripheral systems that are important for full expression of masculine sexual behaviors. This includes activation of putative sensory receptors on the penis as well as anabolic effects on the muscles attached to the penis. These effects are dependent on DHT and indirectly influence neurons that innervate this region.[838]

Neural Integration of Sexual Motivation and Performance

Research into the neural systems mediating male sexual behavior is just beginning to tease apart the components of the system necessary for sexual motivation vs. coital behavior. As explained in chapter 2, the POA is the integrative center thought to be the site of testosterone-induced activation of coital behavior. Motivational components of male sexual behavior are thought to be modulated by olfactory and other inputs to the amygdala. Male sexual behaviors can be thought of as an integrated combination of motivational and coital behaviors.

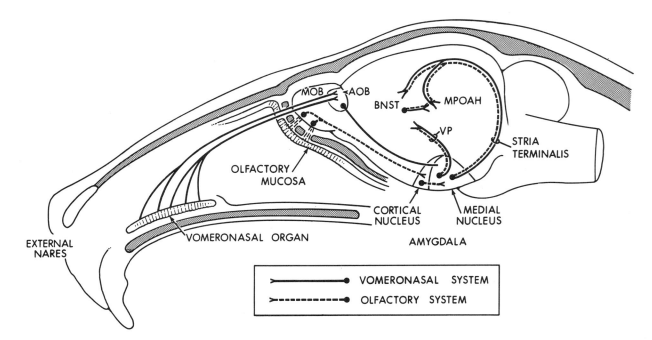

Figure 4.4 Schematic representation of olfactory and vomeronasal pathways that control male hamster mating behavior. Abbreviations: MOB, main olfactory bulb; AOB, accessory olfactory bulb; BNST, bed nucleus of the stria terminalis; MPOAH, medial preoptic area/anterior hypothalamus; VP, ventral pathway projecting from the medial amygdala to the MPOAH. (Adapted from Winans, et al., 1982. Courtesy of S. W. Newman.)

OLFACTORY INPUTS

Olfactory cues are critical to the initiation of sexual behavior in males of several rodent species. For example, the male hamster normally investigates the female's anogenital region and licks the viscous vaginal secretions of estrous females prior to initiating mating.[828] The male then executes a single mount with intromission and intravaginal penile thrusting that, after several minutes, leads to ejaculation. Experimentally interfering with olfactory inputs to both the vomeronasal organs and the olfactory mucosa by plugging the nares (i.e., nostrils, see figure 4.4) prevented males from mounting an estrous female. However, such interference with olfactory inputs failed to disrupt the behavior of males that had already initiated a mating sequence.

Neuroanatomical experiments have demonstrated that the chemoreceptors in the vomeronasal organs project to the accessory olfactory bulb, whereas receptors in the olfactory mucosa project to the main olfactory bulb (figure 4.4; reviewed in Winans et al.[1105]). Both olfactory bulbs project, in turn, to the corticomedial nuclei of the amygdaloid complex. These nuclei project to the bed nucleus of the stria terminalis and onto the medial POA region. An extensive literature[1105] shows that lesioning of any portion of this olfactory projection severely disrupts both chemoinvestigative behavior (i.e., investigative behaviors initiated and sustained by odors) and mating in male hamsters.

Areas of the olfactory projection that are important for these behaviors include both the main and accessory olfactory bulbs, the corticomedial amygdala, and the bed nucleus of the stria terminalis. Although the deficits are less severe, similar sites of neural destruction also reduce mating performance in male rats and mice (reviewed in Sachs and Meisel[896]).

Several early studies suggested that olfactory cues are also instrumental in promoting sexual arousal and performance in male rhesus monkeys.[718] Most observers now agree, however, that this is not the case.[411] There are clinical reports of low sexual drive and erectile performance in men with congenital deficiencies in olfactory system development (Kallmann's syndrome[345]). However, these men also suffer from pituitary hypogonadism due to the inadequate development of neurons in the forebrain that synthesize and release GnRH into the pituitary portal blood vessels. It seems likely that the resulting deficit in the testicular production of testosterone, rather than deficient olfactory function per se, is responsible for the low level of psychosexual function that characterizes these patients. This topic will be discussed in greater detail in the next chapter.

PREOPTIC AREA AND THE ANTERIOR HYPOTHALAMUS
More than 20 years ago Heimer and Larsson[476] showed that electrolytic lesions of the medial POA (see figure 4.7) profoundly disrupted mating performance in adult male rats. Similar observations have subsequently been reported in numerous male vertebrates ranging from garter snakes to rhesus monkeys. Conversely, electrical stimulation of the medial POA activates mating in male rats,[652] provided that testosterone is circulating. Furthermore, localized implantation of either testosterone or estrogen into the medial POA activated mounting and intromissive behavior in castrated male rats.[257, 265] As already described, implantation of an aromatase inhibitor, ATD, into the medial POA of male rats and quail blocked the activational effects of systemic testosterone on the expression of masculine sexual behavior. These data imply that in rat and quail the aromatization of androgen to estrogen in the POA contributes to the activation of masculine sexual behavior. In agreement with this idea, implantation of DHT into the POA failed to activate mating in rats, either in castrated males[536] or in castrates given systemic injections of estrogen concurrently.[85]

Much evidence shows that masculine sexual motivation can persist in animals even when coital performance has been eliminated by destruction of the medial POA. Hansen and colleagues[460] first reported that male rats bearing neurotoxic lesions (made by infusing ibotenic acid) of the cell bodies of the medial POA showed increased levels of anogenital sniffing and climbing over estrous females, even though after lesioning they never mated with these females. In fact, if given access to a water spout, the drinking behavior of males bearing medial POA lesions was dramatically increased in the presence of an estrous female.[459] The authors argued that the frustration of not being able to convert sexual arousal into appropriate coital motoric outputs was somehow

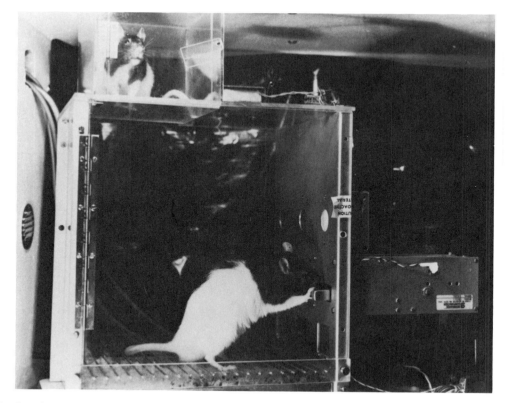

Figure 4.5 Experimental set-up for studies of sexual reinforcement. A male rat is required to press the bar 10 times in order to turn on a light briefly above the lever. Beginning 15 minutes after the onset of the test session, 10 lever presses by the male cause the light to come on and the female rat to drop into the compartment. Copulation then occurs, and the test is terminated after the male ejaculates. After much experience in this test situation, males exhibit consistent, high levels of lever pressing during each 15-minute session. (From Everitt, 1990.[333])

reduced as a result of the redirection of this drive. A related observation was made in male rhesus monkeys bearing electrolytic lesions of the medial POA.[963] These males stopped mounting, intromitting, and ejaculating with sexually receptive females in standard behavioral tests. They were, however, frequently observed masturbating to ejaculation in their home cages while watching females caged across the room. These males were clearly capable of becoming sexually aroused and were able to achieve ejaculation provided actual sociosexual interactions or coital movements were not required in the process.

Perhaps the most rigorous demonstration of the dissociation between performance and motivational aspects of masculine coital function following medial POA lesions comes from the work of Everitt and Stacey.[335] These workers trained sexually experienced male rats to press a lever to obtain access to an estrous female with which they eagerly mated (figure 4.5). It is difficult in such studies to establish a rate of bar pressing that is sufficiently high to allow

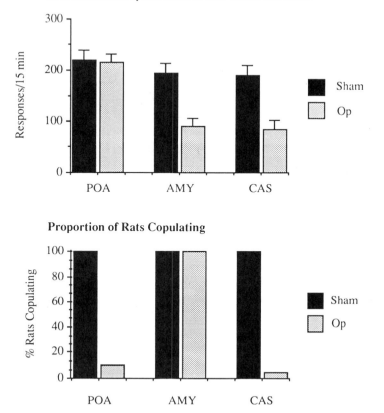

Instrumental Responses under 2nd Order Schedule

Proportion of Rats Copulating

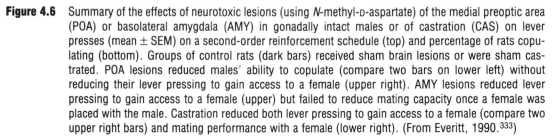

Figure 4.6 Summary of the effects of neurotoxic lesions (using *N*-methyl-D-aspartate) of the medial preoptic area (POA) or basolateral amygdala (AMY) in gonadally intact males or of castration (CAS) on lever presses (mean ± SEM) on a second-order reinforcement schedule (top) and percentage of rats copulating (bottom). Groups of control rats (dark bars) received sham brain lesions or were sham castrated. POA lesions reduced males' ability to copulate (compare two bars on lower left) without reducing their lever pressing to gain access to a female (upper right). AMY lesions reduced lever pressing to gain access to a female (upper) but failed to reduce mating capacity once a female was placed with the male. Castration reduced both lever pressing to gain access to a female (compare two upper right bars) and mating performance with a female (lower right). (From Everitt, 1990.[333])

reliable inferences about the motivational state of the animal whose response to brain lesioning or endocrine manipulation is being monitored. In order to achieve this reliability Everitt and Stacy used a secondary reinforcer (a light flashing on above the lever), which was routinely paired with the presentation of an estrous female during initial conditioning sessions. Males trained in this situation developed very stable, high rates of bar pressing behavior, sustained by presentation of the secondary reinforcer (red light).

The researchers then made neurotoxic lesions (by locally infusing of the excitatory amino acid *N*-methyl-D-aspartate; NMDA) that destroyed cell bodies in the medial POA of sexually experienced, adult male rats (figures 4.6, 4.7). Predictably, this procedure dramatically reduced the proportion of males copulating with an estrous female once access had been gained by pressing a lever. However, the rate of bar pressing, taken here as an index of masculine sexual motivation, was unaffected by these lesions (figure 4.6). This result contrasted with the low rate of bar pressing displayed by other groups of male rats receiving lesions of the basolateral amygdala (see next section on the amygdala) or males castrated after the initial conditioning session. Clearly, castration reduced males' motivation to press the lever in this situation and reduced coital performance in the presence of a female. Other data from this laboratory showed that the lever pressing behavior of castrated males increased significantly within several days after the onset of testosterone injections, implying that sexual motivation was facilitated by this steroid.

AMYGDALA

In 1939 Kluver and Bucy[593] reported that large lesions of the amygdala and overlying temporal cortex caused a "hypersexuality syndrome" in male rhesus monkeys. Questions have been raised about the reliability of this observation because they observed only a limited amount of sexual activity in control animals. The specificity of the lesion effect has also been questioned because the lesions included the entire amygdala as well as the overlying temporal cortex.[333] As already described, lesions restricted to the medial amygdala severely disrupt chemoinvestigatory behavior and mating in male hamsters, presumably due to the interruption of olfactory inputs into brain circuits that mediate masculine sexual arousal. Everitt and co-workers[334] reported that neurotoxic lesions (made with NMDA) of the lateral and basal nuclei of the amygdala significantly impair lever pressing by male rats working on a second-order schedule of reinforcement for access to an estrous female (figures 4.6 and 4.7).

Interestingly, males with basolateral amygdaloid lesions display normal levels of mating, once confronted with an estrous female. They are deficient only in performing operant responses, required to gain access to the female, that depend on environmental cues other than those coming directly from the female herself (e.g., sight of the female including her solicitational behavior, or smell or ultrasounds emitted by the female). Clearly, sexual arousal engendered by these primary cues is unimpaired by basolateral amygdaloid lesions. In these males, lever pressing for the secondary reinforcer resumed when amphetamine was infused into the nucleus accumbens. These workers suggest that the amphetamine-induced release of dopamine from nerve terminals in this region (cell bodies of which are found in the ventral tegmental area) compensates for the lesion-induced disruption of amygdaloid inputs. This idea will be discussed more generally in the next section on neurotransmitters.

To summarize, using a second-order reinforcement paradigm, it has been possible to demonstrate that the amygdala is important for motivational components, while the POA is important for coital components of masculine sexual behavior. The finding that treatment with amphetamine can help to overcome motivational deficits following amygdalaid lesions illustrates, how-

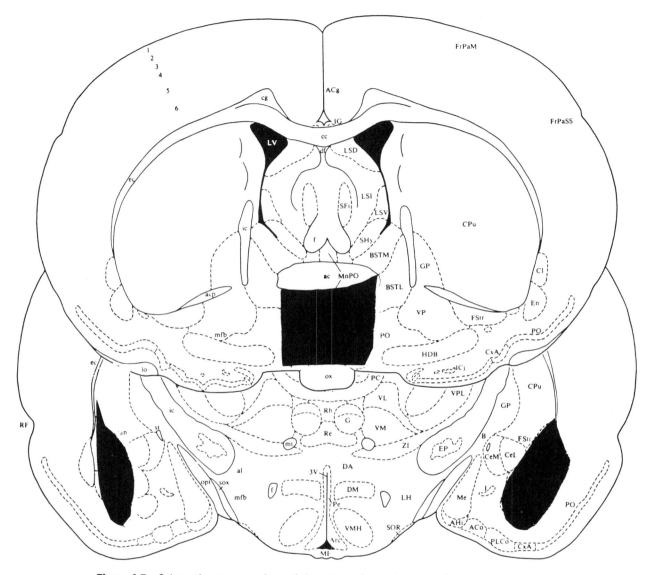

Figure 4.7   Schematic representations of the extent of neural damage (black areas) in male rats that received neurotoxic lesions of either the medial preoptic area (MnPO; midline damage indicated on upper section) or the basolateral amygdala (bilateral damage on lower section). (Adapted from Paxinos and Watson, 1982; Everitt and Stacy, 1987, and Everitt et al., 1989.) Some of the abbreviations used: CC, corpus callosum; AC, anterior commissure; OX, optic chiasm; CPU, striatum; VMH, ventromedial hypothalamus; DM, dorsal medial hypothalamus. For additional abbreviations see Paxinos and Watson (1982).[798]

ever, that these are not the only brain regions involved. Other neural systems that project to the POA or the amygdala can also modulate masculine sexual behavior.

Most neural systems that project from one brain region to another are characterized by their neurotransmitter. In the next section, the role of specific neurotransmitters in the modulation of masculine sexual behavior will be discussed.

Influence of Neurotransmitters and Neuromodulators on Masculine Sexual Behavior

DOPAMINERGIC NEURONS

Dopamine neurons that project from the midbrain to limbic brain regions as well as dopamine neurons in the hypothalamus have been implicated in the regulation of masculine sexual arousal and coital performance. These include the mesolimbic dopamine neurons projecting from the ventral tegmental area to the nucleus accumbens (mentioned earlier), and the incertohypothalamic dopamine neurons projecting from the dorsoposterior hypothalmus to the medial POA. A third group, the tuberoinfundibular dopamine neurons projecting from the arcuate nucleus to the median eminence, is implicated indirectly.

Mesolimbic Dopamine Neurons   As already described, amphetamine-induced release of dopamine from terminals in the nucleus accumbens compensated for the detrimental effects of baso-lateral amygdaloid lesions on the operant responses of male rats to gain access to an estrous female. Other evidence[333] further implicates mesolimbic dopamine neurons in the regulation of masculine sexual arousal and sexual reward.

Selective destruction of these dopamine neurons in male rats through intracerebral injection of the catecholamine neurotoxin, 6-hydroxydopamine, significantly lengthened mount latencies. However, once males had begun to mount, they proceeded to intromit and ejaculate in a normal sequence. This suggests that the consummatory aspects of masculine coital performance were unimpaired by this treatment. These males were tested with estrous females that had been ovariectomized and made fully proceptive (sexually motivated) and receptive (displaying lordosis) through injections of estrogen followed by progesterone (as described in chapter 3). When such females also were treated with the dopamine receptor blocker α-flupentixol, they no longer displayed the proceptive responses characteristic of estrous rats but retained their ability to display lordosis when mounted by the male.

Interestingly, males bearing neurotoxic lesions of the nucleus accumbens rarely mounted these estrous females in which proceptive responsiveness had been largely abolished by α-flupentixol. Control males usually initiated a copulatory sequence despite the absence of overt proceptive cues from their estrous partners. Apparently, other types of incentive cues (e.g., sight or smell of the female) are sufficiently arousing for most male rats to initiate mating.

It seems likely that the deficits in sexual behavior observed in males with lesions of the nucleus accumbens reflect their inability to respond to the motivational cues that normally suffice to arouse the male. Everitt[333] obtained similar results in males following infusion of dopamine receptor blockers directly into the nucleus accumbens.

Two methods have been developed recently to allow an investigator to sample the extracellular concentrations of dopamine in the brain. These are in vivo voltammetry and in vivo microdialysis. These methods have both been used to address the question of whether dopamine release from mesolimbic terminals in the nucleus accumbens is selectively enhanced by sexual stimuli. Voltammetry involves monitoring the pattern of electrical current flow at the tip of an electrode that is thought to reflect oxidation of extracellular dopamine at the electrode tip—the more dopamine there is, the more oxidation will be measured. A complementary method known as microdialysis involves measurement of small amounts of dopamine in extracellular fluid collected through diffusion across a semipermeable membrane at the base of a probe implanted into the nucleus accumbens.

Pfaus and colleagues,[814] using in vivo voltammetry and in vivo microdialysis (in different rats), found that dopamine release in the nucleus accumbens rose sharply when a male was exposed to an estrous female (the female was restrained behind a wire-mesh screen to prevent physical contract). Subsequently, when males were given access to estrous females, this dopamine signal remained elevated throughout a mating sequence, fell after ejaculation, and then rose again near the end of the postejaculatory period of sexual inactivity. By contrast, in vivo release of dopamine from the dorsal striatum, which receives axonal projections from dopamine neurons in the substantia nigra and is concerned with sensorimotor function (see chapter 11), was unaffected by presentation of the estrous female.

These results confirm results obtained from pharmacological studies implicating mesolimbic dopamine neurons in the control of masculine sexual arousal. Such findings, together with reports that testosterone, as well as its metabolites estrogen and DHT, can enhance dopamine transmission in mesolimbic terminal regions[16, 731] further implicate this dopamine system in masculine sexual arousal. It is important to remember, however, that the mesolimbic dopamine pathway has been implicated in the control of a variety of motivated behaviors, including feeding and drinking, as well as in several types of drug-ingestive behaviors. Its role in governing motivated behavior is clearly not restricted to mating.

Incertohypothalamic Dopamine Neurons   Hull and co-workers (reviewed in Bitran and Hull[120]) have implicated dopamine projections to the medial POA in the control of consummatory aspects of mating in male rats. For example, infusion of the dopamine receptor agonist apomorphine into the medial POA facilitated the rate at which males achieved successive intromissions leading to ejaculation without affecting their initial latency to mount an estrous female. This same treatment also stimulated penile erection in males restrained on their backs. Both the behavioral and erectile responses were blocked by pretreatment with a dopamine receptor blocker, affirming that the effects of apomorphine resulted from specific actions on dopamine receptors.

Studies of the effects of castration and testosterone replacment on activity of incertohypothalamic dopamine neurons have yielded conflicting results. Early studies of Simpkins and colleagues[959] suggested that testosterone inhibited the release of dopamine from these terminals, a surprising finding in light of the pharmacological results suggesting that the activation of dopamine receptors in this region enhances mating performance. More recently, Baum and associates[82] found no effect of castration or steroid replacement on dopamine release in the medial POA, regardless of whether or not males were exposed to an estrous female. Although sex steroids, estrogen in particular, are thought to facilitate masculine coital performance by acting in the medial POA, there is no evidence that this effect is mediated by the dopaminergic innervation of this region. The steroidal and dopamine systems in the POA seem to act independently.

NEUROPEPTIDES AND MASCULINE SEXUAL BEHAVIOR
Several circulating as well as centrally formed peptides influence masculine coital performance. In some instances (e.g., prolactin, corticotropin-releasing hormone), the effects are primarily pharmacological and are potentially of clinical relevance. In other instances, particular neuropeptides (e.g., endorphin, GnRH, substance P, neuropeptide Y) are implicated in the normal physiological control of motivational or consummatory aspects of mating in normal males.

Prolactin Clinicians have long suspected that chronic hyperprolactinemia, resulting from the hypersecretion of prolactin from small pituitary tumors or during chronic stress, reduces erectile function and sexual motivation in men. Studies using animals strongly support these impressions. For example, Doherty and colleagues[298] studied adult, sexually experienced male rats in which chronic hyperprolactinemia was induced by transplanting pituitary glands from other rats under the kidney capsule. Normally, the secretion of prolactin by the pituitary is restrained by the action of dopamine released from tuberoinfundibular dopaminergic neurons into the pituitary portal vessels perfusing the median eminence. Pituitary glands placed under the kidney capsule are readily vascularized and, in the absence of any inhibitory dopamine input, secrete large amounts of prolactin into the general circulation. As shown in figure 4.8, insertion of pituitary grafts and the resultant hyperprolactinemia significantly reduced mount and intromission rates in male rats in tests with estrous females while also reducing erectile function in the same males tested while restrained on their backs.[298] In a companion study, the inhibitory effect of hyperprolactinemia on erectile function was completely reversed by severing the spinal cord at the thoracic level. From these results we infer that the inhibitory effect of prolactin on erection is mediated by the peptides' action at some supraspinal site in the CNS that has yet to be determined.

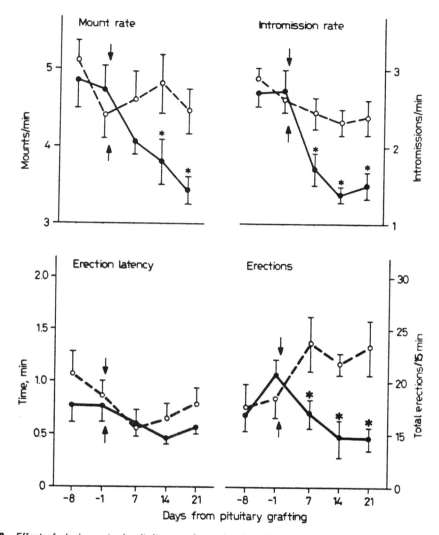

Figure 4.8 Effect of placing ectopic pituitary grafts under the kidney capsule (time of implantation indicated by arrows), and resultant hyperprolactinemia, on mounting and intromission rates in tests with estrous females (upper graphs) and on penile erectile function in tests of the same adult male rats when restrained on their backs (lower graphs). Hyperprolactinemia reduced the rate of mounting and intromission and the frequency of penile erection but not the latency period for erections (lower left). Open circles, control males; closed circles, hyperprolactinemic males. (Adapted from Doherty et al., 1986.[298])

The physiological actions of prolactin are well established in female mammals. In the rat these include the promotion of lactation, enhanced maternal behavior (see chapter 8), and the stimulation of progesterone secretion by the corpora lutea during the first half of pregnancy. Prolactin is also secreted by the male pituitary gland in about the same concentrations as in females. Some evidence suggests that in males prolactin facilitates LH-induced testicular steroidogenesis and increases androgen receptors in the reproductive tract. However, the role of prolactin in the neuroendocrine regulation of masculine sexual behavior is still uncertain.

Endorphins   β-Endorphin-containing neurons project from the arcuate nucleus to the medial POA and seem to inhibit the consummatory aspects of masculine sexual function, including erection. Hughes and colleagues[509] showed that the infusion of β-endorphin into the medial POA caused dose-dependent reductions in males' mating performance. Conversely, infusions of the opioid receptor antagonist naloxone into the same site enhanced ejaculatory performance in sexually experienced male rats. These observations complement the results of an earlier study[714] showing that systemic administration of morphine inhibited mating in male rats at doses too low to affect rats' spontaneous locomotor activity.

The acute inhibition of masculine sexual behavior by morphine should be distinguished from the more pervasive loss of sexual motivation and erectile function that has long been known to occur in heroin addicts.[240] In the latter instance, ingestion of the opioid agonist causes a long-lasting suppression of LH secretion and a resultant drop in testosterone production. This withdrawal of androgen, perhaps combined with the direct effects of heroin in medial POA sites, leads to a striking reduction in all aspects of sexual arousal and coital function in male heroin addicts.

Evidence also suggests that opioid neurons *promote* sexual motivation in the male. Numerous studies have shown that opioid mechanisms facilitate the consumption of sweet substances, even though they may lack any nutrient content. For example, subcutaneous injection of the opioid receptor antagonist naloxone significantly reduced the ingestion of saccharine solution by rats.[646] Naloxone also inhibited "sham drinking" of sugar water by rats implanted with esophageal fistulas that diverted the ingested fluid away from their stomachs.[583] This type of ingestive behavior, which is especially dependent on opioid mechanisms, must be sustained by the taste of the ingested fluid rather than by any metabolic benefit.

Lieblich and co-workers[633] asked whether analogous circumstances exist in the context of masculine sexual behavior. One such example would be the male rat that continues to mate for several weeks following androgen withdrawal due to castration. Such males quickly cease mating if tested with estrous females that display low levels of proceptive behavior.[650] Thus, their sexual arousal and subsequent mating performance are especially dependent on the stimulus qualities of their female partners. Subcutaneous injection of nalox-

Box 4.1 The Coolidge Effect

Farmers long ago noticed that male animals that had recently mated with a particular female would, for awhile, appear uninterested in further copulation. However, if a new female was introduced, the male that had previously seemed sexually sated would investigate and, if the female was receptive, begin copulating. Continued introduction of novel females can further extend the males' copulatory motivation and performance. This phenomenon is known as the Coolidge effect and has been seen in many species including rats, in which the exchange of stimulus females is often part of tests of masculine copulatory behavior. Also, as noted in the text, one can elicit a similar effect in rats by simply removing the female for a few minutes and then replacing her. The increased sexual interest of males for a novel female is called the Coolidge effect because there was a popular joke about former President Calvin Coolidge, whose wife complained (in the joke) about his failing ardor compared to roosters that mate every day. The president then supposedly pointed out that the rooster was allowed to mate with a *different* hen each day. Frank Beach and a student, in giving a conference report about such an effect in rats in the 1950s, decided to refer to it simply as the Coolidge effect to get a chuckle out of the audience. To their surprise, members of the audience simply nodded their heads and acted as though they understood the reference perfectly well (it *was* a popular joke, apparently). The name has stuck since then.

one to males within 2 to 3 weeks after castration significantly inhibited mounting and ejaculation, whereas the same treatment had no effect on mating in gonadally intact male rats. In another study,[726] male rats ejaculated repeatedly with an estrous female until a criterion of sexual exhaustion was reached (see box 4.1). If the female partner was then removed from the test cage for several minutes before being replaced, control males reliably resumed mating. In these circumstances, sexually exhausted males given naloxone were significantly less likely to resume mating, suggesting that an opioid mechanism normally facilitates sexual arousal in such animals.

Sexual arousal in males depends on their interpreting and responding to the incentive motivational cues emitted by estrous females that have previously been associated with the consummatory act of mating or ejaculation. Obviously, it is impossible to ask a male rat what it finds rewarding. As an alternative, the conditioned place preference paradigm has been developed to assess the rewarding properties of different stimuli (such as drugs of abuse and natural rewards, including food and water). For example, rats that normally prefer to spend time in a black chamber of an apparatus will shift their preference to a white chamber after repeated pairing of the white compartment with amphetamine or morphine treatment.[185]

This method has also been used to study masculine sexual reward. In one such study[703] (figure 4.9), a conditioned place preference for the initially nonpreferred chamber was established in sexually experienced male rats by giving them access to an estrous female in this site. Groups of these animals were then either castrated or sham operated. Seven and fourteen days later, the males were placed alone for 45 minutes in the test apparatus, and the amount of time spent in each chamber was recorded. Prior to each of these tests, differ-

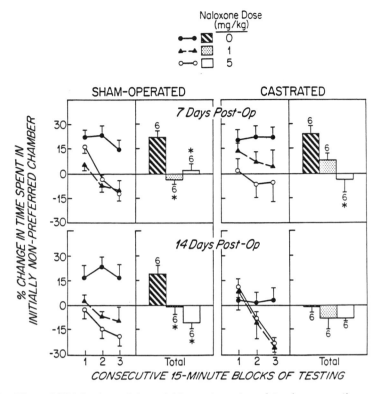

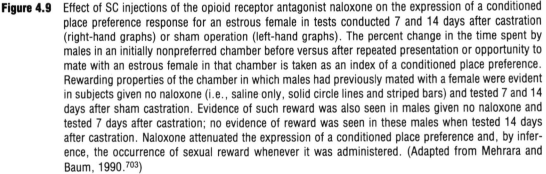

Figure 4.9   Effect of SC injections of the opioid receptor antagonist naloxone on the expression of a conditioned place preference response for an estrous female in tests conducted 7 and 14 days after castration (right-hand graphs) or sham operation (left-hand graphs). The percent change in the time spent by males in an initially nonpreferred chamber before versus after repeated presentation or opportunity to mate with an estrous female in that chamber is taken as an index of a conditioned place preference. Rewarding properties of the chamber in which males had previously mated with a female were evident in subjects given no naloxone (i.e., saline only, solid circle lines and striped bars) and tested 7 and 14 days after sham castration. Evidence of such reward was also seen in males given no naloxone and tested 7 days after castration; no evidence of reward was seen in these males when tested 14 days after castration. Naloxone attenuated the expression of a conditioned place preference and, by inference, the occurrence of sexual reward whenever it was administered. (Adapted from Mehrara and Baum, 1990.[703])

ent subgroups of males were injected with naloxone or saline vehicle to assess the effects of inhibiting neurotransmission in opioid circuits throughout the brain.

Sham-operated (i.e., gonadally intact) males given saline prior to each test showed a consistent 20% increase in the amount of time spent in the previously nonpreferred chamber (the one that had been paired with an estrous female). By contrast, naloxone-treated intact males spent significantly less time in the chamber previously associated with an estrous female. This suggests that the cues associated with the chamber were less rewarding to these groups. This outcome was seen in males when first tested 7 days after castration. When tested 14 days after castration, even saline-injected males had lost their conditioned place preference for the chamber previously paired with an estrous female. This finding suggests that testosterone normally enhances the rewarding attributes of incentive stimuli associated with an estrous female.

Since naloxone was given systemically in this study, the results provide no indication of *where* in the brain the drug acted to inhibit the expression of a conditioned place preference. Hughes and colleagues[511] also found that naloxone injected systemically into male rats inhibited the expression of a conditioned place preference for an estrous female. However, they obtained no such effect after direct infusion of naloxone into the medial POA of gonadally intact male rats. This latter finding is consistent with numerous studies suggesting that the medial POA controls consummatory, as opposed to motivational, aspects of masculine coital function. Neurophysiological evidence[450] shows that opioid peptides activate mesolimbic dopamine neurons when infused into the ventral tegmental area. Mitchell and Stewart[731] showed that infusion of either morphine or another opiate (dynorphin 1–13) into the ventral tegmental region of male rats stimulated orientation toward an estrous female. These findings suggest that opioid inputs to mesolimbic dopamine neurons may participate in males' interpretation of sexually relevant incentive stimuli.

Other Peptides   Dornan and Malsbury[303] reviewed the scientific and clinical literature concerning the effects of a variety of additional neuropeptides on masculine sexual arousal and performance. Oxytocin is synthesized and released by magnocellular (large) neurons of the paraventricular and supraoptic nuclei, which project to the posterior pituitary gland, and by parvocellular (small) neurons in several parts of the brain (see chapter 15). When injected into the cerebral ventricles of male rats, oxytocin significantly shortened mount and ejaculation latencies.[510] Conversely, infusion of a selective oxytocin receptor antagonist increased males' mount latencies and reduced the incidence of mating. These results point to a facilitory role for oxytocin in masculine sexual arousal. Since hypophysectomy fails to reduce sexual arousal or mating performance in male rats as long as they are treated with testosterone,[807] it seems unlikely that oxytocin of pituitary origin plays a major role in controlling masculine coital function. However, centrally projecting oxytocin neurons may facilitate masculine sexual arousal or performance.

Three additional neuropeptides have been shown to facilitate sexual arousal or coital performance when administered to adult male rats. Gonadotropin-releasing hormone (GnRH), α-melanocyte-stimulating hormone (α-MSH), and substance P all exert such effects when administered intracerebrally (reviewed in Dornan and Malsbury[303]). More research is needed, preferably using yet-to-be-developed selective antagonists of these peptides, to determine whether they normally play any role in controlling coital function in males.

It is interesting that substance P–containing neurons projecting from the medial amygdala to the bed nucleus of the stria terminalis are more prevalent in male than in female rats.[653] Also, castration of adult male rats reduces the amount of substance P in this projection, which presumably conducts olfactory information. These observations justify further research into the possible role of substance P in controlling masculine coital activity.

Finally, two additional neuropeptides, corticotropin-releasing hormone (CRH) and neuropeptide Y, have been shown to lengthen mount latencies and reduce the incidence of mating when infused into the cerebral ventricles of adult male rats. This inhibitory action of CRH is particularly interesting because the synthesis and release of this neuropeptide, like prolactin, increase dramatically in stressed animals. Acute as well as chronic stress can disrupt the expression of masculine sexual behavior in rats (see chapter 10). A reduction in sexual motivation and a loss of erectile function commonly occur in clinically depressed men. More research is needed to determine whether centrally released CRH, possibly working in consort with chronically elevated prolactin, contributes to this loss of coital function.

To summarize, mesolimbic and incertohypothalamic dopamine neurons are implicated in the modulation of masculine sexual behavior. The mesolimbic dopamine neurons projecting from the ventral tegmentum to the nucleus accumbens are thought to be important for motivational components of male sexual behavior. In contrast, the incertohypothalamic dopamine neurons are thought to play a role in coital behaviors. Other peptides are also implicated in masculine sexual behavior. Prolactin and opioids are thought to inhibit consummatory components of coital behavior, including erection and ejaculation. Paradoxically, endorphins may also stimulate motivational components of male sexual behavior.

Steroids and the Development of Masculine Sexual Behavior

We have considered some of the neural and endocrine mechanisms that govern masculine sexual arousal, penile erection, and the motoric patterns of mating in adult males. As shown in figure 4.2, adult male and female ferrets differ dramatically in their exhibition of masculine sexual behavior following gonadectomy and treatment with testosterone or estrogen. Likewise, adult males and females display very different responses to testosterone when given a choice between approaching an estrous as opposed to an anestrous female (see figure 4.3). These data, collected using ferrets, resemble the results obtained in several different vertebrate species. Both the motivational aspects of mating, including partner preference, and the capacity to perform the motoric aspects of mating are sexually differentiated. We will now consider the role of prenatal and early postnatal exposure of the nervous system to sex steroids in controlling the differentiation of both motivational and consummatory aspects of masculine sexual behavior. We will consider data from a model system, the ferret. However, the relevance of these results for other mammalian species, including primates, will become apparent.

As described in chapter 2, sex differences in the morphology of the external and internal genital organs, in portions of the central and peripheral nervous systems, and in the capacity to exhibit a range of sociosexual behaviors develop primarily because of the perinatal action of testosterone secreted by the mammalian testes. Ovarian steroidogenesis in female mammals is first initiated well after this perinatal period, and thus the feminine morphologic and behavioral phenotype develops in the presence of low rates of ovarian secretions (although the mother's ovaries are releasing considerable amounts of estrogen and progesterone during this period). As already explained, in many mammalian species including ferrets, circulating concentrations of testosterone are significantly higher in males than in females during certain fetal periods and postnatally within hours and again for several days, weeks, or months (depending on the species). As will be illustrated shortly, sociosexual aspects of maleness develop only after exposure of the male nervous system to testosterone or its estrogenic metabolites during over the sum *total* of these perinatal periods.

Gestation lasts 41 days in ferrets. In males the testes begin secreting testosterone around embryonic day 24 (E24), and continue to do so during the rest of gestation.[604] Although measurable in females, testosterone concentrations are significantly lower than in male fetuses over this embryonic period. At birth, plasma testosterone concentrations rise in males to even higher concentrations for a few hours, then decline to the low concentrations characteristic of females.[331] Small though significant sex differences in plasma testosterone levels occur intermittently during the next 3 postnatal weeks.

Elevations in circulating testosterone during fetal life are responsible for the differentiation of the Wolffian duct structures into the epididymis, vas deferens, seminal vesicles, and prostate glands. At the same time, DHT, formed in the genital skin, promotes the differentiation of a phallus and the fusion of the genital folds into a scrotum that the testes eventually descend into shortly after birth (see chapter 2).

Masculine Coital Behavior

Much evidence also implicates testosterone in the differentiation of both the motivational and motoric features of masculine sexual behavior in male ferrets. Studies by Baum and Erksine[76] showed that administration of testosterone during postnatal days 5 to 20, but not at later ages, strongly facilitated females' exhibition of male-typical sexual behaviors. Following gonadectomy and testosterone treatment in adulthood, these animals exhibited neck gripping, mounting, and pelvic thrusting behaviors when tested with estrous females. Castration of male ferrets on postnatal day 5, but not on postnatal days 20 or 35, significantly attenuated their ability to mate with estrous females when tested in adulthood. From these results, it seems clear that testosterone normally acts in male ferrets during the first 20 postnatal days to promote coital masculinization. Extended *prenatal* exposure of female ferrets to testosterone, achieved by administering the steroid to pregnant ferrets from E16 to E41, failed to duplicate the coital masculinizing action of administering testosterone neonatally. At first glance, this suggests that fetal exposure of male ferrets to testosterone is not essential for coital masculinization. As will be shown below, however, this conclusion turns out to be incorrect.

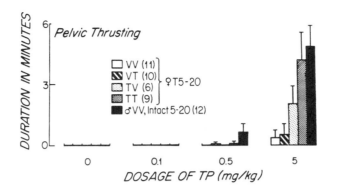

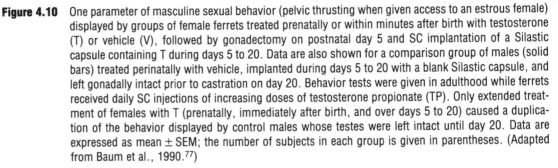

Figure 4.10 One parameter of masculine sexual behavior (pelvic thrusting when given access to an estrous female) displayed by groups of female ferrets treated prenatally or within minutes after birth with testosterone (T) or vehicle (V), followed by gonadectomy on postnatal day 5 and SC implantation of a Silastic capsule containing T during days 5 to 20. Data are also shown for a comparison group of males (solid bars) treated perinatally with vehicle, implanted during days 5 to 20 with a blank Silastic capsule, and left gonadally intact prior to castration on day 20. Behavior tests were given in adulthood while ferrets received daily SC injections of increasing doses of testosterone propionate (TP). Only extended treatment of females with T (prenatally, immediately after birth, and over days 5 to 20) caused a duplication of the behavior displayed by control males whose testes were left intact until day 20. Data are expressed as mean ± SEM; the number of subjects in each group is given in parentheses. (Adapted from Baum et al., 1990.[77])

For testosterone (given to females over postnatal days 0 to 20) to masculinize coital function effectively, the dose had to produce circulating concentrations of testosterone that were considerably higher than those normally found in male ferrets at these neonatal ages. Administration of a lower (more physiological) dose of testosterone produced only marginal long-term behavioral effects in females. Are males more sensitive to the masculinizing effect of neonatal testosterone exposure than females? Baum and colleagues[77] showed this to be the case. Males are considerably more sensitive than females to the masculinizing action of a low dosage of testosterone given for 15 days beginning on postnatal day 5. This enhanced responsiveness to testosterone was best duplicated in females that were exposed to testosterone both prenatally and again immediatley after birth for several hours (figure 4.10). This result suggests that exposure of the developing male nervous system to testosterone must occur over an extended perinatal period to achieve complete coital masculinization. Analogous data have been collected for several other mammalian species, including the rhesus monkey, in which both fetal and early postnatal manipulations of androgen have been shown to affect the adult expression of masculine mating behavior.[827]

Sexual Orientation

Numerous experiments, using ferrets as well as other species (reviewed in Adkins-Regan[4]), show that perinatal administration of androgen to females dramatically augments their later exhibition of masculine coital responses in tests with an estrous female. Far fewer studies have systematically explored the effects of early steroidal manipulations on later patterns of sociosexual preference. In experiments with ferrets,[77, 993] tests of sexual preference were conducted by allowing subjects to approach either a sexually active male or an estrous female in the goal boxes of a T-maze. After each approach, the animals were allowed to interact physically for 1 minute prior to a subsequent test. A pilot study had shown that after gonadectomy in adulthood and treatment with estrogen, males preferred approaching estrous females rather than sexually active males. Surprisingly, when treated with testosterone, castrated male subjects showed an equal preference (i.e., no preference) for either the estrous female or the stimulus male. As one might expect, ovariectomized female subjects, when treated with estrogen but not testosterone preferred the sexually active stimulus male.

We next assessed sexual preference in gonadectomized ferrets while treating them with estrogen. Initially, sexual preference was studied in groups of females that had been ovariectomized on postnatal day 5 and treated with either a high or a low dose of testosterone during days 5 to 20 or days 20 to 35. Control groups of males and females, which had been gonadectomized on day 35, showed the expected pattern of sexual preference when given estrogen and tested in adulthood (i.e., males preferred to approach and interact with estrous females; females preferred sexually active males). Females treated during postnatal days 5 to 20 with a high dose of testosterone showed a significant reduction in their preference for a male. However, the magnitude of the shift in these females' preference was not sufficient to make them resemble control males. No other neonatal testosterone treatments effectively altered females' later sociosexual preference.

We have recently examined the preference behavior of female ferrets that were exposed to androgen over a much longer perinatal period than in previous experiments.[77] As shown in figure 4.11, females given a low dose of testosterone during postnatal days 5 to 20 only, still preferred to approach a stimulus male. Females that were also exposed to testosterone before birth, immediately after birth, and again during postnatal days 5 to 20 showed a pattern of preference for estrous females that was identical to that of control males. This suggests that such prolonged perinatal exposure to testosterone is normally required for male ferrets to develop their sociosexual preference, just as extensive testosterone exposure is critical for the development of motoric elements of masculine sexual behavior.

It is too early to say whether testicular steroids contribute in a similar manner to the development of heterosexual orientation in men, or conversely, whether altered patterns of fetal or neonatal steroid secretion contribute to the etiology of homosexual orientation in human males. Nonendocrine experiential factors may also play important roles in the development of sexual partner preferences in animals and in man. For example, in male rats[445] and dogs[89] social isolation during early postnatal life disrupts the later ability to exhibit

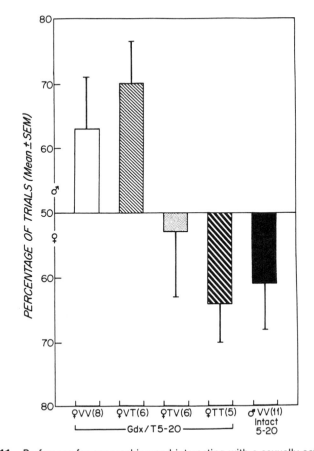

Figure 4.11 Preference for approaching and interacting with a sexually active stimulus male (male symbol) or an estrous female (female symbol) in a T-maze displayed by the same groups of female and male ferrets described in figure 4.10. Tests of sexual preference were conducted in adulthood while ferrets received daily SC injections of estradiol benzoate (15 µg/kg). As for pelvic thrusting behavior (figure 4.10), the masculine pattern of sexual partner preference (represented by males castrated on day P20 far right, dark bar pointing down) was best induced in females by extended perinatal treatment with testosterone (prenatally, immediately after birth, and during days 5 to 20—see TT, striped bar at right). The number of subjects is given in parentheses. (Reproduced from Baum et al., 1990.[77])

motoric components of masculine sexual behavior. However, nobody has systematically studied sociosexual preferences in males after early social deprivation (or restriction of early social partners to peers of one sex or the other). In addition, no one has studied the possible interaction between the perinatal effects of testosterone and the composition of the early social environment on the development of sociosexual orientation in animals. Even with such experimental data in hand, it would be difficult to extrapolate automatically to the human condition because the social environment and the enormous responsiveness to changes in this environment can potentially shape sexual responsiveness.

Sequential Roles of Estrogen and Androgen

The likely role of neural estrogenic metabolites of testosterone in controlling the activation of sexual behavior in adult male ferrets and other species has already been discussed. Much evidence suggests that the organizational action of testosterone on the developing nervous system also depends, in part, on the neural conversion of circulating testosterone into estrogen. Studies conducted in several mammalian species, including rat, rabbit, ferret, and rhesus monkey, show that the activity of aromatizing enzyme in the nervous tissues of the preoptic area, hypothalamus, and temporal lobes is an order of magnitude higher in fetal animals than in adulthood (reviewed in Tobet et al.[1031]). During the final quarter of gestation, male and female ferrets have equivalent high concentrations of aromatase activity in the POA and in the mediobasal hypothalamus and temporal lobes.[604] Males consistently, however, have higher concentrations of circulating testosterone during this period. As a result, the nervous system of the fetal male ferret produces estrogen at a rate that exceeds that of females.

Experimentally induced inhibition of estrogen biosynthesis in fetal male ferrets can be induced by transplacental administration of a drug (ATD) that blocks the activity of aromatase. ATD caused signficant reductions in males' capacity to exhibit masculine coital behavior when they were given testosterone in adulthood and tested with estrous females.[1030] Treatment of male ferrets with ATD during postnatal days 0 to 15, by contrast, failed to disrupt males' later coital capacity, even though neural aromatase activity was strongly inhibited.[74] As described earlier, depriving male ferrets of endogenous testosterone by castration on postnatal day 5 or giving females a high dose of testosterone during postnatal days 5 to 20 caused a striking inhibition and facilitation, respectively, of later masculine sexual behavior. These results show that a testicular steroid, presumably testosterone, plays an important role during the first several weeks of life in masculinizing ferrets' coital potential.

That testosterone itself is neonatally active is further established by the observation that neither estrogen nor DHT nor a combination of estrogen and DHT given to female ferrets during postnatal days 5 to 20 could duplicate the masculinizing action of testosterone on later mating performance.[79, 84] Thus, in male ferrets estrogen and testosterone appear to act sequentially during prenatal and early postnatal development, respectively, to masculinize coital potential. Whether these two steroids act separately or in concert to influence the differentiation of neural mechanisms controlling both motivational and performance aspects of masculine sexual behavior has not been determined.

As was discussed in chapter 2, studies employing other mammalian species, including rat, hamster, and guinea pig, have also implicated estrogens in the differentiation of masculine sexual behavior (reviewed in Baum[73]). Whether testosterone itself also contributes to this process in these species has not been determined. Evidence of estrogenic involvement in the process of coital masculinization of male primates, however, is not as clear.

When considering the comparative data on the hormonal control of coital masculinization, it is important to note that avian species differ from mammals. In birds the female is the heterogametic sex (has two different sex chromosomes), whereas in mammals it is the male that falls into this category (see chapter 2). Numerous experiments (reviewed in Adkins-Regan and Ascenzi[5]) using quail and zebra finch show that the courtship and mating capacity characterstic of adult males will develop in both sexes unless estrogen is present at some early period (prehatching in quail; immediately after hatching in zebra finch) to demasculinize this capacity. That is, in contrast to mammals, in avian species estrogen acts to eliminate, not faciliate, the differentation of masculine coital potential. Normally, this demasculinizing action of estradiol occurs in females.

This fact is especially paradoxical in that estrogen, acting soon after hatching in zebra finches, also plays a crucial role in promoting the development of neural mechanisms that control the learning and production of masculine song during courtship (see chapter 7). In addition, estrogen acts shortly after hatching to ensure that male zebra finches develop the capacity to form pair bonds with female conspecifics. More research is needed to specify the possible sources (gonadal or adrenal secretion; localized neural production through androgen aromatization) and timing of estrogenic stimulation prior to and shortly after hatching in both male and female birds. This information should help to explain how the same hormone can act in both sexes to promote sexually dimorphic aspects of neural and behavioral differentiation.

Some clues to the answers to these seemingly inconsistent results may be found in the literature on invertebrates (see chapter 14). In invertebrates, hormones can have very different effects, depending upon previous hormones the animal has been exposed to and the hormonal milieu at the time the hormone is secreted. The pattern and duration of hormone secretion also codes specific information in invertebrates. Thus, the idea that one hormone has different effects on male and female songbirds may reflect the prior hormone exposure, the hormonal milieu, or the pattern of hormone secretion in these animals.

Relevant Sites of Steroid Action in the Developing Nervous System

Very little is known about the neural sites where sex steroids act during development to control psychosexual differentiation. In quail and in rats, correlations exist between the size of the medial nucleus of the POA, whose volume is sexually dimorphic, and the ability of males to exhibit masculine sexual behavior in adulthood. In quail this particular dimorphism seems to reflect the temporary action of androgen (i.e., the male phenotype is readily eliminated in adult birds by castration and restored after testosterone replacement[795]). Nobody has studied the sites in the female quail where estrogen acts to demasculinize their behavioral potential. Likewise, it is not known where estrogen acts in the male zebra finch's nervous system to promote establishment of pair bonding in adulthood.

As discussed earlier, in rat, ferret, and numerous other species, large lesions of the medial POA profoundly disrupt masculine coital performance (but not motivation). However, lesions that are restricted to *sexually dimorphic* portions of the medial POA in rat and ferret cause only minor deficits in masculine coital performance (reviewed in Cherry and Baum[202]). Until more is known about the neural substrate for the motivational and consummatory components of masculine sexual behavior in adult males, it will remain difficult to specify neural sites at which estrogen and testosterone act during development to influence the differentiation of these behaviors.

General Summary and Conclusions

1. Masculine sexual behavior consists of both motivational and consummatory components. Motivational components include those behaviors engaged in by an animal to gain access to a female. Consummatory components are those behaviors necessary for coitus (i.e., mounting, erection, intromission, and ejaculation).

2. In mammalian species, male sexual behavior is activated by the secretion of testosterone from the Leydig cells of the testes. Both spermatogenesis and testosterone secretion are under the tonic control of LH released from the pituitary in response to GnRH release from the hypothalamus.

3. Testosterone activates masculine sexual behavior through more than one mechanism:

a. Testosterone is converted to DHT in peripheral tissues to stimulate sensory receptors, muscle, and other androgen-sensitive tissues. In rats, this process may potentiate penile reflexes such as erections.

b. Testosterone acts centrally in the POA to activate male sexual behavior. At least some of these effects are androgen dependent (i.e., testosterone itself or DHT acts on androgen receptors).

c. Estrogen, formed intraneuronally from testosterone, induces specific effects on masculine sexual behavior, including sexual motivation or arousal, in several species. In rats, estrogens seem to activate both the motivation and performance of copulation, whereas in ferrets only the latter appears to be affected by estrogens.

4. The POA is the integrative center thought to mediate the effects of testosterone on the performance of coital behavior in the male. The amygdala is thought to be important for organizing the motivational components of masculine sexual behavior.

5. Masculine sexual behavior is modulated by dopaminergic and peptidergic inputs to the POA and amygdala. The mesolimbic dopamine system is thought to be involved in the motivational components of male sexual behavior. The incertohypothalmic dopamine system is implicated in the actual performance of coital behavior. Peptides have been found to modulate both coital behavior and the motivation to mate.

6. Sexual differentiation of masculine sexual behavior in the ferret occurs through the sequential effects first of estrogen and then of testosterone, start-

ing before birth and continuing during the first several weeks of life. These hormone actions influence the development of sociosexual partner preference as well as mating performance.

Acknowledgment

Preparation of this chapter was supported by Research Scientist Development Award MH00392 to the author.

5 *Hormonal Influences on Human Sexual Behavior*

C. Sue Carter

This chapter is intended to provide an overview of a topic of interest to almost all of us: human sexual behavior. Unfortunately, there are relatively few rigorous studies of the ways in which hormones may affect human sexual relations, which is a very difficult and demanding field of study. Gonadal hormones do not seem to affect sexual behavior in humans or other primates as clearly or as strongly as they do in rodents, despite the expectations of many people throughout history. However, there are several indications that hormones have some influence on human sexual behavior and that some of those effects are exerted upon the brain in a manner similar to hormonal influences on the brain in other mammals.

What are the effects of castration upon the sexual behavior of humans and other primates and which hormones appear to be responsible? What are some of the complicating factors that make the study of human sexual behavior difficult?

Introduction

Masters and Johnson[672] divided the "human sexual response" into phases, including sexual excitement, plateau, orgasm, and sexual resolution or satiety. Even individuals with very low levels of sex steroids may experience these responses, suggesting that the basic physiology of the human sexual response is not dependent on gonadal hormones. However, steroid hormones may modulate human sexual behavior, and in particular, androgens or estrogens probably enhance sexual motivation. These ideas will be developed later in this chapter.

Both erotic stimuli and psychological fantasy can induce sexual excitement. During the excitement phase both male and female humans experience psychological sexual arousal and genital vasocongestion (retention of fluid). Sexually aroused individuals may reach a plateau phase, which usually lasts for a period of several minutes or longer. If erotic stimulation continues, orgasm can follow.

Orgasm was described by Kinsey and associates[581] as "the explosive discharge of neuromuscular tensions at the peak of the sexual response. . . . Some, and perhaps most persons may become momentarily unconscious at the moment of orgasm . . ." (pp. 627–628). "Sexual arousal and orgasm involve the whole nervous system and, therefore, all parts of the body. Orgasm in the female matches the orgasm of the male in every physiological detail except for the fact that it occurs without ejaculation" (p. 635).

Temporal patterns of sexual response and the latency period needed before resumption of sexual responding following orgasm may be different in males and females. In general, males require a longer period of resolution before they are able to again reach orgasm.[672] However, the basic phenomenology of the human sexual response and perhaps the basic neurophysiology of sexual responses may be similar in males and females.

Hormonal Influences on Human Male Sexual Behavior

The role of the testes in human reproduction and sexual behavior was recognized in antiquity. At puberty there is a dramatic increase in sexual activity or interest. Concurrent increases in the size of the testes and penis (and other bodily changes) are readily observed and cannot have escaped the attention of any culture. It also was presumably apparent to most cultures that sexual activity by postpubertal, but not prepubertal, males was related to subsequent pregnancy. Domestication of animals and the use of castration to control reproduction and other aspects of male behavior, including aggression, date back thousands of years. Anecdotes abound, but quantitative data and controlled experiments are very rare even in the modern literature on human sexual behavior. The following discussion will examine historical and contemporary perspectives regarding the hormonal mechanisms influencing human sexual behavior.

Testicular Hormones Not Essential for Human Male Sexual Behavior

HISTORICAL BACKGROUND

Removal of the testes (castration) or external genitalia as punishment or tribute in war has been common throughout history. Ancient drawings from Egypt and Ethiopia depict "mounds of severed genitalia gathered from enemies destroyed in battle (p. 739).[581] In Assyria records of castration as punishment date from the fifteenth century B.C. Aristotle (384–322 B.C.) described the effects of both prepubertal and postpubertal castration.

Castration has been and continues to be used in attempts to control human sexual behavior. Castrated men (eunuchs) were preferred as harem guards, but despite popular expectations, many eunuchs continued to engage in sexual behavior. Some religious orders have required voluntary castration of their members in an attempt to facilitate celibacy. More modern attempts to subdue human male sexual behavior have involved the use of "voluntary" or forced castration in the rehabilitation of sex offenders, including individuals convicted of exhibitionism, child molestation, and, in some cases homosexuality. Castration also was used to "cure" masturbation as recently as the early twentieth century. Debate over the usefulness of castration in the treatment of "excessive" or inappropriate sexual activity continues and has been supplemented by the introduction of methods of "chemical castration," discussed subsequently.

ROLE OF THE TESTES IN ADULT SEXUAL BEHAVIOR

Adult castration is usually but not always followed by a decline in sexual activity. Medical records and studies of other primates indicate that castrated males may continue to show sexual behavior for years or even decades following castration. Some castrated men experience a decline or total absence of sexual activity, while others do not. Many reliable reports indicate that castrated men are capable of erections and orgasm.[581] Castrated men are of course infertile but may continue to experience all other aspects of sexual behavior, although usually at lower levels than in gonadally intact men. Levels of circulating androgens are very low following castration or testicular failure. However, the minimal amount of testosterone needed to support the diverse components of sexual behavior has not been established.

DEVELOPMENTAL EFFECTS OF TESTICULAR HORMONES

Infant and prepubertal males can experience nocturnal erections, indicating that the mechanisms needed for erectile "potency" exist even when testicular activity is low. This finding is interesting in light of the fact that nocturnal penile erections are reportedly infrequent in hypogonadal adult men. Hypogonadism refers to various adult conditions in which the gonads are not fully functional or in which the endogenous production of testosterone falls below the normal range (usually defined in men as below 3 ng/ml of serum). In men this condition can occur following castration for medical or other reasons, or individuals may experience testicular failure due to disease or genetic abnormalities.

A myriad of nonhormonal experiential factors confound attempts to detect the role of prepubertal hormones in subsequent adult behavior. The role of testicular secretions in childhood remains poorly understood. It has been generally assumed that prepubertal testicular failure or castration would be more detrimental to male sexual behavior than would postpubertal loss of testicular function.[581] However, as described later, testing this assumption is difficult. Overt sexual activity is usually infrequent in children. The behavioral effects of prepubertal hormones, therefore, have been examined only indirectly in adults with a history of subnormal hormonal exposure.

AGING

Regarding the role of androgens in human male sexual behavior, a major early source of concern arose from the common observation that sexual behavior tends to decline during aging. The testes also decrease in size, and testosterone levels decline somewhat, the most marked changes occuring after age 60. However, various studies[261, 580] have indicated that even men in their 80s or older may continue to be sexually active. Correlations between levels of total testosterone and sexual activity are usually weak.

Changes in the availability or stimulus value of a sexual partner and concurrent declines in free testosterone (due to increased steroid hormone binding with age) could influence sexual motivation and subsequent performance. A number of diseases can also affect sexual function (e.g., diabetes, prostate cancer, and heart disease). It seems most likely, therefore, that age-related changes in partner availability, declines in general health, increases in the prevalence of various diseases, and drugs or other treatments for such conditions may be more important than testosterone in causing age-related declines in sexual activity.

What Hormones Are Important?

NONTESTICULAR SOURCES OF ANDROGENS

Testicular secretions are not essential for either orgasm or "potency"as measured by the ability to show a penile erection.Castrated and hypogonadal men continue to have the "ability" to perform sexually, and some may do so at high levels. These studies, however, do **not** prove conclusively that androgens are not involved in human sexual behavior, since the production of androgens is not limited to the testes. The adrenal glands also make androgens, although these are less potent than testicular androgens. The prostate gland, which is not usually removed with castration, also is capable of synthesizing dihydrotestosterone (DHT). In addition, adipose tissue (i.e., fat) is an important steroid hormone reservoir (in both males and females), containing concentrations of testosterone and DHT up to ten times higher than those in serum. Furthermore, adipose tissue is an important site for the formation of 5α-reduced androgens, including DHT.[276, 803] Therefore, androgens from other sources in the body may contribute to the maintenance of sexual function in some individuals, and body fat may be a significant contributor to individual variation in behavior.[941]

EVIDENCE FROM CLINICAL STUDIES: HYPOGONADISM AND
HORMONE REPLACEMENT THERAPY

One rare genetic condition, termed Kallman's syndrome, results from gonadotropin-releasing hormone (GnRH) deficiency. Kallman's syndrome is especially interesting because its victims are hypogonadal from birth. Their prenatal genital development is relatively normal because testicular hormone secretion during the early developmental stages in not dependent on the fetal pituitary but is supported by the mother's gonadotropin production. Patients with Kallman's syndrome have low levels of testicular hormones during development, and they do not experience puberty without medical intervention. Untreated, these individuals fail to develop masculine secondary sex characteristics (i.e., become **virilized**) and remain youthful in physical appearance, although they usually attain normal adult height.

Untreated hypogonadal adults suffering from Kallman's syndrome or related diseases are not usually homosexual. However, they do report a relative disinterest in sexual behavior, low levels of sexual activity, and mild depression and rarely experience spontaneous daytime or nocturnal penile erections. Hormone replacement therapies (either testosterone or pituitary hormones, which stimulate testicular development) increase virilization. Androgenized hypogonadal men report increases in sexual interest, spontaneous daytime erections, and nocturnal penile erections. However, sexual activity, including autoerotic behavior (i.e., masturbation) does not increase dramatically at least within the first year after exposure to testosterone.[176] These studies, of course, may be complicated by the unusual sexual and social histories of these men and shyness or embarrassment over their medical condition and sexual immaturity.

Sexual Performance versus Motivation   Studies of castrated men or men with adult testicular dysfunction clearly suggest that neither the testes nor high levels of androgens are *essential* for sexual performance when sexual stimulation is provided by a partner or intense erotic stimuli. However, the frequency of sexual activity in normal life is typically lower in men with low levels of androgens.[50, 261]

Until recently it was generally assumed that hypogonadal men were less able than normal men to respond with erections to erotic stimulation. Recent laboratory studies indicate that this is not the case. Strong erotic stimuli including pornography or even self-induced fantasy may elicit erections with latencies similar to those seen in normal men. These studies did not attempt to examine orgasmic responses. However, self-reported frequencies of sexual thoughts or fantasies through diaries suggest that androgens *can* stimulate this component of human behavior. Thus, it has been suggested that a major behavioral effect of testicular secretions is to increase spontaneous sexual thoughts, sexual desire, sexual interest, or libido.[48] Erections elicited by erotic stimuli are apparently not dependent on high levels of androgens. In contrast, in hypogonadal adults, "spontaneous" erections and sexual thoughts (those not requiring external stimulation) tend to increase following androgen treatment (reviewed in Davidson et al.).[261]

Recent quantitative and experimentally controlled studies[50, 261] are of theoretical importance because they suggest that testicular secretions can modulate sexual behavior by increasing thoughts or motivation, thus leading to sexual activity. This hypothesis is, of course, very difficult to test. The occurrence of a "thought" is subject to many nonhormonal processes including experience. The very act of requesting information could alter an individual's frequency of sex-related thoughts. It is relatively simple to describe and measure sexual activity and erections, but much more difficult to define or assess human sexual motivation.

Problems with Assessment of Affective Behaviors   Another major problem in assessing the possible cognitive effects of any hormone relates to the behavioral specificity of hormone action. As described in the context of animal studies, depression or stress might directly or indirectly alter mood or motivation. Androgens with their wide-ranging anabolic effects could alter behavior at many levels and may have broad effects on human motivation or mood, thereby influencing sexuality secondarily. Self-reports and mood questionnaires from hypogonadal men indicate that many men experience general lethargy, a loss of "energy," and depression when androgen levels decline. These effects are seen even when the individual is unaware of whether or not he is receiving hormone-replacement therapy.

Experiments in which men experience a rapid loss of androgen also are confounded by the complexity of hormone "withdrawal." Like menopausal women, adult men experiencing a rapid decline in androgen may have "hot flashes," mood shifts, and other withdrawal symptoms. Prepubertal boys and adult, untreated hypogonadal men who have had minimal exposure to androgen do not experience these symptoms, suggesting that the effects of androgens or androgen withdrawal in an adult are influenced by a prior history of androgen exposure.

In addition to "cognitive" or "motivational" interpretations of the behavioral data described here, it is possible that the perception of sensory stimuli may be altered by the presence of androgens.[259, 262] Psychophysical techniques permit the precise analysis of human sensory perceptions. Using these methods, it was found that hypogonadal men receiving prolonged androgen treatment became progressively less sensitive to vibrotactile stimulation of the penis.[176] The ability of a hormone to modulate sensory input could be important in both sexual motivation and performance.

TESTOSTERONE, DHT, AND ESTROGEN

Early clinical studies in men indicated that relatively large doses of estrogen could inhibit "libido." In addition, estrogen treatment had other side effects including mammary enlargement and female patterns of fat deposition that were not considered desirable in men. Therefore, it was traditionally assumed that estrogen was a "female sex hormone" that would reduce male sexual behavior. However, more recently, the animal studies described in chapter 4 have raised the possibility that estrogens are involved in the behavioral effects of testosterone.

The possibility that low doses of estrogen may facilitate rather than inhibit human male sexual behavior remains largely untested. It is possible that testosterone may serve as a prohormone that delivers the androgen to specific target cells, including the brain. According to this hypothesis, *intracellular* conversion to an estrogen would permit highly local effects of the estrogens, without the undesired "feminizing" actions that would follow exposure to high levels of systemic estrogen. Concurrently, testosterone itself or DHT would function to "virilize" the peripheral tissues such as the accessory sex organs, genitalia, or muscle.

OTHER HORMONES AND HUMAN MALE SEXUAL BEHAVIOR

The work described here has emphasized the effects of steroid hormones on sexual motivation and performance. However, many other hormones and neurochemicals may influence sexual behavior. Synthetic progestins including medroxyprogesterone acetate and cyproterone acetate, have been used in the treatment of sex offenders. These "antiandrogenic" drugs provide a form of chemical castration and are reported in uncontrolled studies to decrease sexual motivation.[49] In addition, oxytocin and vasopressin are released by the posterior pituitary during sexual behavior and have actions on smooth muscle, such as the vas deferens, and blood pressure, both of which are important in erection; both of these polypeptides also have behavioral activity in animals and, as will be described in greater detail later, may also influence sexual behavior.

Hormones released during stress and adrenal activity may also influence sexual behavior directly or indirectly. Hormones released during chronic stress, such as the adrenal corticosteroids or opiates, inhibit sexual behavior and other aspects of reproductive function. This idea is discussed further in chapter 10. However, short-term or acute stress may temporarily increase sexual arousal due to sympathetic nervous system activation.

DRUGS AND SEXUAL BEHAVIOR
Alcohol and marijuana are widely used in the context of sexual behavior. Alcohol or marijuana may reduce social inhibitions, promoting sexual behavior indirectly. High doses of alcohol can directly inhibit the ability to ejaculate. Chronic use of alcohol or marijuana and many other chemicals is typically associated with gradual declines in sexual behavior. Such drugs damage the nervous system directly and may indirectly interfere with sexual behavior by inhibiting steroid hormone production. Chronic use of many drugs (especially alcohol) also has been implicated in impotence and eventual infertility.

Studies of illicit drug use or side effects from drugs used in medical treatment (reviewed in Segraves et al.[935]) suggest that chronic use of depressant drugs, including opiates (such as heroin), barbiturates, antianxiety drugs, antihypertensives and anticonvulsants, usually reduces male sexual behavior. Conversely, acute use of stimulants such as amphetamines and cocaine reputedly can stimulate some components of sexual behavior. Chronic use of stimulants, however, may result in sexual dysfunction. In addition, addicted individuals often become disinterested in both social and sexual interactions. The mechanisms of most of these phenomena remains poorly understood but probably include effects on the autonomic nervous system (needed for erection and ejaculation) as well as effects on the brain and endocrine systems.

Hormonal Influences on Human Female Sexual Behavior

Hormonal Effects on Perfomance versus Motivation

In most primates, including humans, ovarian hormones are not essential for the expression of female sexual behavior. However, to varying degrees, sexual behavior in primates can be influenced by steroid hormones.[1086] When female rhesus monkeys are tested alone with a single male in a small area, they often show sexual behavior throughout the entire menstrual cycle, although the probability of mating may be slightly higher around the time of ovulation, the phase of the cycle when other spontaneously ovulating mammals are most likely to be sexually receptive. In contrast, when females are tested in larger areas or in multifemale groups, most females mate primarily during the mid-cycle, the periovulatory period. Wallen[1086] has interpreted these data and the larger literature on primates to hypothesize that ovarian hormones influence the expression of primate sexual behavior *when female choice is permitted.* Similar conclusions can be drawn from the literature on human females.[3, 1059]

As summarized by Wallen,[1086] in rodents both the ability (performance) and desire (motivation) to mate are hormone dependent. In contrast, in primates, females are capable of engaging in sexual behavior without the benefit of ovarian hormones. However, the sexual motivation or desire of a female primate may vary as a function of the menstrual cycle or other endocrine events.

ESTROGEN

Ovariectomy can produce a gradual decline in female sexual behavior in rhesus monkeys and to varying degrees in other species.[1086] Estrogen, whether secreted by the ovarian follicle or given as replacement therapy, may have broad effects on primate behavior. Estrogen apparently can increase female motivation and may facilitate peripheral changes such as the production of odors that make the female more attractive to a male partner. In human females, estrogen also increases vaginal lubrication and thus can influence sexual behavior indirectly.

PROGESTERONE

Most primates are capable of spontaneous ovulation. During the menstrual cycle, progesterone is secreted around the time of ovulation, and following ovulation progesterone from the corpus luteum is the dominant ovarian hormone. There are some indications that brief exposure to progesterone can facilitate female sexual behavior in primates. However, the most consistent effects of prolonged exposure to progesterone in primates, including humans, are inhibitory. For example, luteal phase inhibition of sexual activity has been reported in monkeys and humans exposed to progesterone.

Baum and associates[78] have suggested that progesterone also decreases female attractiveness in rhesus monkeys. Progesterone could be indirectly inhibitory due to its capacity to act as an "antiestrogen," or it could have direct inhibitory effects on female sexual motivation.

The behavioral effects of progesterone or synthetic progestins in human females remain difficult to interpret. Women taking oral contraceptives, which often contain progestins, may report either increases or decreases in sexual activity.[899] These results are confounded by the associated freedom from concern about pregnancy, which might increase sexual activity. However, a number of reports suggest that declines in sexual interest occur in progestin-treated women. It has been suggested that such effects may be an indirect "antiandrogenic" action of the progestin.[899]

ANDROGENS

There are suggestions in the literature that normal variations in androgens (secreted by the ovary or adrenal) during the menstrual cycle could be responsible for reported cyclic fluctuations in sexual interest.[942] Some women report perimenstrual increases in sexual activity, and androgen levels may show related patterns of fluctuation. However, data on menstrual cyclicity in sexual behavior are rather weak,[899] possibly because sexual activity involves many social factors in addition to the sexual interest of the female.[1086]

The adrenal cortex produces significant quantities of androgens, and adrenalectomy is detrimental to female sexual behavior in humans and monkeys. In monkeys, declines in sexual behavior following adrenal removal were somewhat reversed by treatment with androgen but were not affected by treatment with estrogen. Furthermore, since the 1940s, exogenous androgen treatments have been given to human females for diverse medical purposes. Even in very low doses, androgen treatments can increase sexual motivation in some human females, and it has been suggested by Sherwin[941] that women may be, in comparison to men, more sensitive to the behavioral effects of androgens.

The ability of exogenous androgens to promote female sexual behavior is of therapeutic interest and is being explored in medical research. However, androgenic or anabolic hormones carry potential side effects, including sterility, virilization, male patterns of body hair growth, baldness, and liver and cardiovascular damage. It also should be noted that normal men endogenously produce levels of androgens that are well above those needed to maintain high levels of sexual behavior.[262] Thus, at present, the usefulness of androgens as aphrodisiacs is limited to men with abnormally low levels of androgens, and other applications are potentially hazardous.

Human Sexual Behavior: A Hypothesis for the Coordination of Male and Female Sexual Behaviors

As described above, there is reason to believe that both male and female humans are capable of responding to androgens with increased sexual interest. Furthermore, in the relative absence of sex steroids, at least the reflexive components of the sexual response can be elicited in males and females. Davidson and associates[262] observed that profoundly hypogonadal men were able to experience erections as quickly as normal men if they were presented with highly erotic stimuli. In contrast, in the absence of strong stimuli, hypogonadal men typically show lower than normal levels of spontaneous sexual interest or sexual activity with a partner. In double-blind studies, androgen replacement therapy increases sexual interest and, to a lesser degree, sexual activity in these hypogonadal men. Such data offer further support for a role for androgens in sexual motivation.

A large pharmacological literature has implicated a variety of neurochemicals, including steroid hormones, in the modulation of male sexual interest and erectile potency[935] (see chapter 4). Apart from work on steroid hormones, very little is known about the pharmacology of human female sexual behavior. Perhaps this is not because drugs do not affect women but because women are not dependent on an erection for sexual activity. However, as argued by Kinsey and associates,[581] the major difference in human sexual behavior is based on the presence of ejaculation in the male but not the female: "Ejaculation may constitute a spectacular and biologically significant event which is unique to the male, but it is an event which depends on relatively simple anatomic differences, rather than upon differences in the basic physiology of sexual response in the female and male."

In spite of the scarcity of controlled studies, clinical reports and illicit drug use have implicated most of the neurochemicals described earlier in human sexual behavior, at least in males. One chemical, oxytocin, is of particular interest and has characteristics suggesting that it might play a pivotal role in sexual behavior.[188] Oxytocin is released during the orgasmic phase of the human sexual response in both men and women[184, 770] and during ejaculation in males of several species. Through its contractile effects on smooth muscle, oxytocin could play a role in sperm transport in males. In women, uterine contractions caused by peripherally released oxytocin may facilitate sperm transport and may play an indirect role in sexual satiety.[259]

It is also possible that oxytocin released in the brain has a more direct role in sexual behavior. Activity in oxytocinergic neurons and the release of oxytocin depend upon the interaction of a variety of other hormones and neurochemicals.[573] Steroid hormones, particularly estrogen and testosterone, may facilitate oxytocinergic activity at many levels, including modulation of oxytocin binding[534] and oxytocin release. In general, correlations exist among the pharmacological agents that stimulate the release of oxytocin and those that stimulate sexual behavior.

Breast, genital, or cognitive stimulation can stimulate the release of oxytocin[573]; the central release of small amounts of oxytocin may cascade (over a period of minutes) through positive feedback to cause the pulsatile release of oxytocin in the brain and also into the peripheral circulation.[184, 770] Both central and peripheral events surrounding the release of oxytocin may induce psychophysiological activities, such as changes in genital blood flow, heart rate, or blood pressure, that accompany or follow orgasm. Because high doses of oxytocin inhibit sexual behavior[995, 1109] and oxytocin has been implicated in sexual satiety,[259] it is possible that oxytocin released during orgasm acts on the nervous system to induce a refractory state. There is also evidence implicating oxytocin in the formation of social bonds in animals.[191, 573] Shared sexual experience may thereby facilitate social bond formation in humans.

Little is known about the neurochemistry of human sexual behavior. Based primarily on animal research, we hypothesize that the release of oxytocin or the neural activity accompanying the release of oxytocin could be pivotal events in the phenomenology of the human sexual response and sexual satiety in both sexes. These highly speculative hypotheses have not been tested in humans, but if correct they have clinical implications for the diagnosis and treatment of sexual disorders and may be related to a variety of unexplained sociosexual experiences.

Summary

Human sexual behavior can occur in the absence of gonadal hormones; however, these hormones appear to modulate sexual behavior. Human male sexual behavior, including erectile function, may continue in the absence of the testes and in other men with low levels of testosterone. However, quantitative studies suggest that reductions in testicular secretions are associated with declines in sexual interest or motivation. Testosterone may have effects on diverse processes including those responsible for spontaneous erections, mood, and sensory processing leading to sexual activity. Testosterone within the normal biological range is probably the only true "aphrodisiac." However, even androgens, used in large, chronic doses, for example, during anabolic steroid abuse, may inhibit sexual behavior.

In most primates, including humans, ovarian hormones are not necessary for females to engage in sexual behavior. However, motivation or sexual desire and possibly orgasmic responsivity can vary as a function of the menstrual cycle. Estrogen may facilitate sexual desire and attractiveness. Progesterone is not necessary for human female sexual behavior. However, prolonged exposure to progesterone in women—for example, in the luteal phase or during pregnancy—may actually inhibit sexual interest. Androgen secretion in females also may vary as a function of the menstrual cycle. Although the production of androgens in women is usually much lower than that found in men, there are indications that women are more sensitive to androgens than men.[942] The cellular actions of androgens in both sexes may require intracellular conversion to an estrogen (see chapter 4).

Oxytocin is released during the human sexual response in both males and females. The actions of oxytocin can be modulated by sex steroids and neurotransmitters that have been implicated in sexual behavior. Oxytocin, or neural events associated with the release of oxytocin, might play a role in coordinating sexual excitement, orgasm, and sexual satiety, although at present data supporting this hypothesis are purely correlational.[188]

Most behaviorally active drugs, including many medicines, have some capacity to influence sexual behavior directly or indirectly . In general, depressants diminish sexual interest and performance. The effects of stimulants are more complex and may include transient facilitations of sexual behavior, but chronic drug abuse is often associated with declines in sexual behavior. Chronic stress also may inhibit sexual behavior. These effects of most drugs and stress are complex and may involve direct neural effects or indirect actions on steroid hormone production.

Human research in this field is rare, and the cellular mechanisms of hormone actions can only be inferred from the animal research. Animal studies, such as those described throughout this volume, can be used to model basic biological mechanisms and phenomena. Cross-species comparisons, including human data, facilitate an understanding of the functions, adaptive significance, and mechanisms of a particular behavioral pattern. Knowledge derived from diverse sources permits the development of descriptive and predictive models, which in turn may allow eventual prevention and treatment of biochemically based sexual disorders.

6 Diversity of Hormone-Behavior Relations in Reproductive Behavior

David Crews

Because we are mammals, many people find other mammals more interesting than fish, insects, or snakes. But some of the most fascinating variations in the strategy to reproduce have arisen among the reptiles and fishes, resulting in relations between hormones and mating behavior that are very different from those described in the preceding chapters. These alternative strategies force us to look again at mammals, including ourselves, and ask questions about the evolutionary forces that have produced the hormone- behavior relations described in the previous chapters. We also see that in spite of the variation in the ways in which hormones affect reproduction and sexual behavior, in those species of vertebrates that have been investigated, the same brain regions are important. This rewarding aspect of the comparative approach will resurface throughout the coming chapters.

What are the different strategies animals can use for reproduction, and what are the constraints such strategies must accommodate? Why are the gonads activated in some species long before mating, and what happens to the hormone-behavior relationships in such cases?

Introduction

Without due consideration of the neural and behavioral correlates of differences between higher taxa and between closely related families, species, sexes, and stages, we cannot expect to understand our nervous systems or ourselves.[168]

If you have ever spent time watching animals, either in a zoo or in your home, you have probably noticed that there is an incredible diversity among species in the behaviors they exhibit. Each species engages in some behaviors that are characteristic of and unique to that species. These are referred to as species-typical behaviors. From reading the first few chapters, you have probably also realized that there is also great diversity in the ways in which hormones can affect the nervous system and an animal's behavior. To the student, this diversity might seem like an unwanted complexity, something else to complicate the story and your studying. It is the object of this chapter to convince you that as you gain an appreciation of the diversity in hormone-behavior relations, you can begin to understand more completely the basic mechanisms mediating these processes. In addition, you will gain a greater understanding and appreciation for the evolution of hormone-brain-behavior relations.

At the most fundamental level, the study of diversity provides us with a different perspective from which to view hormone-brain-behavior relations. There has been a tradition in modern times to specialize. The study of the causes and development of behavior is usually separated from the evolution and ecological patterns of behavior. There has also been a trend toward reductionistic investigations of behavior. In other words, scientists have been inclined to investigate the molecular changes in the brain correlated with a behavior rather than to study the actual behavior itself. However, it is important to keep in mind that there are many levels of biological organization and that molecules always function within cells, cells within organs, organs within animals, and, ultimately, animals within environments. Thus, the molecular aspects of hormonal action are important for our understanding of these processes. But they tell us very little about behavior. For this, we must turn to studies of the whole animal. To learn about the evolution of behavior, we must turn to ecological and evolutionary analyses.

Those scientists interested in the immediate causes of behavior tend to be unaware of the great advances that have been made in evolutionary biology. Similarly, most scientists interested in ecological and evolutionary questions ignore advances made in neuroendocrinology and molecular biology. Quite simply, "reductionists see little to be gained from holistic studies, and whole organism biologists do not recognize the value of molecular analysis."[829] This philosophical gap and lack of communication between these two approaches to the study of brain-behavior relations makes it difficult to be a generalist. Yet to understand behavior, we must attempt to integrate the different levels of biological organization. If done with insight, it can lead to new discoveries in evolution and ecology, physiology and molecular biology.

This chapter emphasizes an interdisciplinary approach to behavioral analysis, including an evolutionary approach. Obviously, one can apply Darwinian thinking to behavioral questions without being an evolutionary biologist. For readers who might be encountering an evolutionary or ecological approach for the first time, it is important *not* to assume that evolutionary thinking is confined to the discipline of biology. Indeed, modern Darwinian theory can be a powerful tool for molecular, anatomical, physiological, and behavioral research regardless of one's formal disciplinary home.

The general principles that should guide you in attaining this evolutionary and ecological perspective of behavioral endocrinology will be discussed next. These principles include descriptions of some of the modes and patterns of reproduction present in animals. There are a variety of evolutionary forces that have led to various behavior-controlling mechanisms. These will be discussed first, followed by examples of the diversity in hormone-behavior relations that has been observed to date. These and other studies are at the interface of ecological physiology, evolutionary biology, and behavioral endocrinology. Next, two animal model systems will be described in detail to illustrate how these three fields might be integrated. Finally, some conjectures are offered about a fundamental aspect of biological organization and how hormone-behavior relations might have evolved in vertebrates. We will conclude with some speculations about which came first, sex or sexual behavior.

Overview of General Principles

Modes of Reproduction

In the preceding chapters, the discussion of sexual behaviors and courtship behaviors has focused on species with two sexes. In the animal kingdom, however, this is not the only strategy for propagation of a species. We tend to focus on mammals because their mode of reproduction employs internal fertilizaton of the egg in a female by a male, with the female giving birth to live young. But this is only one mode of reproduction. A remarkable array of reproductive modes have evolved.

Animals can be classified according to (1) division of individuals according to eggs or sperm production (or both), (2) method of production of young, and (3) method of fertilization (table 6.1). Humans and other mammals have two sexes, male and female. As you have already learned, this means that during development, the fetal gonads become testes in males and ovaries in females. This separation of the gonads into separate-sexed individuals is called gonochorism. On the other hand, in some species the same individual has both types of gonad and can produce both eggs and sperm. These individuals are called hermaphrodites. In some hermaphroditic species (e.g., earthworms and sea bass), the production of eggs and sperm occurs simultaneously. In others (e.g., tropical reef fish), the production of eggs and sperm occurs sequentially. It is important to keep in mind that the two forms of hermaphroditism are fundamentally different. In the former instance, individuals are two sexes at the same time, whereas in the latter instance, individuals are only one sex at a time.

Finally, there are some species in which all individuals have only ovaries and produce only eggs. This is called parthenogenetic reproduction. (The word comes from the Greek words *parthenos*, meaning virgin, and *genesis*, meaning birth.) In some of these all-female species, such as the popular aquarium fish, the Amazon molly, the sperm from the male of another species is required to activate development, although the sperm's genome is not incorporated into the genome of the offspring. In other parthenogenetic forms (e.g., aphids and whiptail lizards), sperm are not required for complete and normal development.

Still another important distinction in modes of reproduction is the method by which the young are reproduced—viviparity or oviparity. Basically, viviparity ("live-bearing"), exists when the young develop within the body of the mother as occurs in mammals. An important component of viviparity is that nutrients and waste products are exchanged between the mother and the fetus. Oviparous animals are egg-layers. Eggs may be ovulated and laid singly or by

Table 6.1   Different Modes of Reproduction

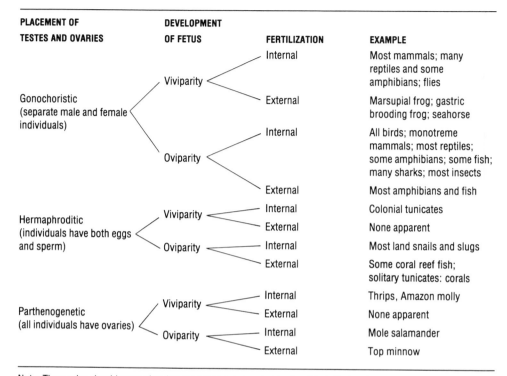

PLACEMENT OF TESTES AND OVARIES	DEVELOPMENT OF FETUS	FERTILIZATION	EXAMPLE
Gonochoristic (separate male and female individuals)	Viviparity	Internal	Most mammals; many reptiles and some amphibians; flies
		External	Marsupial frog; gastric brooding frog; seahorse
	Oviparity	Internal	All birds; monotreme mammals; most reptiles; some amphibians; some fish; many sharks; most insects
		External	Most amphibians and fish
Hermaphroditic (individuals have both eggs and sperm)	Viviparity	Internal	Colonial tunicates
		External	None apparent
	Oviparity	Internal	Most land snails and slugs
		External	Some coral reef fish; solitary tunicates: corals
Parthenogenetic (all individuals have ovaries)	Viviparity	Internal	Thrips, Amazon molly
		External	None apparent
	Oviparity	Internal	Mole salamander
		External	Top minnow

Note: The reader should recognize that the scheme presented is simplified. Each category represents extremes on what is really a continuum; intermediate forms exist. Furthermore, some animals may actually exhibit different reproductive modes at different stages of the life cycle. The interested reader should consult Blackwelder and Shepard, 1981[123] for a more complete survey of the diversity of animal reproduction.

the thousands and may or may not have protective shell coverings. Still another reproductive mode is believed to have led to viviparity called ovoviviparity. In this instance, the fertilized eggs are retained within the body, but there is a reduction in the placental membranes and no nutrients are exchanged.

The last distinction to be made is whether fertilization occurs internally or externally. Mammals, birds, and reptiles all practice internal fertilization. The mode of fertilization in amphibians, fish, sharks, and rays varies from species to species. This distinction is important because hormones can have opposite effects in these two modes of fertilization. It is also important because male and female reproductive behaviors, including mating behavior, can vary dramatically as a function of internal versus external fertilization.

Patterns of Reproduction Among Seasonal Breeders

Multiple patterns of seasonal reproduction exist even within species that have two sexes. As discussed in chapters 3 and 4, many species of animals are seasonal breeders. One important distinction among reproductive patterns lies in

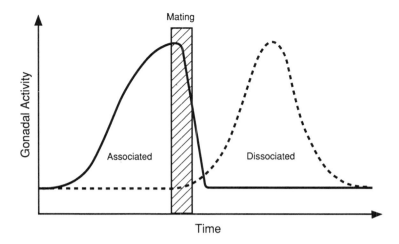

Figure 6.1 Associated and dissociated reproductive patterns exhibited in vertebrates. Gonadal activity is defined as the development of eggs and sperm or increased sex steroid hormone secretion. Note that in individuals exhibiting the associated reproductive pattern (solid line), the gonads are fully developed at the time of mating, and circulating levels of sex hormones are maximal. In individuals exhibiting the dissociated reproductive pattern (dashed line), the gonads are small, and sex steroid hormone levels are low at the time of mating. For the sake of the argument, the dimensions of the reproductive pattern are depicted as mutually exclusive extremes. Intermediate forms exist. (From Crews, 1984.[231])

whether the animal mates in relation to its seasonal gonadal cycle. If the animal produces and releases its sperm or eggs during the mating season, this is known as an associated reproductive pattern. If a species produces sperm and eggs at some time other than during the mating season and then stores them until mating occurs, this is known as a dissociated reproductive pattern (figure 6.1). Humans have developed ways to modify the environment and so have become emancipated from many of the factors that have led to seasonal reproduction in other animals. There is evidence in humans of some vestiges of seasonality, however, as indicated by the seasonal variation in birth rates and hence in the rate of conception. For example, in Hong Kong, the low temperatures in January are correlated with a peak in conceptions (figure 6.2).

The animal model systems most widely used in behavioral endocrinology are the rat, guinea pig, mouse, and hamster. These species as well as many other mammalian and avian species exhibit associated reproductive patterns. That is, periods of sexual behavior are restricted to times when the gonads are active. In species exhibiting an associated reproduction pattern, sexual behavior in the male is activated by elevated serum concentrations of testicular steroid hormones (see chapter 4). In the female it is the pattern and amount of estrogens and progestins produced by the ovary that regulate the periods of sexual receptivity (see chapter 3). In species with dissociated reproductive patterns, breeding activity occurs when the gonads are small and are not producing gametes or steroid hormones. In these species, sexual behavior is independent of concurrent gonadal steroid hormone control but is activated by some other stimulus.

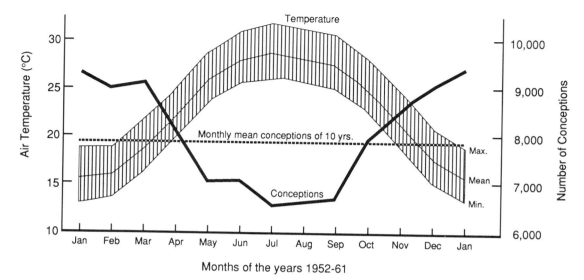

Figure 6.2 Seasonal variation in conceptions in Hong Hong. This is sometimes referred to as the "comfort hypothesis" because it is during the coldest months when people are huddling indoors that the greatest number of conceptions occur. It should also be noted that the peak in conceptions coincides with the Chinese New Year. The mean conception rate for the same period is represented by the horizontal line. (Redrawn from Chang et al., 1963.[198])

Still another pattern of reproduction is spontaneous versus induced ovulation.[220] In many animals gonadal activity is initiated by environmental changes that occurred many weeks or months earlier (see later discussion). Once initiated, the eggs develop and are released spontaneously at a particular time regardless of whether or not mating occurs. This is known as spontaneous ovulation. In other animals, however, mating activity actually induces ovulation or, in some, gonadal growth. Cats and rabbits are examples of animals that are behaviorally receptive during the breeding season but do not ovulate unless mated. As discussed in chapter 3, experiments have shown that the act of copulation in cats and rabbits leads to a neuroendocrine reflex that results in luteinizing hormone (LH) release by the pituitary and consequently ovulation. Other animals show even more extreme variations. In the ferret and mink, the eggs do not undergo final maturation nor does ovulation occur unless the female experiences the violent precopulatory behavior of the male in which he energetically throws her about. In the musk shrew and the garter snake, ovarian activity is not even initiated unless the female is first courted and mated.

Evolutionary Forces Leading to the Reproductive Modes and Patterns Used by Animals Today

A successful strategy for investigating and making sense of diversity in the neuroendocrinology of reproduction is to look for generalities. The comparative method is the traditional approach in biological investigations. It has been shown repeatedly that comparison of various organisms leads to discoveries of themes or traits that recur throughout all animals. Traits are any property of the organism that one is interested in measuring. When closely related species are compared, it becomes possible to trace the progressive specialization of traits and thus illuminate the course of evolution.

While it is important to know what is present, it is equally important to know what might occur but is not present. For example, from table 6.1, we note that there apparently are no examples of hermaphroditic or parthenogenetic viviparous species practicing external fertilization. What is absent usually reflects a basic and sometimes insurmountable conflict among constraints, or limitations inherent in the environment, development, or evolutionary history of an organism. When we understand such constraints, we can account for observed differences and, whatever the cause, predict what might be found in certain circumstances. Such an understanding also can suggest what is unlikely or has not evolved in our world.

Three concepts should guide the reader in learning about these evolutionary forces. The first considers the functions of sexual behavior. The second concerns the distinction between natural selection and sexual selection. The third describes the nature of the constraints that have shaped the evolution of reproductive processes.

REPRODUCTIVE SYNERGISM VERSUS REPRODUCTIVE ISOLATION
In an evolutionary sense, reproduction is the single most important element in an individual's life. It is more important even than the length of an individual's survival. Simply put, if an individual does not reproduce, its genes will not be represented in future generations.

Reproduction has been host to the evolution of many specialized behaviors. We assume that individuals exhibiting these behaviors left more offspring. Detailed analyses indicate that in many species, behaviors associated with reproduction tend to be highly ritualized, stereotyped, and characteristic of a species. However, although they both have focused on sexual behaviors, behavioral endocrinologists and evolutionary biologists traditionally have viewed the function of sexual behaviors differently. Behavioral endocrinologists emphasize the fact that reproductive behaviors serve to coordinate the events that lead to successful reproduction. Evolutionary biologists emphasize the fact that reproductive behaviors serve to isolate a species.

The position that reproductive behaviors have evolved to coordinate hormonal, gonadal, and behavioral events is known as *reproductive synergism*. Proponents of this position point out that reproduction is a carefully regulated process. Each successive phase of reproduction is dependent upon preceding events. At the same time, each phase sets the stage for what follows (figure 6.3). Reproduction occurs only when the participants send and receive appropriate visual, auditory, chemical, seismic, ultrasonic, or electrical signals (see chapter 7). This process results in the appropriate coordination of the maturation and release of each individual's gametes (egg and sperm).

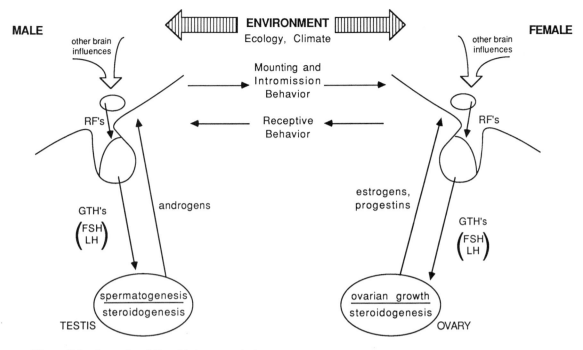

Figure 6.3 Dynamic relationship between the internal and external environments in the control of mating behavior in many vertebrate animals. The behaviors of the male and the female help to synchronize the maturation and release of sperm and eggs so that fertilization occurs. Changes in climate, ecology, or behavior of other members of the species initiate and modulate gonadal and hormonal changes during reproduction. Thus, hormones regulate behavior in the individual animal and are themselves affected by other stimuli, including the behavior and, indirectly, the physiology of its mate. RF, releasing factors; GTH, gonadotropic hormones; FSH, follicle-stimulating hormone; LH, luteinizing hormone. See chapter 1 for details of the hypothalamus-pituitary-gonadal axis.

The position that reproductive behaviors evolved to keep species from interbreeding is known as *reproductive isolation*. Proponents of this position hold that species-typical sexual behaviors serve as reproductive isolating mechanisms to maintain species boundaries. If individuals from different species do mate, fertilization will not occur. If fertilization does occur, viable offspring often will not result because the egg lacks the necessary sets of compatible chromosomes required for normal growth and development. Even when the species are closely related, indicating a recent (in an evolutionary time scale) divergence, the young produced tend to be sterile.

Recently there has been a shift in evolutionary biology away from the isolationist perspective. The argument is that if evolution favors reproductive success, then it is in the individual's interest to focus on selecting the best mate. It is not as important to avoid mating with the wrong species. This recent shift in emphasis in evolutionary biology perhaps resulted from a renewed appreciation of sexual selection as an important evolutionary process.

NATURAL SELECTION VERSUS SEXUAL SELECTION

Darwin considered natural selection and sexual selection as different processes. Both are primary forces driving the evolution of traits. For our purposes, natural selection results in traits that are adaptational responses to changes in the environment. The resulting variation in traits between and within species is shaped by differences in survivorship. In other words, animals that survive are those with traits that are adaptive to their environment.

Sexual selection, on the other hand, arises from interactions among individuals that compete for mating opportunities. Females often choose males on the basis of the morphological or behavioral characteristics they display. Natural selection and sexual selection often act in opposite directions on male traits favoring, for instance, drabber plumage (natural selection), on the one hand, and showier plumage (sexual selection) on the other.

Sexual selection has led to the evolution of extravagant sex-linked coloration, ornamentation, or behaviors with no apparent function in the struggle for survival. Such traits often are sexually dimorphic. Males tend to develop specific traits that are involved in courtship or mating and occur during the breeding season. In this instance, individual variation in these traits is sculpted by differences in reproductive success. The number of offspring an individual produces during its lifetime will determine whether this trait is continued in the species. Thus, "Sexual selection is responsible for most of the characters, morphological, physiological, and behavioral, that are observed as subserving the efficiency of the reproductive act as an important monitor of fitness."[186]

Darwin conceived of sexual selection as arising from aggressive interactions between males (male-male competition) and the female's selection of a mate (mate choice). Males compete among themselves for access to females. A variety of traits such as antlers, horns, and tusks have evolved as a result of male-male competition.

Aggression between males can have a direct effect on female reproduction. It will prevent other breeding males from having access to females (as in elephant seals[615]) or from harming the female (as in dung flies[796]). Aggression among males can also have an indirect effect. It can inhibit or suppress the normal reproductive physiology of the female, as occurs in green anole lizards (figure 6.4).

Mate selection may also be based on the availability of particular resources such as food. Thus, in many species, females choose real estate, and males compete to control access to that real estate.[790] For the purposes of this discussion, however, I will focus on mate choice by females and refer the reader to chapters 7 and 9 for a review of the causes and consequences of male-male aggression.

At least three competing variants of the natural selection hypothesis have been offered to explain the evolution of female preference,[584, 892] each of which emphasizes that females choosing optimally will produce young whose viability and survivorship are enhanced by the female's choice of mate. The "good genes" explanation suggests that females benefit by mating with particular

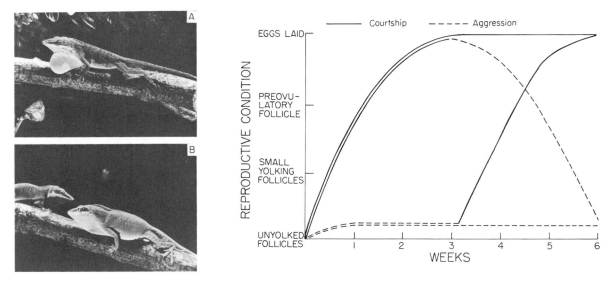

Figure 6.4 In the left panel are pictures of male green anole lizards performing a courtship display (*A*) and an aggressive display (*B*). Note the differences in body posture. The right panel shows how the courtship display facilitates ovarian growth in female green anoles, whereas the aggressive posture inhibits ovarian growth. In this experiment, females were exposed to the courtship or aggression stimulus for the entire 6 weeks or for 3 weeks first and then to the opposite stimulus for the next 3 weeks.

males having traits that enhance survivorship, thereby imparting these benefits to her young. In this case, the quality of the male's displays is assumed to reflect the individual male's genetic constitution. A second variant of the natural selection hypothesis is the "handicap principle," which postulates that females favor males with "expensive" traits. These are traits that put the male at greater risk of predation or have greater energetic cost. It is reasoned that males that can exhibit elaborate traits have a greater handicap and therefore must be better fit than males with less developed traits. Finally, a relatively recent variant is the "parasite load" idea. This idea is that brighter coloration or some other elaborate trait is associated with a genetic resistance to deleterious parasites. Thus, females choose brighter, more colorful males because this coloration indicates heritable disease resistance that can be passed on to their young. In all three forms of the natural selection hypothesis, male traits are regarded as being indicative of high genetic quality. Female preference is thought to evolve because of the advantages the female and her offspring acquire by mating with these males.

The sexual selection hypothesis has two main variants.[584, 892] One is Fisher's runaway sexual selection hypothesis. In this paradigm, male traits that influence mate choice become genetically correlated with female preference by virtue of the mating system. As the traits increase in frequency, the preference for the trait passively increases in the female. Thus, females do not gain directly from choosing particular males. Rather, the preference evolves as a correlated response to selection on the male trait.

A more recent variant of the sexual selection hypothesis that attempt to account for the evolution of female preferences is that of sensory exploitation. Ryan[892, 893] has pointed out that sensory systems are predisposed to specific stimuli. For example, as you will learn in chapter 7, the frog auditory system is tuned to certain frequencies and female *Xenopus* frogs prefer certain qualities in the call of males. The sensory exploitation hypothesis postulates that males have evolved calls to exploit the preexisting sensory biases in the female that themselves evolved for reasons independent of female choice.

The latter two hypotheses present different scenarios to explain evolution of behavior-controlling mechanisms. Fisher's runaway selection hypothesis presumes a genetic linkage between male traits and female preferences. Changes in the female are a passive function of change in the male. The sensory exploitation hypothesis predicts that preference in the female is determined by various constraints. Male behavior then has changed to maximize stimulation of the female's sensory systems. Whatever the evolutionary reason, the act of choosing the correct mate is of utmost importance. We will see how in birds the compatibility of mates has a dramatic effect on whether or not young are produced.

CONSTRAINTS ON REPRODUCTION

You have learned that sexual behavior in vertebrates is dependent on gonadal steroid hormones for its activation. However, as we will see, this conclusion stems primarily from the species that have been studied. It does not reflect a universal truth. Indeed, species differences in hormone-behavior relations often can be traced to adaptational responses to the physical and social environments. This is true because reproduction is constrained by (1) the immediate environment, (2) limitations inherent in developmental and physiological processes, and (3) evolutionary history.

Environmental Constraints   The evolution of reproductive seasons is determined by factors selecting against those individuals bearing young during times of food scarcity or other adverse environmental conditions. Individuals that produce young during optimum conditions have been favorably selected. In other words, these individuals were most likely to reproduce and pass on their genes to the next generation. This has been termed the *ultimate* cause of breeding seasons. Ultimate factors that determine the timing of breeding seasons include adequate food, availability of nesting materials, and predation pressure. *Proximate* causation refers to those stimuli used by the organism to actually initiate and terminate breeding. Well-known examples of proximate factors are seasonal fluctuations in day length, temperature, moisture, and so on. The responsiveness of the neuroendocrine system to proximate cues may vary seasonally. This seasonal variation probably reflects endogenous circadian and circannual rhythms and is discussed in chapter 16.

Environmental constraints on reproduction are especially severe when the environment is harsh. For animals living in a harsh environment there is only a brief favorable period for reproduction. Under these conditions, animals must respond rapidly and directly to physical changes in order to mate. The female must respond rapidly in order to reproduce. The young must grow sufficiently to survive the upcoming harsh conditions. These species exhibit an explosive or opportunistic pattern of reproduction in which all breeding activity is compressed into a few days or weeks.

Developmental and Physiological Constraints   Developmental and physiological processes may also constrain when animals breed. These processes can shape the mechanisms controlling reproduction. For example, mature sperm in most species cannot be produced in less than 6 weeks. Although some mice and ground squirrels can produce mature sperm in as little as 31 days, they appear to be the only exceptions to this rule. A similar time constraint applies to the production of eggs, although some small rodents are capable of generating eggs in less than 1 week. In cold-blooded vertebrates, it is common for egg maturation to take many months or even years.

A second constraint is the temperature-dependence of gonadal activity. Gamete production and steroid hormone secretion will not occur at cold temperatures. This presents a problem for many animals that live at high altitudes or in high latitudes. For these animals, mating must occur as early in the spring as possible so that the young can be born and grow enough to survive the next winter. Some species produce sperm during the summer and then store them through the winter. In this way, the male is able to inseminate females immediately on emergence from hibernation. In many bats, sperm storage lasts for several months, but in some reptiles it can last as long as 17 years.

In many mammals, including some species of bears, the western spotted skunk, and kangaroos, implantation of the embryo is delayed. The embryo goes into a kind of suspended animation called embryonic diapause that can last for as little as 1 week or as long as several years. At the end of diapause, the embryo implants and development resumes. In other species, particularly cold-blooded vertebrates, there simply is not enough time available in one season for gametes to grow, adults to mate, and the young to develop. Cold-blooded animals, or ectotherms, rely more on the external environment for temperature regulation, whereas mammals and birds, often called warm-blooded animals, or endotherms, rely on metabolic energy to produce and maintain an elevated body temperature. This can be an arbitrary distinction, however, because many ectotherms, such as honeybees and lizards, can maintain elevated body temperatures by behavioral means.

Warm-blooded animals living at high altitudes or latitudes typically migrate to warmer areas or hibernate for the duration of the cold months. In species that hibernate, such as small rodents, it was long a puzzle how males could enter hibernation with small testes but emerge with large testes. Recently, it has been discovered that animals such as turkish hamsters periodically arouse from hibernation, warming up for a few hours or days. It is during these arousals that the gonads grow. Cold-blooded animals living in extreme environments, however, do not exhibit periodic arousals, nor do they show any signs of gonadal growth during the cold winter months. In these animals, it is common for gamete growth and steroid secretion to be temporally dissociated from breeding activities.

Evolutionary History The evolutionary history, or phylogeny, of the species is another source of constraints predisposing the evolution of certain mechanisms and not others. Simply put, what has come before determines to a large extent what will follow. We might predict, therefore, that closely related species sharing a similar reproductive pattern but living in different environments will exhibit similarities in the neuroendocrine mechanisms underlying their modes of reproduction. An example of this can be found in garter snakes (*Thamnophis*), a large genus believed to have radiated into the New World after crossing the Bering Strait. All garter snake species that have been examined to date, even those living in Mexico, have a dissociated reproductive pattern and probably have the same neuroendocrine mechanisms controlling mating behavior. We might also predict that distantly related species living together and facing similar challenges would have similar neuroendocrine mechanisms controlling mating behavior. For example, most vertebrates that originated in the tropics but presently live in temperate regions exhibit an associated reproductive pattern. Thus, constraints imposed by both the external and internal environments of a species influence its social displays and their physiological consequences.

Survey of Diversity in Hormone-Behavior Relations

The Importance of Mate Compatibility

Stress can have a profound negative effect on reproduction. Crowding, social domination, and captivity can effectively inhibit reproduction. On the other hand, specific social conditions or behaviors can also stimulate reproduction. Research with species representing every vertebrate class has shown that certain behaviors are necessary for the proper stimulation of the physiological changes that must occur in reproduction. For example, in ring doves and green anole lizards (figure 6.4), the courtship behavior of the male is required if the ovaries of the female are to grow. Indeed, the rate of ovarian growth is determined by how much male courtship behavior the female sees. The male's aggressive behavior has the opposite effect and inhibits ovarian growth.[229]

So, making the correct choice of a mate can have a definite impact on a female's reproductive success. This is seen particularly well in long-lived species where it has been possible to monitor an individual's lifetime reproductive success. For example, for the past 35 years, Coulson has studied a colony of kittiwake gulls. These gulls nest on the windowsills of a riverside warehouse in Northumberland, England. In many instances, they pair for life. Other pairs of kittywakes, however, have a different mate the next breeding season. In about half of the pairs that break up, mates are changed because the original partner has died. In the other half, pairs of kittiwakes "divorce." The cause of divorce can be traced to the failure of the pair to hatch at least one egg the preceding year. Not only do successful pairs fledge more young, they also produce eggs faster, indicating that females in these pairs reach breeding condition earlier.[222, 1027]

Bluhm[126] has studied the reproductive consequences of pair incompatibility using canvasback ducks. The reproductive success of females that were allowed to stay with their self-chosen partner was compared with the reproductive success of females that were separated from their self-chosen partner and paired with another male chosen at random. The results were clear cut. Only females from pairs with self-selected males laid eggs. A similar situation is found in the cockatiel, in which reproductive success is enhanced if females are allowed to choose a mate as opposed to being forcibly paired with a male.[1123]

Bluhm has pioneered this exciting new area of research in behavioral endocrinology that includes the endocrine correlates of mate compatibility. She has found that the female canvasbacks from forced pairings lack specific hormone changes.[127] We know from research with other vertebrates, including humans, that copulation can trigger changes in circulating hormone levels, which can promote sperm transport and implantation. Courtship stimulation can result in more rapid ovarian growth in animals such as ring doves and green anole lizards. Thus, behavior-physiology interactions are an important aspect of neuroendocrine relations. You will learn more about this subject in chapter 7.

Mixed Reproductive Strategies

If environmental, physiological, and phylogenetic constraints can influence reproductive processes, it is likely that the neuroendocrine mechanisms controlling each of these processes must have undergone corresponding adaptations. What evidence is there for this?

First, recall the associated and dissociated reproductive patterns described earlier. Although we know a good deal about the neuroendocrinology of sexual behavior in species exhibiting associated reproductive patterns, we know next to nothing about these mechanisms in species exhibiting dissociated reproductive patterns. This deficit has occurred because scientists have concentrated almost exclusively on species which have associated reproductive patterns. Indeed, even in those species in which we know that gonadal growth is associated with mating, we often do not know whether it is the cause or the consequence of the mating behavior. The importance of this point cannot be underestimated. As you have already learned, in a variety of species mating can initiate gonadal activity in the female or in the male. In other species, copulatory stimuli are known to be responsible for the final stages of gamete development or for successful fertilization or implantation of the fertilized embryo.

Despite these shortcomings, it is possible to discern four basic reproductive strategies in vertebrates (table 6.2). In most domesticated species, both the

Table 6.2 Reproductive Strategies in Gonochoristic Vertebrates

Gonadal activity may be temporally associated or dissociated from mating behavior in each sex. The result is a reproductive strategy in which the sexes have the same or different reproductive patterns.

	MALE	
	Associated	*Dissociated*
FEMALE — *Dissociated*	Many laboratory and domesticated mammals; most birds; many temperate and tropical lizards, crocodilians	Most temperate turtles and tortoises, Indian lizard, timber rattle-snake, rough earthsnake; tiger salamander; pike
FEMALE — *Associated*	Musk shrew; Arctic fulmar; Mexican spiny lizard, Australian skink, mole skink, leaf-toed gecko, European viper, eastern coral snake; shiner perch, catfish	Hibernating bats; several rattlesnakes, cobra, and harmless North American snakes; plaice, common carp

male and the female have an associated reproductive pattern. There also are a number of species in which both sexes exhibit a dissociated reproductive pattern. Most exciting are the species in which the sexes exhibit a mixed reproductive strategies. In these species, one of two things can happen. The male can produce sperm before breeding and store them until mating ocurs. Alternatively, mating occurs, and the female stores the sperm in her reproductive tract for later use. In this instance, the act of mating initiates gonadal growth in the female.

These species that have mixed reproductive strategies hold great promise for untangling ecological and evolutionary forces on reproductive behavior. That is, in species exhibiting mixed reproductive strategies, the sexes must differ in fundamental ways in the organization and activation of behavior-controlling mechanisms. For example, Rissman[856] has shown how in the Asian musk shrew, mating behavior in the male coincides with testicular growth and is activated by increasing testicular androgen secretion. In the female, however, receptivity precedes ovarian growth and is independent of gonadal hormone control.

Mixed reproductive strategies can also be found within the same sex of a single species. A recent discovery suggests that individuals within a species may differ fundamentally in neuroendocrine-controlling mechanisms. For example, in several rodent species, researchers have found that individuals within a population may utilize different proximate cues for regulating gonadal activity. Photoperiod may be important in some individuals, whereas in others it may be temperature or food.[158] Individual differences in the required proximate cue can be adaptive, resulting in a fine-tuning of reproduction in the population in response to its environment.

A recent discovery in behavioral ecology is that individuals within a given population may adopt distinctly different physiologies, morphologies, or behaviors. These are termed alternative life-history strategies. These traits may be heritable, as is the case in bluegill sunfish. There are three types of male bluegill sunfish: a large colorful male that defends territories and solicits females, a small male that sneaks matings when the territorial male is otherwise occupied, and a large but drab male that mimics females in appearance.[444] The sneaker steals fertilizations by streaking in to release sperm as the female releases her eggs. The female mimics effectively insert themselves between a courting territorial male and the female he is courting; in this manner the female is courted by the male but it is the mimic that fertilizes the eggs. These alternative life-history strategies are heritable. Developmental and genetic studies indicate that sneakers grow up into female-mimics, whereas territorial males produce male young that are large and brightly colored. Circulating concentrations of androgens differ in the different types of male bluegill sunfish. Androgen concentrations are higher in territorial males than in sneaker or female-mimics.[579]

Many fish are hermaphroditic. Some have testicular and ovarian tissue simultaneously and trade behavioral roles during the spawning act (simultaneous hermaphrodites). Others undergo a sex change during life (sequential hermaphrodites). There are actually two types of sequential hermaphrodites. Some are first male and then female later in life (protandrous). Others are first female, then male (protogynous[274]). Recently, behavioral endocrinologists have begun to study these unusual reproductive systems. Cardwell's research focused on the stoplight parrotfish.[181, 182] There are two color phases in this protogynous species—a small, drab "initial" color phase and a large, bright "terminal" color phase. Most of the initial color phase individuals are female, but a few are males and practice the female-mimic strategy. All terminal color phase fish are males. The gonadal sex change from ovaries to testes is accompanied by other changes as well. Sex change is accompanied by a sharp decline in circulating concentrations of estradiol and an equally striking increase in plasma androgens. Interestingly, administration of androgens to functional females will induce the formation of testes and the coloration characteristic of terminal color phase males. Also, the terminal color phase males establish territories in the coral reef and actively patrol the borders, attacking any intruding terminal color phase males. The smaller, initial color phase males do not establish territories but do sneak matings.

Proximate Stimuli Activating Sexual Behavior

We know that for a number of vertebrates the steroid hormones secreted by the active gonads are necessary for sexual behavior. This elevated concentration of gonadal steroid hormones is required if proximate stimuli such as the behavior or scent of another individual or some change in the environment is to release sexual activity. In these animals, the sex hormones alter the perceptions of the individual, and stimuli take on new meanings.[93] Other organisms, however, have circumvented this reliance on gonadal steroid hormones. Instead, they rely solely on various proximate cues to activate sexual behavior. Here we will mention some examples of this by considering first the environment as a source of critical stimuli. We will then consider animals in which the behavior or tactile stimuli provided by members of the opposite sex initiate sexual behavior. Finally, we will learn how chemical signals, or pheromones, can trigger complex sexual behavior in vertebrates.

ENVIRONMENTAL STIMULI

If mating behavior can occur when the circulating concentrations of sex steroid hormones are low, does another stimulus activate sexual behavior? In species inhabiting extreme environments that are opportunistic breeders, the use of other stimuli is apparent. Physiological constraints have led to specific stimuli being co-opted as proximate triggers for sexual behavior. For example, in the desert-dwelling zebra finch, the male maintains mature sperm and high androgen levels throughout the year. Similarly, the female's ovaries contain developed ova at all times. In the deserts of western Australia, rain may occur only once in a 3-year period. The falling rain initiates reproductive behavior in the zebra finch. Within 10 minutes after rain begins falling, the zebra finch begins copulating. Nests are built within 4 hours. Eggs are laid within a week. Thus, although the androgen-dependence of sexual behavior in adult male zebra finches is well established,[35] androgens may play only a permissive role. That is, the ability of rainfall to activate sexual behavior depends upon the priming effect of androgen. This hypothesis remains to be tested experimentally. In all studies on the mating behavior of zebra finch, water has been freely available. It is likely, though, that the specialized adaptation to water in the zebra finch will be reflected in the neuroendocrine-controlling mechanisms.

SOCIAL STIMULI

Wingfield has shown that endocrine profiles associated with mating are specific to the social system of a number species of birds.[1106] This probably reflects important differences in the neuroendocrinology of these birds (figure 6.5). For example, in species of birds in which one male pairs with one female to help to feed its young (monogamy), the male exhibits only a brief period of high levels of testosterone when territories are being established in the spring. In species in which males pair with two or more females and do not help feed the offspring (polygyny), the male maintains high testosterone levels and remains aggressive throughout the breeding season. When testosterone was administered to males so that high testosterone levels were maintained, males from monogamous species became polygynous in their behavior.

CHEMICAL SIGNALS

Another example of diversity in hormone-behavior relations concerns the relationship between hormones and chemical signals or pheromones. Classically, the definition of hormones emphasizes internal communication while the definition of pheromones emphasizes external communication. This distinction is becoming blurred as scientists discover that some hormones may also func-

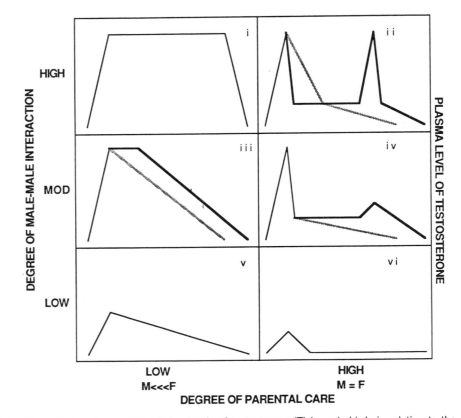

Figure 6.5 Theoretical patterns of circulating levels of testosterone (T) in male birds in relation to the degree of male-male interaction and the degree of parental care (feeding of young, brooding, and so on) provided by the male. The bold line indicates populations in which multiple broods are produced, whereas the light line indicates populations in which single broods are produced. Patterns where there are no distinctions between single and multiple brood populations are indicated by a single line. High male-male interaction and low parental care result in maximum levels of T (stippled line) throughout the breeding season, whereas low male-male interaction and high parental care result in a very low amplitude pattern of T. Note that in populations with multiple broods there may be second surges of T with varying amplitude with each clutch. Only two clutches are represented here, but in species that raise three or more clutches there may be three or more peaks of T. (Redrawn after Wingfield et al., 1990.[1106])

tion as pheromones. A well-known example is found in pigs.[948] Two metabolites of androgen play an integral part of the courtship and copulatory sequence (figure 6.6). As the boar faces the sow, he positions himself in front of her and forcefully breathes into her face. The air current picks up molecules of sex attractant secreted by submaxillary salivary glands in the mouth. This sex attractant has a distinctive odor. If the female is receptive, one whiff of the male will cause her to stand immobile, arching her back in lordosis, and allow the boar to mount and copulate. Application of this discovery to animal husbandry has resulted in the manufacture of an aerosol preparation containing these androgen metabolites called Boar Mate that is used to immobilize sows for artificial insemination.

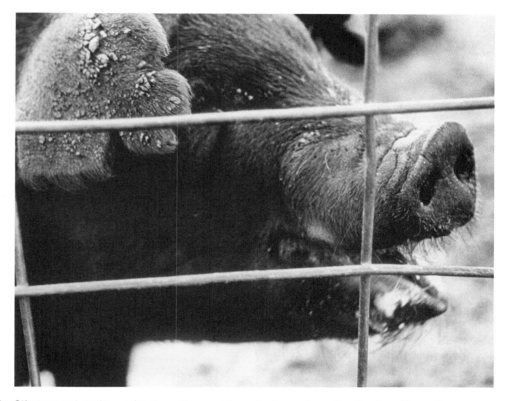

Figure 6.6 Olfactory and auditory stimuli are the most important cues to mating in pigs. Shown is a young, sexually mature Duroc boar salivating. The male typically investigates each female for estrus. On this day, none of the females was in estrus and thus the saliva was not so much as it can be. (Photo by J. McGlone.)

Another example of hormones serving as pheromones is found in goldfish (figure 6.7). Research by Sorenson and Stacey[978] has revealed that the female produces two hormones that have specific but separate actions on the physiology and behavior of the male. One hormone is a progestin produced by the preovulatory follicle. This hormone is involved in the final maturation and ovulation of the oocyte. It is also excreted into the water and has a profound influence on the male's endocrine physiology (figure 6.7). The presence of this hormone in the water leads to increased circulating concentrations of pituitary gonadotropins and testicular progestins, which in turn stimulate sperm production.

Another group of hormones found to activate species-specific reproductive behaviors are the prostaglandins. Administration of prostaglandins elicits female-typical spawning behavior in goldfish and other fishes with external fertilization.[978] During ovulation, prostaglandins are released and receptive behavior is stimulated in the female. In the water, prostaglandins then trigger sexual behavior in males.

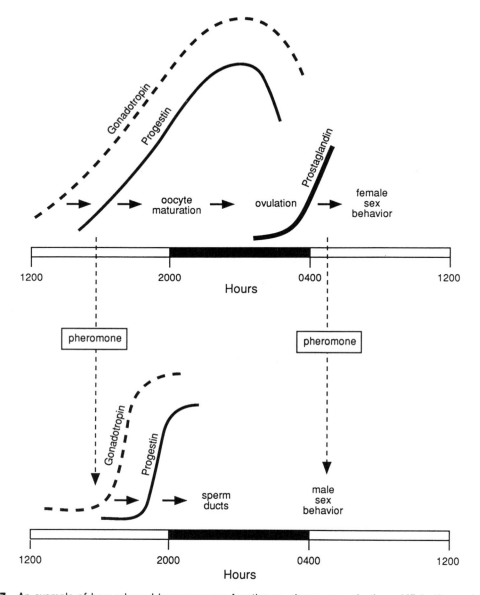

Figure 6.7 An example of how released hormones can function as pheromones. In the goldfish, the ovulating female sequentially releases two hormones with distinct pheromonal effects on male physiology and behavior. This dual pheromone system is set in motion when environmental cues (warm water temperature and appropriate spawning substrate) trigger a preovulatory surge of gonadotropin release from the pituitary. The gonadotropin surge rapidly stimulates ovarian follicle cells to synthesize a progestin, $17\alpha,20\beta$-dihydroxy-4-pregnen-3-one, which acts hormonally on the oocyte to promote maturation (resumption and completion of meiosis). When released to the water, this progestin acts through sensitive and specific male olfactory receptors to rapidly increase plasma gonadotropin, which in turn increases the numbers of sperm in the sperm ducts by stimulating testicular synthesis of this same progestin. Males that detect the progestin pheromone are believed to benefit by being able to release more sperm during the highly competitive spawning. When ovulation occurs, the presence of the oocytes in the reproductive tract stimulates synthesis of a prostaglandin, $PGF_{2\alpha}$, which triggers female spawning behavior. At the same time, the prostaglandin is released to the water and stimulates males to court the ovulated female.

It is of interest that in species with internal fertilization, prostaglandins have very different effects. For example, in crickets, lizards, garter snakes, and guinea pigs, prostaglandins stimulate rejection behavior and the loss of sexual receptivity. If prostaglandins are given to female or male tammar wallabies, a small kangaroo, they will crouch and behave as if they were giving birth.

Studies of fish hormonal pheromones may force us to reconsider some basic concepts of pheromonal function. For example, it is doubtful that the hormonal pheromone system of goldfish functions in true chemical "communication."[175] There is no evidence that the female chemical signal is either "specialized" or released in such a way as to increase female reproductive success directly. Rather, it appears more likely that goldfish hormonal pheromones function in "chemical spying" in a manner consistent with the sensory exploitation theory of sexual selection. In other words, males have evolved the ability to detect these chemicals in response to intense competition among males for access to ovulated females. Such chemical spying almost certainly represents an early stage of pheromonal evolution. This association would be expected to lead to chemical communication when the reproductive success of the signaler could be increased by increasing the efficiency of signaling.

We have sampled just a portion of the diversity in hormone-behavior relations found in animals. Regardless of the mechanics of reproduction, coordination of individuals leads to a synchronization of reproductive processes. This is true even in species that do not reproduce sexually. Particularly in birds and mammals, freedom of choice of a mate is an essential element in successful reproduction. It is evident from this survey that males and females can vary in ways other than producing sperm or eggs. When in relation to mating the gametes are produced and whether they are stored or used immediately varies according to the constraints outlined earlier. Males and females need not respond to these pressures in the same way. This conclusion is clearly is evident in species in which one sex exhibits an associated reproductive pattern and the other sex has a dissociated reproductive pattern. Comparative studies reveal that the "exceptional cases" are less rare and more widespread than is generally realized. Finally, the trigger for sexual behavior can vary from species to species. In some it is a change in a particular physical factor in the environment such as rainfall or even the color green signifying new growth in the vegetation. In other species it can be the sight, sound, or smell of other individuals. In these instances, hormones are affecting the perceptions of the individual.

Insights into the Evolution of the Processes and Mechanisms of Reproduction

An Animal Model System for the Study of the Hormone Independence of Courtship Behavior

As discussed in chapter 1, Berthold demonstrated in 1849 that the testes of the rooster produced a chemical that dramatically changed the animal's behavior.

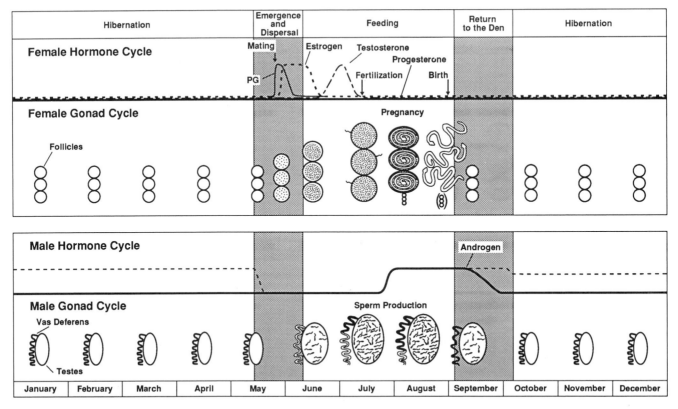

Figure 6.8 The major physiological and behavioral events in the annual reproductive cycle of the red-sided garter snake in Canada. Animals spend most of the year underground. In the spring, they emerge and mate before dispersing to summer feeding grounds. In the female, mating initiates gonadal growth as well as changes in the hormone profile of the female. Young are born in late summer. Since all metabolic processes slow down during the cold months, androgen levels in the male will be elevated in the spring if he entered hibernation with elevated levels (dotted lines); however, androgen levels usually are basal on emergence (solid line). Sperm are produced during the summer after mating and are stored in the vas deferens (heavy squiggle line next to testis) during the winter.

Since that experiment, there have been thousands of studies on a variety of vertebrate species that have yielded similar results. The consistency of the data has led many to presume that mating behavior in all vertebrates is activated by gonadal steroid hormones. Here the dissociated reproductive pattern provides us with a natural experiment. In the red-sided garter snake, a basic conflict between environmental and physiological constraints has created novel neuroendocrine mechanisms.

The red-sided garter snake is found in the northern United States and in Manitoba, Canada. In this region winters are usually severe, and the snakes may spend as long as 9 months in hibernation in subterranean limestone caverns (figure 6.8). With the spring thaw, the animals emerge, and there is a brief 3- to 4-week breeding season. After this there is a summer feeding phase that can last 2 to 3 months. During this time the females also gestate and give birth. Beginning in late August, animals begin returning to the caverns from which they emerged the previous spring.

Emergence from winter dormancy in the spring is stimulated by increasing ambient temperatures. Males emerge *en masse* while the females emerge singly beginning about 1 week later (figure 6.9). As each female emerges, males in the immediate vicinity approach her. A pheromone on the female's back elicits a vigorous response in the male called "chin-rubbing." Chin-rubbing consists of the male coursing up and down the back of the female rapidly and repeatedly with his chin, all the time rapidly flicking his tongue on the female's back. The male next aligns his body along the female's and attempts to intromit a hemipenis. (All male lizards and snakes have two penises rather than one and alternate their use in successive matings.) Since one hundred or more males may be attracted to a single female, a writhing mass of snakes results called a "mating ball" (figure 6.9). After the female mates, usually with only one of the males, she immediately leaves the den area. Approximately 3 weeks after the first emergence, virtually all of the females have emerged from hibernation, and the intensity of male courtship wanes. Males then leave the area and disperse to their feeding grounds, not to return until the fall when the weather cools. The animals return to the den from which they had emerged the preceding spring.

All of these events can be duplicated in the laboratory simply by cooling animals in the fall to 2° to 4°C and maintaining them at this temperature for 12 to 17 weeks. In the laboratory, male courtship initially is intense but also wanes 3 to 4 weeks following emergence. Only prolonged periods of cold temperatures can restimulate male behavior. Indeed, captive males will never again exhibit this same intense and synchronous courtship behavior unless they are hibernated.

Males emerge from hibernation with regressed testes and epididymides enlarged with stored sperm (figure 6.8). The sperm that a male uses in mating were produced during a testicular growth cycle the previous summer. In the adult male, spermatogenesis begins about 6 weeks after emergence in the spring and continues for 10 to 12 weeks. Associated with spermatogenesis is an increase in the circulating concentrations of androgens. Testicular collapse occurs when males return to begin hibernation. If the winter is early, they may enter hibernation while androgen levels are still elevated. If the androgen titer is high in the fall, it will be elevated initially on emergence in the spring due to the slow metabolic clearance rates during hibernation.

Females also emerge with regressed ovaries and low serum estrogen. Unlike sperm, mature ova cannot be stored successfully over winter. Females are attractive and receptive, however, on emergence and quickly mate. As soon as the female mates, she becomes unattractive and unreceptive to males. Mating also stimulates a neuroendocrine reflex that culminates in ovarian growth and ovulation 6 weeks later. Immediately after mating, or perhaps initiated during copulation, there is a significant rise in circulating concentration of prostaglandins. This is followed shortly by a surge in the circulating concentrations of

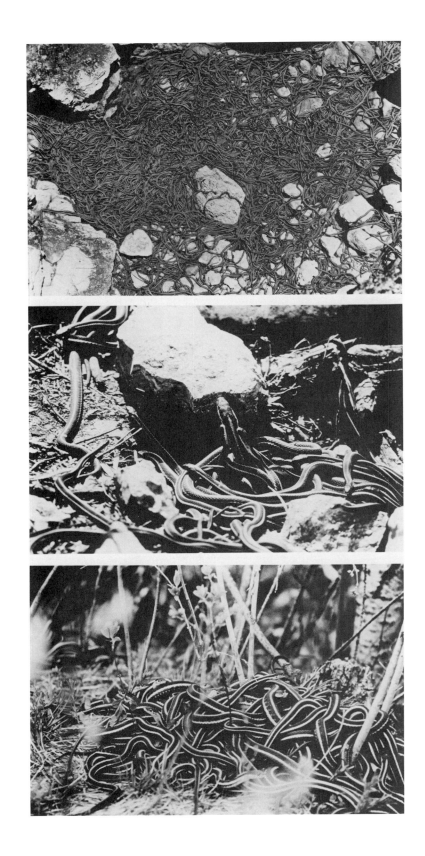

estrogen, which remains elevated for several days before declining to basal level. Estrogens remain low until 3 to 6 weeks later, when the ovarian follicles enlarge.

This mating-induced neuroendocrine reflex is essential for ovulation (figure 6.10). Specific sensory stimulation received during mating initiates this neuroendocrine reflex. It begins with the male's intromission into the female's cloaca. (The word *cloaca* in Latin means "sewer," referring to the fact that in all vertebrates except mammals there is a single urogenital opening.) Anesthetization of the cloaca or spinal cord prior to coplation prevents the transmission of sensory information essential for the reflex.

A question that immediately comes to mind is how can red-sided garter snakes mate when their gonads are regressed and sex steroid hormone concentrations are low? Experiments indicate that the neuroendocrine mechanisms controlling reproduction in the red-sided garter snake are different from those of more commonly studied species that mate when their gonads are fully active. What has been established to date is that so long as males have undergone a period of low-temperature dormancy, they will display courtship behavior on emergence into warm temperatures and in the presence of an attractive female. Further, removal of the testes, adrenals, or even the pituitary will not prevent males from courting when they emerge. Similarly, treatment with androgen will not prevent the waning of chin-rubbing behavior 3 to 4 weeks after emergence nor will it induce courtship in males during the summer months. Taken together, these data indicate that adult male red-sided garter snakes possess a neuroendocrine mechanism controlling courtship behavior that does not rely on the activational effects of sex steroid hormones.

Like the sunfish discussed earlier, male garter snakes have alternative life-history strategies. The majority of male red-sided garter snakes court only females and never are themselves courted by other males. This discrimination is based on sex-typical pheromones. Females typically produce one pheromone, while males typically produce another (figure 6.11). However, in approximately 16% of the mating balls in a season, a male is the object of courtship. These individuals are termed "she-males." The more typical males are called "he-males." The she-males produce the female-typical attractiveness pheromone and have a competitive advantage in the mating ball. In experiments in which 20 he-males and one she-male were placed in an arena with an unmated female, the she-male mated with the female significantly more often than did the he-males. This mating advantage perhaps results from the she-male con-

Figure 6.9 Emergence of male red-sided garter snakes at hibernaculum entrance during the spring. Top panel, Males emerge first and en masse. Middle panel, Females then emerge singly over a 3-week period, resulting in the formation of mating balls. The female is the individual with the large head in the center of the figure; the rest are courting males. In garter snakes, the females are about three times larger than males. Unlike the situation in most mammals, the testes inhibit body growth in male garter snakes. Bottom panel, A mating ball of red-sided garter snakes. There is only one female present, the rest of the snakes are males.

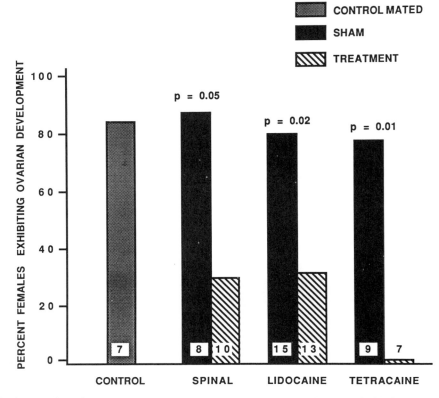

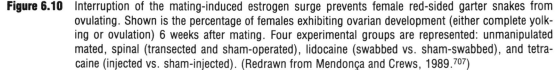

Figure 6.10 Interruption of the mating-induced estrogen surge prevents female red-sided garter snakes from ovulating. Shown is the percentage of females exhibiting ovarian development (either complete yolking or ovulation) 6 weeks after mating. Four experimental groups are represented: unmanipulated mated, spinal (transected and sham-operated), lidocaine (swabbed vs. sham-swabbed), and tetracaine (injected vs. sham-injected). (Redrawn from Mendonça and Crews, 1989.[707])

fusing the other he-males in the mating ball, causing them to ignore the female and court him. That is, in the mass confusion of the mating ball, the she-male is confronted with a single source of the attractiveness pheromone, whereas the he-males are confronted with two sources.

She-males are genetically male. They have fully functional testes and accessory sex structures. They court and mate with females. She-males do not even differ significantly from he-males in length and weight. She-males differ from he-males by producing the pheromones characteristic of adult females but not the pheromones that are characteristic of males. She-males are also different in their endocrine physiology. He-males have testosterone-to-estrogen ratios of 94:1 compared to the female ratio of 3:100. The testosterone-to-estrogen ratio of she-males is about 250:1 (more than 2.5 times that of he-males and more than 3,000 times that of females). This may seem paradoxical at first. However, we recently found that she-males have high levels of an enzyme in their skin. This enzyme converts testosterone to estrogen, a hormone known in females to stimulate production and release of the attractiveness pheromone.

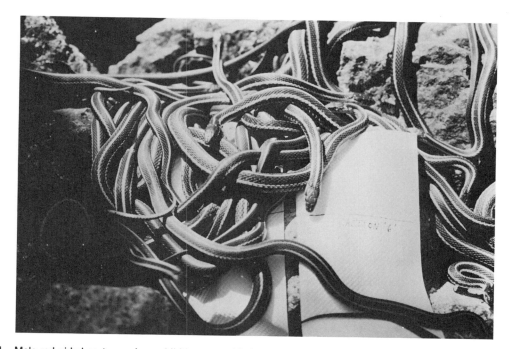

Figure 6.11 Male red-sided garter snakes exhibiting courtship behavior to chemical cues placed on paper towels. Three pheromones control garter snake mating behavior: a female "attractiveness" pheromone that is a methyl ketone, a male "identification" pheromone that is squalene, and a mating "inhibition" pheromone whose identity is still unknown. In this picture, the left paper towel has the synthesized female attractiveness pheromone while the right paper towel contains the solvent only. Tests were conducted by placing the paper towels in the den where courting male garter snakes had access to them. (From Mason et al., 1989.[671])

Interestingly, while administration of estrogen to adult males causes them to produce and carry the attractiveness pheromone in their blood, they do not release it onto the skin surface, and adult males treated with estrogen are not courted. Presumably, this reflects a sex difference in the skin. In the she-males, the high levels of aromatase may convert testosterone to estrogen in the skin, causing production or release of the female-typical attractiveness pheromone.

Chin-rubbing behavior in the male red-sided garter snake is elicited by the tongue-flick delivery of the attractiveness pheromones. One particular area of the brain, the anterior hypothalamus-preoptic area (POA) appears to be involved in the display of chin-rubbing behavior. If the POA is lesioned in males shortly after they have emerged, they will stop courting. Even if the lesions are produced before entering hibernation, males with damage in the POA will not court. The deficits in courtship behavior that result following lesions of the POA are not due to the destruction of hormone-concentrating neurons in the POA. We know this because courtship behavior is not activated by increased concentrations of testicular androgens. Therefore, the role of the POA in chin-rubbing behavior (and copulation?) and the mechanism that triggers the behavior remain to be determined.

The fact that sex steroid hormones do not appear to play a role in the activation of courtship behavior of male garter snakes does not mean they play no role at all. As explained in chapters 3 to 5, in species exhibiting an associated reproductive tactic sex steroid hormones are important both in the adult and during development. Indeed, developmental experiments with male red-sided garter snakes indicate that the seasonal surge in testicular androgens primes the neural mechanisms underlying chin-rubbing behavior.[233] The priming with androgens allows courtship behavior to be triggered by a specific environmental cue—the spring shift in temperature—rather than by a surge in sex steroid hormones.

Why do male garter snakes stop courting females about 1 month after emergence from hibernation? This decline in courtship behavior is not due to the males becoming used to females. Males that have had daily exposure to females exhibit courtship behavior equal to that of males kept isolated after emergence and only later tested with attractive females. The answer may lie in the natural sequence of events. Even after spending many months without food, recently emerged male red-sided garter snakes do not feed. This is not due to a lack of food, because males refuse food even if it is offered. Females, on the other hand, begin to feed soon after they emerge and leave the den areas. Males leave the den to forage for food 3 to 4 weeks after emergence, at the same time courtship begins to decline. The remainder of the summer is spent feeding. Males do not court attractive females during the summer feeding phase. This voluntary abstinence from food is common in species inhabiting marginal habitats. In ground squirrels, pinnipeds, Emperor penguins, the arctic fulmar, and the red-sided garter snake, feeding and mating behaviors are mutually exclusive events in at least one of the sexes.

We have seen how environmental and endocrine factors influence specific reproductive functions and behaviors in the red-sided garter snake. Some conclusions that can be drawn include the following: (1) Gonadal growth and sexual behavior are not necessarily temporally associated, (2) sexual behavior can occur independent of gonadal steroid hormones, and (3) the initiation, maintenance, and termination of sexual behavior are independent of each other and are controlled by different cues.

An Animal Model System for the Study of the Evolution of the Neuroendocrine Control of Sex-Typical Behaviors

Most whiptail lizard species are gonochoristic, having both male and female individuals that reproduce sexually. However, one-third of the 45 species of whiptail lizards are unisexual, consisting only of individuals that reproduce by true parthenogenesis. We know that the parthenogenetic species arose fully formed from the hybrid mating of two sexual whiptail species. Indeed, in many instances, we know which species were involved. For example, the parthenogen, *Cnemidophorus uniparens*, arose from the hybrid union of *C. inorna-*

tus and *C. burti*. Furthermore, we know that *C. inornatus* is the maternal ancestor of *C. uniparens* and *C. burti* is the paternal ancestor.

Unisexual vertebrates may be particularly useful to the behavioral endocrinologist interested in evolution. These species allow the investigator to study brain-behavior evolution in a manner impossible with conventional species. This is true because, in one sense, parthenogenetic whiptail lizards and their related sexual species represent a "snapshot" of evolution. This allows us to compare the neuroendocrine mechanisms that control reproductive behaviors in the descendant species with those of the ancestral species. This ability in turn allows us to address two fundamental issues from a new perspective: First, do the neural circuits that subserve male-typical and female-typical sexual behaviors differ or are they similar? Second, how might the cellular mechanisms that control sexual behaviors have evolved?

As pointed out earlier, reproductive behaviors tend to be unambiguous, characteristic of the species, and critical to the individual's reproductive and evolutionary success. In 1978 we made the serendipitous observation that unisexual whiptail lizards exhibit behaviors remarkably similar to the courtship and copulatory behaviors of related sexual species (figure 6.12). In gonochoristic whiptail lizards the male approaches and investigates the female with his bifid (split) tongue, an action that presumably indicates involvement of chemical senses. If the female is sexually receptive, she stands still for the male, allowing him to mount her back. Usually just before the male mounts the female, he grips with his jaws either a portion of the skin on the female's neck or her foreleg. As the male rides the female, he scratches her sides and presses her body against the substrate. The male then begins to maneuver his tail beneath the female's tail, attempting to appose their cloacal regions. During mating, one of two hemipenes is intromitted into the female's cloaca. With intromission, the male shifts his jaw-grip from the female's neck to her pelvic region, thereby assuming a contorted copulatory posture I have termed the *doughnut*. This posture is maintained for 5 to 10 minutes, after which the male rapidly dismounts and leaves the female.*

---

* The fundamental difference between sexual and unisexual organisms makes it important to have subtle but necessary semantic rules. (1) Strictly speaking, it is inaccurate to refer to "male sexual behavior" (i.e., mounting and intromission behavior) and "female sexual behavior" (i.e., receptive behavior). Each individual usually displays those behaviors characteristic of its gonadal sex (or homotypical behaviors) but has the capacity to exhibit behaviors characteristic of the opposite gonadal sex (or heterotypical behaviors). Thus, it is more accurate to refer to male-typical and female-typical sexual behaviors. (2) Although parthenogenetic whiptails have only ovaries and lack male genitalia, it is not appropriate to refer to them as females. The term female only has meaning in the context of "male." (3) Parthenogenetic whiptails exhibit behaviors seen commonly in sexually active male whiptails during mating. These I term pseudosexual behaviors. Since male-typical and female-typical sexual behaviors can only refer to those behavioral displays associated with males and females in gonochoristic species (e.g., intromission and receptive behaviors, respectively), it is not appropriate to use this terminology when describing the pseudosexual behaviors of parthenogenetic species. Therefore, because two sexes usually do not occur in unisexual organisms, the terms male-like and female-like rather than male-typical and female-typical are used to refer to the appropriate pseudosexual behaviors.

C. inornatus   *C. uniparens*

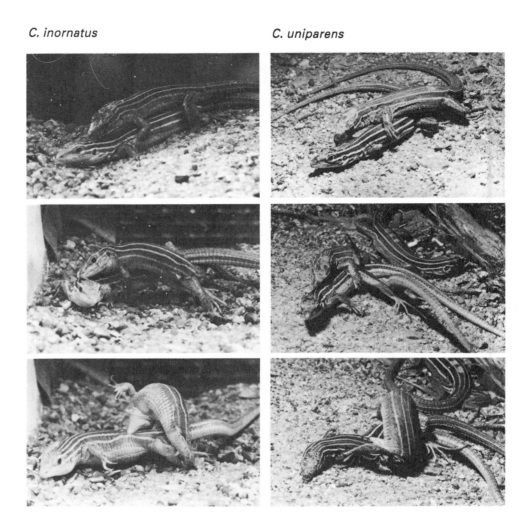

Figure 6.12 Mating sequence (left) in the gonochoristic whiptail lizard, *Cnemidophorus inornatus*, the maternal ancestor to the parthenogenetic whiptail, *C. uniparens*. Pseudosexual behavior (right) the all-female parthenogenetic whiptail lizard *C. uniparens*. Note the similarity in the behavioral sequence to that of its gonochoristic ancestor. (From Crews, 1987.[232])

This same sequence of events is observed in at least five species of unisexual whiptail lizards (see figure 6.12). That is, one individual will approach and mount another individual and, after riding for a few minutes, the mounting (male-like) individual will swing its tail beneath that of the mounted (female-like) individual, apposing the cloacal regions. At the same time, the mounting individual will shift its jaw-grip from the neck to the pelvic region of the mounted individual, forming the doughnut posture. Since parthenogens are morphologically female, there are no hemipenes, and intromission does not occur.

How do we know whether pseudosexual behavior in a unisexual lizard is not just a trivial discovery? (Every scientist should ask themselves this kind of question whenever an unusual behavior or phenomenon is discovered.) First, we know that pseudosexual behavior is not peculiar to *C. uniparens*. Pseudosexual behavior has been observed in at least five other species of parthenogenetic whiptail lizards as well as in the parthenogenetic morning gecko. Furthermore, behaviors similar to pseudosexual behavior have been described in other unisexual or asexual vertebrate and invertebrate species.[230] So this is not an isolated occurrence of the behavior. Second, pseudosexual behavior facilitates ovarian development. Studies show that parthenogens are more likely to lay eggs and will lay more clutches if they engage in pseudosexual behavior.[234, 448] This fact indicates that the behavior has an adaptive function. Is pseudosexual behavior simply the result of the development of parthenogenesis? If this were true, one would not expect females of sexually reproducing species to exhibit male-typical behaviors nor males to exhibit female-typical behaviors. This clearly is not the case. Females mounting or males allowing mounting are normal parts of sexual activity in many species. Importantly, females of the ancestral species *C. inornatus* have been observed to mount other females. Thus, pseudocopulatory behavior is not a newly evolved trait in unisexual whiptails. Rather, the neural circuits underlying these behaviors have been retained from their sexual ancestral. This reflects, in part, the brain organization of the vertebrate behaviors.

Could pseudosexual behavior be a function of captivity? Is this an unusual behavior induced by the stress of the laboratory? If this were the case, we would not expect *C. uniparens* to reproduce at normal levels in the laboratory. Reproduction is an extremely complex process that is sensitive to the organism's environment. Even slight perturbations in certain variables can result in captive animals failing to reproduce, a fact evident in great abundance in many zoos. In my laboratory, however, both unisexual and sexual whiptail lizards reproduce as frequently as do animals in nature. That is, they typically lay three clutches of eggs each containing 3 to 4 eggs during the course of a reproductive season. Also, it is clear that stress does occur in these animals, as evidenced by the fact that in cages containing three or four individuals, there always is one dominant individual who reproduces, and one subordinate individual who fails to reproduce. Finally, it is common in the laboratory to see behaviors not observed in nature. For example, female-female mounting behavior in *C. uniparens* has been observed in the field only once in 13 years of research, and even then not by me! In this same period, however, I have seen only one mating of a sexual whiptail species. The difficulty of observing certain behaviors in nature is not restricted to whiptail lizards. For example, Mount[764] states, "I never witnessed sexual activity among red-tailed skinks in the field, although I spent many hours at the height of the mating season in areas where the skinks were abundant." (p. 370) He goes on to speculate: "This fact may be correlated with the prolonged duration of copula. In many small lizards, if not most, this period lasts no longer than 3 to 5 minutes. Probably, individuals so engaged are considerably more vulnerable to attack by predators than if they are separate and foraging. This would be especially true if mating took place in relatively exposed places. Perhaps (skinks), then, normally mate in sheltered situations such as the burrows and passageways constructed by (tortoises)." Still, there is indirect evidence that pseudocopulation occurs in nature. As in copulation, the jaw-grip of the mounting individual leaves skin abrasions that scar. This characteristic mark is found in nature on both unisexuals and in females of the sexual species.[238]

Why do parthenogenetic whiptails display mounting behavior? Do these animals have high levels of male-typical androgens when displaying male-like behavior? No. Radioimmunoassay of the circulating androgens revealed uniformly undetectable plasma concentrations at all stages of the reproductive cycle. Not only is there no evidence of transient surges in these androgens during the course of the ovarian cycle, but postovulatory animals exhibiting male-like pseudosexual behavior are no more likely to have detectable androgens than are preovulatory parthenogens exhibiting female-like pseudosexual behavior. Also, the nature and pattern of sex steroid hormone secretions in females of the sexual species and the parthenogens are virtually identical. Taken together this indicates that the evolution of parthenogenesis has *not* been accompanied by an alteration of the usual pattern of endocrine changes.

The reproductive cycles of both female sexual whiptails and unisexual whiptails are very similar. Each consists of a series of three to four discrete ovarian cycles 3 to 4 weeks long. The ovaries simultaneously ovulate from one to three eggs each. After ovulation, the ova pass into the oviducts, where shell deposition occurs. Shelled eggs are usually laid 7 to 10 days after ovulation. Production of the next clutch may be initiated within several days of egg-laying.

The temporal patterns of ovarian hormone secretion also are remarkably similar in the ancestral and descendant species. In both, the circulating concentrations of estradiol increase as the follicle grows, peaking around the time of ovulation (figure 6.13). Progesterone levels begin to increase during the latter stages of follicular maturation but are at their peak after the time of ovulation. In both female whiptails and parthenogenetic whiptails, circulating concentrations of androgens are uniformly low and are not detectable by radioimmunoassay.

Female *C. inornatus* are receptive to the courtship displays of the male only in the vitellogenic or yolking stage. Females are highly aggressive to courting males prior to ovulation or during pregnancy. Removal of the ovaries abolishes sexual receptivity, whereas estradiol replacement therapy restores receptivity. Interestingly, postovulatory female *C. inornatus* have been observed to exhibit the heterotypical or male-typical sexual behavior, and there is some evidence that progesterone stimulates female-female mounting.

Pseudosexual behavior in parthenogenetic whiptails is also related to ovarian state. Female-like receptive behavior is limited to the preovulatory stage of the follicular cycle, whereas expression of male-like mounting behavior occurs most frequently during the postovulatory stages of the cycle (figure 6.13). These behavioral roles during pseudocopulations in the unisexual species are paralleled by differences in the circulating levels of sex steroid hor-

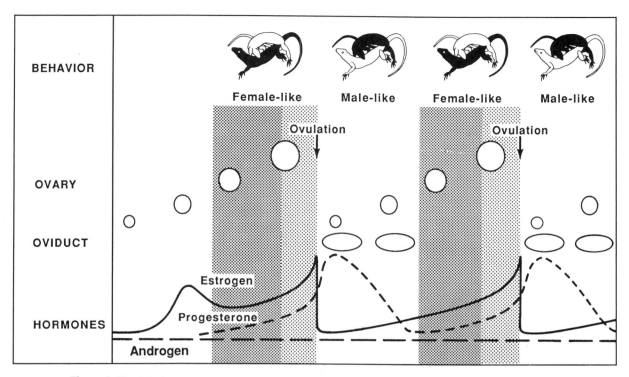

Figure 6.13 Relation among male-like and female-like pseudosexual behavior. ovarian state, and circulating concentrations of sex steroid hormones during different stages of the reproductive cycle of parthenogenetic *Cnemidophorus uniparens*. The transition from receptive to mounting behavior occurs at the time of ovulation (arrow). (Redrawn from Crews, 1987.[232])

mones. That is, individuals show primarily female-like behavior during the preovulatory stage when estradiol concentrations are relatively high and progesterone relatively low. Just the opposite is seen during the display of male-like behavior in the postovulatory phase, when concentrations of estradiol are low and concentrations of progesterone have increased.

We believe that pseudocopulatory behaviors in unisexual whiptails are triggered by ovarian hormones. In support of this idea, pseudocopulatory behaviors have never been observed in reproductively inactive or ovariectomized individuals. This means that in the absence of hormones pseudocopulatory behavior does not occur. In addition, female-like behavior is almost completely restricted to the yolk deposition phase. Male-like behavior, on the other hand, is most frequent in postovulatory or pregnant animals. Also, individuals alternate female-like and male-like pseudosexual behaviors as they progress through the ovarian cycles during the course of the breeding season. Of course, it is necessary to demonstrate that replacing the appropriate hormones will trigger pseudocopulatory behaviors to establish this relationship unequivocally.

The transition from female-like to male-like pseudosexual behavior apparently occurs when hormone concentrations in the blood are changing. At ovulation, estradiol concentrations decrease, and progesterone concentrations increase (figure 6.13). Is it possible that this shift in hormone concentrations plays a crucial role in controlling the expression of pseudosexual behavior? To test this, animals were ovariectomized and then treated with progesterone, estradiol, or a sham (control) operation. The results were clear cut. Pseudocopulations occurred only in pairs in which both individuals were treated with hormones but in a complementary fashion. In other words, animals treated with estradiol exhibited the female-like role, and the progesterone-treated parthenogen assumed the male-like role. In the absence of the appropriate hormones, pseudosexual behavior was not exhibited.

Unisexual vertebrates enable us to address this fundamental question of the neural basis of sex-typical behaviors from a new perspective. The idea that there are dual neural circuits in the brain of all vertebrates, one mediating mounting and intromission behavior and the other mediating receptive behavior, is not new. Researchers have long commented on males that exhibited female-typical sexual behaviors or, conversely, females that exhibited male-typical sexual behaviors. The bulk of modern research, however, has focused on the neuroendocrine mechanisms controlling homotypical behaviors, namely, mounting behavior in gonadal males and receptive behaviors in gonadal females. In other words, each neural circuit has been studied extensively but almost always in isolation from its complement. The parthenogenetic whiptails allow us to study these circuits operating together. Comparison studies will indicate allow us to say what is common to both and what is specific to each.

An opportunity to study sexually dimorphic dual neural circuits together in the same individual is provided in the whiptail lizards. We have found complementary sexual dimorphisms in two hypothalamic regions of the ancestral species *C. inornatus* (figures 6.14 and 6.15). The POA is larger in males than in females, whereas the ventromedial hypothalamus (VMH) is larger in females than in males. Other research has shown that the POA is involved in mounting behavior whereas the VMH controls sexual receptivity, as is true for rodents and other mammals (see chapters 3 and 4).

The brain of the all-female parthenogen is more similar to the female than to the male of its sexual ancestor (figures 6.14 and 6.15). However, implantation of androgens into the POA elicits mounting behavior in both bisexual and unisexual whiptails. Implants of androgens into the VMH fail to elicit mount-

Figure 6.14 Sexual dimorphisms in two hypothalamic areas in three representative whiptail lizards: male *C. inornatus* (top), female *C. inornatus* (middle), and *C. uniparens* (bottom). Presented are photomicrographs of coronal brain sections at comparable levels of the preoptic area (POA, left) and the ventromedial hypothalamus (VMH, right). Drawings are made on the mirror image and trace the perimeter used at that level for size measurement. Selected areas used as landmarks are abbreviated as follows: LFB, lateral forebrain bundle; M, medial POA; L, lateral POA; OC, optic chiasm; PH, periventricular region of the hypothalamus. The arrow points to the subcommissural organ. The OC was detached from the brain of the photographed male *C. inornatus* (top left). The LFB of this animal was lateral to the region included in the figure. (From Crews et al., 1990.)

AH - POA

VMH

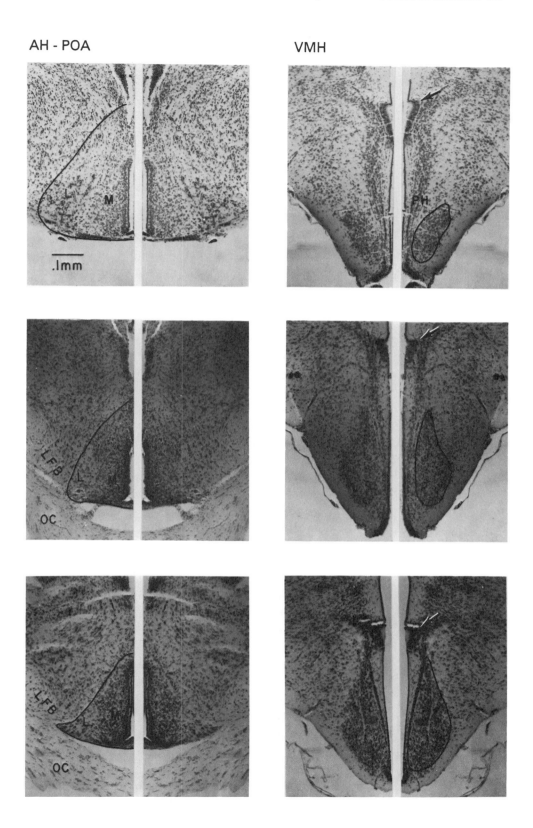

AH-POA/SVL   VMH/SVL

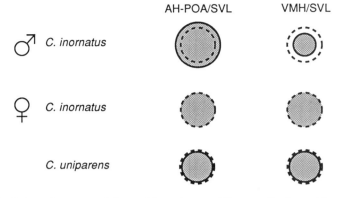

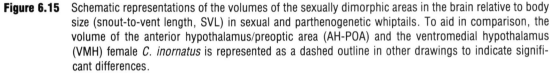

Figure 6.15 Schematic representations of the volumes of the sexually dimorphic areas in the brain relative to body size (snout-to-vent length, SVL) in sexual and parthenogenetic whiptails. To aid in comparison, the volume of the anterior hypothalamus/preoptic area (AH-POA) and the ventromedial hypothalamus (VMH) female *C. inornatus* is represented as a dashed outline in other drawings to indicate significant differences.

ing behavior and have no effect on receptive behavior. Conversely, implantation of estrogen in the VMH activates receptivity in both species, but estrogen implants in the POA have no effect on receptive or mounting behavior. Thus, the parthenogen clearly retains the ability to express male-like behaviors. It does so not because it has developed a masculinized POA but because it has apparently coopted a naturally occurring progesterone surge to trigger the masculine behavioral potential remaining in a feminized brain.

How have the cellular mechanisms subserving sexual behaviors evolved? Again, unisexual organisms provide an unusual opportunity for study. In all instances, with the single exception of blue-green algae, parthenogenetic species arose from gonochoristic species. In the case of whiptail lizards, we even know the species responsible. This allows us to compare the ancestral and descendant species to discover how the mechanisms regulating behavior might have changed. Specifically, did the progesterone activation of male-like pseudosexual behavior in the parthenogen evolve from a sexual species in which male-typical sexual behavior was androgen-dependent?

Whiptail lizards are seasonal breeders, with male *C. inornatus* courting and copulating only during the spring and early summer months. At this time, the circulating concentrations of androgens in males are elevated. The circulating concentrations of progesterone during this period are low and unchanging. Estradiol is undetectable. As in other vertebrates exhibiting an associated reproductive pattern, the courtship and copulatory behaviors of the male *C. inornatus* depend upon testicular steroid hormones. Castrated males court females significantly less often than do intact, sexually active males, and, as expected, treatment of castrates with exogenous androgens reinstates courtship and copulatory behaviors. However, administration of exogenous progesterone also *restores* the complete repertoire of sexual behavior in about one-third of castrated males. Indeed, these progesterone-sensitive males actively court and copulate with females with an intensity equal to that shown by castrates treated with androgen. While not all exogenous androgen-sensitive males are sensitive to progesterone, all progesterone-sensitive individuals are sensitive to both progesterone and exogenous androgens, suggesting that progesterone-sensitive males are a subset of exogenous androgen-sensitive males.

It is always possible that progesterone is being converted to another hormone or metabolite to produce the results described above. To test whether progesterone was acting directly to activate mounting behavior, we used various ligands, or synthetic agonists and antagonists that bind to the hormone receptors. In mammals, R5020 acts as an agonist and simulates the effect of progesterone at its receptor, whereas RU486 acts as an antagonist and prevents receptor activation. In castrated male *C. inornatus*, administration of R5020 stimulates sexual behavior in a similar proportion of castrated males as does progesterone, whereas RU486 prevents sexual behavior in castrated, progesterone-treated males. Since R5020 and RU486 cannot be converted to a progesterone metabolite, these experiments suggest that progesterone may be exerting its stimulatory action (1) as a progestin, not through conversion to other sex steroid hormones, and (2) through progesterone receptors and not through androgen receptors.

These findings are exciting for at least two reasons: First, the behavioral effects of progesterone are opposite those found in studies performed with domesticated rodents and birds. In these species, progesterone uniformly *suppresses* androgen-dependent sexual behavior. Second, studies done with agonists and antagonists suggest that the progesterone receptors may be functionally linked to male-typical sexual behavior. This latter possibility represents a novel or at least formerly undetected relationship between progesterone receptors and neurons involved in male-typical sexual behaviors.

How might this evolution from an androgen-dependent, male-typical behavior in the sexual ancestral species to a progesterone-dependent, male-like behavior in the unisexual descendant species have occurred? Gould and Vrba[430] have pointed out that existing features can be produced by two distinct historical processes. One of these is adaptation, or the gradual selection of traits that results in improved functions. Some traits, however, evolved from features that served other roles or had no function at all, and only later were co-opted for their current role because they enhanced current fitness. The latter process, in which a useful feature is not built by selection for its current role, has been termed exaptation. The difference between the two is that, in adaptation, traits are constructed by selection for their present functions. In exaptation traits are co-opted for their present use. In the present case, the variation in sensitivity to progesterone may be the substrate on which selection operated. This resulted in the novel hormone-brain-behavior relationship observed in the parthenogen. That is, the elevation of progesterone following ovulation presented an appropriate stimulus that, given the low circulating concentrations of androgens, was co-opted to trigger mounting behavior in the parthenogen.

Table 6.3 Some Examples Illustrating the Principle of Complementarity in Behavioral Biology

LEVEL OF BIOLOGICAL ORGANIZATION	COMPLEMENTARY PROCESS	EXAMPLE
Species	Co-evolution of plants and animals	Figs and fig wasps
Organism	Sexual behaviors	Intromission and receptive behaviors
Physiology	Signal receiver	Feedback control in neuroendocrinology
Molecule	Hormone receptor	Steroid hormones and their receptors

Note: At every level of biological organization there are fundamental complementary processes.

Conjectures and Speculations

The Principle of Complementarity

Evolution of a species, a behavior, or a hormone does not occur in a vacuum. Complementarity, or the combination of parts required for completion, is evident at all levels of biological organization (table 6.3). Animals and plants have evolved in the presence of other plants and animals. In many ways, the survival of many plants and animals has become dependent upon, or is modulated by, the presence or behavior of others within the environment. For example, figs depend on fig wasps for pollination; the fig wasps oviposit in the fig, and the resulting young feed on the fruit. Herbivores depend on plants for sustenance. Plants depend upon the animals to disperse seeds. Sexual reproduction requires two kinds of gametes, eggs and sperm. In mating, two individuals must interact in a complementary fashion if fertilization is to occur. In reproductive physiology, there are feedback relationships and the interaction of hormones and their receptors such as those discussed in chapter 1. Thus, complementarity is fundamental to biological systems.

This perspective is useful when considering complex systems such as reproduction. Anyone who has ever watched carefully how animals mate will be struck by the complementary nature of the actions that lead up to and include copulation. Normally, copulation is a behavior made possible only by mutual consent. This consent is a reflection not only of the satisfactory nature of the external stimuli provided but also of the internal milieu that motivates each individual to seek a partner. Beach[92] referred to this as the principle of stimulus-response complementarity. According to this principle, successful mating will occur only if both partners are in the appropriate physiological and behavioral condition and the behavior of each partner elicits the appropriate behavioral response from the other. This principle can be restated in two simple sentences: Mounting will not be successful if the mounted animal is not receptive. A receptive animal will not be mounted unless there is a willing partner.

The principle of stimulus-response complementarity, however, has broad implications. For example, the principle can be applied to all animals regardless of their mode of reproduction. The principle is also independent of the genetic or gonadal sex of the participants. Female-associated responses tend to evoke masculine responses in both males and females. Similarly, male-associated responses tend to evoke feminine responses in both males and females.

This principle may also affect our understanding of sexual selection. Just as there is variance in male displays, so also is there variance in female preference. Could this statement underlie an important phenomenon waiting to be investigated? As Bluhm[126] has documented, female canvasback ducks forced into pairs with males they did not select fail to lay eggs. Could this phenomenon be generalized to other species? If we refer to a successful pairing as a "resonance" between the preference behaviors of the partners, might this concept reflect a similar resonance at a physiological level? That is, when females choose their mating partners, are they selecting males whose physiology will stimulate maximum reproductive success? As Bluhm has shown, such a hypothesis is relatively easy to test. The answer should reveal itself best in those species exhibiting strong mate choice or having evidence of assortative mating.

The concept of complementarity in biological systems is useful because it makes one think of units rather than single elements. In biology it is often said that the whole is more than the sum of its parts. This is readily seen in mating behavior in which two individuals must coordinate and synchronize reproductive processes. Only with such interactions will reproduction be successful. This logic can be extended to all levels of biological organization. Still, the trend in behavioral neuroendocrinology is to focus on a single sex, a single behavior, or a single hormone. This is evident in studies in which the investigator may spend years determining the reproductive cycle in the male (or female) while ignoring the potential contribution of the partner.

On the other hand, at the genetic level, individuals are far from being complementary. Differences in reproductive interests lead one to expect something very different from "harmony" and "mutual coordination" in courtship and mating behavior. Thus, another metaphor for male-female relations is the conflict of reproductive interests. Put simply, no two sexually reproducing individuals, other than monozygotic twins, share identical genetic (reproductive) interests. In this framework, courtship behavior by males and mate choice by females may represent "salesmanship" and "consumerism," respectively.

Hypothetical Scenarios of the Evolution of Behavior-Controlling Mechanisms

Evolution is the cumulation of successful outcomes. How might a steroid hormone-dependent neuroendocrine mechanism have evolved (table 6.4)? There appears to be an ancient functional relationship between gamete (i.e., sperm and or eggs) production and gonadal steroid secretion.[552] Gametes are

Table 6.4 Hypothetical Scenario in the Evolution of Hormone-Brain-Behavior Relationships in Vertebrates

Presented are the major steps envisioned in this process. The first four are probably shared by all vertebrates and hence are more ancient than the last two, which probably vary among species.

1. Functional association between gametogenesis and steroid hormone production.
2. Functional association between steroid hormones and nervous system responsiveness.
3. Functional association between higher neural centers, the pituitary, and gonadal activity.
4. Functional association of gonadal steroid production and development and later activation of gamete delivery systems.
5. Recruitment of integrative (limbic) areas influencing behavior through expansion of steroid-sensitive hypothalamic areas involved in the control of pituitary gonadotropin.
6. Functional association of specific sexual signals and secretion of gonadal steroids.

never produced without a concomitant rise in gonadal steroid production. It is often the case, however, that gonadal steroids are secreted without production of sperm or eggs. It is clear that the sex steroid hormones have come to serve as activators of sexual behavior in a wide variety of vertebrate species. I purposely am avoiding consideration of the equally interesting question of how hormones and their receptors evolved.

As a first step, the nervous system might have become responsive to hormones during development. This could have been followed by development of a structure to regulate gonadal activity—in vertebrates, the anterior pituitary gland. Because the anterior pituitary is situated directly beneath the hypothalamus, a second step might have involved hypothalamic modulation of pituitary activity. As the animal perceived change in its environment, this information could have been integrated at the level of the hypothalamus.

Development of a feedback control system involving the hypothalamus, pituitary, and gonads is the foundation of the functional association between gonadal hormone secretion and reproductive behavior. An exansion of the brain regions involved in the feedback control of pituitary function to include the adjacent behavioral and integrative areas could have mediated the development of these mechanisms. A further step in the evolution of hormone dependency of sexual behavior is seen in some species in which specific sexual signals elicit the secretion of reproductive hormones.

However, it should be emphasized that the presence of sex steroid hormone-concentrating neurons in behavioral integrative areas is not evidence a priori of a functional association between sex steroid hormones and sexual behavior. As pointed out earlier, neither female garter snakes nor female Asian musk shrews exhibit hormone-dependent sexual receptivity, yet sex steroid hormone-concentrating neurons have been identified in both species. As described earlier, species exhibiting dissociated reproductive patterns appear to have evolved alternative neuroendocrine mechanisms.

Reconstructing evolutionary scenarios is useful in that they help to place systems in a larger context. Such scenarios can also lead to predictions or point the investigator toward potential areas of research. For example, a complete understanding of the role of the pituitary in vertebrate reproduction is aided by studies of primitive chordates in which the pituitary is exposed directly to the environment through a hole in the roof of the mouth. Such exercises also help to place in perspective apparent anomalies such as dissociated reproductive patterns or environmental sex determination. Are these phenomena specialized adaptations, or are they representative of more primitive conditions?

Chicken-and-Egg Questions

An evolutionary perspective not only provides new avenues of research but also raises new questions about old answers. This is especially true of chicken-and-egg questions. Consider the evolution of sexual behavior relative to the evolution of sex itself. We can ask the question "Which came first, sex or sexual behavior?" A more precise phrasing would be "Which came first, sexual reproduction or the behavioral facilitation of reproduction?" This leads to the question, "Why are males important?" As discussed earlier, the male plays not one, but two essential roles. The first, of course, is to provide sperm necessary for fertilization of ova. The second is to provide the behavior necessary to ensure normal gonadotropic hormone secretion in females. Experiments with representative species of every vertebrate class have indicated that behavioral interactions are crucial in linking together the stages that comprise the reproductive cycle.

What if we look for this aspect of sexual behavior in asexual organisms? This idea evidently has not occurred to anyone before. If we do look, we find surprisingly clear evidence that the behavioral facilitation of reproduction is widespread and fundamental to reproduction in all kinds of animals. For example, population growth in bacteria is more rapid in colonies that begin with two individuals compared with colonies that begin with one individual; the immediate facilitation in the former ensures a more rapid population growth trajectory. The entire reproductive cycle of the slime mold is predicated on the behavioral interaction of individual organisms. The fact is that the ancestors of most unisexual species today probably reproduced by sexual means, and so they cannot be used as ammunition in an argument on the origin of sexual behavior. Still, in the one organism believed to have always been asexual, the blue-green algae or cyanobacteria, behavioral interactions appear to underlie the reproductive "blooms."

Behavioral facilitation of reproduction may be more ancient than sexual reproduction itself for two reasons. First, behavior is the leading edge of evolutionary change. Reproductive behaviors in particular are thought to have a "disproportionate influence on brain evolution" (Bullock, 1984). It is through behavior that species evolve. Second, the advantages of synchronous reproduction, one of the consequences of behavioral facilitation, are just as great in asexual organisms as they are in sexual species. That is, by reproducing within a restricted period of time, the environment is "flushed" with new offspring, thereby reducing the probability that any single individual will be preyed upon. When combined with periodic availability of resources, the result is coordinated reproduction. There is no reason why a similar explanation may not apply as well to a grunion as to a bacterium.

Let us return to the original question of "what came first." By posing the question as "Which came first, sex or sexual behavior," we encounter a problem inherent in the term sexual behavior. That is, the question has meaning only for species having sexes or practicing sexual reproduction. Such a question is unanswerable. But if we restrict our definition of sexual behavior to the behavioral facilitation of reproduction and not to fertilization, we might be able to provide an answer. I have argued that behavioral facilitation came first.[230] This claim is based on the fact that behavioral facilitation of reproduction occurs in a great variety of organisms, ranging from blue-green algae to mammals. The diversity of organisms exhibiting behavioral facilitation is greater than the diversity of organisms exhibiting meiosis. This makes it likely that behavioral facilitation is more fundamental than sexual reproduction.

Other experiments of nature raise equally interesting questions. For example, Russert-Kraemer[890] describes a *Hydra* that challenges our assumptions about the nervous system and behavior. The behavior of this small freshwater organism has long been studied, being a classic preparation in experimental zoology developed by Trembley in 1744. As in other organisms, behavior is an integral part of reproduction in *Hydra*. In this instance, behavior is the manifestation of the activity of a nerve net, a primitive nervous system.

In *Hydra*, the interstitial cells are the stem cells for both neurons and gametes. Russert-Kraemer[890] describes how two investigators, Burnett and Diehl, discovered in the mid-1960s that application of a particular dye destroyed the nerve cells, rendering a *Hydra* behavior-less. Eventually, such treated animals regenerate their nerve cells and hence their behavior. If this regeneration of nerve cells is prevented, however, the interstitial cells produce huge masses of gametes. This is a remarkable finding because it suggests that even with the loss of a nervous system and hence behavior, these "nerveless" animals continue to reproduce.

Indeed, new frontiers of our understanding of behavioral neuroscience can be found in the study of other microorganisms. For example, Crespi[226] has discovered that tiny (5 mm) tree-living thrips actually switch reproductive modes depending on when they were born and what they eat (table 6.5). The spring generation lay eggs and produce female offspring. The summer generation bear live young and produce male offspring. The trigger for the switch appears to be something in the summer leaves, but exactly what is still unknown. This ability to alternate modes of reproduction provides an opportunity to test hypotheses regarding the evolution of egg-laying and live-bearing. Other animals known to be capable of something similar are aphids and *Daphnia*, which alternate between parthenogenesis and sexual reproduction. As Seger[934] has pointed out, "Large animals easily excite our emotions; small ones probably would if we knew them better."

Table 6.5 The Alternation of Reproductive Modes in Thrips

| *Leaves* | GENERATION | |
	Spring	*Summer*
Spring	Oviparous	Oviparous
Summer	Oviparous	Viviparous

Note: The different generations either lay eggs (spring generation) or give live-birth (summer generation). Oviparity produces all females, whereas viviparity produces all males.

Animals such as these present scientists with new model systems with which to test theories of the ecological and social factors important in the evolution of different modes of reproduction and their attendant behaviors. It is preparations such as these that will give credence to Ghiselin's[398] suggestion that "we have evolved a nervous system that acts in the interest of our gonads, and one attuned to the demands of reproductive competition."

Summary and Conclusions

One of the first things we are impressed by is the great variety of animals, particularly their behaviors and their physiologies. With so many differences, are there any generalities? With the establishment of evolutionary theory, evidence that there is "unity in diversity" has come with discoveries of common anatomical features, the cell cycle, conservation of intermediary metabolism, and the genetic code, to name but a few. Although in vertebrates there appears to be a conservation of the neural circuits underlying sex behavior, it is still too early to state the extent to which this concept can be extended to the hormonal mechanisms underlying behavior.

This particular chapter has documented how some widely held assumptions are generalities only in a very restricted sense. I have shown how much of our conceptual understanding of behavioral endocrinology stems from extensive studies on relatively few species. According to Beach,[92] there are

two cardinal rules that should govern not only the construction of animal models for human behavior, but for all interspecific comparisons regardless of the behavior and the species involved. The first rule is that meaningful comparisons are based not upon the formal characteristics of behavior, but upon its causal mechanisms and functional outcomes. . . . The second rule is that the validity of interspecific generalization cannot exceed the reliability of intraspecific analysis. Significant comparison of a particular type of behaviour in two different species is impossible unless and until the behavior has been adequately analyzed in each species by itself. Only after independent, intraspecific analysis is achieved can we properly interpret the nature and degree of interspecific similarities and differences (pp. 113–114).

To these two rules, a third and fourth might be added. Third, make the consideration of the organism's natural history the first and last step in any biological study of behavior. Fourth, open the way to new insights by questioning traditional paradigms.

When an evolutionary perspective is applied to behavioral endocrinology, we challenge the breadth and validity of our assumptions about the mechanisms that control species-typical behaviors. This is not the same thing as saying that there are no unitary explanations that apply to all mammals (versus nonmammals), endotherms (versus ectotherms), or even vertebrates (versus invertebrates). As this volume testifies, we have gathered considerable information about the neuroendocrine bases of behavior in a few species. To uncover truly broad generalizations, however, we must begin looking with equal intensity and rigor at other organisms.

Thus, the ecological and evolutionary perspective points the way to a variety of natural experiments or "experiments of nature." The pattern of evolution is best illustrated in the diversity of organisms. By studying closely related species that live in different habitats, we can see how each has become adapted. By studying distantly related species that live in the same habitat, we can see whether the solutions to similar problems are different or analogous.

The unique qualities of each species also give us a deeper understanding of the constraints and potential for change in fundamental processes (the interested reader should also see Bartholomew,[59] Bern,[113] Bullock,[168] Crews and Moore,[235] Diamond,[287] Prosser[830]). Where basic conflicts exist, control mechanisms adapt or the species goes extinct. To echo the beginning admonition of Bullock, to ignore comparative research would greatly limit our understanding of the evolution of hormone-behavior relations.

Acknowledgments

Preparation of this chapter was supported by a NIMH Research Scientist Award. Discussions with the following people helped much in development of the ideas expressed here: J. Becker, J. Bull, E. Charnov, P. DeVries, D. Hillis, W. Holmes, J. Lindzey, M. Ryan, S. Sawabini, N. Stacey, F. Stevens, G. Wade, and two anonymous reviewers.

7 *Hormonal Influences on Courtship Behaviors*

Darcy B. Kelley and Eliot Brenowitz

Almost all vertebrates engage in some kind of courtship as part of mate selection. This chapter examines the neural and hormonal control of courtship in three different groups: electric fish, clawed frogs, and songbirds. Electric fish use unusual kinds of signals, brief electrical discharges from modified muscle cells, as sexual advertisements. Electrical discharges propagate well in turbid, underwater habitats where visual signals, for example, would be hard to distinguish. Another very beautiful, to human ears, example of courtship is birdsong. In temperate zones, seasonal song is usually produced only by males, while in the tropics both sexes of some species sing highly coordinated duets. The springtime chorus of croaking frogs also functions as a courtship song to attract potential mates and to advertise the qualities of the signaler. Fortunately for behavioral endocrinologists, these complex behaviors are strongly affected by gonadal hormones and provide an opportunity to explore how steroidal effects on the nervous system influence behaviors.

What are courtship displays, what is their function, and why are they more often performed by males than by females? How do hormones influence the development and adult function of courtship signals? These themes underly our exploration of three diverse and fascinating courtship systems.

Introduction

Courtship behaviors are critical for successful reproduction. During courtship a member of one sex produces a series of signals that induce a member of the other sex to mate. In addition to attracting and stimulating potential mates, courtship signals convey information that can be used in selecting a reproductive partner. Some examples of the sorts of information conveyed are the species to which the signaler belongs, the sex of the signaler, his or her readiness to mate, the size and age of the signaler, and the kind of territory he or she holds.

Evolution of Courtship Behavior

Identifying the sex of a potential mate is obviously critical, and courtship behaviors that differ markedly between males and females can function in this way. Charles Darwin attempted to account for these and other features of courtship behaviors through his theory of sexual selection described in chapter 6. Sexual selection operates when individuals of a species differ in their ability to compete for resources critical for successful reproduction. Darwin believed that sexual selection accounted for some extreme differences between the sexes, such as the peacock's tail. These extreme effects are balanced by natural selection. Natural selection favors the integration of reproductive behavior and physiology with other sorts of behavior (like foraging) and physiological adaptations (e.g., metabolism) that are essential for survival.

In most species, courtship is initiated by males. Recently, Trivers[1040] has helped to explain why males usually compete for access to females while females usually choose among males. His explanation involves the relative investment of energy and time made in reproduction by each sex. First, each sex produces different gametes. Males produce sperm and females produce eggs. Females make a greater energetic investment in the production of their gametes because, in addition to containing the female's chromosomes, eggs generally contain a high energy nutritive substance, the yolk. The yolk sustains the early development of the fertilized embryo. Sperm, on the other hand, consists simply of the male's chromosomes surrounded by a protein coat with an attached flagellum to provide mobility (figure 7.1). Each sperm cell of a male is smaller and therefore energetically much "cheaper" to produce than an egg.

The large difference in energy invested in gamete production is reflected in a sex difference in the number of gametes produced over a lifetime. Females usually produce mature eggs in numbers that range from tens to thousands (egg numbers for human females are a few hundred). Males, however, produce sperm in nearly astronomical numbers. During a single ejaculation, for example, a human male releases about 100 million sperm cells! Differences in investment by males and females are not confined to the gametes. Once the egg is fertilized by a male's sperm, females of many species continue to make a greater investment in the offspring than do males. For example, in mammals the female nourishes the developing embryo throughout a gestational period that may last many months. In addition, female care of the offspring may even persist after it has hatched or been born, until it becomes fully independent. Hormonal involvement in parental behavior will be discussed in greater detail in chapter 8.

Thus, in most animal species, females make a greater investment of energy and time in the production of offspring than do males. A consequence of this difference in investment is that males and females differ fundamentally in the strategies that will maximize reproductive success over their entire lifetime. Since sperm are relatively cheap for the male to produce, his reproductive success is not limited by the numbers of sperm that he can make. Instead, the male's reproductive success will be determined by the numbers of females' eggs that he can fertilize. Males will usually maximize the number of eggs fertilized by mating with as many females as possible. We therefore expect males to compete fiercely for access to females.

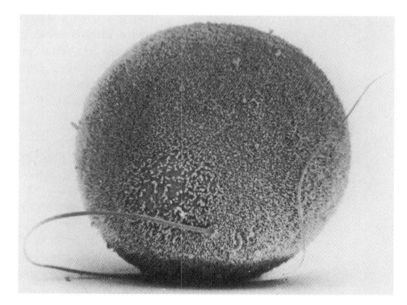

Figure 7.1 Hamster sperm fertilizing a hamster egg. Note the size difference between the sperm and the egg (magnification ×1640). (Photograph by David M. Phillips, reprinted with permission.)

The number of offspring that a female can produce during her lifetime will be severely limited by the costs of making eggs and rearing young. Each egg, then, is of relatively greater importance to a female's reproductive success than each sperm is to a male. A female can maximize her reproductive investment by ensuring that each egg fertilized has a good chance of producing an offspring that will itself survive to reproduce. The female's best means of accomplishing this is to mate only with males of high genetic quality or with males that contribute through care or territorial defense to the survival of offspring. Consequently, females will tend to be choosy about which males they allow to fertilize their eggs. By choosing among competing males, females in effect force males to demonstrate their comparative quality. This selective force has led to the evolution of courtship by males.

Production of Courtship Behavior

How then is a particular courtship behavior produced? Usually the behavior is triggered by a particular stimulus, for instance, hearing the sons produced by a member of the opposite sex. Stimuli are detected by sensory receptors and conveyed into the central nervous system by sensory neurons. Because some stimuli are very complex, different components of the stimulus (for instance, sound pitch and the location of the sound source) are processed by separate groups of interneurons working in parallel. Different sensory stimuli evoke activity in different brain nuclei; this activity then affects interneurons dedicated to producing patterned motor output. The final step is a change in the activity of motoneurons, resulting in contraction and relaxation of the muscles that produce the courtship behavior. Synaptically interconnected brain nuclei that participate in producing courtship behavior have each been identified for the three courtship systems discussed in this chapter.

When males are responsible for courtship, brain nuclei and muscle groups involved in the behavior can differ dramatically in structure and function from those found in females.[562] In some insects, house flies and moths, for example, sensory receptors and neurons associated with detecting sexual signals are different in males and females. In some birds, the brain nuclei that affect motor patterning can also differ. In certain frogs, the motoneurons and muscles that produce attraction calls are different in the sexes. These sensory, neural, and muscular behavioral effector systems are thus sexually dimorphic, as are the behaviors they produce.

The hormonal and neural bases of sexually dimorphic courtship behavior will be the focus of this chapter. We will concentrate on three model courtship systems spanning various vertebrate classes and sensory modalities of communication. These are electric communication in fish, vocalizations in clawed frogs, and song production in birds. Hormones influence the production of courtship signals by acting at different levels of the nervous system in these three groups. In electric fish, hormones act directly upon cells at the most peripheral level of the neural circuits involved in the production and reception of electric mating signals. Hormones are essential for organization of the sexually dimorphic vocal organ in clawed frogs and play an important role in the activation of regions of the hindbrain in the central nervous system that control mate calling. In songbirds, hormones are critical in both the organization and activation of nuclei in the forebrain that regulate song behavior. In considering these systems, we will also see that hormones act on the nervous system as the proximate agents for sexual selection.

Courtship in Weakly Electric Fish

In the tropics of Africa and America are found species of freshwater fish that use electrical signals both for orientation in murky water and in their courtship displays. These fish belong to two taxonomic groups, the mormyriforms of Africa (figure 7.2) and the gymnotiforms of Central and South America. In both groups, courtship is triggered by environmental changes correlated with the onset of the breeding season.[452] Electrical activity in courtship is usually most pronounced in males. In some species, courtship is triggered when the male detects the electrical signals generated by females. Subsequent pairing involves changes in the electrical signals of both sexes much like the duets that characterize pair bonds in tropical birds (see the last section in this chapter).

It has been difficult to study electrical courtship in the wild because mormyrids and gymnotids are nocturnal and elusive. Fortunately, electrical fish can be successfully bred in the laboratory by mimicking the natural conditions

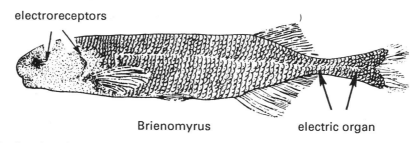

electroreceptors

Brienomyrus   electric organ

Figure 7.2 Overview of mormyrid electric organs and electroreceptors. Line drawing of *Brienomyrus* showing the electric organ, located in the tail, and electroreceptors concentrated in the head region. (Modified from Bass and Volman, 1987.[167])

(pH, water electrical conductivity, "rain," and water depth) that characterize the start of the breeding season. Hagedorn and Heiligenberg used these methods to observe the mating behavior of the glass knife fish, *Eigenmannia virescens*, in laboratory aquaria. Hagedorn observed, "The night of spawning is an electrical extravaganza, males will fight for many nights for [dominance in the mating hierarchy], the females defend spawning territories (floating plants) and the dominant male will spawn only with the dominant female. The female hangs almost vertically in the plants, while the male courts her with a barrage of [electrical] "chirping" (60 to 80/minute) that may last all night. As the female lays her eggs, she produces low amplitude chirps; then the male rubs through the plants fertilizing the eggs. Peripheral, subordinate females try to sneak their eggs into the spawning territory, often turning off their EOD [electric organ discharge] as they rush towards the plant, only to be driven away by the dominant pair." The electrical signal is so powerful in reproductive behavior that gravid females will lay eggs in response to a recording of male chiping.[452]

As might be expected, the electrical signals given by mature males differ from those of females and juveniles that are not yet reproductively mature. In this section, we will consider how sex differences in the electric organ discharge (EOD) are generated and detected. As is the case for frog and bird song (see below), much evidence implicates sex-specific hormones in electrical signaling during courtship. In some cases we are beginning to understand the cellular bases for these hormone effects.

The Electric Channel of Communication

Some electrogenic fish (like *Torpedo*) are capable of delivering sizeable electric shocks of up to 600 volts to stun their prey. The gymnotiforms and mormyrids, however, generate much weaker signals, in the range of a few millivolts to a few volts. These electrical discharges are produced by modified muscle cells called electrocytes (figure 7.3) located in the fish's tail. The electrical signals are received by specialized receptors (called electroreceptors) scattered on the fish's body surface.

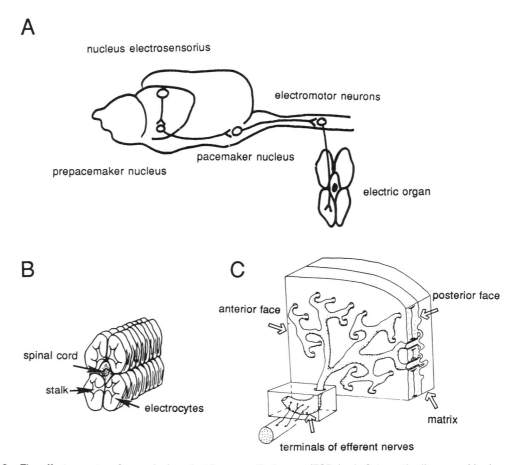

Figure 7.3 The effector system for producing electric organ discharges (EODs). *A*. Schematic diagram of brain nuclei involved in generating EODs. In gymnotiforms, prepacemaker and pacemaker cells are located in the same brain nucleus. *B*. A Magnified view of the electric organ (see figure 7.2). The electric organ consists of columns of serially stacked, disk-shaped cells, the electrocytes. A stalk lies on the anterior side of each electrocyte (see details in *C*). C. Line drawing showing a cut-away view of half of a *single* electrocyte. The three action potential-generating membranes of the electrocyte are the anterior and posterior faces and the stalk. The stalk is innervated in a restricted zone by nerve terminals that arise from axons of the electromotor nerve. The entire cell is enclosed in a compartment containing a gelatinous matrix. (*B* modified from Bass and Volman, 1987[67]; *C* modified from Bass, 1986.[62])

How far away from another electric fish can a signal producer be and still have its electric organ discharges detected? In other words, how big is the signaling fish's **active space?** The answer depends somewhat on the type and size of fish and the electrical characteristics of the water; best estimates are in the range of 70 to 100 cm.[502] As the water's electrical conductivity is lowered (as would happen, for example, when it rains), the active space of the electric signal increases dramatically.[983] On the receptive side, a noisy electrical environment (lightning for example) can interfere with another fish's ability to locate the source of a signal. Thus, electrical signaling is a short-range form of communication; the fish generally have to be within 100 cm (several feet) of each other to interact using this modality. Unlike vision, in which the receptor organs have to be oriented towards the signal source, electroreception does not require directed attention to be effective. The electroreceptors will be stimulated, although to varying degrees, no matter what the orientation of the receiving fish with respect to the signaler.

INFORMATION COMMUNICATED IN ELECTRIC SIGNALS

The basic unit of electrical signaling is the EOD. The EOD is made up of individual pulses that can have a simple or a complex waveform depending on the geometry of the electrocyte that generates them (reviewed in Bass[63]). Individual pulses can be strung together in trains with particular rhythms. If the interval between pulses is very regular and short compared to the pulse duration itself, the signal is called a wave EOD. If the interval between pulses is variable and long, the signal is called a pulse EOD (figure 7.4).

During the first phase of courtship, EODs are used to locate a conspecific of the other sex. The other fish is easy to locate because most electric fish continually discharge at low rates. In addition to location, these spontaneous EODs convey information about the age and sex of the signaler because, in many species, the EOD is different for adult males, females, and juveniles. For example, in *Sternopygus macrurus* (a wave discharging species), mature males discharge at a characteristic frequency of 50 to 90 Hz (cycles per second), mature females at 100 to 150 Hz, and juveniles are intermediate between these two.[500] Since the EOD is correlated with the breeding condition of the animal, it can also convey information about reproductive state.

Some fish use specific EOD discharges as courtship signals. A good example is the "chirp" used in the male courtship. Chirps consist of brief and rapid increases in the EOD frequency. There is no audible component to this electrical signal but when it is played through a loudspeaker it sounds like a chirp. In some species males do most of the chirping. In others, females also chirp as eggs pass through their reproductive tract. In *Sternopygus*, adult males respond to female (but not to male) EOD frequencies by chirping.[501] Thus, in different species of electric fish EODs can be used to attract and stimulate females, to synchronize reproductive behaviors of males and females, and to convey information about the sex of the signaller.

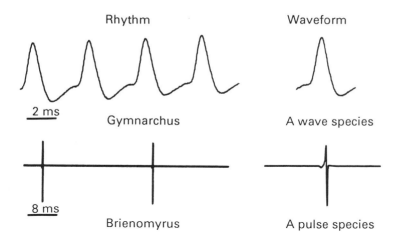

Figure 7.4 Comparison of the EOD of a "pulse" and a "wave" species of electric fish. The EOD rhythm is the rate at which the waveform pulse is produced. The EOD waveform describes individual pulses generated by the electric organ. For the pulse fish, the interval between successive pulses is long compared with the pulse duration itself. For wave species, the rhythm has a wave-like appearance because the interpulse interval is similar to the pulse duration. (Modified from Bass, 1986.[63])

METHOD OF GENERATION AND RECEPTION OF ELECTRIC SIGNALS

As mentioned earlier, electric signals (with rare exceptions) are produced by specialized muscle cells called electrocytes. The electric organ is located in the tail and consists of stacks of disc-like electrocytes. The electrocyte has two sides or faces: anterior and posterior. In addition, the electrocyte has a thin protrusion, the stalk, which in many species, passes through the main body of the electrocyte and connects the anterior and posterior faces. These morphological elements are believed to contribute to the EOD waveform.[67, 108] Electrocytes generate electrical signals in response to activity in their motoneurons. In mormyrids, these electromotor neurons in the spinal cord discharge synchronously in response to a command signal emanating from a nearby relay nucleus (figure 7.3). The relay nucleus received is synaptically connected to an adjacent command nucleus which in turn is driven by nuclei in the midbrain.[106] In gymnotiforms, pacemaker and relay cells are located in the same nucleus.[312]

Electrical signals used in courtship are detected by specialized sensory receptors that are located just below the skin surface. Electrical current gains access to these electroreceptors through a canal that is open to the external water. Electroreceptors are modified hair cells, a type of sensory receptor found also in the ear. When electrically stimulated, electroreceptors release a neurotransmitter that stimulates sensory neurons. Axons of these sensory neurons form the lateral line nerve. Incoming lateral line axons terminate in a nucleus of the hindbrain (the electrosensory lateral line lobe), which in turn projects to a midbrain nucleus (the torus semicircularis).

Sex Differences in Electroproduction and Reception

Sex differences in the form and function of electrocytes have been described in both mormyriforms and gymnotiforms. In many species, the EOD waveform differs in males and females. Typically, the waveform is longer in males. Sex differences in EOD waveform are correlated with the thickness of the electrocyte membrane, which is greater in males than in females. Increases in membrane thickness should increase the ability of the electrocyte to store electrical charges and thus prolong the EOD waveform. In addition, the membrane ion channels that are responsible for the electrocyte action potential are probably different in the sexes.[67, 727]

In addition to the waveform itself, the EOD rhythm can be sex specific. For example, male *Sternopygus macrurus* discharge at much lower rates than females.[500] Sex differences in pulse rhythms also occur and may be due to sex differences in the command signals coming from the brain. We do not yet have a clear understanding of how such sex differences in pulse rhythms and rates are generated by brain interneurons dedicated to producing patterned motor output.

Each fish's electroreceptors are most sensitive (tuned) to specific characteristics of electrical stimuli, typically those associated with the fish's *own* EOD. This is because the EOD is also used for orientation, and the fish must monitor how EOD transmission is affected by nearby objects. When the EOD is different in males and females, the tuning of the electroreceptors is also different in the sexes.[1133] Note that even though the fish's receptors are most sensitive to its own frequencies at low amplitudes, they can also detect the frequencies used by the opposite sex at higher amplitudes.

How does the sensitivity of the electroreceptor come to match the fish's own EOD? The EOD could tune the receptor or receptor tuning could be achieved independently. These alternatives have been studied by removing a piece of skin containing the original electroreceptors in *Sternopygus* and following the tuning of the new receptors that appear as the skin regenerates.[1132] Even if the fish experiences no electrical field at all during regeneration, the new receptors become tuned to the same frequency as the EOD. This result implies that receptor tuning occurs independently of external stimulation by a particular EOD; the actual mechanism that produces receptor tuning is not known. In mormyrids, however, retuning *does* depend on intact electric organ discharge.[65]

HORMONAL CONTROL OF THE EOD AND ELECTRORECEPTORS
Several lines of evidence suggest that sex differences in EODs are controlled by hormones. The primary clue is that the EODs of males and females differ; in many vertebrates, such sex differences are controlled by gonadal hormones. However, field observations of EOD variation by sex often failed to find any sex differences at particular times of the year, suggesting that hormone effects (if indeed they are present) are of the transitory or activational sort.[61, 503] This

observation led to studies in which steroid hormones were given to adult fish, results showed that both the waveform of the EOD and its temporal pattern were affected.

In the mormyrid *Brienomyrus brachistius* (triphasic), either of two major androgenic steroids, testosterone and dihydrotestosterone, will broaden the EOD of adult females or juveniles to a form resembling that of the adult male.[65] In the gymnotid *Sternopygus macrurus*, dihydrotestosterone will prolong the EOD pulse duration and decrease the rate at which the pulses are given.[710, 727] The changes produced by androgens are in the male direction for each species.

Changes in the opposite direction are observed following castration. In male *B. brachistius*, castration causes a shortening of the EOD pulse.[61] Gonadectomy of adult *S. macrurus* causes the EOD rate to increase in males and decrease in females.[710] (Recall that both the waveform of individual EOD pulses and the temporal pattern with which pulses are produced can differ in males and females.) The effect of ovariectomy on EODs of adult female fish suggests that hormones secreted by the female gonad also contribute to the EOD. In *Sternopygus*, administration of estradiol induces an increase in the rate at which pulses are given.[710] The amounts of hormones given in these experiments produced serum concentrations roughly comparable to those measured in individual fish during the breeding season.[1134] It is thus reasonable to suppose that changes in circulating hormone concentrations that are experienced by adult fish are responsible for sex differences in electric organ discharges.

Are sex differences in the tuning of electroreceptors also attributable to gonadal hormones? In *Sternopygus*, dihydrotestosterone has been shown to shift the tuning curve of individual electroreceptors in females to lower frequencies.[711] A similar effect is seen in *Brienomyrus*.[65] These androgen effects shift the tuning of electroreceptors in the masculine direction. It is not known whether individual differences in circulating hormone levels contribute to the individual differences in electroreceptor tuning described earlier.

RETUNING OF ELECTRORECEPTORS AFTER HORMONE EXPOSURE
Androgenic hormones change both the EOD and the sensitivity of the electroreceptor. If, as was suggested in the study of regenerating electroreceptors in a gymnotid fish, the tuning of receptors is independent of changes in the EOD, then electroreceptors in hormone-treated fish should retune even without exposure to an altered EOD. To test this possibility, male fish were given dihydrotestosterone and their EOD was silenced by removing neural input to the electromotoneurons or by lesioning the medullary nucleus that drives the EOD. The sensitivity of electroreceptors was shifted downward by the androgen treatment, as would have occurred in an intact, electrically discharging fish.[349, 560] It is not clear what cellular mechanisms are responsible for this hormone-induced change in receptor tuning. One hypothesis is that the sen-

sory receptor cells themselves contain intracellular receptors for steroid hormones that are capable of changing the cell's electrical properties through changes in membrane ion channels.[67]

Summary and Conclusions

Thus we see that gonadal hormones have very powerful effects on the generation and reception of electric courtship signals in electric fish. All of the hormonal effects observed are reversible and can be readily obtained in adult animals. These two characteristics suggest that the effects are "activational" because they are not permanent and are not confined to a particular developmental period. Many of the effects of hormones on the form of individual pulses in the EOD are closely related to changes in the morphology and excitability of the electrocytes themselves. The rate of EOD discharge is also hormone sensitive. EOD discharge patterns are determined by the rate at which neurons in the motor pattern generator fire. Because some neurons that appear to be part of this circuit concentrate androgenic steroids, hormones could exert effects on the EOD by acting on brain nuclei that produce the EOD motor pattern.[66] Another exciting possibility is that the electroreceptors are directly affected by hormonal secretions.[67] Understanding how hormones affect these sensory cells could yield important insights into the cellular and molecular basis of steroid actions.

Vocal Courtship in Frogs

In temperate zones frog songs are the vocal harbingers of spring. These songs are acoustic signals from males to females and to other males. Why do frogs use sounds rather than visual displays, for example, in their courtship activities? What kinds of information are sent and received? How are the sounds produced and heard? Are acoustic signals different in males and females and how are these differences generated? These questions form the focus of this section on frog courtship behavior.

The Acoustic Channel of Communication

Frog songs attract members of the same species to the breeding site. At the start of the breeding season, males and females are often far from each other and from the breeding site. A problem that such dispersal poses is how to bring males and females together at a good site for tadpole development while conditions are favorable. The choice of a breeding site is dictated by the physiological limitations of **anurans** (frogs and toads): tadpoles usually require fresh water in order to survive and develop. Some species have developed strategies to transcend this limitation. For example, in some tropical species the male carries the developing tadpoles on his back from pond to pond. In other species (*Pipa pipa*), the male presses the fertilized eggs into the spongy back of the female where the tadpoles develop before "hatching" as miniature frogs. These unusual strategies are largely confined to the tropics with their potentially longer breeding seasons. The great majority of anurans, particularly those in temperate zones, face the problem of locating a body of water and a potential mate during a short time period.

Frogs aggregate at breeding sites by using vocal communication. Why do frogs sing rather than, for example, flash a visual signal? Sound has many advantages as a communication signal. Songs are broadcast; the auditory receptors do not need to be in a certain orientation relative to the sound source in order to receive stimulation. Loud songs, particularly those made by choruses of frogs calling together, can travel long distances and thus attract distant frogs. Sounds travel around large obstacles. These advantages are not found in the visual modality; the receiver must be attentive and have its visual receptor apparatus oriented in the right direction. Further, most frogs and toads breed at night when light levels are low but sounds can be easily localized. We can conclude that the auditory channel of communication is utilized by frogs and toads because it can be effective over long distances at night.

INFORMATION COMMUNICATED IN FROG SONG
Male frogs do all of the courtship calling. Other male frogs can respond by adding their voices to form a calling chorus. Male frogs can also vocalize to each other as part of aggressive displays. Aggressive calls are different from the mate calls used to attract females. Females can respond to male songs by moving toward the sound source or by selecting certain males as reproductive partners. Predators may also cue in on calling frogs as potential prey.

Frog songs contain several potentially important pieces of information about the calling male. First, sound **amplitude** can indicate the size of the individual that is calling. Since many frogs exhibit indeterminate growth (i.e., they keep getting bigger as they get older), size is a good predictor of relative age. In many species, call **loudness** is increased by specialized vocal sacs that can enlarge as the animal grows; thus, older frogs produce louder calls. The males's age matters to females because older frogs have successfully survived the environmental hazards that the offspring they sire will soon be facing. Loudness can also convey information on how far away the calling frog is or, for choruses, how many frogs are calling together. A loud chorus may indicate a particularly favorable breeding site.

Sound **frequencies** (or pitch) can also convey information about the calling male because the vocal apparatus grows larger as the frog grows older. A larger vocal apparatus is capable of producing lower frequency sounds. In some frogs, the pitch of individual sounds varies with age, so that older and larger males give lower pitched calls. Finally, the **length of time** that an individual male can afford to spend calling is a good indicator of his health. Many frogs invest considerable energy in calling both because they do not feed and also because it is a physically demanding behavior that relies on rapid muscular contractions of the vocalization apparatus. This effort can be debilitating in a male frog that is not in top physical condition. Calling in tree frogs is said to be the most energetically expensive behavior yet measured in any vertebrate.[1019]

Sound frequencies and the **overall temporal pattern** of the song can also reveal the species of the calling male. The frequencies of frog sounds and their temporal patterns (rhythm and speed) are species-specific "trademarks." The species of a potential mate is extremely important to the female. Females that choose to mate with partners of another species risk losing all the energy invested in their eggs because the hybrid offspring will usually not survive and reproduce.

Taken together, we can see that the information present in a male frog's song could serve as an advertisement of his reproductive state. A male that calls rapidly, in a deep pitch, and for many hours is likely to be a large, old, physically fit male in a location without many predators or other rivals. A short, higher pitched series of calls might be given by a smaller male, frequently chased away from an attractive breeding site by predators or other males.

Not all species have evolved systems for mate choice. In some frogs, the environmental conditions favorable for breeding may be present for such short periods of time that females have no chance to be picky. In such "explosive breeders," the main job is just to find the breeding site and a member of the opposite sex to mate with so that the resulting tadpoles can develop before the pond dries up.[1096] The evolution of mate choice strategies will be discussed in the next chapter.

METHOD OF GENERATION AND RECEPTION OF ACOUSTIC SIGNALS
The vocal organ for frogs and toads is the larynx, a muscular and cartilagenous structure located in the airway, just before the trachea branches into the two bronchi that enter the lungs. Sounds are produced in most frogs by interposing muscular or membranous elements into the air flow. As air moves through the larynx during expiration, air expulsion can be shaped (altered in frequency or temporal pattern) by sound-producing elements. In some frogs (including *Xenopus laevis*, the species discussed below), sounds are produced in a simpler way. The larynx has developed into a cartilaginous "clicker" (figure 7.5). When the muscles that flank the laryngeal cartilages contract, they pull on tendons connected to the sound discs. These discs then pop apart, producing a click.[855, 1119] Repeated click trains make up the trills that male and female *Xenopus* use in courtship signaling.

Male and female frogs have externally located ears; there is no ear canal as in mammals. Sounds are detected by transducers or hair cells located in two organs, the amphibian and the basilar papillae. Nerve cells convey information from the hair cells into the central nervous system (figure 7.6). The first relay station is a nucleus in the hindbrain dorsal acoustic medulla (DAM). Sound information is sent to the auditory midbrain (torus semicircularis [TOR] and then on to specific nuclei in the forebrain (auditory thalamus [ATH] and ven-

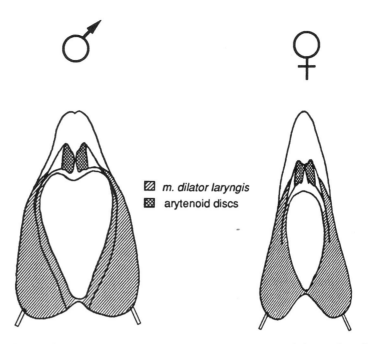

Figure 7.5 Schematic views of the larynx in male and female clawed frogs. Sounds are produced when the arytenoid discs are "popped" apart by the contraction of laryngeal dilator muscles. The female larynx can produce the ticking vocalization (a release call). The male larynx can produce both ticking and mate calling, the song given by male *Xenopus laevis.*.

tral striatum [VST]). Similar brain pathways for receiving auditory information are present in all vertebrates.

Sex Differences in Song Production and Reception

As in many courtship behaviors, song in frogs is usually the exclusive province of the male. How are sex differences in vocal ability established and maintained? In theory, there are four ways to produce sex differences in vocal behaviors. (1) The sexes might differ in whether or not they can receive the stimulus responsible for evoking song (sex differences at the level of the **sensory receptor** or **sensory neuron**). (2) The brain circuitry responsible for processing the incoming sensory information and producing the vocal pattern might differ between males and females (sex differences at the level of brain **interneurons**). (3) Perhaps the vocal producers—motoneurons and musculoskeletal effectors—are so different in males and females that males can sing while females cannot (sex differences at the level of the **motoneurons** and **muscles**). (4) Finally, all of the above could be the same in both sexes, but the system might require a **sex-specific hormone** to function.[562]

In the Kelley laboratory, we have explored possible sex differences in vocal circuitry through studies of song in the African clawed frog, *Xenopus laevis.*

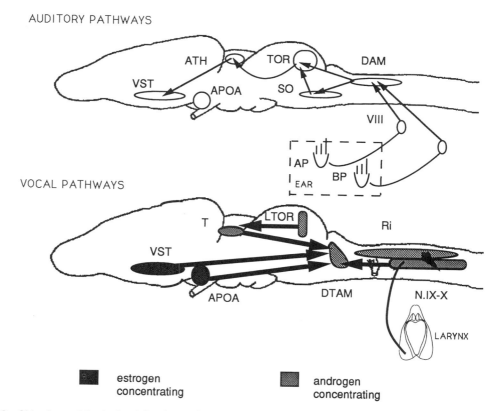

AUDITORY PATHWAYS

VOCAL PATHWAYS

estrogen concentrating

androgen concentrating

Figure 7.6 Side views of the brain of the clawed frog. The regions of the nervous system involved in processing auditory information are shown in the top panel, and those that produce the vocal pattern are shown in the middle panel. Many of these nuclei concentrate steroid hormones (bottom panel). Abbreviations: VST, ventral striatum; ATH, auditory thalamus; APOA, anterior preoptic area; TOR, torus semicircularis; SO, superior olive; DAM, dorsal acoustic medulla; VIII, eighth (auditory) nerve; AP (amphibian papilla); BP, basilar papilla; DTAM, dorsal tegmental area of the medulla; N. IX–X, cranial nerve nucleus IX to X (contains laryngeal motor neurons); LTOR, laminar nucleus of TOR; Ri, nucleus reticularis inferior.

These anurans are native to the southern part of Africa where they inhabit muddy ponds, lakes and even sewers. *Xenopus* is a member of the Pipid family that includes the frog described earlier (*Pipa pipa*) in which the mother incubates the tadpoles in her back.

Clawed frogs become dormant during the dry season by burrowing into the mud. When the rainy season starts, shallow pools of water fill up, and the male frogs emerge and start to call. This song, the mate call, is a metallic-sounding trill with alternating slow and fast phases. The mate call attracts females to the vicinity of the calling male and also excites the female so that she moves around more than she normally would. The female's movement is important because it helps the male to locate her in the muddy water where his vision is not of much use. The male senses water movement through a specialized set of hair cell receptors located within the lateral line organs that cover his body in a precise array. Once the male locates a female, he attempts to clasp her. If the female is sexually receptive, she tolerates his clasp (directed toward her "waist" region). The pair remain in this clasping position while the female extrudes her eggs and the male fertilizes them by spraying the eggs with sperm as they leave her cloaca. If the female is sexually *unreceptive*, she produces a slow and monotonous trill (this sounds like a watch ticking), and the male releases her (figure 7.7).

The mate calls of the male are so loud that although they are made only while he is underwater (and there is a great loss of sound energy at the water-air interface), his song can be heard clearly in the air. The loudness of mate calls and their ability to travel long distances underwater suggest that they serve as an advertisement call that helps females locate the male. Ticking is a much quieter vocal behavior, suggesting that it represents a close range, relatively private channel of communication between the male and the female.

If one male clasps another, the clasped male will tick (and thus be released). Thus both males and females can and do tick. A normal female, however, never produces the fast, metallic trills of the mate call. Why? To answer this question we have examined the way the larynx produces calls and the way the central nervous system controls the larynx.

CENTRAL AND PERIPHERAL MECHANISMS OF CALL PRODUCTION
Laryngeal muscles contract and relax in response to activity of the laryngeal motoneurons located at the very end of the hindbrain in cranial nerve nucleus IX–X. The axons of these motoneurons travel to the vocal organ as the laryngeal nerve. Because laryngeal motoneurons control only vocal muscles, we can identify other brain regions that participate in calling by identifying nuclei whose interneurons synapse on laryngeal motoneurons. These brain regions include two nuclei in the hindbrain (DTAM and the nucleus reticularis inferior [Ri].) Nucleus DTAM is probably responsible for generating the mate call pattern in frogs;[925, 936] it receives input from auditory nuclei in the thalamus (dorsal forebrain) and from ventral forebrain regions (the preoptic area [POA] and the ventral striatum [VST]). The preoptic area has been implicated in controlling behavioral motivation in many species. Like the thalamic nuclei in this pathway, the ventral striatum contains cells that respond to sound.

SEX DIFFERENCES IN VOCAL NEUROEFFECTORS IN THE CLAWED FROG
Are there any differences in the vocal organ or in the brain that can help to explain why male clawed frogs produce a mate call but females do not? Yes; in fact at both levels males differ from females in ways that can be related to vocal abilities. For example, the male larynx contains a large number of muscle fibers that are capable of contracting and relaxing at very rapid rates (up to 100 times/second). The muscle fibers in the female larynx are fewer in number; furthermore, most of them can only contract and relax slowly (up to 40 times/second).

Mate Calling   **A**

Ticking   **B**

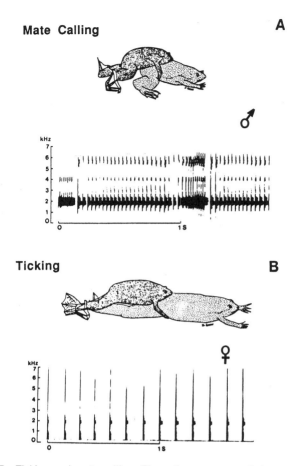

Figure 7.7 Ticking and mate calling. The calls are represented as sound spectrographs in which frequency is shown on the vertical axis and time on the horizontal axis. The basic sound unit for both ticking and mate calling is a brief click in which most sound energy is between 1 and 2 kHz. Mate calling has fast and slow trill phases, whereas ticking is a slow monotonous trill. Male mate calls attract and excite sexually receptive females (top panel). Ticking is given by sexually unreceptive females (bottom panel) and results in the male releasing the female from a clasp.

In the brain, males have more laryngeal motoneurons and interneurons.[563, 564] The vocal pattern generator (DTAM) appears to be more active metabolically in males than in females. Axonal connections between the POA and DTAM and from cranial nerve IX to X to DTAM are robust in males but weak in females.[1097] Do these sex differences in circuitry and muscle fibers contribute to differences in behavior?

To separate the contributions of sex differences in the brain from those of the vocal organ, we devised a way to produce mate calls from the larynx while it is isolated from the brain.[1032] If the nerves that control laryngeal muscle contractions are stimulated in a male with a pattern that mimics the mate call, actual sounds very similar to those of intact males are produced. If the same pattern of stimulation is applied to the laryngeal nerves in the female, mate calls are not produced because the muscles cannot contract and relax rapidly enough. The larynx produces only the temporal pattern that is supplied to it (if it can!). We infer that the temporal pattern for the mate call is produced by the brain. In the female, the vocal organ cannot respond to the mate call pattern because of limitations in the muscle and in the synapses made by laryngeal motoneurons.[918, 1033] It is possible that both male and female brains generate the mate call pattern, but females do not actually call because their vocal apparatus cannot produce fast trills. Alternatively, the female brain may not normally generate the mate call motor pattern or motor command. Females appear to lack certain connections within the vocal motor circuit, providing some support for this suggestion (see later discussion).

HORMONAL CONTRIBUTIONS TO SEX DIFFERENCES
IN VOCAL BEHAVIOR
What other factors contribute to sex differences in the vocal behavior of clawed frogs? In adult males, mate calling depends upon the presence of the testes; castrated males that have stopped mate calling will resume if treated with androgen (testosterone and dihydrotestosterone).[1098] Perhaps exposure to high levels of androgen could induce adult females to give mate calls. However, even after many months of androgen treatment, adult females still do not mate call.[458] Why doesn't androgen work in females? One reason is that it is very difficult to masculinize the larynx in adult females. As we have seen, without a masculine larynx, a female cannot generate the rapid trills of mate calling (no matter what her brain produces). In males, the larynx is masculinized by the secretion of testicular androgens during the first 6 months after metamorphosis.[656, 1034, 1035] If a female is supplied with the appropriate hormones during this period, she will later generate mate calls under appropriate behavioral circumstances. Her larynx is almost fully masculinized and has the right kind of fast twitch muscle fibers,[656, 1035] thus permitting the vocal expression of the masculine call patttern produced by her brain.

The *adult* vocal organ does not require the continued presence of androgen in order to mate call. The *developing* larynx, on the other hand, has an absolute requirement for androgen for it to undergo postmetamorphic masculinization. Thus, during postmetamorphic development, androgen *organizes* the sexual differentiation of the vocal organ in clawed frogs.

MASCULINIZATION OF BRAIN REGIONS THAT GENERATE MATE CALLS
We have identified a number of brain regions that participate in the production of different vocal patterns. Many of these regions are different in males and females (reviewed in Kelley and Tobias,[566] Kelley and Gorlick,[565]). While it seems obvious that some of these sexual dimorphisms must contribute to sex differences in vocal ability, we do not yet have direct proof that this is so. For example, certain connections of interneurons in the vocal circuit (POA to DTAM; laryngeal motoneurons to DTAM; figure 7.6) appear to be missing in

females.[1097] These connections might be essential for stimulating or generating the mate call vocal pattern; without them, the female may be unable to sing. Until we know more about how the vocal pattern is produced by the brain, we cannot test these ideas.

All of the brain regions that affect vocal behavior contain cells that have intracellular receptors for sex steroid hormones (testosterone, dihydrotestosterone, and estradiol; figure 7.6). Expression of steroid hormone receptors characterizes the neurons in the calling circuit. Castrated males do not mate call even though their larynx is fully capable of producing this vocalization.[1032, 1098] We suspect that the action of androgen on the brain is neccessary for it to produce the male vocal pattern in the adult. If true, the *activational* effects of androgen on song would be accomplished in the brain. It is possible that both sexes have the neural elements required to generate the mate call pattern but that only males have the requisite hormones to activate this brain pathway and a masculinized larynx to produce sounds in response to brain commands. Alternatively, steroid hormones could also organize the brain circuitry that produces the masculine vocal pattern, much as they masculinize the larynx. The sexual dimorphism seen in brain vocal circuits is compatible with this latter idea.

Summary and Conclusions

In *Xenopus*, the clawed frog, sex differences in a peripheral vocal organ, the larynx, make important contributions to sex differences in courtship song. Because the female does not have enough fast twitch muscle fibers, she cannot produce the fast, prolonged trills of mate calling, but she can produce the short, slow trills of ticking. The masculine pattern of muscle fiber number and type is established during early postmetamorphic development under the influence of androgens secreted by the testes. If a female is provided with androgenic hormones during this period, her larynx is permanently masculinized and she can mate call. Once masculinized, the larynx does not become demasculinized if deprived of androgens. Thus, masculinization of the vocal organ in *Xenopus laevis* is a clear example of the **organizational** effects of hormones secreted early in development. The neural pathway for vocal behavior is also different in male and female frogs. Because males require androgens to mate call even though their larynx remains masculinized, it seems likely that androgen action on the brain is responsible for **activating** male-specific vocal behavior. It is also possible that androgens organize the neural circuitry for mate calling. Because females given androgen during early postmetamorphic development can mate call, this time period may be essential for organizing the effects of androgen on vocal circuitry in the central nervous system.

Vocal Courtship in Songbirds

There are approximately 8700 species of birds living in the world today. The great majority of these species produce vocal sounds. Vocal behavior is most elaborate among members of the oscine suborder of the Passeriforme birds, more commonly known as the songbirds. More than half of all living species are found in this successful suborder.

The most distinctive trait of songbirds, as the common name suggests, is their ability to produce complexly structured songs. Songs generally consist of a series of syllables, or brief sounds, arranged in a rhythmic sequence that lasts for seconds to minutes. Successive renditions of a particular type of song are usually stereotyped—i.e., they are very similar in structure. The songs produced by each species have a unique structure that sets them apart from the songs of other species found in the same location. A consequence of this **species-specific** nature of song is that there is tremendous diversity in the structure of songs produced by the different species of birds found around the world. In addition, species often differ in the complexity of their song behavior. For example, the white-throated sparrow produces only one very simple song, whereas the rock wren has been estimated to have a repertoire of over 100 song types.[606] Such extreme interspecific diversity provides excellent opportunities for comparative studies of the adaptive function and physiological control of song behavior.

Functions of Song

Song serves two main functions in birds. It can play an important role in aggressive behavior, usually between members of the same sex. This function of song is most often seen in defense of a territory. The second main function of song occurs in the context of courtship. In most songbird species males use song to attract females to their territories. Females may select among many potential mates on the basis of individual song characteristics.[799] The male's song may directly stimulate reproductive behavior in females.[605] In addition to these two main functions, song may act in other behavioral contexts. For example, song may be important in mediating dominance behavior among members of a social group.

SONG AND THE SEASONS

Breeding occurs seasonally in most species of birds that live in temperate and subtropical latitudes. It generally occurs at times of the year when the resources necessary for successfully rearing offspring are most abundant. In such species, song is also seasonal in occurrence. Males sing at high rates early in the breeding season when they first establish territories. Once males have mated with one or more females, who then lay eggs in nests, the rate of song production drops considerably. Outside the breeding season, males may sing only occasionally or not at all.

In tropical latitudes (23.5°N to 23.5°S), seasonal cycles in environmental factors are not as pronounced as at other latitudes. The availability of critical resources for rearing young birds, therefore, does not vary as much with season in the tropics. A consequence of this relative lack of seasonality is that breeding in many tropical species may occur at almost any time of the year. Birds of such species may defend territories and attempt to attract new mates throughout the year. Therefore, it is not surprising that in tropical species, song production is often much less seasonal in occurrence than in temperate and subtropical species.

SONG AND THE SEXES

In most temperate and subtropical species, only the male normally sings. There are, however, numerous exceptions to this observation. In the red-winged blackbird, females produce a relatively simple song that is used in aggressive behavior directed at other females.[104] In the cardinal, late in the breeding season, females sing a song similar to that sung by males during the breeding season.[621]

Among tropical species of birds there is much greater diversity in sexual patterns of song production. Females of many species normally sing. The most complex form of female song is heard in tropical species in which the male and female join together to produce elaborate song duets. Duets are distinguished by precise temporal coordination between the songs of males and females. To a naive listener, these duets may sound as though they are produced by only one bird! Among duetting birds there is much interspecific variability in the complexity of female song compared to that of conspecific males. In an African species, the white-browed robin chat, males produce about eight times as many song syllables in duets as do females.[1036] On the other hand, in the bay wren of Central America, females produce as many different types of songs in duets as do males.[626]

SONG LEARNING

Songbirds learn how to sing. If a young bird is raised in isolation from other birds, he will never produce a normal song.[657, 1028] Some species of birds learn to sing only if they are exposed to song (either from a live tutor or from a tape recorder) during their first year of life. We refer to these species as **age-limited learners**.

One age-limited learner is the swamp sparrow. Male sparrows must hear song between 20 and 60 days after hatching.[658] With repeated exposure to the tutor song, males form a sensory memory or template of the song. At about 8 months of age males first start to translate this sensory template into a motor program. Initially, male sparrows emit sounds that bear only a remote resemblance to the tutor song. This first phase of **subsong** is marked by the production of crude sounds that are highly variable in structure. The young male improves his vocal performance during the next few months. With practice, he comes to produce more polished sounds that bear a closer resemblance to the tutor song. This period of **plastic song** begins at about 10 months of age and is marked by variability in the order in which song syllables are combined. Over the next 1 to 2 months, the male continues to improve his performance so that by 12 months of age he produces a **crystallized song** that has a well-defined, invariant structure. This progressive improvement in performance of singing depends upon the bird being able to hear himself sing. If a bird is deafened before the onset of subsong, he will never develop the ability to produce normal song.[598] If deafened after he has developed crystallized song, however, he continues to be able to sing.

In contrast to age-limited learners, other bird species are able to learn new songs even as adults beyond their first year. These species are referred to as **open-ended learners**. An example is the canary. A young male canary begins to produce subsong about 40 days after hatching.[781] Plastic song begins at about 60 days. A male starts to produce stereotyped adult song by about 8 months of age. Throughout the first breeding season, song remains stable in structure. After the breeding season ends, however, the song becomes extremely variable. In the late summer and early fall, the adult male's vocalizations are similar to those of juvenile subsong. During this period, some song syllables are lost from the bird's repertoire, others are modified, and new syllables may be added. The result is that by his second breeding season, the number of song syllables in a male's repertoire may increase by up to 40%. Unlike age-limited learners, deafening an open-ended learner like a canary as an adult causes song to regress dramatically.

We should note that vocal learning is not restricted to the songbirds. Parrots (order Psittaciformes) show highly developed vocal behavior, which plays an important role in the complex social behavior observed in many parrot species. As known by any one who has taught a pet parrot to speak, members of this order excel at learning to modify their vocal behavior. Hermit hummingbirds (order Trochiliformes) also learn to vocalize.[51]

Sex Differences in Song Behavior

Like other reproductive behaviors, song is strongly influenced by circulating hormone levels. In seasonal breeders, hormones provide a **proximate mechanism** to restrict song production to appropriate times of year. For such species, production of song outside the breeding season may waste much-needed energy and expose the bird to an unnecessary risk of predation. In temperate zone species there is generally a correlation between circulating hormone levels and the degree of song activity.[831]

Arnold[35] demonstrated that the rate of song production by male zebra finches is dependent upon the presence of steroid hormones derived from the testes (figure 7.8). An intact male sings about 45 songs during a 15-minute observation session. Castration of a male reduces his rate of song production to only about eight songs during this same period. If this male then receives an implant of a pellet that releases testosterone propionate, his rate of singing increases once again to about 27 songs in 15 minutes. Removal of this hor-

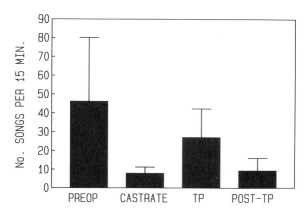

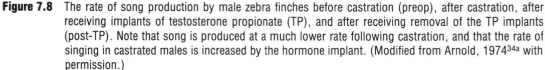

Figure 7.8 The rate of song production by male zebra finches before castration (preop), after castration, after receiving implants of testosterone propionate (TP), and after receiving removal of the TP implants (post-TP). Note that song is produced at a much lower rate following castration, and that the rate of singing in castrated males is increased by the hormone implant. (Modified from Arnold, 1974[34a] with permission.)

mone pellet results in another decline in his song production to about nine songs in 15 minutes. These results indicate that song is directly influenced by circulating hormones.

Harding[463] asked what specific hormones regulate song production. Testosterone may act upon target cells either directly or through one or more of its metabolites. For example, testosterone may be metabolized to several different androgens or may be aromatized to various estrogens (see chapter 2). Harding castrated male zebra finches and implanted them with different combinations of testosterone metabolites. She found that only males receiving hormone treatments that provide both estrogenic and α-androgenic metabolites (testosterone, androstenedione, or estradiol plus 5α-dihydrotestosterone) sing to females. Either estradiol or α-dihydrotestosterone, by itself, fails to reinstate song behavior to its precastration level.

It is interesting that estrogen is necessary for song in **males**. Recall from chapter 2 that estrogen is also necessary to masculinize song control regions in the brain of juvenile female zebra finches. Together, these observations suggest that estrogen plays an important role in both the organization and activation of the song system.

Up to this point we have considered only species in which courtship behavior is directly activated by circulating steroid hormones. There are, however, bird species in which courtship behavior is dissociated from the hormonal state. For example, white-crowned sparrow males will attempt to mate with females even if they have been castrated.[743] In the African stonechat, seasonal patterns of reproductive behavior may not be reflected in seasonal changes in circulating levels of gonadal steroid hormones.[296] For such species, other cues may activate courtship behaviors such as song.[235] These cues could be environmental stimuli, such as the arrival of seasonal rains, or social stimuli, such as the sight of a member of the opposite sex. Under these conditions, we might expect that the activation of song behavior will not be dependent directly upon steroid hormones. The proximate control of song behavior in such species is only beginning to receive attention.

HORMONAL INFLUENCES ON THE DEVELOPMENT OF SONG CONTROL REGIONS OF THE BRAIN

In chapter 2 we described the network of brain nuclei that controls song production in songbirds. Cells in several of these nuclei contain receptors for androgenic and estrogenic hormones. Gurney[447] demonstrated that when newly hatched female zebra finches are treated with estrogen, the neuroanatomy of their song control system is masculinized. Such estrogenized females will produce male-typical song if they receive testosterone implants as adults. In addition, Nordeen and colleagues[775] found that early estrogen treatment of female zebra finches causes them to have more androgen-accumulating cells in song control brain regions. Bottjer[135] showed that in normal male zebra finches, the proportion of cells that accumulate androgen in two song control nuclei, hyperstriatum ventrale (HVc) and magnocellular nucleus of the anterior neostriatum (MAN), increases during the time when song becomes crystallized.

Hormones also influence the incorporation of newly generated neurons into song control nuclei. As you will remember from chapter 2, we can identify newly born neurons by injecting animals with a radioactive form of the nucleotide thymidine. Female zebra finches implanted with estradiol soon after hatching and injected with radioactive thymidine show many more newly generated neurons in HVc and area X than do females that do not receive hormone implants.[775] We do not yet know, however, whether hormones affect the birth of new neurons, the migration of these neurons from the ventricular zone where they are born, or the survival of these cells.

These studies indicate that steroid hormones are important in the masculinization of song control brain regions. Furthermore, these hormones are accumulated by receptors in the nuclei of target cells in these regions. Therefore, hormones may act upon target cells in song regions through a classic steroid receptor mechanism (see chapter 1). However, masculinization of song system anatomy may also occur by other mechanisms. As an example, area X in the forebrain of female zebra finches is masculinized in size by early systemic treatment with testosterone or estradiol. But autoradiographic studies indicate that area X itself lacks receptors for these hormones. We can hypothesize that the size increase in area X occurs in response to afferent input to this nucleus from HVc (figure 7.9).

According this model, early exposure to testosterone or estradiol increases the number of neurons in HVc. This in turn may lead to an increase in the number of HVc neurons that successfully form synapses with area X neurons early in development. The increase in synapse number may result in survival

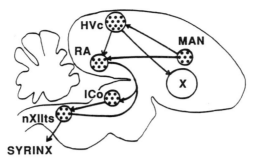

Figure 7.9   Schematic sagittal view of the bird brain, illustrating synaptic connections of the major song control nuclei. Shading indicates nuclei that accumulate testosterone or its metabolites. Abbreviations: HVc, hyperstriatum ventrale, pars caudalis; RA, robust nucleus of the archstriatum; MAN, magnocellular nucleus of the anterior neostriatum, X, area X; ICo, intercollicular nucleus; nXIIts, tracheosyringealis portion of the hypoglossal nucleus. The syrinx is the vocal production organ in birds.

of a greater number of postsynaptic neurons in area X. In support of this hypothesis, area X fails to develop in juvenile female zebra finches in which HVc is lesioned just before the birds receive implants of estradiol.[485] It is a general principle of neural development that the survival of many neurons in vertebrate brains depends upon the formation of a trophic relationship with other neurons.[832] In this way, hormones can exert an indirect effect upon neurons in the brain.

Hormones may also act directly upon neurons through nonclassic mechanisms. Rather than exerting their effects only after binding with receptors in the cytoplasm, steroids may alter the cell's electrical activity by opening or closing ion channels in the cell membrane.[763] Such a mechanism could play a role in hormone-induced masculinization of HVc in zebra finches. As stated above, estradiol increases the size of HVc in female finches. But autoradiographic measurements indicate that only about 7% of cells in HVc of juvenile female finches have receptors for estradiol.[777] It is possible, therefore, that estradiol affects the development of HVc by acting upon the electrical activity of its neurons.

HORMONAL INFLUENCES ON THE DEVELOPMENT OF SONG BEHAVIOR
Hormones are important for the acquisition of song. This has been studied in swamp sparrows by Marler and his colleagues.[659, 660] As we discussed above, swamp sparrows are age-limited song learners. During the first 60 days after hatching, male sparrows learn a sensory model of their species' song. Starting at about 8 months of age, males go through a process of sensorimotor learning in which they translate the sensory template of song to a motor program. Marler and his colleagues measured circulating concentrations of steroid hormones in young male sparrows during different phases of song learning. They found that there are two periods of high circulating testosterone concentration. These testosterone peaks coincide with the times of the sensory and

sensorimotor learning phases of song development. Estradiol levels are also high during the sensory learning phase. To test whether steroids are necessary for song learning, males were castrated at 3 weeks and then tutored with tape-recorded song. The surprising result of this study was that castrated males acquired a sensory model of song and subsequently produced subsong and early plastic song. However, these castrated males did not produce crystallized song unless they received implants of testosterone. Within 3 weeks of receiving testosterone, castrates achieved crystallized song. Apparently, testosterone is not necessary for the sensory and early motor phases of song learning but is essential for the final motor phase. Marler and his co-workers observed that while castration eliminated testosterone in males, estradiol continued to be present during the early phases of song learning. Such estradiol must arise from nontesticular sources in castrates and may play a role in the sensory acquisition of song.

Circulating concentrations of sex steroids are also correlated with song development in open-ended learners. Remember that male canaries are able to learn new songs even as adults. The development of songs by adults occurs in a seasonal manner. Rates of song production are highest in the spring, when testosterone concentrations are highest. When the breeding season ends, testosterone concentrations drop and song becomes unstable. Starting about 1 month after testosterone concentrations reach their lowest yearly level, male canaries show pronounced plasticity of song behavior. Song syllables are modified or replaced at a high rate, resulting in a net increase in song repertoire size. Testosterone concentrations begin to rise during this period of greatest song learning. When testosterone concentrations rise to their highest point, the male's song repertoire stabilizes and new syllables are no longer acquired. This cycle repeats itself each year.[781]

Hormones can produce dramatic changes in the behavior and song control brain nuclei of adult female canaries. Females normally do not sing. Treatment of adult females with testosterone, however, causes them to sing.[780] In response to such testosterone treatment, HVc and robust nucleus of the archstriatum (RA) increase in size by about 90% and 50%, respectively. The increase in the size of HVc may be at least partly due to an increase in the number of neurons. Gonadectomized females implanted with testosterone have a greater number of newly generated neurons in HVc than do females implanted with estradiol, dihydrotestosterone, estradiol plus dihydrotestosterone, or blank pellets.[782] Part of the increase in RA is due to an increase in the length of female dendritic fibers to a value comparable with that seen in male canaries. This leads to the formation of new synapses.[279, 280] Despite this androgen-induced growth of RA, the volume of this nucleus in adult females does not reach male values. Also, the songs produced by testosterone-treated adult females are much simpler in structure than those of males. These observations indicate that hormones may also need to act during the juvenile organization of the song system to produce complete masculinization of song nuclei in the brain and of song behavior.

COMPARATIVE STUDIES OF SEX DIFFERENCE IN SONG BEHAVIOR

As discussed earlier, there is considerable interspecific variation in the structure, complexity, learning, and sexual occurrence of song behavior. We can ask whether such variation in behavior is accompanied by concomitant variation between species in the neural and hormonal control of song. This question can best be addressed through **comparative** studies of bird species whose song behavior differs along an interesting continuum. The goal of such studies is to correlate components of song system structure with vocal behavior.

There is dramatic variation among species in the degree of sexual dimorphism in song behavior. As mentioned earlier only male **zebra finches** sing. In **canaries**, females are capable of singing but do so only rarely. Females of the **white-browed robin chat** of Africa routinely sing in duets with males. However, female chats include only about one-eighth as many different types of song syllables in their repertoires as do males. Another duetting species in which males have more complex song repertoires is the **rufous-and-white wren** of Central America. Males of this species sing about twice as many different types of songs as do females. In two other species of Central American wrens that sing duets, the **buff-breasted wren** and the **bay wren**, there is no sexual difference in the size of song repertoires. As we proceed from zebra finches to bay wrens in this group we find, therefore, a continuum of decreasing incidence of sex differences in song behavior.[36, 147]

Several interesting observations emerge from comparisons of the neural song control systems of these six species. In all species in which females are normally capable of singing, we find the same network of song control nuclei in the female brain as we observe in males. Thus, only female zebra finches lack a well-defined area X. As males and females become more similar in song behavior across species, the similarity in size of the song control regions in their brains also increases (figure 7.10). The same pattern is observed for the number of neurons in these regions.

The pattern of hormone accumulation by cells in song control brain nuclei also varies across these species. This pattern has been examined in the zebra finch, canary, rufous-and-white wren, and bay wren using steroid autoradiographic techniques. Birds are gonadectomized and injected with radioactively labeled testosterone. Cells that accumulate the radioactive testosterone or its metabolites are referred to as testosterone target cells. Comparison of these species shows that the more alike the sexes are in song behavior, the more alike they are in the number of testosterone target cells in the song control nucleus HVc (figure 7.11).[146]

These comparative studies indicate that singing females develop song control systems in their brains that are similar in basic structure and hormone sensitivity to those of males of their species. This observation suggests that the network of brain regions has been conserved during the evolution of new species of songbirds. As you can see, comparative studies provide a powerful means of testing hypotheses about the relationship between neural function and behavior.

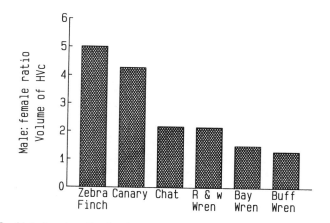

Figure 7.10 Male-female ratios for the volume of hyperstriatum ventrale (VHc) in the zebra finch, canary, white-browed robin chat, rufous-and-white wren, bay wren, and buff-breasted wren. The more alike the sexes of a species are in the volume of HVc, the smaller the male-female ratio. There is a continuum of decreasing incidence of sexual differences in song behavior and a corresponding decrease in the sexual dimorphism of HVc among these species.

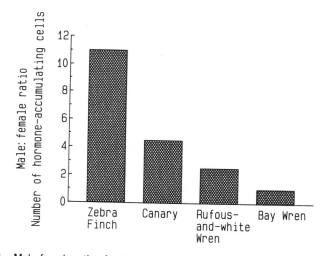

Figure 7.11 Male-female ratios for the numbers of cells in HVc that accumulate testosterone or its metabolites in the zebra finch, canary, rufous-and-white wren, and bay wren. The more alike the sexes of a species are in the complexity of vocal behavior, the smaller the difference between the sexes in the number of testosterone target cells.

Summary and Conclusions

Song is a learned behavior that plays a critical role in courtship by birds. The production of song is regulated by a network of discrete nuclei in the brain. The organization and activation of the neural song control system are each strongly affected by gonadal steroid hormones. Both androgenic and estrogenic hormones play a role. Cells in several song nuclei have receptors for these steroids.

There is extensive interspecific diversity in the degree of sexual dimorphism in song production. Comparative studies indicate that this behavioral variation is accompanied by concomitant variation between species in the neural and hormonal control of song.

General Summary

During courtship a member of one sex produces a series of signals that induces a member of the other sex to mate. These courtship behaviors are interesting for three reasons. First, in species in which individuals are widely dispersed at the beginning of the breeding season, courtship signaling brings the sexes together. In closely related species that share similar territories, courtship rituals can aid in species recognition. Courtship is also a way for individuals to assess or influence each other's reproductive readiness.

A second interesting feature of courtship signals is that they are not produced to the same extent by both sexes. Typically, males initiate courtship and engage in showy and energetic courtship behaviors, songs, or visual displays. This behavior occurs because for males of many species, the resource most critical to their reproductive success is access to females. In terms of energy expenditure, sperm are relatively cheap to produce, whereas eggs are expensive. Males compete for access to eggs and, in mammals and birds, for the maternal care that increases the chances of survival of their offspring. In an attempt to attract females, males of many species have evolved courtship behavior. This behavior involves production of a communicatory signal. In this manner, sexual selection has repeatedly led to the evolution of sexually dimorphic communicatory behavior in animals.

Finally, what information is conveyed by courtship signals? Can females make use of information contained in the courtship signal to choose a male? Do males learn anything about the female's readiness to reproduce from the courtship ritual? Male courtship signals can be read for signs of vigor or longevity, desirable attributes that may be transmitted to the young. Females can also use male courtship signals to assess possible paternal contributions to survival of their offspring through direct paternal care protection from predators, and maintenance of a feeding territory. Females maximize their reproductive success by selectively mating with males of high genetic quality or with males that contribute care or resources to the survival of offspring.

Hormone secretion can alter the development of brain pathways and muscles that are involved in the production of courtship signals. In males, androgens and their metabolites can permanently change the structure and function of neurons and muscles that produce courtship signals. These changes reflect the *organizational* actions of steroid hormones. Hormones also strongly control the production of courtship signals in adult animals. Hormone effects in adulthood typify the *activational* effects of androgens.

The production of communication signals in diverse sensory modalities is regulated by discrete circuits of brain nuclei. In species in which communication behavior is sexually dimorphic, the associated brain nuclei also differ in structure and function between the sexes. In fact, the most dramatic sex differences yet observed in vertebrate brain structure are found in nuclei involved in the production of courtship behavior in various species. Steroid hormones play a crucial role in establishing these sexual dimorphisms in brain structure. These hormones provide a proximate mechanism for the organization and activation of neural circuits associated with the production of communication signals. Study of disparate animals such as electric fish, clawed frogs, and songbirds point to the dominant role of androgenic hormones and their metabolites in the development and adult production of male courtship. This is a striking example of evolutionary conservatism.

Closely related species with differing social systems may show pronounced variation in the pattern of courtship behaviors. Such behavioral variation may result from subtle differences between species in the balance of steroid hormones secreted. Species differences may also result from the timing of hormone secretion, both during critical stages of early development and seasonally in adults. The presence of such extensive interspecific variation in the neural and hormonal bases of courtship shows that there is considerable evolutionary flexibility in the interaction between hormones and the nervous system. Thus, comparative studies of courtship systems provide rich opportunities to integrate behavioral, endocrinological, and neurobiological approaches.

We now explore other, nonsexual behaviors that are altered by hormones. Some of these behaviors, while not sexual, are still closely linked to reproduction, and thus perhaps the importance of gonadal, hypothalamic, and pituitary hormones in such behaviors is to be expected. For example, we begin in chapter 8 by considering parental behavior, clearly an extension of the reproductive process. You may notice that this chapter heavily emphasizes maternal rather than paternal behavior, but that is a reflection of the fact that it is the mother's behavior that is predominantly influenced by hormones. Maternal behavior is, for the most part, initiated by the hormones of pregnancy. Paternal behavior is more prevalent among birds, where very altricial young and a high metabolic rate often keep both parents busy gathering food for nestlings, but even in birds the role of hormones in initiating or maintaining the behavior is not clear.

Conversely, chapter 9 covers aggression with an emphasis on aggression between male rivals. Male-male competition for mating is prevalent among vertebrates, especially in mammals, and so this behavior is also quite relevant to reproductive success. Therefore, it might make some sense that the same androgens that prepare the animal for reproduction by altering growth, spermatogenesis, and sexual motivation at puberty might also prepare the animal for aggressive encounters. Although we will find several unexpected complications in this rather convenient view, and you will find the evidence that androgen increases aggressiveness weaker than commonly expected, it nonetheless seems clear that gonadal steroids can have some influence on aggression. Chapter 10 continues on the related theme of stress, including stress as a result of aggression. Variables such as experience, personality, and social rank within a dominance hierarchy, however, seem to affect directly how an animal reacts to stressful events. Chapter 10 also explores the beneficial short-term effects of hormones released during stress and the dire consequences caused by these same hormones when they are released chronically, and introduces the reader to interactions among the immune system, endocrine system, and the nervous system—a new field of research known as *psychoneuroimmunology*.

Chapters 11 and 12 deal with behaviors that seem far removed from reproduction—motor patterns, learning, memory, and cognitive function. Indeed, the effects of hormones on these behaviors are more subtle than those on the other behaviors we have considered so far. Despite the more modest influence of hormones, these are important processes that have wide-ranging consequences for many behaviors. Chapter 12 may prove especially challenging because it deals with the controversial issue of how men and women differ in cognitive abilities and whether hormones contribute to such differences.

8 Hormone-Behavior Relations in the Regulation of Parental Behavior

Jay S. Rosenblatt

After courtship, copulation, and fetal development have ended, successful reproduction hinges upon whether the offspring will ever reach reproductive age. In response to this requirement, parental behavior has evolved in many species, especially among the mammals and birds. Once again, hormones, perhaps as a result of their preexisting roles in sexual physiology and behavior, have come to coordinate these efforts by preparing the nervous system to display nurturing and defensive behaviors. Among mammals, the many different hormones required to maintain pregnancy and nursing seem to play a part also in maternal behaviors. Some of these same hormones also support reproductive physiology and parental behavior among birds.

What are the varieties of parental behavior, and why do most mammals require extensive maternal care? What are the hormones supporting pregnancy and lactation, and how do those hormones affect behavior? What parts of the nervous system mediate these hormonal influences upon parental behavior?

Introduction

In the evolution of reproduction, hormones have come to play a most important role. They are especially important in parental care. There are many physiological systems involved in parental care that need to be integrated with parental behavior over a prolonged period. Parental care, in addition, must be coordinated with the social and ecological environment because it involves other individuals and depends upon a finely tuned relationship with the environment for the resources the parents need to rear their young.

Although this is the broader evolutionary and social-ecological context in which parental behavior occurs, in this chapter the main concern will be with the hormones that stimulate parental care and how they act to produce their behavioral effects. The first section will review how parental care has evolved in relation to modes of reproduction among the lower vertebrates, fishes, amphibia, and reptiles. The second section will describe the variety of parental behavior patterns and several of the determinants found in the two most advanced vertebrate classes, the mammals and birds. In the third section what is known about the hormonal basis of parental care and associated functions in selected mammalian and avian species will be presented. The hormonal basis of maternal behavior in the rat will serve as a case history that will be discussed in some detail.

Several considerations dictated the choice of animal groups that will be discussed. Chief among these was the availability of research on the hormonal basis of parental care in the different mammalian and avian groups. A second consideration was the desirability of presenting a diversity of parental behavior patterns. Among both mammals and birds, species have diverged in their patterns of parental care. The developmental status of their young at birth may be either altricial or precocial in different species, and this determines to a large extent their pattern of parental care. Altricial newborn are immobile at birth and are fed by the parent, while precocial newborn are mobile at birth and feed by themselves shortly after birth. There is a third group of species among both mammals and birds in which the young are semialtricial or semiprecocial at birth. They are largely mobile but are dependent upon the parent for feeding. Among the mammals, this group is represented by the primates, and among birds by many of the shorebirds (e.g., gulls, terns). However, since little research on the hormonal basis of parental care has been done on these latter species, they will not be discussed in this chapter.

Evolutionary Aspects of Parental Behavior Among the Vertebrates

FISHES, AMPHIBIA AND REPTILES
Not all animals take care of their young by exhibiting parental care. Among most species of fishes, amphibia, and reptiles, females disperse their fertilized eggs, lay them at specially selected sites, or lay them in nests they have built. The eggs are then left to hatch with no further care. In most species that do not exhibit parental care the females lay many more eggs than are hatched. Many more young hatch than usually survive beyond the first few few days or even hours. Reproduction, in these species, therefore, involves a minimum of parental care.

Parental behavior most likely arose in evolution to supplement the physiological mechanisms of reproduction. In other words, parental behavior is thought to have evolved when fertilized eggs did not develop, hatch, and result in survival of enough young to ensure survival of the species. It is closely related, therefore, to hormonally controlled reproductive processes. Parental behavior appears in species exhibiting the two principal modes of reproduction among the vertebrates, egg-laying or oviparity, and live-bearing either through the mechanisms of oviviparity or viviparity. Among the lower vertebrates (i.e., most fishes, amphibia, and reptiles), females are oviparous, and both male and female may exhibit parental care of eggs during incubation and hatching; in several species they may also display care of the hatchlings. Examples are found in many species of fishes, particularly among the mouthbreeders and other teleost fishes. Examples of parental care of eggs and young are also found among frogs and among several species of reptiles.

There are progressive stages in the evolution of parental care in egg-laying species of fish. Many species display external fertilization by males of ova released by the female but no further care of the fertilized ova. The second stage appears in species in which the parents remain with the fertilized ova after they have been deposited. This pattern has many variations in different species. One or the other parent fans the eggs to aerate them, prevent them from being covered by silt, and protect them from predators.

Males predominate in brood care among the most common fishes, the teleosts. This situation has been attributed to a preadaptation in males, which defend territories in which spawning takes place. The males then go on to protect the fertilized eggs that have been deposited in their territories. A further advance occurs in mouthbreeding species, in which the male or female picks up the eggs after they have been fertilized and carries them in the mouth, either for short periods to transport them from one nest site to another or for longer periods until they are hatched. In some species, after releasing the young, females pick up the freely swimming hatchlings in their mouth when a disturbance occurs and then releases them when the disturbance has passed.

Among the lower vertebrates are species of fishes, amphibia, and reptiles in which eggs are retained in the female's reproductive tract (ovoviviparity). Others have developed specialized internal or external organs that have been modified (among males as well) to retain the fertilized ova until the young have completed their embryonic development. Examples of this are the gastric brooding frog[1057] in which the young are incubated internally by the female in her stomach, which is converted into a uterus. Another is the marsupial frog,[310] in which the male assists the female in stuffing fertilized eggs into a vascularized pouch located on her back where they are incubated. In these species one or the other parent often exhibits parental behavior toward the young after they have hatched and been released.

The most advanced patterns of parental care among the fishes are seen in those species in which the ova are released internally into the oviduct. The ova are fertilized by the male while still in the oviduct. Gestation also occurs internally, and live young are released into the environment. Once released, the young are guarded and in some species are provided with nutrition for a period afterwards.[194]

Like many, perhaps all, innovations in organic evolution, parental care arose to supplement existing reproductive processes. Since it also bestowed sufficient adaptive advantage, it became the starting point for the elaboration of the wide variety of behavior patterns devoted to parental care seen among animals today. As a general rule, species that exhibit parental care give birth to fewer young. These individuals develop more slowly and are more likely to survive to reproductive age. Almost all species in the two most highly evolved animal classes, mammals and birds, exhibit parental care of their young. There are some bird species, species of cowbirds and cuckoos, that are exceptions to this rule. These birds deposit their fertilized eggs in the nests of other species, and their young are raised by the host species.

MAMMALS

Parental behavior varies with mode of reproduction in mammals. The primitive mammals, the monotremes (e.g., echidna and platypus), form a bridge between the oviparous reptiles and the viviparous mammals. They are oviparous and incubate their eggs in nests, but following hatching of the young, the female exhibits parental behavior including lactation and nursing of the young.[336]

The establishment of gestation among the more advanced mammals is based upon the evolution of neuroendocrine mechanisms that extend the sexual cycle beyond its normal duration.[87] An earlier stage in the evolution of these mechanisms is seen among the marsupial mammals (e.g., kangaroos, wallabies, opossums). The duration of gestation in almost all marsupials does not extend beyond the length of the sexual cycle, and in several species females give birth midway during the sexual cycle. Although the female Virginia opossum become pregnant, there is no clearly defined hormonal state of pregnancy in this species that differs from that of the estrous cycle: Circulating levels of the ovarian hormones estradiol and progesterone in pregnant females are identical with those of nonpregnant females.[461, 938]

Among the true or placental mammals, the duration of gestation ranges from four times the length of the sexual cycle, as in the hamster, to nine times, as in women, and even longer in other species. Sexual cycling is generally suspended during pregnancy, and there are distinct patterns of ovarian secretion of estrogen and progesterone and pituitary and placental secretion of their hormones during pregnancy that differ from those during the sexual cycle.[475]

Parental behavior among the mammals has retained its close relationship to the physiological and particularly the endocrine and neuroendocrine processes that govern reproduction. Its appearance in the female is synchronized with the end of pregnancy. It is signaled by parturition and the onset of lactation, the hallmark of the mammals. As we shall see, parental behavior, particularly among females, is a hormone-dependent behavior pattern. The endocrine secretions of late pregnancy provide an internal milieu of circulating hormones in a temporal pattern that regulates the synchronized onset of parturition, lactation, and parental behavior. Hormones act on the reproductive tract to stimulate parturition and on the mammary gland to initiate lactation. They also act on the central nervous system to stimulate parental behavior in the female. Males are not stimulated hormonally to exhibit parental behavior; nevertheless, in many species they exhibit it either at the birth of the young or later.[589] In most instances this behavior is likely to be nonhormonal in nature.

Parental behavior is most highly evolved among the true mammals. After internal fertilization the ova become attached to the female's uterine wall, where they undergo embryonic development during pregnancy or gestation. The embryo is joined to the mother by the placenta. There is an exchange of nutrients, gases, and hormones, among other substances, through the highly vascularized tissues of the mother and embryo that are in close proximity.

Table 8.1 Removal of the Ovaries or Pituitary in Pregnancy and its Effect on the Maintenance of Gestation in Various Species

ANIMAL AND LENGTH OF GESTATION (DAYS)	APPROXIMATE STAGE OF PREGNANCY WHEN OPERATION PERFORMED			
	Ovariectomy		*Hypophysectomy*	
	First Half	Second Half	First Half	Second Half
Woman (267)	+	+	+	+
Rhesus monkey (165)	+	+	+	+
Tammar wallaby (29)*	+	+	+	+
Quokka (27)*	+	+		
Guinea pig (68)	±	+	+	+
Sheep (148)	−	+	−	+
Horse (350)	−	+		
Brush-tailed opossum (17)	−	+		
Rat (22)	−	±	−	+
Cat (63)	−	±		±
Ferret (42)	−	±	−	±
Cow (282)	−	±		
Dog (61)	−		−	±
Rabbit (28)	−	−	−	−
Mouse	−	−	±	+
Hamster (16)	−	−	−	+
Goat (150)	−	−	−	−
Pig (113)	−	−	−	−
Virginia opossum (13)	−	−		
Armadillo (150)	Implantation may occur	−		

Key: +, fetuses survive; ±, some fetuses survive; −, fetuses aborted or resorbed. * indicates time from ovulation to birth, excluding the period of diapause.

This table illustrates that maintenance of pregnancy is dependent upon hormone secretions from the ovaries and pituitary gland in some mammals but not all. Species in which fetuses survive removal of the ovaries and/or pituitary gland are dependent upon hormonal secretions from the placenta. (From Heap and Flint, 1986,[475] reprinted by permission.)

Most important is the influence exerted by the embryo and fetus on the reproductive physiology of the mother. The organ through which this influence is exerted is the placenta, which secretes substances that enter the female's circulation. These substances then act to regulate the female's physiology in relation to the developing fetus. In the evolution of the mammals, the fetus has gained increasing control over the reproductive processes of the mother (table 8.1), and in primates the fetal placenta controls the pregnancy from the end of the first month.[263, 475] The female gives birth to live young at parturition or delivery.

BIRDS

An alternative mode of reproduction has evolved among birds, in which all known species reproduce by oviparity or egg-laying after internal fertilization. Among the selective factors that have acted against the evolution of viviparity among birds or, expressed positively, have made oviparity so effective a means of reproduction among birds, is their highly developed pattern of parental care.[122, 570] The duration of parental care extends from the laying of eggs and their incubation to the care of the hatchlings; care of hatchlings is distinguished from incubation by the term *brooding*. Kendeigh[570] has, in fact, suggested that "parental care has reached its highest and most elaborate development in birds." Not only has parental behavior evolved to take care of the young, as among the mammals, it has evolved to take care of the eggs also, a problem not faced in the evolution of parental care among mammals.

The hormonal regulation of egg incubation and parental behavior among birds parallels hormonal regulation of pregnancy and parental behavior among mammals. This is particularly evident among those birds that feed their young with crop milk; the parallel with mammalian lactation is striking. In pigeons and ring doves the pituitary hormone prolactin stimulates the production of crop milk. In mammals, prolactin stimulates lactation. More generally, in females ovarian hormones and prolactin stimulate incubation behavior. It is not known what stimulates males to incubate eggs in species in which males exhibit this behavior. During incubation the parents warm the eggs, thus enabling the embryos to develop. Among the mammals the ovarian hormones prepare the wall of the uterus for the attachment of the fertilized ova. Together with pituitary and placental lactogenic hormones, these hormones maintain gestation during which the embryo undergoes its prenatal development. Parental care is as prominent and varied a behavior pattern among the birds as among the mammals. The hormonal basis of parental care has not, however, been studied extensively among birds, although there has been considerable research on a few species.

Varieties of Parental Behavior Among Mammals and Birds

Among the mammals there is a wide variety of parental behavior patterns. They can be divided into three main types based chiefly upon the developmental status of the young at birth. They are the *nesting* pattern in species with altricial newborn, the *leading-following pattern* in species with precocial newborn, and the *clinging-carrying pattern* characteristic of species with semialtricial or semiprecocial newborn. Exceptions are the marsupials, in which the young are extremely altricial at birth but nevertheless are carried by the mother.

Among the birds a similar division occurs between species with altricial and precocial newborn. Nesting as a feature of parental care is common to both types of species in contrast to mammals, in which only altricial species have nests as a rule. Nesting is imposed upon the avian parents by their oviparous mode of reproduction. In all bird species the eggs are layed in nests that may be very elaborate, as in weaver birds, or just scratches on the ground, as in many gulls. The differences between altricial and precocial hatchlings begin during egg formation, when females of altricial species deposit a smaller proportion of yolk to albumin, which also is less rich in protein and caloric content than the yolk in eggs of precocial species. At hatching, the precocial young, which are not fed by their parents, have twice as large a yolk store as altricial young, enabling them to regulate their body temperature earlier (i.e., to become homoiothermic) and to move about more readily, allowing them to follow the parent and to find food. More than 80% of bird species are altricial.[31]

The newborn hatch in altricial or precocial condition, and it is at this time that different patterns of parental care become evident. Examples of bird species with altricial newborn and prolonged nesting after hatching are robins, canaries, and doves and pigeons. Chickens, turkeys, and ducks are examples of species with precocial hatchlings that leave the nest and follow the mother shortly after hatching.

Another factor that determines the pattern of parental care is the availability and distribution of food in the species habitat. This controls whether parents can remain at one site or must continually or seasonally forage over a large territory to obtain adequate nutrition. If the parents can remain at one site to forage, they can contruct a nest or use a single site to deposit their young while they forage in the area. Parents then return to their young periodically to feed and take care of them. The young of these species are typically altricial or semialtricial. If parents must travel over a large territory to forage, the young must be able to follow the parent (as among many ungulates) or to cling to or be carried by the parent as it travels (as among many primates and several marsupials). Precocial young are able to perform these behaviors.

Among mammals there is an interaction between the composition of the milk and the nursing behavior of the mother. The proportions of the major nutrients, protein, fat, and water, vary with the frequency of nursing in different mammals.[109] In species that nurse less frequently, the nutritional value of the milk is greater than in those that nurse more frequently (figure 8.1). Young that cling to the mother or are carried by her nurse very frequently because the mother's nipples are constantly available. Those young that are left in a nest or at a nest site nurse less frequently at intervals determined by the mother when she returns to the nest. Among rats, mothers nurse their young at 2 to 3 hour intervals. On the other hand, hooded seal pups nurse almost continuously. They double their weights in 4 days of nursing post partum and then are weaned.[137] In contrast, in rabbits and hares, mothers nurse their young only once each day, usually at dusk. More extreme cases are found in tree shrews, in which mothers nurse their young every 48 hours.[665] Among many species of seals, mothers may remain away from their young for a week while they forage at sea during the pup's second week.[366]

SPECIES WITH ALTRICIAL YOUNG

Altricial young among the mammals are very immature at birth. They cannot see or hear and are unable to move well (figure 8.2). They are also unable to regulate their body temperature (i.e., to achieve thermoregulation) or to feed themselves. Parental care usually conforms to a *nesting pattern*. Monotremes

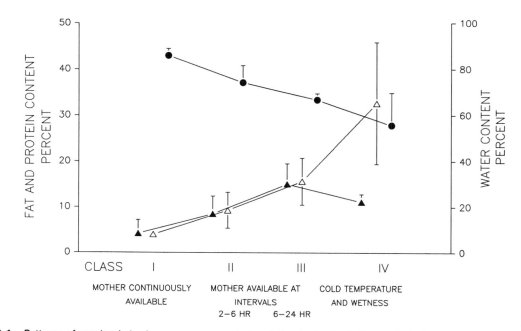

Figure 8.1 Patterns of nursing behavior among mammals in relation to the fat ($\triangle$), protein ($\blacktriangle$), and water ($\bullet$) content of the milk. Examples of class 1 species are marsupials, bears, and primates; class II species are mouse, rat, dog, hamster; class III species are lion, deer, rabbit; class IV species are dolphin, whale, otter. Note increase in fat content in species living in cold habitats and in water. (Data from Ben Shaul, 1962.[109])

are included among these species because their young hatch in an altricial condition.

In altricial species the mother selects a site at which to build a nest. This can be underground, as in many rodent species and rabbits, at ground level, as among carnivores, or in trees, as in squirrels and many species of primates (i.e., prosimians). Mothers nurse their young in the nest. They also usually stimulate them to eliminate, often by licking them. In many nesting species, they retrieve them back to the nest, and exhibit nest defense against conspecific or other potential predators.

Kangaroos, wallabies, and opossums and all other marsupials are exceptions to the general pattern because their young are very altricial but nevertheless are carried by the mother. Among kangaroos and wallabies, for example, the embryonic young at birth crawl into the mother's pouch, where they spend as long as 8 months. They emerge as well-developed, mobile animals with vision and hearing. Although they continue to suckle at regular intervals, the joeys begin to forage for themselves but remain close to the mother for more than a year. Other marsupials exhibit a mixed pattern in which the young are initially carried in a pouch and then cling to the mother's fur (e.g., squirrel-like flying phalanger, koala) or are deposited in a nest (e.g., marsupial mouse). In still other species lacking pouches, the young cling to the mother's nipples, and when they are older they may ride on the mother's back (e.g., wooly opossum, numbat, murine opossum) (Morris, 1965).[758]

Species with altricial young predominate among the birds, although this mode of parental care is derived from the ancestral precocial mode of parental care.[31] Parents of altricial young brood their young for several weeks and feed them special food they have collected and, in some cases, partially digested, which is regurgitated when the parents are stimulated by hungry nestlings (figure 8.2). Parents may continue to feed their young for some time after the young leave the nest until they have begun to feed themselves and are able to fly and hide from predators. Representative altricial species that have been studied are the canary, pied flycatcher, and ring dove.

SPECIES WITH PRECOCIAL YOUNG

A second major pattern is the *leading-following pattern*, which is characteristic of species in which the young at birth are precocial. These young have vision, hearing, locomotive ability, and the ability to achieve thermoregulatation. They are still, however, dependent upon the mother for nursing and protection. The mother leads the young, who follow her. In several species the mother selects a nest site, and the young remain at that nest site for the first few days. The mother returns periodically to feed them. Although they nurse for some time, the young are able to feed by themselves quite soon after birth. Many ungulates (i.e., sheep, goats, cows, horses, deer, and elk) exhibit this pattern of parental care. Some features of this pattern are also seen among smaller mammals such as guinea pigs and kangaroo rats. Sea mammals (i.e., whales and porpoises) exhibit a similar pattern of maternal behavior with their precocial marine young, the young following the mother by swimming alongside her.

Precocial avian species, about 10% of all species of birds, exhibit an abbreviated pattern of parental care compared to altricial avian species. Parents protect their young from predators and emit feeding calls, which attract the young to sources of food. The young hover around the female and follow her when she walks or swims (figure 8.2; hence, the phenomenon of "maternal imprinting," which is found in many precocial avian species). Initially, the parent may provide a source of warmth for the young, but they develop thermoregulation rapidly and become independent of her in this regard. Representative precocial species that have been studied are chickens and turkeys.

SPECIES WITH SEMIALTRICIAL OR SEMIPRECOCIAL YOUNG

The third major pattern is the *clinging-carrying pattern*. This pattern is exhibited by many primate species including humans. In these species the young at birth are semialtricial or semiprecocial and require a great deal of assistance in locomotion. Eyes and ears are open, but the young cannot keep up with the mother as she moves with the social group. They cling to her, and when she rests they walk around and climb nearby branches. They depend upon the mother for nursing and for defense in addition to transportation. Human

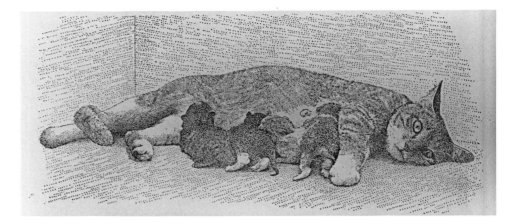

A

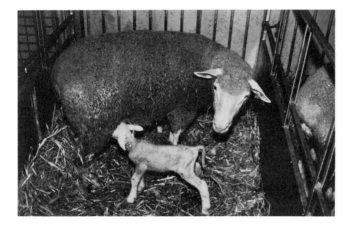

B

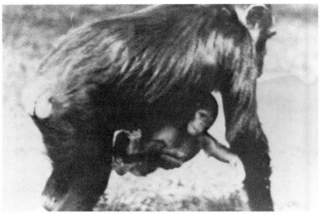

C

Figure 8.2 Types of mother-young interactions in different mammals and birds. Examples of species with altricial, precocial, and semialtricial-semiprecocial young among the mammals and birds *A*, Altricial kittens nursing in the home site. (From Rosenblatt, J., Learning in newborn kittens. *Sci. Am.* 227:18–291.[872] Copyright 1972 by *Scientific American* Inc. Reproduced by permission.) *B*, Newborn lamb less than 1 hour after birth standing and suckling from its mother. (Courtesy of Pascal Poindron) *C*, Semiprecocial-semialtrical chimpanzee infant partially clinging to its mother and partially being carried by her. (From Plooij, F. [1979][823]; Reproduced by permission.) *D*, Altricial newborn yellow-tailed thornbill being fed by mother in the nest. (Reproduced with permission of M. F. Sofer.) *E*, Precocial ducklings following behind the mother who is leading them. (Reproduced with permission of G. R. Roberts.) *F*, Herring gull semialtricial-semiprecocial newborn pecking at the red spot on the female's bill that causes mother to regurgitate semi-digested food. (Reproduced with permission of William D. Griffin.) *G*, Wood pigeon regurgitating "crop milk" into nestling. (From Skutch, A. F. [1976][962]; reproduced by permission.)

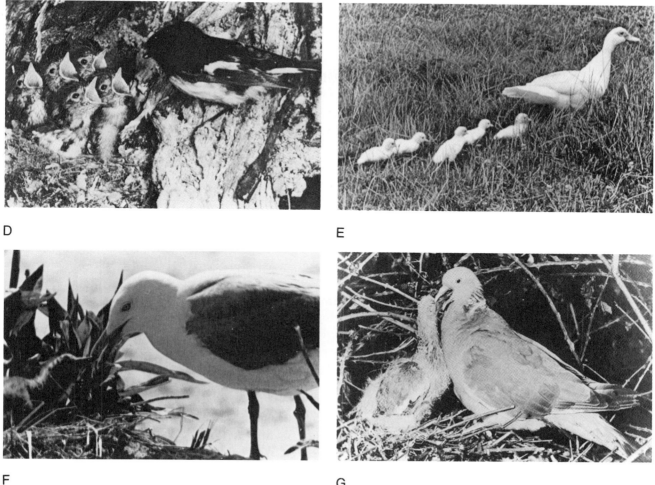

D

E

F

G

mothers carry their infants, but among subhuman primates the infants must cling to the mother and often ride on her back, side, or chest. Human mothers also place their infants in nests (i.e., cribs) and return to feed and clean them periodically like mothers with altricial newborn.

About 10 per cent of all avian species are semialtricial or semiprecocial. These species are considered transitional between altricial and precocial species in many characteristics. Gulls and terns are examples of this type of species (figure 8.2). Nestbuilding is minimal, in general, and the young are exposed. They are, therefore, more mobile than altricial young and can leave the nest by the first day, often in response to parental warning calls given when predators are close. Parents feed the young special food, which is often regurgitated. It is several weeks before the young can obtain food by themselves. Parental care involves complex interactions between the parents and the young, often mediated by special vocalizations.[31]

Hormonal Basis of Parental Behavior in Selected Species of Mammals

Rat

THE HORMONAL REGULATION OF PREGNANCY

Following mating, the female rat undergoes hormonal changes that initiate the processes of implantation of the fertilized ova, suspension of estrous cycling for 22 days until postpartum estrus, and establishment and maintenance of the progesterone-secreting corpora lutea. In addition, the mammary glands begin to proliferate secretory tissue that will produce milk and ducts that will carry the milk to the nipples, and the nipples become enlarged. Many endocrine glands and their hormonal secretions are involved, including a new one that appears only during pregnancy, the placenta. These hormones include the anterior pituitary hormones, luteinizing hormone (LH) and prolactin, and the posterior pituitary hormone oxytocin. The ovaries secrete mainly progesterone but also small amounts of estrogen and testosterone. The placenta secretes prolactin-like hormones called luteotropins and a chorionic gonadotropin, which is luteinizing hormone. There are additional hormones and substances that play a role during pregnancy, such as relaxin and prostaglandin $F_{2\alpha}$.

Following mating, there is a rise in progesterone secretion by the ovaries as corpora lutea form under the influence of LH and prolactin secreted by the pituitary gland. These hormonal changes are a direct response to the sensory stimulus of mating and can be prevented by blocking the neural transmission of this stimulus to the brain.[980,981] Progesterone acts on the uterus, which has previously been prepared by estrogen, to enable the fertilized ova to become attached to the wall of the uterus (implantation). A placenta is formed by each embryo that becomes embedded in the wall of the uterus. The richly vascularized placentas lie in close proximity to the mother's circulatory system. This system enables nutritive and other substances carried in the mother's blood to diffuse to the embryo and provides a means for the embryo to rid itself of metabolic waste products.

During the first half of the 22-day pregnancy, the secretion of progesterone by the ovary is regulated by LH and prolactin (secreted by the anterior pituitary gland) (figure 8.3). A shift takes place on days 12 to 13, and regulation of progesterone secretion is transferred to the placenta. Two placental hormones may be involved in regulating the ovaries, placental lactogen and chorionic gonadotropin. These hormones regulate the secretion of estrogen by the ovaries, in turn stimulating the synthesis and secretion of ovarian progesterone. The female's pituitary gland no longer regulates the secretion of progesterone, which maintains the pregnancy, and the pituitary gland can be removed without terminating the pregnancy (table 8.1). If the placenta is removed by hysterectomy, however, the pregnancy is terminated. Shortly before parturition, pituitary gland secretions and prostaglandin end the pregnancy by terminating the ovarian secretion of progesterone and increasing the secretion of estrogen. Following parturition pituitary gland secretions stimulate the postpartum estrous cycle.

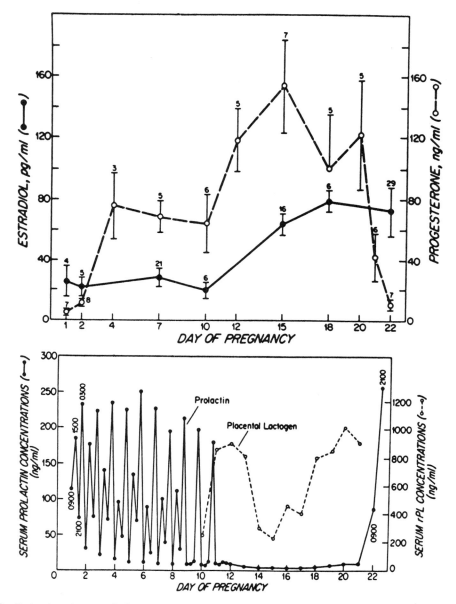

Figure 8.3 Endocrine changes during pregnancy in the rat. *Upper figure* shows circulating concentrations of estradiol and progesterone; *lower figure* shows circulating concentrations of prolactin and placental lactogen. (From Bridges, R.S. [1990][151]; reproduced by permission of The Endocrine Society.)

NEUROENDOCRINE RESPONSES DURING PREGNANCY AND POSTPARTUM

Mammary gland development during pregnancy and postpartum estrus exemplify an aspect of hormone-behavior relationships involved in parental care. In both cases behavioral stimuli or stimuli received during behavior play an important role in regulating the female's endocrine sytem. During pregnancy the female licks her ventral body region, including the nipples and genital region. This causes the release of hormones that stimulate development of the mammary glands. Similarly, during parturition, the fetuses passing through the birth canal stimulate the release of hormones that initiate postpartum estrus and ovulation.

SELF-LICKING AND MAMMARY GLAND DEVELOPMENT

The mammary glands develop during pregnancy under the influence of ovarian hormones and prolactin. Estrogen stimulates duct development, and progesterone stimulates the proliferation of secretory cells located in the alveoli of the mammary gland. Prolactin plays the principal role in the synthesis of milk by the secretory cells.[224]

The development of the glands does not depend solely upon endogenously regulated secretion of these hormones. It was found that the duration of the female's licking of the nipples along the chest and the abdomen increased from midpregnancy onward.[878] To test the possibility that licking of the nipple region might stimulate mammary gland development, pregnant females were fitted with rubber collars that prevented them from licking their nipples and genital region throughout pregnancy. When their mammary glands were removed and examined on day 21 of pregnancy, 1 day before parturition when nearly full mammary gland development normally has occurred, it was found that they had undergone only half the normal extent of development.[879] The amount of secretory tissue was reduced, and milk production was severely limited compared to females that had licked themselves during pregnancy. Using a biochemical measure of gland development (deoxyribonucleic acid, DNA), collared females were also found to have reduced gland development.[700] Full mammary gland development could be produced in another group of collared females by stimulating them with a brush along the nipples and genital region.[484]

UTERO-CERVICAL-VAGINAL STIMULATION AND POSTPARTUM ESTRUS AND OVULATION

Postpartum estrus follows parturition by about 8 to 11 hours, and ovulation occurs about 18 hours after delivery. Females can mate and become pregnant during this estrus, although implantation is delayed because suckling inhibits ovarian secretion of estrogen to synergize with the action of progesterone on the uterus. The occurrence of postpartum estrus behavior followed by ovulation several hours later is a neuroendocrine response to parturition in the rat. Normally, estrous cycles are timed by the light-dark cycle. The estrous cycle that occurs following parturition is an exception. It is stimulated by the process of delivery and specifically by the uterine-cervical-vaginal stimulation the female receives during delivery of the fetuses. By cutting nerves (the pelvic and hypogastric nerves) that innervate the genital region (cervix and vagina) and the uterus,[239] this stimulation was blocked. This prevented sensory stimulation accompanying cesarean-section delivery (made necessary for delivery of the fetuses by cutting these two nerves) from reaching the brain. This, in turn,

REGULATION OF MATERNAL BEHAVIOR IN THE RAT

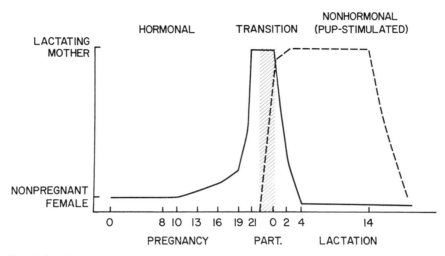

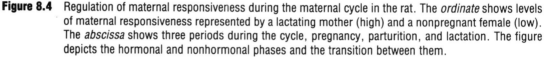

Figure 8.4 Regulation of maternal responsiveness during the maternal cycle in the rat. The *ordinate* shows levels of maternal responsiveness represented by a lactating mother (high) and a nonpregnant female (low). The *abscissa* shows three periods during the cycle, pregnancy, parturition, and lactation. The figure depicts the hormonal and nonhormonal phases and the transition between them.

prevented the activation of neuroendocrine responses leading to postpartum ovulation. Ovulation occurred normally in cesarean-delivered females that had not had these two nerves cut.

HORMONAL AND NONHORMONAL PHASES IN THE REGULATION OF MATERNAL BEHAVIOR

The rat has served as a representative mammal in the study of the hormonal basis of maternal behavior. The rat is representative because the pattern of ovarian hormones and prolactin secreted during pregnancy (figure 8.3) and in the prepartum period is similar to that found in many other mammals, although not all.[873] The mother exhibits maternal behavior for 3 to 4 weeks after parturition. The important hormonal events for maternal behavior occur during pregnancy and around parturition when maternal behavior is initiated. After the mother has initiated maternal behavior, the principal sources of the steroid hormones and prolactin (i.e., the ovaries, pituitary gland, placenta, and even the adrenal glands) can be removed without affecting maternal behavior.[875] Lactation is prevented, however, in females without pituitary gland secretion of prolactin and oxytocin.

After parturition, the mother depends upon stimulation from her young to maintain her maternal behavior. If the young are removed at parturition and mothers, therefore, are deprived of suckling and other forms of stimulation by the pups, maternal behavior declines during the next 4 days.[871] There is, however, a gradually waning influence lasting for 7 days, of the hormonal stimulation that made the female maternal.[791]

The course of maternal behavior after parturition is not altered by removing of hormones or by injecting hormones that might inhibit the behavior at other times (e.g., progesterone). This has led to the proposal that the *maintenance of maternal behavior after parturition* in the rat is not under hormonal control. This theory suggests that the regulation of maternal behavior is divided into two main phases (figure 8.4). There is a *hormonal phase* during pregnancy and in the prepartum period during which maternal behavior is initiated. As noted, this phase gradually wanes during the first week postpartum, and the *nonhormonal phase* follows, in which the female depends upon pup stimulation to maintain her maternal responsiveness. There is also a *transition phase* joining these two phases. During the transition phase hormonal regulation wanes and nonhormonal regulation becomes established. It is, therefore, a critical phase. In other species (e.g., sheep, goats, and humans) the transition phase has been singled out as a "critical period."

HORMONAL STIMULATION OF MATERNAL BEHAVIOR DURING PREGNANCY AND THE PREPARTUM PERIOD

Pregnant female rats have been tested for maternal behavior by presenting them with test pups during the second half of pregnancy (i.e., on days 13 to 22) and especially during the last 24 to 48 hours before parturition. These tests have shown that the number of females that perform maternal behavior gradually increases.[874] Females perform all of the components of maternal behavior, including adopting a nursing posture over the pups, licking and retrieving them to the nest, and nestbuilding[14] (figure 8.5). They also display maternal aggression toward other adults that might harm their young.[676] Earlier during pregnancy females may also show maternal behavior, but they require a longer period of pup stimulation. Females gradually become more responsive to pups during pregnancy, but they need the hormonal stimulation that occurs at the end of pregnancy to enable them to display maternal behavior almost immediately.

These hormonal changes have been studied by artificially terminating pregnancy by removing the fetuses with placentas and the uterus (i.e., performing hysterectomies) at various times before parturition. This procedure causes a rapid reduction in the secretion of progesterone by the ovaries, which signals the premature end of the pregnancy. During the next 48 hours there is a gradual increase in the secretion of estradiol. This is then followed by a rise in progesterone secretion. The female, therefore, resumes estrous cycling. If females are given pups 48 hours after hysterectomy, many of them exhibit maternal behavior immediately. Those that fail to do so are likely to exhibit maternal behavior after 24 to 48 hours with the pups. If the ovaries are removed at the same time that hysterectomy is performed, the females show a delayed onset of maternal behavior. Injecting these females with estradiol benzoate, however, restores short-latency maternal behavior.

In applying the results of these studies to the normal onset of maternal behavior, it was found that there is a prepartum onset associated with the prepartum decline in progesterone and increase in estrogen.[872] Nestbuilding, re-

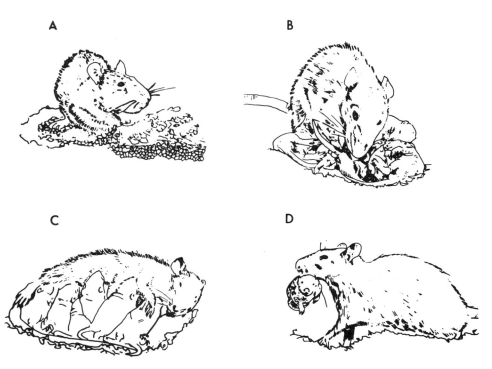

Figure 8.5 Maternal behavior in the rat. The four components of maternal behavior are *A*, nestbuilding, *B*, licking, *C*, nursing, and *D*, retrieving pup to the nest. (From Alberts, J. R. and Gubernick, D. J. [1983][14]; reproduced by permission.)

trieving, crouching over young, and maternal aggression can be elicited from females during the 24 to 48 hours that precede parturition. Uterine contractions also play a role in the onset of maternal behavior. After the initiation of regular and strong uterine contractions 3½ hours before parturition, there was a marked increase in the number of females exhibiting maternal behavior when tested with pups or with intruders.[677] Moreover, the vaginal-cervical stimulation that accompanies delivery of the pups contributes to the onset of maternal behavior, particularly in females undergoing parturition and maternal behavior for the first time.[1125]

In addition to what might be called the care behaviors of the female rat, which are directed at her young, there is another pattern of behavior that is directed at intruders whether of the same or different species that is called *maternal aggression*. When faced with a nest site intruder with her litter nearby, the mother approaches and sniffs the intruder and then launches an attack aimed at its neck and head region. The female bites at the neck of the intruder, climbs its back and pins it in place. The intruder usually flees, but if escape is not possible, it becomes immobile and may turn over on its back: this freezing and submissive behavior usually terminates the female's aggression until the next episode, which may occur only seconds later.

Maternal aggression arises during late pregnancy. It is shown in the laboratory when females are tested by introducing intruders into their home cages.

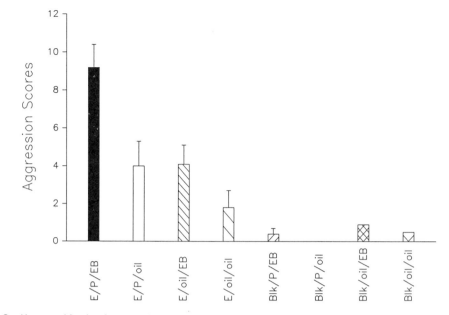

Figure 8.6 Hormonal basis of maternal aggression in ovariectomized, hormone-treated female rats. Silastic capsules 5 mm long containing estradiol (E) or blank (Blk) were implanted subcutaneously on day 0 and left in place through day 16. From days 3 to 15 animals also received either 4 mg progesterone (P) each day or oil as a control. On day 16, animals received an injection of either 5 μg estradiol benzoate (EB) or oil. Group E/P/EB had a higher maternal aggression score than all other groups, group E/P/oil had higher scores than Blk/P/oil, and E/oil/oil had higher scores than all those without E implants. On the ordinate, higher aggression scores indicate more intense aggressive behavior exhibited by females in 10-minute tests with unfamiliar, ovariectomized intruders.

Maternal aggression is maintained during lactation by the presence of the pups and declines during the middle of the third week as the pups begin to be weaned. It is an important aspect of maternal behavior because it protects the young from attacks and cannibalism.

As might be expected, the hormonal basis of maternal aggression is similar to that of maternal behavior, but there are differences. Hysterectomy during late pregnancy stimulates the onset of aggression, and prolonged treatment with estrogen and progesterone followed by estradiol benzoate also elicits maternal aggression[675] (figure 8.6). Maternal aggression differs from other components of maternal behavior, however, in that it does not require pituitary gland secretions (i.e., prolactin). Also, while progesterone inhibits the onset of maternal behavior, high levels of this hormone do not inhibit aggression.

In comparing mice to rats, it was found that the development of aggressive behavior during pregnancy and the early postpartum period follows somewhat different patterns. Mice of the common laboratory strains increase in aggressiveness during the last half of pregnancy, but this pregnancy-induced aggression differs from that of maternal aggression; threats are common, but attacks are infrequent. Immediately after parturition, female mice are not aggressive. Postpartum maternal aggression is initiated during the first 48 hours after parturition. The female needs to be suckled for aggression to be stimulated.[388] It is not, however, the hormonal consequences of suckling (i.e., prolactin and oxytocin synthesis and release) but the sensory stimulation alone that is effective.[1013] Once females have shown maternal aggression, suckling can be prevented by removing the nipples, and such females will remain aggressive at nearly normal levels. Lactating females remain aggressive for as long as they have their young pups nearby. If the pups are removed for 4 hours, maternal aggression wanes. It can be restored by returning the pups to the mother. During the second or third week aggression declines naturally.

ESTROGEN STIMULATION OF MATERNAL BEHAVIOR

Estrogen can also stimulate maternal behavior in nonpregnant female rats that have been hysterectomized and ovariectomized. Because they have not been pregnant they require larger doses than pregnancy-terminated females. Estrogen also stimulates maternal behavior when it is applied directly to the brain. This can been done by implanting bilateral cannulae containing estrogen at the tips in the medial preoptic area (POA) of the diencephalon.[784]

It can also be shown that estrogen stimulates maternal behavior by the opposite procedure of preventing estrogen from acting on the brain. Females are first given an injection of an antiestrogen (i.e., tamoxifen or CB-154) and are then given a systemic injection of estrogen. The antiestrogen blocks estrogen action on the CNS, and this prevents the appearance of maternal behavior.

Antiestrogen (4-hydroxytamoxifen) can be implanted directly in the brain. This procedure has been used to show that the rise in estradiol at the end of pregnancy stimulates the normal onset of maternal behavior. Cannulae containing the antiestrogen are implanted bilaterally in the POA 2 days before parturition. This prevents the normal *prepartum* onset of maternal behavior. If females are delivered by cesarean section and therefore have no contact with their pups, the antiestrogen also prevents a significant number of females from exhibiting maternal behavior toward the pups *postpartum*.[8]

HORMONAL PRIMING AND TRIGGERING OF MATERNAL BEHAVIOR

A lower dose of estrogen is able to stimulate maternal behavior in pregnancy-terminated females than is required in nonpregnant females. This occurs because the pregnancy-terminated females have been stimulated by estrogen and progesterone during pregnancy, whereas nonpregnant females have not received this hormonal stimulation. This is an example of hormonal priming, in which the action of one or several hormones prepares the way for a later hormone to produce its effect. A low dose of estrogen (5 μg/kg estradiol benzoate) stimulates maternal behavior in ovariectomized nonpregnant females that have been primed with estrogen and progesterone. By contrast, a high dose (100 μg/kg estradiol benzoate) is necessary in females that have not been primed with these hormones. This suggests that the rise in estradiol at the end of pregnancy is able to stimulate maternal behavior because the female has been hormonally primed throughout pregnancy.[875]

The longer females have been pregnant before their pregnancies are terminated by hysterectomy, the more rapidly they become maternal. They also respond more rapidly to the endogenous release of estradiol that follows hysterectomy. This phenomenon can be explained by the priming action of pregnancy hormones.

In addition to the concept of *hormonal priming*, there is an equally important concept of *hormonal triggering*. After the female has been hormonally primed she responds to estrogen by the rapid onset of maternal behavior; this is referred to as triggering. The analogy is with the action of a gun: Priming corresponds to cocking the gun that prepares it to fire. The action that follows is rapid and complete in one moment. In maternal behavior, triggering refers to the rapid behavioral response to estrogen. Hormonal priming by itself is not capable of stimulating maternal behavior. It provides the basis, however, for an additional estrogen stimulus that will trigger its onset. It will be shown later that priming and triggering may represent different underlying hormonal actions in the CNS.

NEURAL-HORMONAL BASIS OF ESTROGEN PRIMING AND TRIGGERING OF MATERNAL BEHAVIOR

Maternal behavior in the rat is largely an estrogen-dependent behavior pattern, even when other hormones are involved (see below). The effect of estrogen on maternal behavior is mediated to an important extent by its action on cells within the medial POA.

The concentrations of estrogen receptors in the POA and the hypothalamus (HYP) can be correlated with estrogen stimulation of maternal behavior. This was first shown in females whose pregnancies were terminated on day 16. They were also ovariectomized and given a low dose of an estrogen. Females treated with estrogen exhibit maternal behavior when tested at 48 hours, while females given oil fail to do so.[404] The effect of the estrogen on the onset of maternal behavior lasts about 72 hours and then wanes. Other females that were not pregnant that were given the estrogen or oil following ovariectomy did not become maternal. This is thought to reflect the induction of estrogen receptors by the hormones secreted during pregnancy. In fact, estrogen receptors have been found to be elevated in the POA of females whose pregnancies were terminated before they were hysterectomized and received the low dose of estrogen. In contrast, nonpregnant females that failed to exhibit maternal behavior had low initial estrogen receptor concentrations. After the estrogen injection from 6 hours onward, however, all groups showed a rapid increase in estrogen receptor concentrations.

Just the presence of high concentrations of estrogen receptors at time zero before pregnancy termination is not sufficient to stimulate maternal behavior. Pregnancy-terminated females that received an oil injection instead of estrogen also had high estrogen receptor concentrations in the POA at time zero before pregnancy termination, but they did not show short-latency maternal behavior. Both the initial high estrogen receptor concentration in the POA and the subsequent increase in receptors are the necessary conditions for stimulating short-latency maternal behavior. It is thought that the initial high concentration of estrogen receptors in the POA represents the cellular basis of hormonal priming. The subsequent increase in estrogen receptor concentration after estrogen treatment is believed to represent the triggering effect of estrogen on maternal behavior.

Endogenous hormonal priming of maternal behavior arises during the second half of pregnancy when both estrogen and progesterone levels are elevated. When estrogen receptor levels in the POA were studied in females at various stages of pregnancy from the eighth to the twenty-second day, it was found that they reached the priming level around day 13 and maintained this level until day 22.[403] When specific regions of the POA were microdissected and assayed for estrogen receptors, it was found that the specific nuclei within the POA and adjacent to it, the periventricular preoptic area, the medial preoptic area and the periventricular anterior hypothalamus showed estrogen receptor concentrations similar to these in the entire POA on days 8, 16, and 22 of pregnancy.[405] This corresponds to the period of priming during pregnancy found in the behavioral studies. An additional finding was that estradiol and progesterone treatment for 16 days established estrogen receptor levels in the POA equal to those found in pregnancy-primed females.

The consistently lower estrogen receptor concentrations in the HYP compared to the POA are believed to have behavioral significance. During pregnancy the hypothalamus is relatively insensitive to estrogen. At the same time pregnant females do not show sexual behavior even when they are injected with estrogen. Immediately after parturition, on the day of delivery, however, they spontaneously exhibit sexual behavior during postpartum estrus. Low estrogen receptor concentrations in the HYP were found throughout pregnancy until day 22 just before parturition. On day 22 of pregnancy estrogen receptor levels in the HYP suddenly rose to the level found in the POA. The low estrogen receptor levels in this area may explain why the pregnant female does not respond to estrogen by exhibiting sexual behavior. The rise in estrogen receptors in the HYP just before parturition, therefore, primes the female to respond to the postpartum increase in estrogen by showing sexual behavior.[405]

For comparison with the rat, the brain mechanisms underlying estrogen stimulation of retrieving in ovariectomized female *mice* have been studied by immunocytochemistry. In mice, estrogen receptors were found in the same brain regions as those seen in the rat and several additional ones. When mice with maternal experience were compared with inexperienced mice, the experienced females showed labeling in brain regions mediating olfactory stimulation that were absent in the brains of inexperienced females.[594] Experienced females also showed an increase in estrogen receptors in the ventromedial hypothalamus. Females without experience had reduced concentrations of estrogen receptors in the anterior hypothalamus and the ventromedial hypothalamus and generally reduced concentrations in all labeled brain areas.

Sensory stimuli of biological significance can alter the brain's responsiveness to estrogen and in that way can affect reproductivebehavior. The study cited above may be an example of this because exposure to pups for 5 days increased estrogen receptor concentrations in several brain regions in experienced female mice. In the prairie vole, closely related to the mouse studied above, females exposed to sexually experienced males show increased brain uptake of estrogen in cell nuclei of the preoptic area.[217]

PROGESTERONE FACILITATION AND INHIBITION OF MATERNAL BEHAVIOR

The high circulating concentrations of ovarian progesterone during pregnancy play an important role in the hormonal priming of maternal behavior. Equally important is the role played by the decline of progesterone seen at the end of pregnancy. The withdrawal of progesterone from circulation initiates labor through its effect on the uterus.[385] It also triggers the initiation of lactation because progesterone inhibits prolactin stimulation of the mammary glands.[608] It is the withdrawal of progesterone from circulation that enables the terminal rise in estrogen to stimulate maternal behavior. If high plasma levels of progesterone are maintained following hysterectomy-ovariectomy in females, in late pregnancy, maternal behavior is delayed.[875] Therefore, it appears that progesterone can both facilitate maternal behavior as well as inhibit it. The timing of progesterone secretion in relation to estrogen action is critical. Where progesterone acts in the brain to facilitate and inhibit maternal behavior is not known.

PROLACTIN AND MATERNAL BEHAVIOR

Plasma prolactin levels increase at the end of pregnancy in response to the increased release of ovarian estradiol. Bridges and his colleagues (Bridges, 1990) have established that prolactin is involved in the initiation of maternal behavior. Several different experimental paradigms have been used. Ovariectomized females treated concurrently with estrogen and progesterone for 11 days showed a rapid onset of maternal behavior. Removing the pituitary glands at the start of steroid hormone treatment significantly delayed the onset of maternal behavior. Successive treatment first with progesterone from day 1 to 11 and then with estradiol from day 11 to 22 stimulates short-latency maternal behavior in ovariectomized, nonpregnant females. Maternal behavior can be blocked in animals that have been hypophysectomized or treated with bromocriptine to prevent prolactin secretion. Short latencies are restored by injections of prolactin or by prolactin-secreting pituitary gland transplants.[151]

For prolactin to stimulate maternal behavior in the rat, it must act on the central nervous system. However, prolactin is a large protein molecule, and it is prevented from entering the brain by the blood-brain barrier. However, if it is infused into the lateral ventricle cerebrospinal fluid (CSF) or if it is infused directly into the POA (thus circumventing the blood-brain barrier) of females that have been primed with estrogen, they exhibit short-latency maternal behavior.[150] This clearly establishes that prolactin can act in the POA and perhaps other CNS sites as well, since prolactin in the CSF can reach many circumventricular sites to stimulate maternal behavior.

There is another source of prolactin that has recently received experimental study, namely, cells within the brain itself. This source was found by using radioimmunoassay and immunocytochemical methods and methods for determining messenger RNA (mRNA) for genetic control of the synthesis of prolactin. Investigators have localized prolactin in cells of different brain regions and have traced projections of fibers from these regions to many distant brain regions, several of which are involved in maternal behavior (e.g., POA, anterior hypothalamus, amygdala, nucleus accumbens).[464] As in the studies of maternal behavior cited earlier, infusion of prolactin into the midbrain of female rats increases lordosis behavior, which, like maternal behavior, isalso estrogen dependent.

It is not yet clearly established whether *pituitary prolactin* normally enters the brain and, therefore, whether it is able to stimulate maternal behavior. On the one hand, it has been shown that prolactin in circulation has access to the CSF and presumably the brain by means of a receptor transport system located in choroid plexuses in the lateral, third, and fourth ventricles.[1087] Direct measurements of CSF prolactin concentrations using push-pull cannulae have shown increases following either estrogen or suckling stimulation during lactation, both of which cause the release of pituitary prolactin. On the other hand, there are times when circulating levels of pituitary prolactin are low or absent, as following hypophysectomy, or very high, as after ether stress or haloperidol, yet CSF and brain levels of prolactin are unaffected. Most striking is the finding that on day 22 of pregnancy, when maternal behavior is readily elicited from females, prolactin is not detectable in the CSF despite moderately high circulating prolactin levels.[887] Whether these contradictory results stem from technical difficulties in measuring CSF prolactin or from unknown factors has not yet been settled.

Little is known about how the synthesis of prolactin and its release from cells within the CNS are regulated. Estradiol receptors have been localized in the same cells of the female rat hypothalamus that contain prolactin.[945] Estradiol, therefore, may regulate prolactin action in the CNS. For example, hypophysectomized females exhibited a 50 per cent decrease in CSF and brain prolactin that can be restored to normal levels by injecting them with estrogen.[278] The prolactin must have come from brain cells because the females were hypophysectomized.

In addition to the issues discussed above, there is the question of the interrelationship between estradiol and prolactin at the onset of maternal behavior. This relationship has been described by Bridges[148] as follows: estradiol stimulates the synthesis and release of prolactin, which in turn acts on cells within the POA and perhaps in other brain sites to stimulate maternal behavior. Estradiol may also modulate brain prolactin receptors, but there is no evidence for this.[151] There is an alternative possibility, namely, that prolactin, after its release by estradiol, facilitates the action of estradiol on cells in those brain areas in which estradiol has been shown to stimulate maternal behavior (e.g., the medial POA). It has been shown in non-neural tissues that prolactin regulates the concentration of estrogen receptors and causes increased sensitivity of the cells to an estrogenic stimulus.[400, 767] Similar effects of prolactin may occur in estrogen-sensitive cells of the CNS and particularly in the preoptic area that is involved in maternal behavior.[9]

We can say, therefore, that it is clearly established that prolactin is involved in maternal behavior. The studies that have established a role for prolactin have focused on the pituitary gland as the source of the prolactin that acts on the POA to stimulate maternal behavior. It is not clear, however, that fluctuations in circulating levels of pituitary prolactin directly affect either CSF levels of prolactin or the concentrations of prolactin at various brain sites. Estrogen, which freely passes the blood–brain barrier, may play a role in regulating brain prolactin. It restores normal levels of prolactin in the CSF and in the hypothalamus, and its receptors have been co-localized with prolactin in the cells of the hypothalamus. The interrelationship between estrogen and prolactin may be a reciprocal one: Estrogen may stimulate the synthesis and release of prolactin, and prolactin may in turn increase the sensitivity of estrogen-sensitive cells to the estrogen stimulus.

OXYTOCIN AND MATERNAL BEHAVIOR

A role for oxytocin in maternal behavior was first proposed by Klopfer,[592] who observed its effect in goats. However, it was in the rat that the original studies were done that supported this proposal. Estrogen-primed ovariectomized females received injections of oxytocin directly into the CSF of the lateral ventricles. These animals exhibited maternal behavior within 2 hours of the injection.[802] Systemically injected oxytocin did not stimulate maternal behavior. Females that had not been primed with estrogen also failed to respond to the oxytocin. These experiments suggested that oxytocin acting in the brain in previously estrogen-primed females influenced maternal behavior. Similar findings were reported by Fahrbach and colleagues.[337, 801]

In support of the CSF injection study, a selective oxytocin antagonist (d (CHL2L)L5L-8 ornithine vasotocin) has been administered to pregnancy-terminated females, which were ovariectomized, hysterectomized, and given estrogen as described earlier. The onset of maternal behavior was significantly delayed in these females.[338, 800] Similarly, when given to parturient females that had begun to deliver, the oxytocin antagonist delayed the appearance of maternal behavior for up to 24 hours.[1071] Antiserum to oxytocin has also been used to block estrogen-induced maternal behavior in pregnancy-terminated females.[339]

Oxytocin has been found to influence maternal behavior in the mouse also. In laboratory-raised wild mice (as opposed to domesticated strains) females normally cannibalize pups that are presented to them before parturition. As parturition approaches, they inhibit this behavior. If they are injected with oxytocin systemically while they are still cannibalizing pups, they terminate this behavior and begin to show maternal behavior toward them.[680, 681]

In rats, additional support for a role for oxytocin in maternal behavior comes from creating a lesion of the paraventricular nucleus (PVN) during pregnancy. This destroys the majority of brain oxytocin-secreting neurons and results in an increase in cannibalism and in the latencies for retrieval. It also produces deficits in other aspects of maternal behavior (e.g., nestbuilding, grouping young, licking and crouching over them[524]).

Several factors have clouded the issue of the role of oxytocin in maternal behavior in the rat. First, it is not effective in all strains of rat. In the United States it is effective in females of only one strain. In addition, very specific caging conditions are required for oxytocin to stimulate maternal behavior. The cage in which the female is given oxytocin and in which she is tested for maternal behavior cannot be one with which she is familiar, yet it cannot be one that is entirely novel to her.[340] Finally, in recent years (since 1985), it has been difficult to elicit maternal behavior with oxytocin in the original strain of rats. Oxytocin, however, has proved to be effective in females of other strains that have been made anosmic with intranasal zinc sulfate. Zinc sulfate treatment by itself, however, stimulates short-latency maternal behavior in virgins.[524]

Studies have investigated the neuroanatomical and neurochemical basis of oxytocin action in the CNS of female rats. Oxytocin acts on cell membrane receptors (rather than on receptors in cell nuclei), and these have been localized in brain regions that mediate maternal behavior (e.g., the anterior olfactory nucleus, the bed nucleus of the stria terminalis, the central nucleus of the amygdala, and the ventromedial nucleus of the hypothalamus.[524] Sources of oxytocin transmitted to these areas, identified using immunohistochemical methods, are the paraventricular nucleus and the anterior commissural nucleus, the principal sources, and the POA and the supraoptic nucleus.

During the latter half of pregnancy, when maternal behavior normally arises, only one brain region, the bed nucleus of the stria terminalis, shows an increase in oxytocin receptor number. This brain region is involved in the maternal behavior shown by nonpregnant females and hormonally stimulated females.[361] This increase may be based upon an increase in estrogen, which regulates oxytocin action in the brain by causing its release from the anterior commissural nucleus, and by increasing oxytocin receptor concentrations.[218]

In summarizing the studies on the role of oxytocin in maternal behavior in the rat, it is difficult to reach a clear conclusion on this issue. The neural substrate for oxytocin action on CNS areas involved in maternal behavior exists, and the release of CNS oxytocin in these areas has also been demonstrated. The behavioral studies of oxytocin stimulation of maternal behavior at best limit the effect to only one or two strains. Even in the original strain it may no longer be possible to replicate earlier reported oxytocin effects on maternal behavior. In this strain constraints on the conditions under which oxytocin stimulates maternal behavior in estrogen-primed females (e.g., duration of residence in cage) are not well understood.

Rabbit

The pattern of hormone secretions during pregnancy in the rabbit is similar to that seen in other mammals[873] (figure 8.7). Although it is a nesting species, its

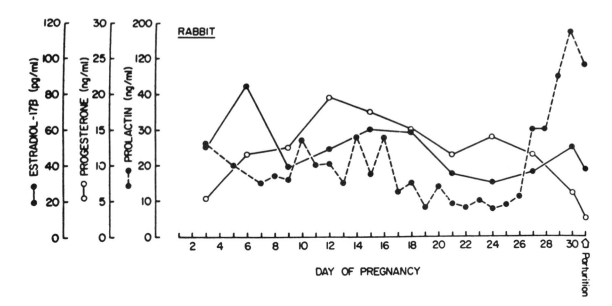

Figure 8.7 Hormone secretions during pregnancy in the rabbit. Graph shows circulating levels of estradiol, progesterone, and prolactin from day 0 to parturition on day 31. (From Rosenblatt, J. S. and Siegel, H. I. [1981][873]; reproduced by permission.)

postpartum maternal behavior is strikingly different from that of other small mammals with altricial young. Like other mammals, at parturition the mother deposits her young in a nest. Nests are built at parturition or shortly before, underground in burrows in some species and above ground in others. After parturition the mother returns to nurse her young only once each day and for only a brief period lasting about 3 minutes.[1135] Mothers exhibit licking of the young but do not retrieve them to the nest (it is very unlikely that the young would be out of the nest and need to be retrieved). In addition, the mother produces a nipple pheromone during pregnancy and lactation.[508] This enables the young to locate and grasp the nipple rapidly. The hormonal basis of maternal nestbuilding at parturition and pheromone production, but not of postpartum nursing and nest defense, have been studied in the rabbit.

Nestbuilding in the rabbit consists of two behavior patterns. First, the hair on the female's ventrum gradually loosens during late pregnancy, and she plucks it from her chest to line her nest. In addition, she picks up leaves, hay and other materials to construct a nest. Nestbuilding and hair loosening and pulling are always closely linked. Among the methods used to determine the hormonal basis of these behaviors was termination of the normal 30 to 32-day pregnancy at midpregnancy with either estrogen injections, hysterectomy, or ovariectomy. Investigators also studied rabbits at the termination of 20-day pseudopregnancies. All of these procedures resulted in the onset of nestbuilding and hair loosening. These conditions have in common a decline in progesterone and a rise in estrogen secretion. Females were, therefore, ovariectomized and injected with various schedules of estrogen and progesterone. The schedule most effective in stimulating nestbuilding was treatment with estrogen lasting at least 18 days and progesterone treatment terminating 3 days before estrogen ended. In the rabbit, as in other mammals, estrogen stimulates the release of prolactin. During the hormone treatments prolactin could, therefore, mediate estrogen and progesterone stimulation of maternal nestbuilding. This, in fact, was shown to be the case. When estrogen-progesterone treated females were hypophysectomized or late-pregnant females were treated with the dopamine agonist ergocornine to prevent prolactin release, maternal behavior failed to appear.[26, 1136]

Brain regions have been located in the rabbit that are responsive to prolactin and estrogen.[25, 294] Tissue from several regions of the entire hypothalamus exhibit responsiveness to prolactin, but areas such as the olfactory bulb are devoid of prolactin responsiveness. Prolactin injected into females alters neuronal firing in the medial preoptic area, the brain site at which prolactin stimulates maternal behavior in the rat.[211]

With respect to estrogen, Anderson[25] has mapped estrogen-sensitive areas in the rabbit brain by autoradiography. The regions are very similar to those found in the rat and include several that are involved in rat maternal behavior. In the rabbit these include the medial preoptic area, medial amygdaloid complex, nucleus accumbens, and bed nucleus of the stria terminalis.

Behaviorally, the unusually brief daily contact between mother and young during lactation has been of particular interest. Other mammals would not be able to maintain their maternal behavior or continue to lactate with such brief daily contacts with their young; yet the rabbit is able to maintain these functions. One way to study the underlying mechanisms for the maintenance of maternal behavior and lactation in the rabbit is to see whether the mother is at all dependent on stimulation from her young to maintain them. Young were removed from mothers at parturition, and each day the female was anesthetized and the pups were allowed to suckle her. This was done to stimulate prolactin release and to maintain lactation. Since anesthetized females do not treat suckling by their young as "nursing," they were, in effect, deprived of pup stimulation. For example, when females are suckled in this way they do not remain away for 24 hours but return to their young to nurse them several hours later when they are again awake.[350] This occurs despite the fact that their mammary glands are empty. After a week of being suckled in this way it was found that the female's lactation was maintained, but she no longer approached her young for nursing. Nursing behavior, therefore, could not be maintained if pup suckling occurred while the female was not awake. Prolactin released during suckling was not able to maintain the female's nursing behavior if she was anesthetized during the nursing.

When this study was done with females that had already nursed their young for nearly two weeks, the results were quite different.[1029] At the end of a week during which nursing only occurred while females were anesthetized, all of the females approached and nursed their young when given the opportunity. This indicates that the female is less dependent on stimulation from the young to maintain her nursing once she has had experience nursing them. It may be, as in the rat, that once the female has established her nursing behavior, nursing can be maintained for a period without daily nursing contact with her young.

In the rat, females that have had experience taking care of their young for as little as 3 days are able to maintain their maternal behavior over a 4-day period without young.[871] If they are separated from their young at birth they are unable to do this. They do not respond immediately to their young when reintroduced to them 4-days later. A similar situation seems to exist in the rabbit.

Production of nipple pheromone, upon which the young depend for rapidly locating and grasping the nipple, is dependent on hormones. Estrogen and progesterone induce pheromone production in ovariectomized females. Nipple pheromone is normally produced shortly after mating, and during pregnancy and lactation when progesterone secretion is high.

Another pattern of reproductive behavior observed in female rabbits is chin rubbing, which is also under hormonal control.[975] The female places her chin on an elevated surface and rubs it along the surface, depositing an odorous substance. She does this repeatedly. Estrogen injected into ovariectomized females stimulates both the production of the pheromone and chin rubbing behavior. Unlike nipple pheromone production, chin rubbing and production of the pheromone which the female deposits are inhibited by progesterone. This behavior is elevated in estrous females but declines after mating and remains low during pregnancy and lactation. The decline after mating is one of the few early signs of conception in the rabbit. The function of chin rubbing has not yet been established. It may serve to designate the female's territory and repel other rabbits or it may enable the female to locate her own burrow.

Summarizing, the female rabbit shows an abbreviated pattern of maternal behavior compared to most other mammals. Nursing occurs only once a day, retrieving the young to the nest is absent, and there is no contact between mother and young apart from the brief daily nursing. Nestbuilding occurs before parturition, and during parturition the female licks the young and defends them. Nestbuilding and hair loosening are under the control of estrogen, progesterone, and prolactin. Production of nipple pheromone is stimulated by estrogen and progesterone (prolactin has not been studied). Chin rubbing is stimulated by estrogen and is inhibited during pregnancy and lactation by progesterone. Nursing is probably initiated by hormones but is soon regulated by daily nursing contact with the pups. Later in lactation it is less dependent upon daily nursing of pups. Sites of action of estrogen and prolactin in the brain have been located and correspond to the sites found in the rat.

Sheep

Sheep are herd animals like many other ungulates including goats, horses, cows, and elk. Their maternal behavior is adapted to the special requirements of this mode of social life. Parturient females separate themselves from the

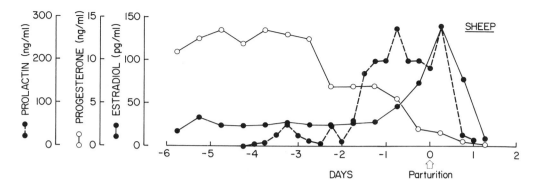

Figure 8.8 Hormone secretions during the last 6 days of pregnancy in sheep. Graph shows circulating levels of estradiol, progesterone, and prolactin from day 144 of pregnancy to parturition on day 150. (Data from Chamley et al., 1973.[197])

herd and give birth to their young in a clearing, where they remain for several days periodically nursing their lambs. The mother and young rejoin the herd soon afterward where she and her offspring are less vulnerable to predation. The precocial young at birth must be well developed in their locomotory abilities, and their sensory capacities at birth to enable them to follow the mother as she travels with the herd foraging for food. Mothers nurse only their own young and reject the lambs of other mothers. There must be mutual recognition, therefore, between mother and young for the young to be fed. Mothers identify their lambs by their odors and their appearance. Vocalizations by mothers and young also play a role in mutual recognition. Mother and young, therefore, develop individual recognition and form a special social bond. A special hormonal mechanism based upon oxytocin may have evolved to enable females to establish the bond with their young at parturition.

Maternal behavior in sheep arises at parturition. It includes licking the lamb thoroughly, vocal exchanges with the young, and nursing it. Since the hormonal changes at the end of pregnancy are similar to those occuring in the rat and in most other mammals (figure 8.8), studies have explored the possibility that estrogen and prolactin stimulate maternal behavior in ewes. Only experienced ewes exhibit maternal behavior in response to experimental treatment with hormones, although there are exceptions that will be described. Estrogen has been identified as one of the hormones that stimulates maternal behavior, whereas progesterone is only minimally effective and prolactin is ineffective.[824]

Oxytocin has proved to be important for stimulating maternal behavior in the ewe during parturition. Its role in maternal behavior may have arisen in sheep (and perhaps goats as well, as noted earlier), to enable mothers to establish a bond rapidly with their young at parturition. There is an interesting relationship among three reproductive processes in the stimulation of maternal behavior in sheep. These are cervical-vaginal stimulation, which the female receives as the fetus passes through the birth canal during parturition, hormonal stimulation of maternal behavior by oxytocin, and the role of olfaction in the ewe's early and rapid attachment to her newly born lamb.

Cervical-vaginal stimulation influences maternal behavior in two ways. It influences the hormonal stimulation of maternal behavior and also influences the female's response to the odor of amniotic fluid shared by her lamb and its placenta during parturition. These two types of influences will be discussed separately and then it will be shown how they are related to one another.

Cervical-vaginal stimulation enables subthreshold doses of estrogen to stimulate maternal behavior in nonpregnant ewes. Despite the subthreshold dose of estrogen, which is ineffective in nonstimulated ewes, maternal behavior is elicited if estrogen is accompanied by cervical-vaginal stimulation.[574] The effect of cervical-vaginal stimulation is caused by oxytocin secreted either by the posterior pituitary gland into the general circulation, from which site it then enters the brain, or by the brain itself. During cervical-vaginal stimulation, CSF concentrations of oxytocin in ewes increase to levels found during labor and delivery.[573] When oxytocin is administered directly into the CSF in ovariectomized, estrogen-primed, multiparous ewes and they are then tested for maternal behavior with young lambs, they exhibit the principal components of maternal behavior.[572] This behavior includes, on the one hand, approaching and following the lamb, low-pitched bleating, permitting suckling, and sniffing and licking the lamb, and on the other, the absence of butting the lamb and withdrawing from it. Maternal behavior elicited by oxytocin does not last long, however; it arises rapidly following the injection of oxytocin but declines within 1 hour. Some component of the normal hormonal stimulus is lacking.

It is important to note that estrogen priming, which the ewe would normally receive during pregnancy, is necessary for oxytocin to stimulate maternal behavior, whether oxytocin is injected or secreted endogenously in response to cervical-vaginal stimulation. Without estrogen priming, females fail to show maternal behavior, butt the lambs, and withdraw from them.

One way to prevent maternal behavior would be to prevent the female from receiving the cervical-vaginal stimulation normally received during parturition. This was accomplished by giving ewes an injection of a local anesthetic in the dura of the spinal cord (i.e., peridural anesthesia). This treatment blocks neural transmission between the cervical-vaginal area and the brain.[826] One group received the injection about $1\frac{1}{2}$ hours before parturition to block this stimulation completely, and a second group was given the injection only 10 minutes before expulsion of the fetus and therefore received most of the normal amount of uterocervical stimulation. Nearly 90 per cent of primiparous ewes receiving the earlier treatment failed to show maternal behavior within 30 minutes of expulsion of the fetus, and this was also true in more than 25 per cent of multiparous ewes. Delaying the peridural injection until 10 minutes before expulsion of the fetus produced no interference with maternal behavior. As evidence that the effects of the peridural neural block resulted from preventing the release of brain oxytocin, it was shown that maternal behavior could be restored to near normal levels by injecting oxytocin into the CSF.

Other factors such as endogenous opiates also play a role in the effects of cervical-vaginal stimulation on maternal behavior. Blocking the release of oxytocin with naltrexone injected directly into the CSF of estrogen-primed ewes with maternal experience prevents cervical-vaginal stimulation from stimulating maternal behavior.[571] Naltrexone prevents cervical-vaginal stimulation from causing the release of endogenous opiates into the CSF and therefore prevents the release of oxytocin.

Olfaction plays an important role in the ewe's maternal behavior. It aids her in her response to the amniotic fluid that bathes the newborn and the placenta. It also plays an important role in her identification of the newborn, which provides the basis for her highly specific attachment to it.[826] Ewes gradually learn the odors of their newborn lambs during the first 2 hours postpartum. As time passes, they increasingly reject alien newborn lambs with different odors.

Females are repelled by the odor of amniotic fluid bathing the placenta until just before expulsion of the fetus. As parturition approaches, they begin to find it attractive. During parturition they lick the placenta and eat it. Ewes continue to find the placenta attractive for about 2 hours after the fetus has been expelled, and then the attraction virtually disappears at about 4 hours postpartum.[631] Anosmia produced by intranasal infusion of zinc sulfate and procaine chlorydrate (substances that destroy the olfactory receptors and anesthetize the olfactory neurons) eliminates both the repulsion to and the attraction of amniotic fluid, demonstrating that these responses are based on its odor.

The effects of cervical-vaginal stimulation on oxytocin secretion are related to both the ewe's response to her newborn and her responses to olfactory stimuli. Cervical-vaginal stimulation is capable of extending the period during which ewes will accept alien newborn lambs. It is also capable of extending the period during which ewes find amniotic fluid attractive.[825] Both of these effects of cervical-vaginal stimulation may represent the action of brain oxytocin on the olfactory bulb as well as on CNS structures mediating maternal behavior. There are oxytocin receptors in the olfactory bulbs of sheep,[54, 379] and oxytocin injected into the CSF stimulates maternal behavior as described earlier, but it has not been shown that it affects responses to amniotic fluid. An additional mechanism underlying the female's response to her lamb may be the action of noradrenaline in the olfactory bulb of early postpartum females. Depletion of this neurotransmitter blocks the extrinsic innervation of the olfactory bulb and results in the absence of selective nursing of her own lamb by the ewe.[630, 820]

Summarizing this section, sheep exhibit a pattern of maternal behavior in relation to their precocial young that is adapted to their mode of social living in a herd and their wide-ranging foraging behavior for food. Important features are the onset of maternal behavior at parturition and the rapid formation of a selective behavioral bond with their own offspring. Oxytocin may have evolved in sheep to enable the female to form a maternal bond with newly born lambs rapidly at parturition. Cervical-vaginal stimulation, like that received during parturition, plays an important role in maternal behavior. It facilitates the action of estrogen, causes the secretion of oxytocin, and alters the female's olfactory repulsion to alien young and to the odors of the placenta. This is very likely due to the action of oxytocin on the olfactory bulbs and the CNS. Cervical-vaginal stimulation may also affect olfaction by causing noradrenaline release in the olfactory bulb.

Hormonal Basis of Parental Behavior in Selected Species of Birds

Among birds parental care consists of two principal components: there is a period of **incubation** followed by hatching of the young, and a period of **care of them or brooding behavior** until they fledge. Although *brooding* behavior technically refers specifically to sitting on or covering the young, it will be used here in a broader sense to refer to all parental care including feeding and leading the young to food.

These two closely related phases of the reproductive cycle in birds will be discussed separately in this section. The main issue is the hormonal basis for each of these parental behaviors. A second issue is whether there are differences in the hormonal basis of incubation and care of the young in avian species with altricial young and in those with precocial young. There are behavioral differences between these two types of species in care of the young, although their incubation behavior is quite similar. Species with altricial hatchlings have extended periods of nest occupation, sitting on the young and warming them, feeding them, and protecting them from conspecific and other predators. Birds with precocial young have a short initial period of nest occupation and a more extended period of care outside the nest when the young feed by themselves but remain close to the parent and follow it, being protected by the parents. Representatives of species with altricial young are the ring dove and canary,[962] and representatives of those with precocial young are the chicken and turkey.[171, 452]

Ring Dove and Canary

INCUBATION AND BROOD PATCH FORMATION

Incubation arises out of the earlier phases of courtship and nestbuilding and is initiated following egg-laying. The ovarian hormones estrogen and progesterone are involved in these earlier phases and may contribute simultaneously to the formation of a *brood patch*.[540] The brood patch is a defeathered, highly vascularized, and edemic area on the ventrum that is pressed against the eggs during sitting. This area is particularly sensitive to tactile and thermal stimulation. Brood patches occur in a large number of avian species, in the parent that incubates the eggs, or in both parents when they share in sitting. Even in those species in which the brood patch is not fully developed, there is often defeathering of the ventrum.

In the vast majority of species with brood patches, estrogen and prolactin and sometimes progesterone are responsible for its formation. In the canary estrogen and progesterone during the nesting period stimulate formation of the brood patch, and its increased sensitivity to tactile stimulation is instrumental in subsequent nestbuilding.[488] Whether prolactin is also involved in brood patch formation in the canary is not known.

It is interesting that the parasitic brown-headed cowbird, which does not incubate its own eggs, does not form a brood patch. Prolactin secretion in this species shows a seasonal pattern similar to that characteristic of parental species, yet the ventral skin is unresponsive to the combination of estradiol and prolactin that induces brood patch formation in other species.[494, 936] In two species of phalarope birds (Wilson's and northern), only males exhibit nestbuilding, incubation, and brooding of the young. They develop brood patches, and females do not. When both sexes were injected with estradiol, testosterone, prolactin, or various combinations of these hormones, only males developed brood patches, and it was in response to prolactin and testosterone.[533]

INCUBATION BEHAVIOR

Incubation behavior in the ring dove and other altricial species has two phases (figure 8.9).[199, 416, 949] In the first phase, at the start of incubation, progesterone may stimulate incubation in both parents, although the need for hormonal stimulation of incubation is not well established for males.[199, 201] Progesterone synergizes with estrogen in the female but is not as effective in stimulating incubation behavior in inexperienced birds as it is in birds with breeding experience.[720] Specifically, *incubation* experience enhances the effects of progesterone on incubation. Nestbuilding, which establishes a site for incubating the eggs, also is effective, but courtship experience is not.

Sitting on the eggs induces a decline in progesterone secretion and a rise in prolactin secretion around the time of midincubation. While the parents continue to sit undisturbed, a transition from progesterone to prolactin occurs in the hormonal regulation of incubation (figure 8.9). Prolactin then maintains incubation behavior until hatching occurs.[417, 950, 951] Experienced ring doves make the transition more rapidly than parents breeding for the first time.[741] Even more interesting is the fact that both male and female ring doves with previous breeding experience can maintain their own readiness to incubate without any contact with the eggs merely by watching their mate incubate the eggs.[721] Birds breeding for the first time are unable to do this. Seeing the mate incubate appears to stimulate the release of prolactin, since experienced birds also show full-crop gland development.

Like other members of the order Columbiformes (e.g., pigeons and doves), both ring dove parents feed their young by regurgitating material from their crop glands (i.e.,"crop milk") into the squabs' throat.[620] Development of the crop gland and crop milk secretion are dependent on prolactin secreted by the pituitary gland. The crop gland begins to develop around the time of midincubation after the parents have been sitting on the eggs for about a week.

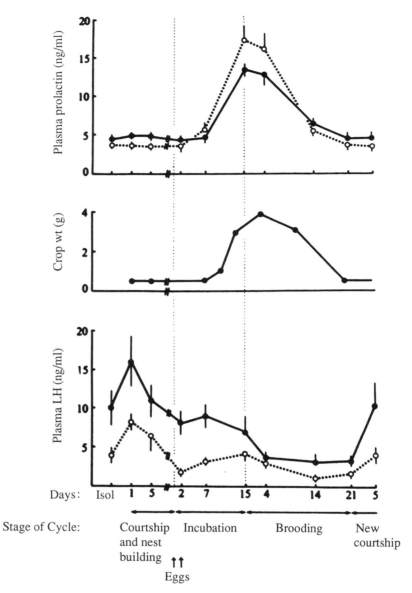

Figure 8.9 Concentrations of plasma prolactin and LH in male (filled circle) and female (open circle) ring doves during a breeding cycle. Crop weights are also shown. The time scales are for courtship and nest-building, then for incubation, and then for brooding young. Birds were in isolation (Isol) before they were paired at the start of the cycle. Concentrations of estradiol (E), testosterone (T), and progesterone (P) are high during courtship and nestbuilding and decline after egg laying (not shown). (From Goldsmith, et al., [1981][417]; reproduced by permission.)

As noted above, there is rise in prolactin secretion around midincubation. This is the result of tactile and perhaps visual stimulation provided by the eggs. It depends, therefore, on the earlier initiation of incubation by progesterone.

In other species with altricial young, the canary, starling, and pied flycatcher, prolactin levels rise early in incubation and remain high throughout.[619, 954] Prolactin also stimulates incubation behavior in the budgerigar, and steroid priming, particularly with estrogen, is necessary.[514] Although prolactin may stimulate incubation behavior in these species, contact with the eggs is required by inexperienced parents to maintain both prolactin secretion and incubation for the duration of incubation. In all species studied, including both altricial and precocial species, removing the eggs or separating inexperienced females from their nests during incubation leads to a rapid decline in prolactin secretion and incubation behavior.[416]

The brown-headed cowbird, a parasitic species, lays eggs in the nests of other species and does not exhibit incubation behavior. It is interesting, therefore, that although prolactin binding sites in the brains of males and females of this species are similar in distribution to those in starlings, a parental species, binding density in the preoptic area was less in the brown-headed cowbird.[46] This might indicate that they are less responsive to prolactin in the brain areas involved in parental care.

The onset of *incubation behavior* in the hen and turkey is correlated with a rise in the circulating levels of prolactin and a decline in steroid hormones. This has led investigators to propose that prolactin stimulates incubation in these species. Prolactin was injected into turkeys and hens and was successful in stimulating incubation. To be effective, the hormone had to be injected in hens that were laying eggs or hens that had been ovariectomized and given estradiol. Incubation normally occurs after this phase of the reproductive cycle. Laying hens have already passed through the steroid-regulated phases of the reproductive cycle. Estrogen or progesterone, or both hormones, therefore, prime females to initiate incubation in response to prolactin.

BROODING: CARE OF YOUNG

Parental care among birds has been studied most extensively in the ring dove and the hen, species with altricial and precocial young, respectively. Whether these species are typical of other altricial and precocial species with respect to the hormonal stimulation of parental behavior is difficult to assess because so few species have been studied. We shall discuss these two species in this section.

The ring dove is similar to the hen in the high level of prolactin present at the end of incubation and at hatching[417] (figure 8.10). This provides the basis for the early brooding of the newly hatched squabs. Brooding or sitting on the squabs in the ring dove may be considered a continuation of incubation behavior now directed at the squabs instead of the eggs.[619] There is, however, a strong tendency for inexperienced incubating males and females, when presented with a choice during the normal cycle, to sit on a nest with eggs as

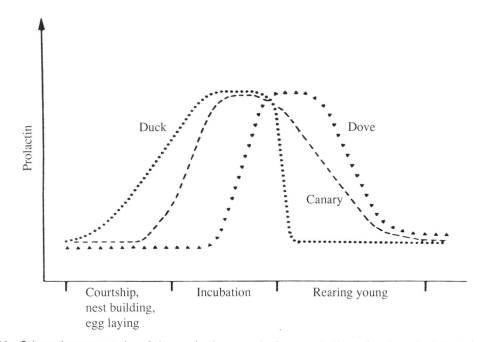

Figure 8.10 Schematic representation of changes in plasma prolactin concentration in female mallard ducks (*Anas platyrhynchos*), canaries (*Serinus canarius*), and ring doves (*Streptopelia risoria*) during the breeding cycle. Prolactin concentrations in the hen are similar to those in the mallard duck. (From Goldsmith, A. R. [1983][416]; reproduced by permission.)

opposed to a nest with squabs.[742] This preference changes dramatically when the squabs are hatched. With breeding experience, parents presented with a choice show a tendency to sit on a nest with squabs rather than a nest with eggs during incubation. This shows that prolactin can mediate the transition from incubation to brooding behavior that normally occurs at hatching.

Other aspects of parental care in the ring dove are either specific to this and related species, such as feeding the squabs by regurgitation of crop milk, or are common to altricial species, such as defending the young in the nest. In species with precocial young, the parent may defend the young at the nest, but more often the young respond to her alarm call at the approach of a predator by dispersing and hiding in brush or becoming immobilized. Unlike the young of precocial species, the ring dove young remain in the nest for nearly 2 weeks after hatching and continue to provide the brooding parents with ventral tactile stimulation as well as visual stimulation. This causes the release of prolactin, which induces the production of crop milk, which is used by both males and females to feed the young.[417] The crop gland continues to increase in weight from the time of hatching until about 4 to 5 days after hatching and then declines in weight over the next 7 days when the young begin to feed themselves.

Young ring dove squabs are able to induce crop gland development in foster parents.[172] They do this through the release of prolactin by the pituitary glands of both male and female ring doves, as shown by the parents' response to exposure to hungry 3-day-old squabs for 1 hour. The question arises whether this reciprocal relationship between parents and young in which the squabs stimulate the release of prolactin and the production of crop milk, which is then fed to them, also includes the maintenance of parental behavior by the prolactin that is released.

It was initially believed that prolactin stimulated ring doves with previous breeding experience to feed 7-day-old young by producing a milk-engorged crop gland that provided the main source of motivation for feeding.[618] It was shown, however, that incubating ring doves, under the influence of prolactin, attempted to feed squabs despite the absence of crop milk and an engorged crop. Feeding behavior occurred in response to persistent ventral stimulation by newly hatched squabs and occurred as rapidly in inexperienced as in experienced prolactin-stimulated parents.

Prolactin can act directly on the CNS, and several prolactin-concentrating sites have been located.[173] It can reach the brain from the peripheral circulation possibly through a prolactin receptor mechanism located in the choroid plexus.[174] As noted above, even without previous parental experience up to two-thirds of females fed squabs when they were injected systemically with prolactin. However, Lott and Comerford[640] found that inexperienced male ring doves required both progesterone and prolactin to initiate sitting on the squabs and feeding them. When prolactin was infused directly into the CSF where it could act directly on the CNS without producing crop gland development, one-third of the females showed squab-feeding behavior, and many more exhibited bill-opening toward them, which is a signal to the squab to stimulate the parent to regurgitate food. Systemic injections of prolactin are, therefore, more effective in eliciting parental feeding than prolactin injected into the CSF. This suggests either that not all of the prolactin reaches the CNS or that there are multiple sites of prolactin action, not all of which are reached by CSF administration of prolactin.

Squab-induced release of prolactin most likely maintains parental behavior in the ring dove as well as stimulating the crop gland. However, prolactin levels gradually decline after the first week despite the fact that feeding the squab continues into the second week. Moreover, there is less and less crop milk in the material regurgitated into the squabs and more and more seed. Either prolactin continues to maintain parental care throughout the 2-week period of parental care in this species, or parental behavior is maintained nonhormonally by squab stimulation beginning around the end of the first week.[949]

In other species with altricial young (e.g., canary, starling, and pied flycatcher) parental behavior may also be initiated by prolactin secreted during incubation. The behavior is then maintained by prolactin released in response to stimulation by the young, and feeding behavior is exhibited without the intervening processes of crop gland development and regurgitation of crop milk.

At different intervals after hatching in different species, parental care may be maintained nonhormonally by stimulation from the young.

Hen

The hen initiates parental care of her chicks immediately after hatching following a 21-day incubation period. The behavior consists of fluffing out her feathers and settling over the young, allowing ventral contact that serves to keep the young warm and quiet. When the chicks are separated from her, the mother emits two types of calls, clucks and tidbits, which attract the chicks to her, often for feeding, although the mother herself does not feed them. From the beginning, the chicks feed by pecking at food on the floor, but they can survive for a period of time after hatching on their yolk stores.

Studying nonincubating hens and stimulating their parental behavior has enabled us to understand how hormones play a role in the parental care of hens. Parental care can be induced in nonincubating hens by exposing them to newly hatched chicks. The chicks are placed under the hen in the darkness, and both are confined in an enclosed area for about 9 hours.[848, 849] Of particular importance is the ventral skin contact that occurs between the hen and the chick.[651] The following morning a large number of hens exhibit tidbitting and clucking, and during the next 2 days nearly all exhibit these parental behaviors. If, on the other hand, chicks are given to hens during the daylight, parental care is slower to develop, largely because the hen, responding to them visually before tactile contact takes place, pecks at and often wounds or kills the chicks, treating them as intruders. As aggression subsides, parental care develops, and 3 to 4 days later these females are also exhibiting parental care. In females receiving chicks in darkness rather than in daylight, physical contact between the hen and chicks is greater, and this accelerates their onset of parental care.

At hatching, prolactin levels in the hen are high. The role of prolactin in parental care may be to facilitate contact between the mother and the chicks for the first several hours after hatching as a continuation of incubation behavior. It may also alter ventral skin sensitivity and so facilitate contact with the chicks.[651] When the parental behavior of incubating hens with high levels of prolactin was compared to the behavior of nonincubating hens with low levels of prolactin, the incubating hens showed parental behavior sooner. They remained in contact with the chicks nearly all of the time, much longer than the nonincubating hens. More of them also emitted food calls, and none of them pecked at the chicks. Prolactin, therefore, mediates the onset of parental behavior in the chicken.

Exposure to chicks, eliciting the performance of parental behavior, does not, however, maintain the initial high level of prolactin in incubating hens. Also, in nonincubating hens that exhibit parental behavior, exposure to young does not stimulate an increase in prolactin levels. A study showed that in both groups prolactin levels decreased over 8 days, during which the hens exhibited parental behavior. One reason for this may have been that the chicks became more active after the first few days, and contact time between mother and chicks decreased to less than half of the time maintained at first. Nevertheless, tactile stimulation by chicks of the mother's ventrum, even at reduced levels, is necessary to maintain brooding.[651] Parental care in hens appears to be maintained on a nonhormonal basis after its onset. Moreover, it is unlikely that even ovarian hormones play a role because they do not contribute to any aspect of postincubation parental care in chickens.[849] Similar findings concerning the decline of prolactin levels during parental care have been reported in turkey hens, female mallard ducks, and female ring-necked pheasants.

Summarizing this section on avian parental behavior, we find that the oviparous mode of reproduction gives rise to two parental phases among birds. The first is the incubation phase, which, in most species, both precocial and altricial, is stimulated by prolactin. Prolactin is also involved in the transition to the second phase. This phase of brooding behavior involves crouching over or sitting on the newly hatched young. The similarity of behavior patterns of incubating and brooding suggests that they are closely related, and experimental evidence confirms this. Among precocial species, prolactin levels decline rapidly after hatching, and parental behavior appears to be maintained on a nonhormonal basis. Among altricial species, prolactin levels decline more slowly after hatching, following the cessation of nest occupation and crouching over young, and significant levels may still be present 1 or 2 weeks later. The presence of prolactin may maintain parental behavior. On the other hand, parental behavior may be maintained on a nonhormonal basis in these species also.

The ring dove differs from most species with altricial young because it feeds its squabs with a "milk" produced by the crop gland. This gland develops during incubation, and its growth and secretion are stimulated by prolactin. Incubation in the female ring dove is stimulated by estrogen and progesterone. Evidence is conflicting about the hormonal basis (if any) for incubation behavior in males. During incubation, tactile stimulation from the eggs elicits the release of prolactin. After hatching, prolactin secretion is maintained at a declining rate for nearly 2 weeks by tactile and visual stimulation from the squabs. Although prolactin continues to stimulate crop gland activity, parental care may be maintained nonhormonally in this species as well. There are brain sites in the ring dove that are responsive to prolactin, and prolactin injected into the CSF of the brain is capable of eliciting parental behavior.

General Summary

The following are the main points that summarize the content of this chapter on hormone-behavior relationships in the regulation of parental behavior in mammals and birds:

1. Parental behavior is most highly developed among the mammals and birds. Among the mammals the hormonal basis of parental care evolved in relation to the viviparous mode of reproduction. The hormones that regulate

pregnancy and parturition play a crucial role in the onset of maternal behavior and the initiation of lactation. Among the birds the hormonal basis of parental care evolved in relation to the oviparous mode of reproduction. This dictated two phases of hormonal regulation of parental care, care of the eggs during incubation and care of the young after hatching. There are parallels between female mammals and birds in many aspects of parental care. While not as clearly defined behaviorally as the corresponding periods among birds, the prepartum and postpartum periods among mammals bear a relationship to the periods of incubation and care of the young. Late pregnancy prepares the female mammal to take care of the young by seeking isolation from the social group and by establishing her readiness to exhibit parental care just as incubation behavior prepares avian females to brood the hatchlings. Males among mammals and most birds do not undergo the same physiological changes as females, yet many exhibit parental care. The causes of parental care are more varied among males than females.

2. Parental behavior is adapted to the developmental status of the young at birth among both mammals and birds. Among both mammals and birds three kinds of patterns have evolved in relation to the altricial, precocial, and semialtricial or semiprecocial status of the young. These patterns among mammals are the nesting pattern, the leading-following pattern, and the clinging-carrying pattern. Among birds the nesting pattern is present during incubation in nearly all species, but parental care after hatching differs in species with altricial and precocial young and in the few species with semialtricial or semiprecocial young. In altricial species the nesting pattern is of longer duration, and there is extended parental feeding of the young. Precocial species exhibit a leading-following pattern. Parents do not feed their young but often lead them to food. Semialtricial species show parental feeding of the young and early mobility by the young but not leading-following.

3. Among the mammals that have been studied, the hormones important for maternal behavior are the ovarian hormones estrogen and progesterone, and prolactin either from the pituitary or the brain. These hormones maintain pregnancy in all species, but there are species differences in the patterns of secretion of these hormones and in their regulaton during pregnancy. Estrogen and progesterone prime females to respond to triggering stimulation by estrogen or estrogen in conjunction with prolactin and/or oxytocin. Too few species have been studied to be able to state whether there is uniformity in the hormonal basis of parental care among the mammals. There may be specializations—for example, it is likely that oxytocin plays a role in the onset of maternal behavior in sheep to ensure that the mother forms a selective bond with her lamb rapidly at parturition.

4. Among the birds, ovarian hormones in females and perhaps testicular hormones in males combine with prolactin as the hormonal basis of incubation and parental care. In species that feed their young with crop milk, incubation is divided into two hormonal phases in females, stimulated first by progesterone and then by prolactin. In species with altricial young, prolactin continues to

stimulate parental care for several days after hatching, whereas in species with precocial young prolactin stimulation of parental care very likely terminates soon after hatching.

5. There is an indication among females in several species of mammals and birds that hormonal stimulation plays a role mainly in the initiation of parental care. The maintenance of parental care appears to be based upon stimulation provided by the young. Parental behavior among both mammals and birds, therefore, may be organized into two principal phases—a hormonal phase during pregnancy and parturition in mammals or incubation and hatching in birds and for a short period after parturition or hatching, and a nonhormonal phase following this. In mammals the nonhormonal phase arises soon after parturition during what may be called a transition period. Among birds the nonhormonal phase appears earlier after hatching in precocial species than in altricial species.

6. Hormones stimulate parental behavior in females by their action on the central nervous system. Sites of action of estrogen, progesterone, prolactin, and oxytocin have been studied in mammals, and several of the sites have been found to play roles in mediating maternal behavior. Among the birds, possible sites of action of prolactin in parental care have been identified.

9 Hormones and Aggressive Behavior

Edward P. Monaghan and Stephen E. Glickman

There are plenty of reasons to suspect hormones are involved in aggressive behaviors. After all, among humans there is clearly a sex difference in the commission of violent crimes, and the two sexes have very different concentrations of hormones. Might not the latter fact be responsible for the former? Several animal models support the idea that androgens increase aggressiveness and ovarian hormones decrease aggression. There is a surprising complexity, however, in the relations between androgens and aggression, not the least being that aggressive encounters can alter androgen secretion. In addition, in some species females are more aggressive than males, but gonadal steroids are implicated in this difference, too.

What is aggression and why is it particularly difficult to study? Can androgen treatment affect the likelihood that an individual will be aggressive or will itself be attacked? How can the experimental context overshadow any hormone effect, and what happens to hormonal secretion after participating in an aggressive encounter?

Introduction

However regrettable it may seem, aggressive encounters occur in the lives of most individuals in most species. Often the outcomes of these aggressive interactions determine whether an individual will successfully reproduce or survive. Clearly, understanding the causes and effects of aggression is important to understanding the natural history of any species, including our own. As we will see, there is also little doubt that hormones can affect the probability of an aggressive encounter. However, four problems complicate our discussion of hormonal influences on aggression: (1) the difficulty in defining aggression, (2) the related issue of the importance of the natural history of a species for the normal context of aggression, (3) the necessarily dyadic nature of aggressive behavior (i.e., we must analyze at least two individuals), and (4) the fact that aggressive encounters can themselves have a profound influence on hormonal secretions. We will continue to return to these points throughout our discussion of aggression.

We begin this chapter with a discussion of the problems that require solution and the decisions that need to be made before hormone aggressive behavior relationships can be explored. We then turn to a consideration of two examples, each offering distinctive insights. Intermale aggression in domestic mice (*Mus domesticus*) has provided an unusually stable and sensitive system for the detection of hormonal effects. This will be contrasted with aggression in primate social groups, which can reveal the complexity of hormone-behavior interactions. Such studies of hormone-aggression relationships in rhesus monkeys emphasize the extent to which modulating effects of hormones are limited by the social context in which they are expressed, and the fact that the effects of social interaction on hormones are often more prominent than the effects of hormones on social interaction. We conclude with a brief discussion of human issues relevant to hormones and aggression.

The Definition of Aggression

In their natural habitats, animals fight or threaten one another to defend resources or gain access to new resources. However, aggression appears in a variety of situations, and the response topographies that characterize aggression can vary or be quite subtle. This has made the development of a satisfactory definition of aggression troublesome. In fact, substantial confusion has arisen in the literature because of the diversity of definitions of aggression.

Biologists, approaching the problem from an evolutionary perspective, have tended to focus on aggressive behaviors as one route to successful **competition for limited resources** (e.g., food, mates, or territories that permit successful foraging, reproduction, and rearing of offspring). Such a definition could logically include defensive-aggressive behaviors that result in protection of one's own reproductive potential, or that of one's offspring (e.g., maternal defense of infants). Few biologists would classify predation on another species as aggressive behavior, instead viewing it as more closely related to feeding, although possibly having independent motivational properties.

The most widely accepted psychological definitions appear to be more inclusive, but more difficult to measure. There are two key elements: the presence of behavioral sequences that could result in one animal injuring or killing a second animal, and "intent" to achieve that end.[765] The latter element is included to distinguish true aggression from the incidental killing that results when an elephant steps on a dung beetle, although the assessment of intent is problematic. If one includes "psychological" injury, this definition is sufficient to encompass most any class of behavior that might be viewed as aggressive. In this chapter we have opted to examine aggression primarily in the context of the narrower, biological definition, although our examination of human aggression will consider the more inclusive psychological components.

Another common confusion in the aggression literature results from the failure to distinguish between aggressive or submissive behaviors and dominance-subordinance relationships, the latter representing a potential *consequence* of aggression. But it is important to recognize that there are other potential routes to the emergence of dominance. For example, we will learn in chapter 10 that there may be marked individual differences in the extent to which aggression is used to maintain dominance within a primate group. Moreover, the behaviors of subordinates can be critical elements in maintenance of dominance relationships, without need for any actions by the dominant animal.[883] These distinctions are particularly important in hormone-behavior studies. First, they force the recognition that dominance in a particular situation can exist without aggression, and second, they raise the possibility that aggressive and submissive behaviors may be modulated by different endocrine systems.[622]

How to Evaluate Aggression

Translating broad concepts of aggression into particular measurements is a challenging affair. Those interested in the neural and endocrine mechanisms of aggression must explore the possibility of common modulating mechanisms underlying quite different aggressive behaviors, as well as unique systems that control particular sequences of aggression. The investigator must first select the particular category of aggression to examine. In the most widely used classification of aggression (by a psychologist oriented toward the animal literature), Moyer[765] listed eight categories of aggression, based on the situation in which the aggression is observed: predatory, intermale, fear-induced, irritable, territorial, maternal, instrumental, and sex-related. Brain[140] later advocated including intermale, territorial, and sex-related aggression under the single heading of "social aggression." Some of Moyer's categories may be more appropriate than others, depending on the species studied.

Selecting Combatants: Species and Sex

Two implicit assumptions made by many investigators studying aggression are that males fight more frequently and persistently than females and that testosterone is the significant hormone. As a result, the overwhelming majority of studies of mammalian aggression between two individuals (i.e., **dyadic** aggression) involve male-male pairings. However, in many species there is extensive female-female competition. For example, in social canids (dogs, wolves, etc.), reproductive inhibition by the alpha (i.e., the most socially dominant) female is a potent determinant of ultimate entry to the breeding system, and female-female aggression is probably as common as male-male aggression.[348] Male-female aggression between wolves, however, is relatively rare.

The research literature is also biased toward a limited set of mammalian species. Traditionally this has been those species studied in psychological laboratories, in which males are substantially larger and often more aggressive than females (i.e., laboratory mice and rats, and rhesus monkeys). As a result, there are excellent descriptions of the postures involved in aggressive interactions between males of these species. A great deal is also known about the neural and endocrine systems of these species, permitting concurrent studies of physiological mechanisms. Aggression varies considerably across species, and when aggression is studied in females, the appropriate conditions may be

Box 9.1   An example of a species in which females are more aggressive than males: the spotted hyena

Spotted hyenas, inhabiting the plains of sub-Saharan Africa, are among the most successful social hunters on earth (Kruuk, 1972; Mills, 1990). They live in complex social groups and feed on a variety of prey, including animals as large as zebra (figure 9.1*A*). They also display a set of behavioral and morphological characteristics that have drawn the attention of endocrinologists. Within hyena social groups, adult females are highly aggressive, dominating adult males during competitive feeding and during other aspects of daily life (Frank, 1986). This female dominance enables mothers to ensure adequate nutrition for their offspring (Hamilton, Tilson and Frank, 1986). Female spotted hyenas are also slightly larger than males and have external genitalia that are very similar to those of the male. The hypertrophied clitoris (figure 9.1*B*) has a central urogenital sinus through which the female spotted hyena urinates, receives the male during copulation, and gives birth. There is no external vagina, as the vaginal labia have fused to form a pseudoscrotum.

This suite of what are usually considered masculine characteristics mimics the effects of androgens administered to a variety of female mammals during fetal-neonatal development (see chapter 2). However, the natural genital "masculinization" of the female hyena is remarkably complete. According to our current understanding of sexual differentiation, the form of the external genitalia of the female hyena requires the presence of androgens during sensitive stages of development. The circulation of such androgens during appropriate periods of development might also be expected to increase body weight, enhance aggression, and promote the appearance of rough social play.

Studies of maternal and fetal endocrinology in spotted hyenas are currently under way using a colony of animals maintained at the University of California, Berkeley. Results to date suggest a novel mechanism may be operating to androgenize the female fetus. Androstenedione, secreted by the maternal ovary, is converted to testosterone by the placenta and passed to the developing fetus through the umbilical circulation (Glickman et al, 1987; Yalcinkaya, Glickman and Licht, 1991). Such placental testosterone may be the critical agent responsible for the "masculinization" of the female spotted hyena during fetal life. In addition, the ovaries of hyenas secrete substantial quantities of androstenedione throughout the lifespan and this steroid has been found to facilitate aggression in rodents (Erpino and Chappelle, 1971). Removal of the ovaries reduced the aggressiveness of adult female hyenas toward males (Baker, 1990). However, since ovarian secretions include a variety of androgens and estrogens, all of which might facilitate aggression (Simon and Whalen, 1987), it is not yet clear which ovarian products are responsible for enhancing female aggressiveness toward males. The emergence of female dominance in nature is also affected by nonhormonal factors. For example, male hyenas disperse at puberty, whereas females reside their entire lives within a single clan. Since resident hyenas tend to form coalitions against intruders (Zabel, Glickman, Frank, Woodmansee and Keppel, *in press*), individual dispersing males are confronted by groups of large, aggressive, allied females. It is not surprising that males behave in very subordinate fashion (Frank, Glickman and Zabel, 1989).

Finally, there are extraordinary levels of intense aggression that occur shortly after birth between the twins that generally constitute a hyena litter (Frank, Glickman and Licht, 1991). This aggression, which is accompanied by high levels of plasma androgen, commonly results in the death of one sibling if the twin hyenas are of the same sex (figure 9.1*C*). It is possible that, in the course of selecting high androgen levels for both sexes during fetal life, conditions arose which promoted violent neonatal aggression. The influence of fetal androgens on neonatal aggression remains to be determined. It seems likely that in the course of solving the enigma posed by female spotted hyenas, we will also clarify the role of hormones on aggression in other complex mammals.

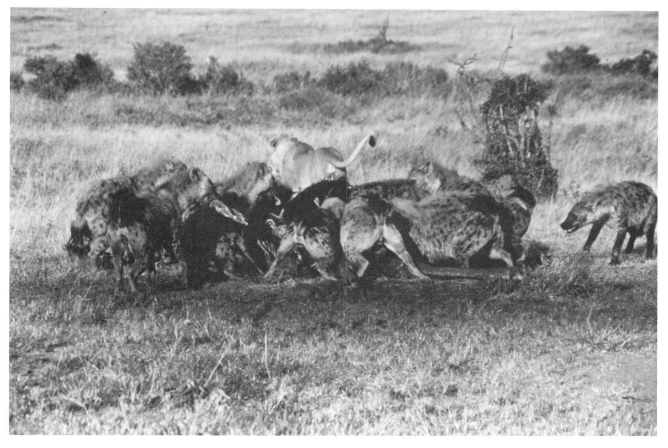

A

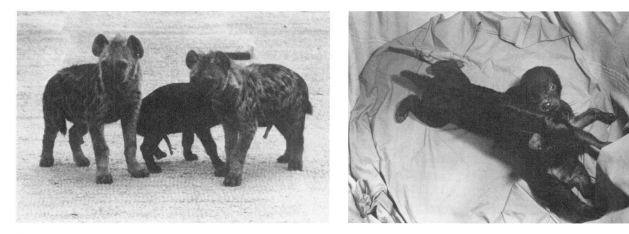

B

C

quite different from those that are appropriate for males. For example, as discussed in chapter 8, females tend to show the greatest amount of aggression postpartum, in the presence of pups (i.e., maternal aggression).

We know less about species where the female is the larger of the two sexes, despite the fact that in 25% of mammalian species females are larger than males.[836] For example, hamster females are often as aggressive as males and are capable of dominating males in a variety of social situations.[362] Among nonlaboratory species, the female spotted hyena represents an extreme case of female aggressiveness and dominance in a highly social mammal, indicating the possible range of variation in sexually dimorphic aggression (box 9.1).

Selecting Test Situations and Conditions of Housing

THE DUSKY-FOOTED WOODRAT

Consider a concrete example of the importance of selecting the appropriate test situation and housing conditions for aggression testing from the case of the dusky-footed woodrat. These are rats of moderate size (adults weigh 200 to 500 gm) found in oak woodland and stream-related habitats along the Pacific coast of the United States. They are technically solitary animals; that is, they normally reside in independent dwellings (called houses, often 2 to 6 feet in height) that have been constructed of branches or twigs. Individual rats construct and maintain these shelters, gnawing small or medium-sized branches from trees or locating fallen branches on the ground, and carrying them to their house. Houses generally outlive their occupants, sometimes lasting for decades, while individual woodrat tenants come and go from one year to the next. It is generally agreed that possession of a house is crucial for survival in the world of the woodrat. It provides shelter from predation and extremes of climate. Moreover, the houses are repositories of food collected by the occupants, providing a hedge against bad weather or prowling predators (including owls, coyotes, badgers, weasels, and a variety of snakes). The number of houses in any given habitat is limited by the availability of good sites.

Although there is just one adult woodrat in each house, each individual knows its neighbors as individuals, meeting them in the vicinity of particular houses, and also in more neutral areas while foraging. Wallen[1085] was able to demonstrate this by linking individual woodrats to particular houses in the field, trapping and transporting them to a laboratory setting and observing interactions between neighbors and between strangers (i.e., rats that lived so far apart that it was reasonable to infer that they had never encountered each other). Neighbors demonstrated clearly defined dominance relationships. There was little fighting and only cursory investigation. Strangers engaged in a great deal of social investigatory behavior.

Woodrats also have a sharply defined breeding season in the winter and spring. At this time adult females confront the problem of producing infants who will be able to find a house of their own, a requirement for survival. Part of the maternal "strategy" involves production of small (two-rat) litters, which receive a great deal of maternal nourishment in a short period of time. Female woodrats are highly aggressive during this time, excluding males from the vicinity of the house.[638] Some highly favored offspring are able to take over their mother's house while she moves elsewhere, although even in this case, there is direct competition from a sibling. Despite houses and mothers, it is all a risky business. Survival rates of newborn woodrats to the next breeding season (one year later) are probably no better than 1 in 3. Male woodrats fight to maintain possession of a house and exclude other males from surrounding houses. Although it is difficult to observe aggression in the field, the incidence of wounds increases dramatically during the breeding season, coincident with a rise in testosterone levels.[178]

Thus, as the breeding season proceeds, there is intense competition for houses between all woodrats and intermale competition for a place in the breeding system. This perspective provides a rationale for manipulating several variables that reflect natural seasonal changes in hormone levels and aggression. It also suggests test conditions that incorporate such features of the habitat as possession of a house. Finally, knowledge of the natural habitat situation directs attention to the variable of genetic relatedness, which is generally ignored in captive studies, and forces the realization that competition is frequently "unfair," involving opponents who are not matched for age, size and sex.

Experimental data bear out the importance of understanding the natural context in which aggression occurs. In the course of examining aggression between woodrats in the laboratory, we found that when paired in a neutral arena during the breeding season, castrated males fought as vigorously as intact males and were as successful as intact males in dominating encounters.[178] However, when woodrats were permitted to construct and defend individual houses, intact animals had a clear advantage.[407] In this case, the emergence of a major effect of gonadal hormones on aggression and dominance depended on the presence of the appropriate defensible resource in the test situation.

LABORATORY RATS

Even in the domesticated albino rat used in the laboratory, testing conditions can affect whether hormone-aggression relations are found. For example, laboratory rats show fairly low levels of aggression when they are simply paired in a neutral (open) arena. Some investigators have used electrical shock, social isolation, or both in order to increase the display of intermale agression in rats, and hormones often seemed to have only weak effects on this behavior. Recently researchers have begun to look at behavior in the ethologically more meaningful context of mixed sex housing. The approach employed is the colony intruder model in which animals are housed in small mixed sex groups, then at testing, an unfamiliar animal is introduced to the colony.[125] Under such conditions, rats display high levels of aggression depending on their hormonal condition. Normally, the dominant male attacks the intruder. After castration a previously dominant male will show little aggressive behavior, and defense of the colony will be taken over by other males who assume a dominant role. However, if the animal is treated with testosterone after castration, he will continue to display high levels of aggression.[13] Thus, under the conditions of the colony intruder model, the display of aggression in rats is dependent on the presence of testosterone and somewhat independent of experience. Under other conditions, effects of experience often rival hormonal influences.

EXPERIENTIAL AND SOCIAL GROUP EFFECTS
Many years ago, Ginsburg and Allee[402] demonstrated that the behavior of mice in aggressive dyadic encounters was markedly affected by whether they had won or lost prior encounters in the test situation. We have seen similar effects in woodrats.[177a] Later in this chapter we describe variation in the effects of hormones on aggression in rhesus monkeys depending on prior experience and social context. In general, among long-lived mammals with highly organized social systems, variation in social context often overrides any hormonal effects on aggression.

Measurement of Aggression

The measurement of aggression begins with good description of the natural sequences of aggressive interactions displayed by the species in question. For example, in 1963 Grant and Mackintosh[437] provided a detailed description of such interactions in three commonly used species of laboratory rodent: guinea pigs, rats, and mice. The sequence of approaches, investigatory behaviors, upright/lateral defensive postures, and biting attacks were illustrated and made available for other researchers. The detailed use of such ethological descriptions enabled others[125] to conclude that shock-elicited aggression in rats, which has been a commonly used procedure, is better characterized as shock-elicited defense. As Conner and colleagues[221] observe, it is probably not surprising that such behaviors are less sensitive to manipulations of androgens than those involving intermale aggression.

To this point, research on hormones and aggressive behavior has largely involved a focus on the final, "consummatory" phases of aggressive interactions. However, there is also an appetitive (motivational) component to aggression that is often overlooked in contemporary studies. Under certain conditions, rats will run a maze for the "reward" of attacking another member of their species.[610, 1022] Wallen's[1086] recent studies of sexual behavior in rhesus monkeys indicate major differences in the endocrine mechanisms controlling consummatory and appetitive behaviors; chapter 4 discusses similar distinctions regarding sexual behavior in rats. It seems likely that similar distinctions will appear in the case of aggressive behavior when the appropriate investigations have been completed.

A study of hermit crabs[223] indicates the kind of result that might be anticipated. The test situation simulated a problem commonly solved by aggression in nature. Hermit crabs live in shells discarded by other animals as residences, with individual crabs changing homes as they grow in size. Possession of a shell that is neither too large nor too small is required for survival in nature, and contests for such a resource are a natural part of existence for hermit crabs. After determining the detailed pattern of hermit crab contests for possession of a shell, Courchesne and Barlow found that isolation increased the frequency of aggression in hermit crabs, much as in rats and mice. However, the changes were only in the final, consummatory phases of aggressive interactions. Early appetitive/investigatory behaviors proceeded in similar fashion in isolated and nonisolated animals. Such awareness of the phases of aggressive behavior, coupled with concurrent measurement and manipulation of hormonal substrates is needed in order to provide a complete account of the endocrinology of aggression.

Hormones and Aggressive Behavior

The organizational/activational hypothesis of hormone action (see chapter 2) proposes that early exposure to hormones permanently organizes the central nervous system in such a way as to increase the likelihood that certain behaviors will be activated by later hormone exposure.[817] If this applies to aggressive behavior, then exposure to hormones during the perinatal period should increase the likelihood that later exposure will result in high levels of aggression. We will review data addressing the role of organizational and activational effects of hormones on aggression in both mice and monkeys in the following sections.

When people discuss hormonal effects on aggressive behavior, they often assume that there are modifications in the sensitivity of some brain system mediating aggression. However, hormones can modify aggressive behavior in very diverse ways,[2, 622] including changing the signaling properties of the "intruder" (e.g., through changes in secretion of pheromones; see chapter 13), or by changes in body size that permit or inhibit the expression of aggression as well as shifts in the sensory and perceptual sensitivities of the recipient. In addition, there are indirect routes, for example, changes in ability to learn and remember details of prior social interactions that permit distinguishing kin from non-kin, and so on. Research that would truly disentangle these alternative routes of action is very rare.

Hormonal Substrates of Aggression in Mice

Domestic mice display a fairly high level of spontaneous aggression, and so have been used extensively in this area of research. Here we will consider only one form of aggression: physical combat between conspecifics. This is usually thought of as intermale aggression.[1080] Female mice will engage in agonistic behaviors under certain conditions, such as postpartum aggression in defense of pups, when mounted if in a nonreceptive state, or in fear-induced situations.

However, the spontaneous aggression seen between two unfamiliar mice in the laboratory is generally considered to be primarily a male trait. Toward the end of this section we will review some recent work with female mice that is refining our view of the sexual dimorphic nature of aggressive behavior.

Natural History and Social System of Mice

The house mouse is a nonseasonal breeding nocturnal animal. In the field, mice establish territories, called demes, where food and water is readily available. Each deme is founded by a single male and one or two females. Males routinely patrol the borders of their deme and will attack strange male or female mice who attempt to enter. Most of the offspring, especially males, are eventually forced to immigrate.[1072] In the wild, most fighting would therefore be classified as a form of territorial aggression. One suggested role for the aggression is to ensure maximal dispersal of mice so as to take advantage of a favorable environment.[882]

Tendencies to display aggression vary among individuals. When encountering an unfamiliar mouse, some males attack quickly and others show extended delays. Based on the interval between encountering and attacking another animal, mice can be divided into short- and long-attack latency groups. These traits are genetically influenced, since both short- and long-attack latency animals can be selectively bred. It appears that in an established community, short-attack latency males have an advantage both in defending their own deme or in invading another male's territory. However, when migrating to an entirely new area, the long-attack latency animals are probably more successful because they expend less energy in random attacks.[1072] In addition to a genetic component to this behavioral difference, we will later see that aggressive behavior in the two groups has different hormonal requirements.

Aggression Between Males

In the laboratory, aggression tests with mice usually involve three main elements: (1) a stimulus or opponent, (2) the test arena, and (3) a criterion for measuring the behavior.

1. Most tests are conducted with two animals of the same treatment condition or with a test animal and a stimulus animal. The stimulus animal is often a male whose olfactory bulbs have been lesioned and therefore cannot smell. Such mice elicit aggression as would an intact male, but they are said to neither initiate fighting nor retaliate when attacked.[275] Other researchers use the "bully test," in which prepubertal males serve as the stimulus animals. The obvious concern in these tests is that the stimulus for the behavior is another animal whose behavior cannot be completely controlled. Mechanical stimuli such as a moving bottle brush have been used in an attempt to gain greater control, but interpretation is more difficult.

2. The test arena often consists of a neutral cage in which the animals are initially separated by a barrier that is removed and the behavior recorded. A variation on this paradigm is placing one animal in the home cage of another. The key point is that in most situations there is limited space with no means of escape, and therefore the option to retreat, normally available in the wild, is eliminated.

3. Probably the element that varies the most between studies is the measurement of aggression. The most complete method is to record the frequency and latency of various behavior patterns such as biting, lunging, and mounting. Some researchers simply look at the latency at which a given behavior first occurs, or the amount of time an animal engages in a behavior during the test. In some cases tests are terminated after the first attack to minimize wounding, whereas others use the severity of wounding as their criterion for behavior. Other researchers focus on the outcome, namely who wins or loses. The behavior a researcher chooses to record will undoubtably influence the results.

HORMONES AND AGGRESSION DURING DEVELOPMENT

Since spontaneous aggression in mice is more easily elicited between two males than two females, behavioral endocrinologists suspect testosterone to have a role in mediating this behavior. Developmental studies that looked at testosterone concentrations revealed that the initiation of aggressive behavior in intact males coincides with the prepuberal rise in testosterone.[55] This correlational data suggests an activational role of testosterone in male aggression. However, in adults there was no correlation between testosterone concentrations in blood and various measures of aggression including success or failure in an aggressive encounter. Thus the presence of a minimal concentration of testosterone reached during puberty may increase the display of aggression, but differences in testosterone concentrations beyond this point are not good predictors of an individual's aggressiveness.

EFFECTS OF TESTICULAR HORMONES IN ADULTS

Early work demonstrated that prepubertal or adult castration of male mice essentially eliminates fighting.[103] After several reports of difficulty in replicating these results, the role of testosterone in mediating male aggression was qualified. Males with fighting experience were not as dependent on testosterone for expression of aggressive behavior, but previous findings were replicated in studies using males with no prior fighting experience.[932] Subsequent researchers have often kept subjects isolated after weaning in order to control for the effect of experience. Such interplay between hormones and experience is a theme which we will address repeatedly.

In addition to experience, genetic factors can also influence the role of testosterone in the activation of behavior. The maintenance of aggressive behavior in the short-attack latency group is not dependent on the presence of testosterone, whereas long-attack latency animals need testosterone to maintain aggressive behaviors.[1072]

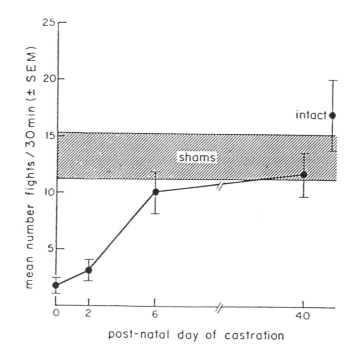

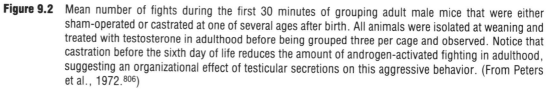

Figure 9.2 Mean number of fights during the first 30 minutes of grouping adult male mice that were either sham-operated or castrated at one of several ages after birth. All animals were isolated at weaning and treated with testosterone in adulthood before being grouped three per cage and observed. Notice that castration before the sixth day of life reduces the amount of androgen-activated fighting in adulthood, suggesting an organizational effect of testicular secretions on this aggressive behavior. (From Peters et al., 1972.[806])

ORGANIZATIONAL EFFECTS OF HORMONES ON AGGRESSIVE BEHAVIOR
Early reports that testosterone treatment did not elicit aggression in adult ovariectomized (OVX) females[1037] suggested an organizational sex difference in aggressiveness (see also below). Subsequent studies varied perinatal hormone exposure to determine whether hormonal manipulations could decrease, or "feminize," the hormone sensitivity of adult males and increase, or "masculinize," hormone sensitivity of adult females (see chapter 2).

To investigate the sensitive period for early hormone actions, male mice were castrated or sham operated on day 0, 2, 6, or 12 after birth. On day 40, neonatal castrates were sham operated and previously sham operated animals were castrated. With testosterone treatment in adulthood, day 0 and 2 castrates showed less aggression than shams (figure 9.2). Animals castrated later in life showed no difference in adult performance compared to shams.[806] These findings suggest that the sensitive period for the organizational effects of testosterone terminates between days 2 and 6. This conclusion was confirmed by work with females, in which early neonatal exposure to testosterone was most effective in producing aggressive behavior in adulthood, and exposure after day 11 had little effect.[160] Manipulations earlier in development demonstrated that prenatal hormones can also sensitize mice to later hormone exposure, but the early neonatal period seems more critical for the differentiation of aggressive behavior.[1079]

Is the effectiveness of neonatal testosterone in masculinizing aggressive behavior in females due to a decrease in sensitivity to the organizing effects of testosterone? If this were the case, then chronic testosterone exposure after the perinatal period might behaviorally masculinize females at a time when acute treatment had no effect. To test this hypothesis, female mice were ovariectomized on day 30 and then given a large injection of testosterone propionate (TP) or oil daily for 20 days. After a 45-day interval, all mice received TP treatment and weekly aggression tests. By the end of testing, 75% of the TP-pretreated animals fought compared with only 25% of the oil-pretreated animals.[313] These findings demonstrate that even after neonatal development, chronic androgen exposure *can* sensitize females to the aggression-arousing effects of testosterone exposure later in life.

These findings cast some doubt on an organizational/activational role of androgen in mediating aggressive behavior, since a strict interpretation of the hypothesis would predict a limited perinatal period during which the developing system must be masculinized by androgen for subsequent exposure in adulthood to activate a sexually dimorphic behavior. More damage was done to the model by findings that large daily injection of TP for 2 to 6 weeks was capable of masculinizing aggressive behavior even in adult OVX females.[141, 1012, 1081] Since the proper dosage and duration of testosterone treatment can activate aggressive behavior in normal adult females, early organizational action of testosterone is not a *prerequisite* for the androgenic induction of aggressive behavior in adulthood.

The possibility remained that the sensitive period for the organizational effects of a hormone never completely disappears. Chronic testosterone treatment may organize, or reorganize, a neural substrate in females such that later or continued testosterone exposure elicits male-like aggressive behavior, or chronic testosterone may somehow increase aggression without *permanently* altering the response to testosterone. If the former hypothesis is correct, then once a female begins to show male-like levels of aggression in response to chronic testosterone treatment, she might be expected to be more sensitive to subsequent testosterone exposure even after a hormone-free interval. To test this hypothesis, adult OVX females were treated with chronic TP until they showed male-like aggression. After a 60-day rest from hormone, the females again received TP and aggression tests. There was no difference between the amount of TP needed to induce aggression in the first and second trials. In other words, the testosterone pretreatment did not result in long-term changes in aggression in OVX females.[1081] Therefore, chronic testosterone exposure in adulthood seems to act in an activational, rather than a "late-organizational" manner.

Because these experiments used pharmacological doses of androgen, the organizational/activational model could still be valid normally. Barkley and Goldman[56] induced aggressive behavior in adult OVX females by implanting a

Silastic capsule containing testosterone, resulting in circulating blood levels of testosterone that were within the range of intact males. Furthermore, aggression could be maintained with a smaller dose of testosterone, which could not maintain the weight of seminal vesicles in castrate males. This finding demonstrates that long-term adult testosterone treatment can sensitize neural systems in females to the aggression-inducing effects of testosterone, but this effect may not be permanent.

Taken together, these findings suggest that a strict organizational/ activational model of aggression is inappropriate. Early androgen exposure can permanently alter an organism's responsiveness to later treatment, but this "sensitive period" has been demonstrated to extend at least into the second month of life in mice. Even without previous exposure, chronic testosterone treatment can activate male-like aggressive behavior in adult female mice. Thus it would be better to think in terms of a system becoming progressively less sensitive to testosterone as the organism develops. Such a model accounts for the necessity of extended androgen exposure late in development to produce the same effects as minimal exposure very early in life. Although chronic testosterone treatment can elicit aggression in adult females, it has not been demonstrated to permanently alter neural systems mediating aggression.

EFFECTS OF METABOLITES OF TESTOSTERONE

Thus far we have only dealt with the effect of androgens, specifically testosterone, on aggressive behavior. In adult male mice, both the aromatized and 5α-reduced metabolites of testosterone, estradiol, and 5α-dihydrotestosterone (DHT), can restore high levels of aggression in castrates.[474] This finding eliminates any simple explanation of hormone action. The decreased aggression in intact males treated with antiestrogens provides further evidence for the role of aromatized metabolites.[136, 142, 471] However, unlike chronic testosterone treatment, extended treatment with estradiol does not elicit aggression in adult female mice.[57] This suggests an organizational difference between males and females in their ability to respond to the aggression-promoting properties of estrogen.

Aromatized metabolites have early organizational effects on aggression. Female mice treated neonatally with either estrogen or TP and then tested in adulthood were masculinized such that their aggressive behavior did not differ from control males.[314] These and other findings suggest that the aromatized metabolites of testosterone are responsible for the early androgen influence on aggression in mice.[159, 958]

PERIPHERAL EFFECTS OF HORMONES

One way to make some sense out of the effects of the different metabolites of testosterone is to consider the peripheral effects of hormones. Hormones can affect the appearance of an individual and the extent to which it serves as an aggression-eliciting stimulus for other animals (box 9.2). Olfactory cues from the urine of other animals serve as important social signals between rodents.[968]

Mice use odors to recognize individuals, determine sexual receptivity, and distinguish between dominant and submissive males. A male mouse rubbed with the urine of a strange male elicits much higher levels of aggression when introduced into the cage of another male than one which was rubbed with a female's urine. The aggression-eliciting factor in urine is hormone dependent since urine from castrated males does not elicit higher levels of aggression. If the castrates are treated with testosterone, their urine will again elicit higher levels of aggression. So in addition to acting centrally, testosterone may act peripherally, that is through pheromonal cues, to affect aggression.

One possible explanation for the effects of the metabolites of testosterone on aggression is that the aromatized metabolites have a predominantly central effect. For estrogen treatment to elicit aggression in adulthood, it may be necessary for the animal to have an preexisting neural substrate that the hormone can activate. This could explain why estrogen treatment does not elicit aggression in OVX females but can increase aggression in castrated male mice. On the other hand, the reduced metabolites, such as DHT, may act on the periphery to alter pheromonal cues that will elicit more attacks from opponents. Thus chronic testosterone treatment of adult females may act by altering the pheromonal cues she emits.

Aggression in Females

Thus far, we have been considering aggressive behavior from a masculine point of view, that is, what hormonal manipulations cause female mice to behave aggressively under conditions that elicit aggression in males. In most studies on aggression, mice are housed singly after weaning. This eliminates prior fighting experience and tends to increase overall aggression when such males are paired in a neutral arena. However, females raised under these conditions show very little fighting when paired; thus, spontaneous aggression has long been considered a primarily male phenomenon. Recently researchers have begun to look at seminatural conditions to determine when and why females fight. The approach employed is the colony intruder model.[125] In this model, animals are housed in small groups, and at testing an unfamiliar animal is introduced to the colony. Many females raised under these conditions indeed show high levels of aggression directed at the intruder.[498]

EFFECTS OF OVARIAN HORMONES ON AGGRESSION IN THE ADULT
To look at hormonal influences upon such aggressive behavior in females, Hood[497] used the colony intruder paradigm to determine the tendency of rats to fight at various times throughout the estrous cycle (figure 9.5). Female rats showed more aggression when hormone levels, especially progesterone, were low. Developmental studies provide further evidence that hormones tend to inhibit the expression of aggression in female mice. Prepubertal females fight as readily as similar aged male mice, but at puberty, when hormone levels rise, male aggression increases whereas female levels decline. Furthermore, where-

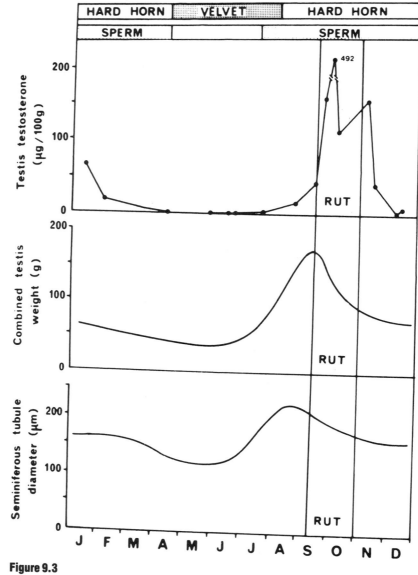

Figure 9.3

Box 9.2   An Example of Effects of Peripheral Structures on Aggression

Many mammals are seasonal breeders. In such species, there are drastic differences in hormone levels throughout the year. Often there is a correlation between these changing hormones and the frequency and intensity of aggressive interactions. Along with the hormonal and behavioral changes, the appearance of these animals can be very different. For example, red deer breed in early autumn. Testosterone levels in stags begin rising in the summer and peaks in early autumn. Among the many effects of the hormone is the stimulation of antler growth (figure 9.3). Aggressive behavior also shows a rise in early autumn (figure 9.4). To test for the influence of testosterone on the increased fighting, some animals were castrated in late summer (Lincoln et al., 1972[635]). This caused a decrease in frequency of agonistic encounters involving that animal. One possible explanation is that lower testosterone levels decreased the animals motivation to engage in agonistic behavior. However, there are several alternative explanations which could account for the change in behavior. Castration also resulted in the loss of the deer's hard antlers and growth of the sensitive velvet antlers. This male would be at a severe disadvantage in any aggressive encounter and would thus rapidly learn to avoid agonistic encounters. Furthermore, the deer's appearance may not elicit an aggressive response from other animals. Thus the change in behavior could be due to the loss of weaponry necessary to initiate or provoke attack just as likely as to some effect on a neural mechanism mediating aggression. This example is meant to illustrate that we must be cautious in interpreting the results of studies which manipulate hormone levels in one animal.

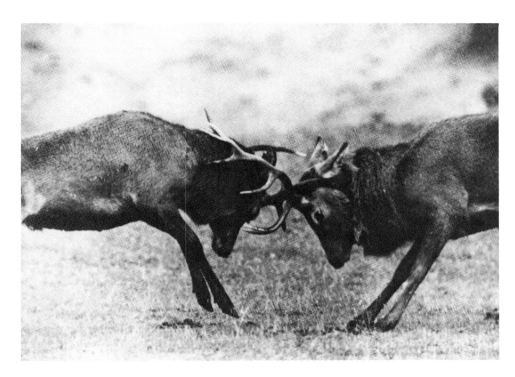

Figure 9.4

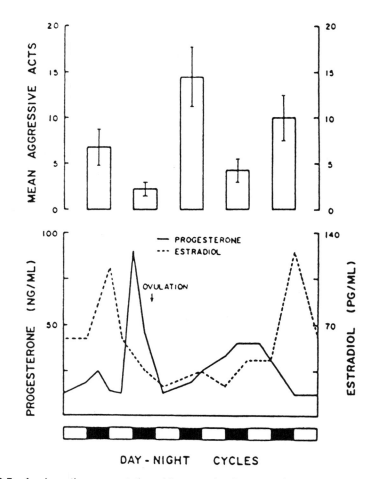

Figure 9.5 A schematic representation of hormone levels across the estrous cycle of female rats (lower graph), and the mean number of aggressive acts produced by females at different times in that cycle (upper histograms). The females were tested in an "intruder model": subject animals lived together in a large colony cage, and their behavior was measured after a previously unknown rat (a diestrus female) was placed in the cage for 15 minutes during the dark phase. Note that the lowest amount of aggression is seen during the night in which mating would normally take place (second bar from the left), and the highest level of aggression is seen the next night, when ovarian hormone levels are lowest. (From Hood, 1984.[497])

as gonadectomy tends to *decrease* aggression in male rats, it does not in females. In fact, treatment of females with replacement estrogen and progesterone reduces attacking behaviors.[267] Thus, at least for rats and mice, evidence suggests that gonadal hormones have an opposite effect on aggressive behavior in males and females: Testicular hormones play a permissive role in males and ovarian hormones inhibit the expression of aggressive in females.

MATERNAL AGGRESSION

As mentioned earlier, female rodents show high levels of postpartum aggression.[1013] This maternal aggression peaks during the first postnatal week and is characterized by immediate attack towards the flanks and neck of any animal attempting to enter the nest area. During the late gestational and lactational periods, females undergo drastic hormonal changes. However, since maternal aggression is maintained following gonadectomy and adrenalectomy, steroid hormones are suspected to play only an auxiliary role in its expression. The suckling of pups appears to be the key stimulus for inducing increased levels of aggression in the dams. Suckling affects circulating prolactin levels, but postpartum manipulations that alter prolactin activity do not alter levels of aggression. Effective manipulations for reducing postpartum aggression are removing the pups from the dam or preventing suckling by removing the dam's nipples (thelectomy). Thus suckling must produce a biochemical change independent of the pituitary–gonadal/adrenal axis, which is responsible for induction and maintenance of maternal aggression. Changes in ovarian hormones during gestation aid in the expression of maternal aggression in that they increase the nipple size, thus enabling the pups to suckle.

ORGANIZATIONAL EFFECTS OF HORMONES ON AGGRESSIVE BEHAVIOR
There are also subtle effects of neonatal hormones on aggression in female mice. Vom Saal[1080] examined the effect of intrauterine position on maternal aggression, interfemale aggression, and androgen-induced aggression. Each fetus in a litter of mice is located between two other fetuses within the U-shaped uterus of the mouse (except for the two fetuses at the end of each leg of the U). Fetuses were delivered by cesarian section and then categorized by the sex of the individuals adjacent to them in the uterus. A female in between two males was called a 2M female, one between two females was called a 0M female. Vom Saal then examined aggressive behavior in these mice. 2M females exhibited greater aggression than did 0M females on all measures: postpartum aggression, interfemale aggression, and androgen-induced aggression. This suggests that androgen exposure in utero does not simply change the sensitivity of female mice to androgens, since aggression was enhanced in all testing situations, but may instead predispose individuals to aggression.

Hormonal Substrates of Aggression in Rhesus Monkeys

Natural History and Social System of Rhesus Monkeys

Primate social systems range from the relatively solitary existence of certain nocturnal, insectivorous species, through the complex multi-male, multi-female social groups found in selected old world monkeys and apes. Eisenberg and colleagues[322] noted that the critical development in the evolution of the most complex primate social groups was the emergence of sufficient male-male tolerance to permit multiple adult males to coexist and cooperate while competing within a stable social group. He further suggested that the presence of a subgroup of males, graded according to age (as in gorillas), was a key intermediate step in such evolution. Rhesus monkey troops, comprising multiple adult males and females and their offspring, reflect the highest levels of subhuman primate social organization.[24] There are complex dominance relationships among males within such troops, as well as female dominance relationships organized along matrilines.[636]

To examine the effects of hormones on aggressive behavior, scientists have generally worked with small groups of captive monkeys. This approach has revealed the effects of early hormonal manipulations on later aggressive behavior and permitted analysis of correlations between such things as testosterone levels and aggressive interactions. However, in some cases, such hormonal effects would never be detected in the social context of the normal rhesus monkey troop.

Organizational Effects of Hormones

Young male rhesus monkeys typically exhibit more frequent threats, rough social play, and mounting behavior than females of similar age. Goy and colleagues[433, 434] have carried out a number of studies concerned with the impact of androgens during fetal life on the subsequent behavior of female rhesus monkeys. In their original experiments, androgens were supplied to pregnant females during days 40 to 110 of a 160-day gestation. Provision of such androgens increased the frequency of mounts, threats, and rough social play in these pseudohermaphroditic female monkeys. In subsequent work, Goy and his collaborators[431] were able to demonstrate that these effects are timed during fetal development, with effects on genital morphology and sexually related mounting behavior mediated by androgens present during the early phases of sexual differentiation (days 40 to 64), while effects on play result from the presence of androgens during later stages of gestation (days 115 to 139). This separation of morphological and behavioral effects (i.e., the later androgen treatment which increased rough-and-tumble play without altering genital appearance) enabled Goy and coworkers to rule out indirect effects of androgens on rough play mediated by differential maternal treatment of male infants. However, these effects were originally analyzed in reduced social groups with animals of similar age. Lovejoy and Wallen[642] have recently examined the basic sexual dimorphisms in threats, play, and mounting behavior in more natural, complex rhesus social groups. Under these conditions, sex differences in mounting behavior and play persist. However, sex differences in aggression are eliminated by the social context. Presumably any effects of hormones are overriden by other powerful social variables, for instance, social dominance status of one's mother.

Activational Effects of Hormones

Although aggression studies involving hormonal deprivation and replacement have not been done in primates, some excellent correlational work has been carried out by a group of researchers at Yerkes.[116] The highly developed social system of rhesus monkeys provides an excellent opportunity to investigate the relationship between hormones and aggression in a social context. The basic approach of these investigators was to measure hormone levels before and after arranged, and in some cases naturally occurring, aggressive interactions. In such a paradigm, it should be possible to determine if hormone levels predict the outcome of an aggressive interaction and how the interaction itself affects hormone levels. All the work is done in the context of social groups. As the researchers point out, more precise control over extraneous variables could be obtained by arranging dyadic encounters between previously isolated animals. However, it was within a social system that primate aggression evolved, and therefore this approach should have higher validity and may offer insight into functional significance of the hormone-behavior interactions.

Naturally Occurring Variation in Hormones

As mentioned earlier, rhesus monkeys have well-defined dominance hierarchies. Early work suggested a positive correlation between dominance status and plasma testosterone levels.[868] To test if testosterone levels were predictive of rank in newly formed groups, several small all-male groups were formed from previously unfamiliar males. The monkeys' testosterone levels prior to group formation did not correlate with the rank they would later attain in the group. However, once dominance ranking was stabilized, a significant rise in testosterone levels (as much as tenfold) was consistently noted in the alpha males. In several of the groups, the alpha male attained the highest testosterone levels, and in all cases there was a prompt increase in testosterone levels upon becoming the alpha male. However, in long-existent stable groups no correlation was seen between rank and testosterone levels. These findings suggested that although testosterone levels do not determine success or failure in an aggressive situation, the outcome of the encounter may affect testosterone levels. Further support for this theory comes from the response of males when exposed to females. Normally males show a significant rise in testosterone levels upon introduction of females. However, in one case, when upon introduction the group of males were attacked and defeated by the females, there was no rise in testosterone levels. Again this suggested that the outcome of an experience affects testosterone levels (see chapter 13).

Effects of Aggression on Hormones

These researchers proceeded to test the hypothesis that success or failure in an aggressive encounter will determine testosterone levels, that is, defeat will result in depressed testosterone levels and victory will result in elevated levels. Testosterone levels of individual males were measured before and after introduction to an unfamiliar group. After attack and defeat, the animal was removed. In each case, a significant depression in testosterone levels to 10% to 15% of baseline was seen within 24 hours. The testosterone levels of defeated males kept isolated would remain low for several weeks. Introduction of a female or placement within a familiar social group aided in recovery. On the other hand, alpha males who successfully defended against overthrow attempts showed elevated testosterone levels. Such observations led to the conclusion that it was not the aggressive interaction or the physical harm experienced by the animal, but the cognitive interpretation of the event that determined the resultant change in hormone levels. In order to test this conclusion, researchers used a group of monkeys which were routinely captured and blood tested. After one sampling, researchers held up two infant monkeys outside the cage. Seeing the struggling infants, the males charged the fence in attempts to attack the investigator, who did not respond. After 40 minutes of continued vicious attack attempts, the investigator departed, and others proceeded to recapture the males and take blood samples. No change in testosterone levels was observed. The males had expressed high levels of aggressive behavior, but since they neither won nor lost, the experience had no effect on testosterone levels.

Hormonal Substrates of Aggression in Humans

Many researchers who enter the field of aggression do so for humanitarian reasons, namely, to gain an understanding that may help alleviate some of the suffering which humans inflict upon each other. It soon becomes evident what an overwhelming venture this is. The task of defining and measuring aggression in rodents was problematic. Most researchers agree that an "intention" of the animal to inflict harm is a key component. But what of human interactions? Most of our agonistic encounters occur on the verbal level: Is this aggression? Is corporate backstabbing the human form of conspecific aggression, or should we focus on true physical harm such as what occurs in the course of a war? But does such massive, organized aggression have any relation to what occurs between two men in a barroom brawl? The point is that many human behaviors are so greatly influenced by societal pressures (not necessarily a bad thing) as to make them almost impossible to recognize and define. If we choose to focus on spontaneous physical combat, then we ignore the vast majority of what many of us consider to be aggressive interactions. Even if we satisfactorily define our behavioral measure, how then do we conduct our research? Obviously, putting subjects in a threatening situation is unethical. It is evident that research into human aggression is extremely difficult, and although we will point out the shortcomings in the existing literature, we believe it is a worthwhile endeavour.

Clinical and Institutional Research

Clinical research involving hormone manipulations has been conducted on men convicted of violent crimes. Most of the participants in these studies were sexual offenders. The use of such subjects makes interpretation difficult because of the combination of sexual and aggressive components of the act. Nonetheless, some interesting and consistent conclusions have been reached.

In several studies participants were treated with drugs that act as anti-androgens either by reducing testosterone levels or by interfering with hormone receptor dynamics.[138, 617] Recidivism in subjects treated with anti-androgens was significantly lower than in those individuals who did not receive drug treatment. While on the drug, the men reported a reduction in the frequency and intensity of fantasies and urges related to sexually deviant, aggressive activities. Researchers have concluded that the antiandrogens act to reduce an individual's motivation to engage in deviant behaviors, thus allowing for the adaptation of socially acceptable alternatives.

Genetic Variables

The importance of considering the appearance of an individual when assessing behavioral interactions is often neglected by researchers in behavioral endocrinology. We are often too eager to jump to conclusions about neural substrates and motivation. For example, reports indicate a higher than expected proportion of XYY individuals involved in violent crimes.[888] These individuals tend to develop faster and have higher testosterone levels than their adolescent peers. Genetic and hormonal explanations have been offered to explain this high level of aggression. An alternate explanation might take into account the appearance of XYY adolescence. Actions that might be interpreted as adolescent pranks when committed by a normal 15-year-old may be viewed as violent when committed by an XYY individual if he looks more like an adult. Also, some of these individuals are mentally retarded and therefore have been institutionalized, and both of these factors could lead to antisocial behavior. Thus in humans, if we exclude sexually related actions, it is difficult to see a direct effect of hormones on aggressive behavior.

Hormone-Aggression Relations in Normal Individuals

In normal adult males, no clear correlation has been found between plasma testosterone levels and non-sexually related aggression,[713, 740] although some evidence exists for such a relationship in adolescents.[788, 1011] Studies of high-school-aged males have reported a greater incidence of hostile acts and aggressiveness among individuals with high testosterone levels. Such studies show a correlation—that is, there is some relationship between testosterone and aggression in adolescents—but they do not demonstrate that testosterone causes an increase in aggressive behavior. Testosterone may indeed increase the motivation to engage in aggressive behaviors or permit the expression of such behaviors in individuals predisposed to aggression due to social factors. Another possible explanation involves the peripheral effects of the hormone, namely, the appearance of the individual. Peripheral effects of testosterone include increased muscle mass and body hair and this more mature or intimidating appearance may influence the way peers or authorities interpret and respond to that individual and the response of others may in turn affect his view of himself.

A great deal of attention has recently been focused on steroids in sports. A controversy has arisen as to the role androgens may play in physical performance. As for endogenous steroids, androgens reportedly rise prior to competition and remain high in the winners relative to the losers. However, the hormone levels both before and after a match appear to correlate more closely with the individual's mood than with his performance: the contestants with the highest spirits prior to a match had higher testosterone levels and, among the winners, those who were most satisfied with their performance had the higher post-match testosterone levels.[132] Thus, as we saw with rhesus monkeys, it is the cognitive or affective interpretation of the experience that affects hormone levels rather than hormones affecting the outcome of the interaction.

Exogenous (Anabolic) Steroid Use

As for exogenous steroid use, much clinical research suggests that it does little to improve fitness or performance. Why then is its illicit use so widespread in sports? Some researchers suggest that it is because the dosage used by many body-builders is 10 to 100 times that used in clinical studies and that at these levels, a significant effect on training may be seen. At such high doses, steroid use is exceedingly dangerous: In addition to the cardiovascular and liver damage that may result, individuals may show affective dysfunctions, such as depression, mania, hallucinations, and paranoid delusions. In a recent report, more than 20% of the subjects showed significant behavioral problems while on steroids.

Summary

Aggression is a social behavior, and therefore it is—not surprisingly—also is a very context-dependent behavior. The sex, reproductive condition, social history, species, even the strain of the individual being studied (and those same characteristics of its opponent) can all affect the likelihood of an aggressive encounter. Other factors that can have a major influence on whether or not aggression will take place are somewhat species-specific (houses for woodrats, an outgrown shell for a hermit crab, horns for deer, olfactory stimuli for mice, etc.) and cannot be understood without a consideration of the animals natural history. From this perspective, gonadal hormones are simply one of many influences. It appears that the presence of testosterone and its metabolites can increase the display of aggression, but that some minimal level is sufficient. We have seen that prior experience and the testing condition can alter whether testosterone will in fact increase aggressiveness. Furthermore, the aggressive encounter will alter subsequent testosterone secretion. For those species with a complex social system, such as monkeys and humans, the cognitive interpretation of the interaction, as opposed to the experience itself, appears to determine an individual's hormonal response to an aggressive encounter.
Some important points to remember:
1. Many different kinds of aggression and many different contextual factors

(some of which are species-specific) affect the likelihood and/or extent of aggression displayed.

2. Androgen can facilitate aggressive behavior in several species (e.g., rats, mice, deer, and monkeys), leading to a sex difference in aggression. However, there are times, such as around parturition, when the females of these species become very aggressive and there are many species (e.g., hamsters, hyenas) in which females are usually more aggressive than males. These exceptions indicate that other factors can activate aggression in the relative absence of androgen.

3. Low concentrations of androgen seem to be sufficient to effect the androgenic facilitation of aggression. Thus, in every species that has been studied, including humans, endogenous concentrations of plasma testosterone of individuals do not correlate with the extent of their aggressiveness nor predict their success in aggressive encounters.

4. Aggressive encounters between male monkeys can profoundly alter their subsequent testosterone secretion, and there is evidence that androgen production in humans is similarly sensitive to social events.

5. In mice, perinatal androgen may also have an organizational influence on the responsiveness of animals to future androgen stimulation, but there is evidence that prolonged androgen exposure of females in adulthood can overcome that effect. Aggression in mice is also strongly influenced by olfactory stimuli: Animals whose urine indicates previous testosterone exposure are more likely to provoke attacks, and mice incapable of smelling odors show very little or no aggressiveness even if they are males with their testes intact.

10 Neuroendocrinology of the Stress-Response

Robert M. Sapolsky

We all know that life can be difficult, but evolution has provided mechanisms to protect the body during crises. Such protection requires many different changes in many different parts of the body, and, as usual, hormones coordinate these widespread and diverse efforts. When the crisis is past, ebbing hormone levels signal the all-clear, and the body resumes other interests such as eating, body repair, and reproduction. But if the crisis persists, or if the individual's perception of crisis persists, hormones continue to drive the body to take desperate measures, sometimes with disastrous consequences. Stress and the interaction between stress and the immune system are the focus of this chapter.

What are the hormonal responses to stress and how do they normally provide help for the immediate future? What are the physiological consequences of long-term stress and why does stress seem to affect some individuals more than others?

Introduction

Ours is not an ideal world. If it were, nations would beat their swords into plowshares, there would always be enough parking spaces, and we'd always have exact change for pay phones. But it is not an ideal world, and our bodies are constantly challenged by this imperfection. We can get a serious illness or an injury. The rains may fail, locusts may swarm, and we must spend a season malnourished, walking miles daily to forage. We may be menaced by predators, or by the aggressiveness of members of our own species. Our hearts may be broken by loss. We are even smart enough to fear these things. In fact, we sometimes anxiously anticipate them before they happen.

Normally, our bodies are in a state of physiological balance, but so pervasive are the challenges and imperfections of the world that we have evolved an entire physiological system to buffer us from those perturbations. Stress physiology is the study of the perturbations that upset our physiological balance and of our bodies' efforts to reestablish balance. Stress pathophysiology is the study of how, when we are knocked out of balance severely enough, disease emerges.

Some Definitions and Some History

It is an obligation of all stress physiologists to begin by reviewing some of the confusion of terms. The word stress was borrowed by biologists from engineers in a fairly imprecise way. Stress can mean *the thing* that creates an imbalance, or *the response* of your body to it, or both. Two terms have since been adopted to distinguish between the two. A **stressor** is anything that disrupts physiological balance. It can be a physical insult—famine, for example—or a psychological insult—the expectation of famine. The **stress-response** is the body's adaptations designed to reestablish the balance. **Stress** will be used informally to refer to the general state of stressors provoking stress-response.[208, 670, 937]

While these terms are recent, the ideas underlying them go back millennia. Hippocrates, in 400 B.C., postulated that disease did not represent divine will but rather arose from logical antecedents. This rationalist view is the foundation of modern medicine. He emphasized that health consisted of a harmonious balance with the surrounding world, while disease arose from challenges to that balance. This notion of balance ran through the works of many subsequent investigators. For example, Claude Bernard coined the phrase "internal milieu." He emphasized that organisms have evolved to become more independent of the outside environment, and that a goal of physiological systems was to buffer the internal environment or milieu from environmental perturbations. By our century, this stability of the internal milieu was termed **homeostasis**.

Stress physiology emerged as a real discipline primarily owing to the work of Walter Cannon (1871–1945, who coined the term homeostasis) and Hans Selye (1907–1982). By the beginning of this century, it was clear that maintaining homeostasis was indeed a high priority of the body, but there was little understanding of how our bodies accomplished this balance.

Two endocrine systems dominate the stress-response. Both involve the adrenal gland. The core, or medulla, of the adrenal gland secretes the most famous hormone of the stress-response, adrenaline (also known as epinephrine). Cannon demonstrated the role of epinephrine in stress physiology. The outer layer of the adrenal, the cortex, secretes a class of hormones called glucocorticoids. Selye was the first to discover their role. Cannon and Selye also made critical contributions to the theoretical framework of stress physiology. They both emphasized the nonspecificity of the stress-response. In other words, the magnitude of a stress-response is determined by the magnitude of the imbalance, not by the direction of the homeostatic imbalance. To give a concrete example, imagine a scenario from the savannah. A zebra is mauled by a lion. The lion has not hunted successfully in days and is near starvation. The zebra's stomach is ripped open, yet for the next hours, it has just enough strength to evade the lion. The bodies of that lion, near starvation, and that zebra, terrified and in pain, are having very similar stress-responses. Somewhat similar responses would be triggered whether someone is too hot, too cold, about to make a first terrifying parachute jump, or about to go to a first terrifying high school dance. Cannon termed this nonspecific reaction the **flight or fight response** because such very different situations trigger the same response. He found that various stressors all trigger secretion, of the epinephrine. Cannon thought that he was studying how the body successfully coped with a stressful situation. To some extent, this is true.

Selye noted that stressors also provoked glucocorticoid secretion, and he termed this nonspecific response the **general adaptation syndrome**. Both terms are basically synonymous with the stress-response. Selye frequently recounted the story of how he came to think about the nonspecificity of the stress-response. As a young scientist, he was investigating the physiological effects of a potential new hormone (which turned out not to really exist). Every day rats received injections of ovarian extracts containing this putative compound. He found that the rats developed peptic ulcers, enlarged adrenal glands, and shrunken tissues of the immune system. His tremendous excitement collapsed when he found that the same symptoms were occurring in his control rats. Rats receiving extracts from other organs or with saline alone had the same symptoms. Clearly, the changes could not have been caused by his putative hormone. Selye intuited that the experience common to all the rats, experimentals and controls alike, was the unpleasantry of daily injections. Perhaps, he thought, he was observing the nonspecific response to unpleasantry itself. He tested this by subjecting rats to other unpleasantries—cold, heat, hemorrhage, illness, and so on. The rats showed the same changes. The stress-response appeared to be nonspecific; it did not matter what the emergency was so much as that there was an emergency.

Selye initially had thought that the stress-response was beneficial, as reflected in his use of the word adaptive as his phrase for the stress-response. Yet Selye's rats were getting sick—they had peptic ulcers and their immune systems were collapsing. The answer was clear: Under some circumstances, the body's adaptations in the face of stressors are not perfect. Stress pathophysiology had been founded.

In the first half of this chapter, I review the complex physiology of the stress-response. Which hormonal and neural systems are stimulated by stressors, which are inhibited? What physiological adaptations do these bring about, and why do they make sense? Why do these adaptations fail at times, and bring about a variety of diseases? In the second half of the chapter, I consider why psychological stressors are stressful and why individuals differ in the quality of their stress-response and their vulnerability to stress-related disease.

The Neural and Endocrine Mediators of the Stress-Response

To understand how the body adapts to stressors, we must begin by cataloguing the mediators of such adaptation; this is, in effect, an introduction to the actors.[30, 867]

Systems Stimulated by Stressors

As noted, glucocorticoids and adrenaline (hereafter called epinephrine) are the two most critical hormones released during the stress-response (figure 10.1).

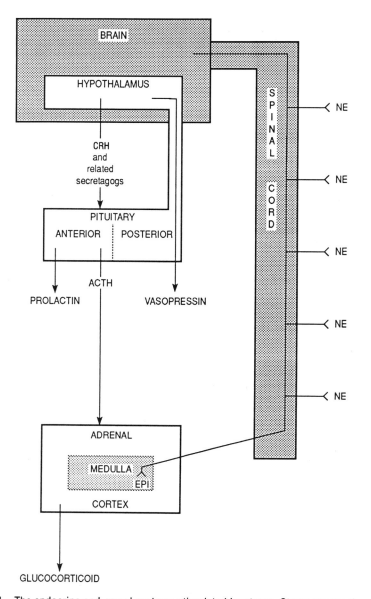

Figure 10.1 The endocrine and neural systems stimulated by stress. Stress causes the release of CRH and related secretagogs by the hypothalamus, which enter the hypothalamic-pituitary portal circulation. This triggers anterior pituitary release of ACTH, which in turn stimulates glucocorticoid release from the adrenal cortex. Prolactin is also released by the anterior pituitary during stress; as with ACTH, its secretion is ultimately under complex hypothalamic control, but those hormones are deleted here for simplicity. Vasopressin is released by the posterior pituitary; in this case, hypothalamic control is neural rather than hormonal in that the cell bodies for the vasopressin-releasing neurons are actually located in the hypothalamus. In addition, the sympathetic nervous system is activated, releasing norepinephrine (NE) from most of its nerve endings; the sole exception is the release of epinephrine (EPI) from the sympathetic projection that terminates in the adrenal medulla. For simplicity, pancreatic release of glucagon has not been portrayed.

Glucocorticoid secretion by the adrenal cortex is just the final step in a cascade of events beginning in the brain.

A stressor is perceived by the brain. The hormone corticotropin-releasing hormone (CRH) is released from the base of the brain, the hypothalamus. CRH stimulates the pituitary gland to release adrenocorticotropic hormone (ACTH), which stimulates the adrenal to release glucocorticoids. Glucocorticoids are steroid hormones, and a number of different forms occur. In humans and primates, the dominant form released is **cortisol** (also known as **hydrocortisone**), whereas in rodents it is corticosterone. During stress, there is an increase in secretion of CRH within a few seconds, of ACTH within perhaps 15 seconds, and of glucocorticoids within a few minutes. Predictably, the picture is actually far more complicated than this. CRH, which was isolated only recently after decades of work, is only one of probably a half dozen hypothalamic hormones that modulate ACTH release from the pituitary. Recent work shows that different stressors cause different patterns of these hormones to be released by the hypothalamus.

The other main branch of the stress-response is the **sympathetic nervous system**. Neural control of peripheral bodily functions is generally divided into voluntary and involuntary (or autonomic) control. The former allows you to make intentional muscle movements: You sign checks, make silly faces, tap dance, and so on. The latter mediates responses like blushing, gooseflesh, orgasms, and getting breathless. This involuntary **autonomic nervous system** has two components with opposing roles. The parasympathetic nervous system mediates calm vegetative functions such as growth and digestion, slow heart rate, and breathing. It is typically stimulated during sleep or after a large meal. In contrast, the sympathetic nervous system is stimulated by arousal, vigilance, or emergency. When something scares us, the sympathetic response triggers the "adrenaline" surge that we feel. Sympathetic relays originating in the spine terminate in the adrenal medulla and stimulate the release of epinephrine within seconds. Other projections go to essentially every organ in the body and release the closely related hormone norepinephrine. Epinephrine and norepinephrine both belong to the class of compounds known as **catecholamines**. As will be seen, glucocorticoids and catecholamines together mediate most of the changes that form the stress-response.

Other hormones typically are secreted during stress as well. **β-Endorphin** is secreted by the pituitary gland and is part of a class of opiate compounds that regulate pain perception and reproductive physiology during stress. Reproductive physiology is also affected during stress by the pituitary hormone **prolactin**. **Vasopressin** (also known as antidiuretic hormone), is a posterior pituitary hormone involved in the regulation of renal function and water volume. Finally, **glucagon**, a pancreatic hormone, helps to regulate carbohydrate trafficking. This does not represent a complete list of the endocrine systems stimulated, but these are the ones that will be referred to most frequently. All of these systems help to marshall and conserve body resources in preparation for a crisis.

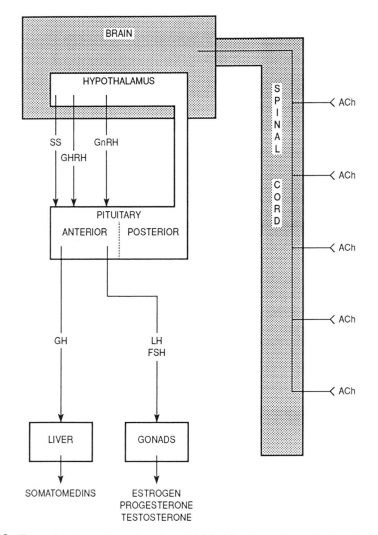

Figure 10.2 The endocrine and neural systems inhibited by stress. Normally, hypothalamic GnRH stimulates the pituitary release of LH and FSH, which in turn stimulate gonadal secretion of steroid hormones. During stress, the secretion of all these is inhibited. Pituitary release of GH is stimulated by GHRH and inhibited by somatostatin (SS). During stress, GHRH release is inhibited, whereas there is no clear evidence that secretion of SS is changed. The result is decreased GH release and in turn, decreased somatomedin release. As discussed in the text, the inhibition of this growth axis is somewhat species-specific. Finally, parasympathetic nervous system activity (as represented by the release of acetylcholine [ACh]) is inhibited. For simplicity, the inhibition of pancreatic release of insulin is not included.

Systems Inhibited by Stressors

As noted, the sympathetic and parasympathetic branches of the autonomic nervous system usually work in opposition (figure 10.2). Thus, the parasympathetic system is inhibited promptly by stress. There is also inhibition of the numerous hormones involved in reproductive physiology and behavior. The secretion of gonadotropin-releasing hormone (GnRH), luteinizing hormone (LH), follicle-stimulating hormone (FSH), and the gonadal steroids are inhibited by stress. Finally, the secretion of **insulin**, the pancreatic hormone concerned with glucose storage, is typically inhibited.

A more confusing picture is seen with **growth hormone** (GH). Its release from the pituitary is under neural control. The hypothalamus secretes both growth hormone–releasing hormone (GHRH), which stimulates GH release, and somatostatin, which inhibits it. These work like an accelerator and a brake, respectively. GH, in turn, exerts many of its effects by stimulating the secretion of **somatomedins** by the liver. In rodents, the secretion of GH, and consequently of somatomedins, is promptly inhibited by stressors. In contrast, in humans, most short-term stressors stimulate GH release transiently, whereas more sustained stressors tend to inhibit release.

The Logic of the Stress-Response: A Descent into Teleology

What good are these hormonal changes? It seems particularly reasonable to ask this in the context of the variety of stressors that elicit this relatively consistent set of responses. As physiologists, we are trained to understand what the body does when it is too hot and when it is too cold. Intuitively, it seems that the responses to each should be fairly different, if not downright opposite. Similarly, it seems to us that being frightened and injured (like the zebra) should be a rather different physiologic state from being hungry and predatory (like the lion). Why, then, should there be a whole set of physiologic changes, the stress-response, that is elicited whether you are too hot or too cold, whether you are the zebra or the lion? Is there a logical explanation for these changes?

Much of biology has a logical structure that can be discerned. The disparate endocrine and neural changes that comprise the stress-response actually make a fair amount of sense. Such differing states as being too hot or too cold, injured or hungry, can all elicit similar responses because there is a common thread to all of them. Even though the different stressors throw the body out of homeostasis in different directions, the task of reestablishing the balance, however disrupted, is still fairly similar.[768]

First and foremost, both the zebra and the lion have an immediate need for energy. The metabolic hallmark of the stress-response is the need to mobilize energy for immediate use. Energy storage is inhibited. Preexisting stores of energy are broken down into simpler, more readily utilized forms in the bloodstream. This represents the metabolic equivalent of going to the bank in a time of financial crisis and emptying your savings account in order to have cash in your pocket.

The net result is increased concentrations of glucose in the bloodstream. The glucose, along with oxygen, must be delivered more rapidly to the muscles that are being worked heavily in the zebra and lion. Thus, the breathing rate increases to facilitate the exchange of oxygen in the lungs. Cardiovascular tone also increases. Blood pressure and heart rate rise. Water is retained in the circulation to increase the blood volume. In addition, parts of the circulatory system are shut down to ensure that blood is preferentially shunted to the organs and muscles that really need it.

This pattern of curtailing nonessentials is seen in many other ways. If a hurricane appears to be heading for your town, this is not the afternoon to decide to paint the kitchen, or to finally replant the tulip bulbs in the garden. It is an emergency, and long-term building projects can wait for tomorrow. By this logic, numerous **anabolic** processes are inhibited by the stress-response. Digestion is curtailed. While the digestive process will eventually provide the body with needed nutrients, it will not do so rapidly enough to help that lion or zebra in the coming minutes, and it is an unnecessary expense in the meantime.

By the same logic, reproductive physiology and behavior are usually inhibited by stressors. Reproduction is certainly one of the most expensive, optimistic things you can do with your body (especially if you are female), and it simply cannot be a high priority when you are sprinting for your life. Similarly, growth and tissue repair are typically inhibited. The former is dramatically the case in young, growing organisms. The immune system is also inhibited during the stress-response. This is the system that is responsible for detecting a tumor that could kill you in 6 months or for generating antibodies during the next few weeks to fight a novel infectious agent. Given that time span, the expensive task of immune surveillance can be postponed until after the emergency.

Another feature of the stress-response is the suppression of inflammation and pain perception. Suppose in the initial attack on the zebra, its knee was injured. In most circumstances, the logical next step would be an inflammatory response. Capillaries dilate to allow fluid to rush into the extracellular space, leukocytes migrate into the region to scavenge damaged tissue. The knee swells and becomes painful and difficult to use. This is a way to convince the organism to rest the knee and allow it to repair. But this is a luxury that the zebra cannot afford. True, the knee joint may become even more injured if the zebra continues to use it, but the consequences will be far worse if the animal stops. Thus, inhibition of the inflammatory response makes a fair amount of sense. In addition, pain perception can be blunted as well. For example, at the height of battle, soldiers are occasionally grievously injured and do not even notice the pain at the time. Such "stress-induced analgesia" has been documented in many circumstances.

Thus, when subjected to a physical stressor, it is adaptive for the organism to mobilize energy and deliver it to the parts of the body that need it, to curtail non-essential physiological processes, and to blunt pain and inflammation. As will be detailed in later sections, these are precisely the consequences of the various endocrine and neural responses.

Some investigators have begun to view these hormonal shifts not only as a way to understand how the organism **initiates** its response to the emergency but also how it eventually **terminates** the response. This can potentially explain some puzzling features of the stress-response. For example, some of the many metabolic consequences of the shifts in glucocorticoids, catecholamines, glucagon, growth hormone, and insulin wind up appearing to be contradictory; precisely opposing responses are triggered. The resolution of this puzzle may be that the various hormones work at different speeds. Catecholamines, for example, produce their effects upon target tissues within seconds, whereas some of the effects of glucocorticoids or growth hormone can take hours. Thus, two opposing endocrine signals may be given simultaneously, yet they may exert their effects at different times. The slower responses may not be mediators of the stress-response as much as "counterregulatory" signals that prepare the organism for eventually recovering from that stress-response.

The Illogic of the Stress-Response: The Emergence of Stress-Related Disease

The stress-response seems ideal for aiding the zebra or the lion in their stressful encounter. Energy is mobilized and delivered where it is needed, pain is blunted, costly anabolism is deferred until more auspicious times. In some ways, their bodies are even already gambling that the stressor will be survived and are preparing for a return to normal. From this perspective, the system seems quite adaptive. Yet, from the first day of Selye's work, it was apparent that the stress response is not perfect; his rats had peptic ulcers and atrophied immune systems. Viewed in retrospect, we know that Selye had discovered the tip of the iceberg of stress-related disease. If the stress response is so logical and adaptive, why do such diseases emerge?

The answer lies in the sort of disclaimers that one gets with the instructions for a new applicance: The stress-response, just like a new microwave oven, must be used properly. It is an ideal system for allowing an organism to deal with short-term physical stress, and that is exactly the sort of stressor that most organisms face most of the time. Stress-related disease appears most likely to emerge when the stress-response is activated for **too long**, or **too frequently** (i.e., **chronic stressors**) and when it is activated for **no physiological reason** in the first place (i.e., **psychological/social stressors**).

Selye noted the seeming paradox that the physiological system he had discovered, so logical and adaptive under some circumstances, could cause disease. He was among the first to guess that prolonged stressors could cause disease. His explanation for the phenomenon, however, was mostly incorrect. Selye conceptualized the stress-response as coming in three stages. The first, **alarm**, involved noting the challenge to homeostasis, the stressor. The second, **resistance**, consisted of successfully dealing with the short-term physical insult. The third stage was when disease started, when the stressor went on for too long. Selye termed this stage **exhaustion**.

In his view, at some point, the capacity to mount a stress-response fails. The adrenal runs out of glucocorticoids to secrete. The sympathetic nerve endings become depleted of catecholamines, and so on. In effect, the army defending the body from the external stressor runs out of ammunition, and the stressor can now assault the body unhindered. In actuality, this scenario of exhaustion does not really occur very often. With sustained stressors, for example, the adrenal increases its capacity to secrete catecholamines by increasing the concentrations of the rate-limiting enzyme for catecholamine synthesis, tyrosine hydroxylase. In addition, the adrenal cortex, the zone in which glucocorticoids are synthetized, increases in size (explaining why Selye's original rats had hyperplastic—enlarged—adrenals). In some circumstances of sustained stress, the hormonal output decreases over time, but this is because the organism has become habituated to the stressor (i.e., it views the event as less stressful) rather than because it has become depleted of the hormones. This theory can be proved by showing that when the catecholamine response to a sustained stressor decreases, a novel stressor still elicits a large catecholamine response.[603, 670, 937]

Thus, there is little evidence that sustained stressors deplete the system of the hormones needed for the stress-response. The army does not run out of ammunition. The problem is that with sustained stress, the stress-response can eventually be as damaging as the stressor. To extend the military metaphor, if you keep spending your budget on bullets instead of on bread or education, you can ultimately destroy your country just as utterly as could an invading enemy. Most features of the stress-response are damaging, inefficient, and even dangerous. Yet, that zebra and that lion must activate the stress-response; it is an emergency. If the body constantly decides it is an emergency and activates the stress-response, disease eventually emerges. In subsequent sections, I will review how the hormones of the stress-response bring about the logical, helpful adaptations to acute physical stressors and how the same hormones, secreted over time, are pathogenic.

The Metabolic Stress-Response

When faced with an acute physical stressor, there are two logical metabolic responses.[418] First, the body makes sure that none of the energy substrates in the bloodstream are stored away. Second, it gets access to previously stored energy and converts it back to circulating energy substrates.

The first task is accomplished quite readily. In times of plenty, when there are surplus energy substrates in circulation, the body stores them in complex storage forms. Circulating fats (in the form of fatty acids and glycerol) are stored in adipose tissue as triglycerides. Amino acids are stored throughout the body as proteins, and glucose is stored as glycogen. The critical hormone in this storage process is insulin, which is secreted by the pancreas in response to a logical signal—increased circulating glucose concentrations. At fat cells, insulin promotes glucose uptake, fatty acid synthesis, and blocks the breakdown of triglycerides. All of these steps promote the formation and maintenance of triglyceride stores. In muscles, insulin promotes glucose and amino acid transport, glycogen and protein synthesis, and blocks the breakdown of proteins and glycogen. Finally, in the liver, insulin promotes the formation of glycogen and blocks the breakdown of preexisting glycogen. Insulin is the prototypical hormone signaling that there is no metabolic crisis looming on the horizon.

With the onset of a stressor, insulin secretion is typically inhibited, and storage of substrates is halted. The process of gaining access to substrates already stored is more complex, principally involving glucocorticoids, catecholamines, and glucagon. Collectively, they reverse all the effects of insulin. In fat cells, glucose uptake, protein synthesis, and fatty acid synthesis are halted. Preexisting triglycerides are broken down (lipolysis), and free fatty acids are flushed into the circulation. In muscle, the uptake of glucose and amino acids, and the synthesis of glycogen and proteins are halted. Preexisting glycogen and proteins are degraded (glycogenolysis and proteolysis), and glucose and amino acids are flushed into the circulation.

Stored energy has now been turned into cash—circulating glucose, amino acids, and fatty acids. As a final step, glucocorticoids, catecholamines, and glucagon stimulate the liver to convert fatty acids and amino acids to glucose ("gluconeogenesis").

Thus, in the face of an acute stressor, there are increased concentrations of glucose available to whichever tissue needs it. How do these metabolic adaptations cause disease when activated chronically? Quite simply, if you constantly mobilize energy at the cost of energy storage, it will ultimately prove disastrous (see chapter 15). Constantly breaking down stored proteins in order to flux amino acids into the circulation produces myopathy, the wasting away of muscles, a prime storage site for protein. This causes weakness and fatigue. Fatigue will also arise from the fact that, collectively, the processes of lipolysis, proteolysis, glycogenolysis, and gluconeogenesis are inefficient. One can use a surprisingly apt metaphor from the economic world. If you open a long-term savings account, in which money is put away for a stipulated period, you receive a lot of interest for keeping the money in the account and a penalty if you break the agreement and withdraw the money early. Similarly, the body is penalized for constantly mobilizing energy from storage sites and transforming it, as described above; each biochemical step is inefficient, and in toto, approximately 30% of potential energy is lost.

The Cardiovascular Stress-Response

In the presence of a physical stressor it is logical to increase cardiovascular tone in order to deliver more of the mobilized glucose and oxygen to the tissues that need it. This is mostly accomplished through the sympathetic nervous system. It stimulates the heart to beat faster. Blood pressure is increased through vasoconstriction, which indirectly increases the force of cardiac contractions. Blood flow to some organs (for example, the digestive tract) is decreased; this is part of the strategy of shutting down nonessentials. Blood volume is also increased by vasopressin, which increases water resorption by the kidneys, a process described further in chapter 15.

The pathogenic results of these changes are obvious when they continue for too long. If you are sprinting across a field with a lion on your heels and your blood pressure is 160/95, this is good for you. If you have the same blood pressure whenever you have to stand in a line, you are dangerously hypertensive. Chronic hypertension will damage heart muscle, weaken vessel walls, and promote the deposition of cholesterol and the formation of atherosclerotic plaques. It is well established that chronic stress and certain behavior patterns (the Type A behaviors of competitiveness, impatience, and hostility) are risk factors for coronary heart disease.

The Gastrointestinal Stress-Response

As discussed, it makes sense to inhibit the gastrointestinal (GI) tract during an acute physical stressor; digestion can wait for later. These changes are principally mediated by the autonomic nervous system through its shift from parasympathetic to sympathetic tone. Normally, the former stimulates digestion. In the mouth, saliva is secreted, while in the stomach, acid, pepsinogen, mucus, and gastrin are secreted. In the intestines, secretion of a large array of digestive enzymes and hormones is stimulated, including lipase, trypsinogen, chymotrypsin, enterokinase, cholesystokinin (CCK), and vasoactive intestinal polypeptide (VIP). Furthermore, stomach churning and the relaxation and tightening of sphincters are all coordinated to promote digestion.[858]

With stress, all of these processes are inhibited, due both to the decreased parasympathetic tone and to the increased sympathetic outflow. We are all familiar with the first sign of the shutdown—our mouths become dry when we are nervous because we have stopped secreting saliva. In addition, the sympathetic nervous system decreases blood flow to the GI tract.

With prolonged stressors, a number of gastrointestinal pathologies emerge, including gastric ulcers. The causes of stress ulceration are poorly understood, but several theories have been proposed: (1) Because blood flow to the GI tract is inhibited, the delivery of oxygen and nutrients is curtailed. If this situation is prolonged, erosions and ulcers may form in the gastric mucosa. (2) Normally, the stomach expends considerable energy in building and thickening stomach walls and secreting mucus. Both protect the stomach walls from the potentially ulcerative effects of the powerful gastric acids. When the stress-response is prolonged (and acid secretion is inhibited chronically), the stomach curtails both of these housekeeping activities. In effect, the stomach decides that it is a waste of energy to thicken walls and make mucus if there is only minimal exposure to gastric acids anyway. Then, when the stressors abate and acid secretion resumes at its normal heavier rate, the stomach walls are vulnerable to erosions and ulcers. In this scenario, damage occurs not so much during a stressor as during its aftermath. (3) Ulcer repair is aided by a class of compounds called prostaglandins. Glucocorticoids, however, are powerful inhibitors of prostaglandin synthesis. Thus, prolonged stressors may not only cause ulcers but may also disrupt their repair.

The Reproductive Stress-Response

While it may be logical to reproduce if you are that zebra or lion, the presence of prolonged stressors will wreak havoc with reproductive physiology and behavior. This response is seen throughout the animal kingdom.[834, 905, 1089] In many species, increased population density or decreased food resources are stressors that inhibit ovulation in females. This forms an elegant means by which populations self-regulate their growth rate. In some species (notably, some New World primates), reproduction is often inhibited not so much by the stressor of food shortages as by the stressor of social subordination. A high-ranking monkey ensures that she is the only member of her group to reproduce by physically harassing subordinates into anovulation. Male reproductive physiology is also vulnerable to chronic stress in varied species. Stressors such as surgical incisions, drought, sustained exercise, or defeat in social competition will suppress testosterone secretion. And among humans, there are endless psychological stressors that disrupt reproduction. To give some sense of the magnitude of our sensitivity to stress, it has been estimated that some 80% of complaints of reproductive dysfunction by men in this country turn out to be psychogenic rather than organic in origin.

Much is known about how stressors disrupt reproduction in both sexes. The summary presented here represents a consensus from studies of various mammalian species; there is, of course, phylogenetic variability. Among females, the points of inhibition are numerous. At the hypothalamus, the secretion of GnRH is inhibited by stress-induced secretion of β-endorphin and CRH upon the brain. One step below that, pituitary responsiveness to GnRH is also inhibited, decreasing LH and FSH secretion. This is due to the inhibitory actions of glucocorticoids or prolactin. Glucocorticoids also inhibit ovarian sensitivity to LH. The net result of these steps is to make the secretion of estrogen and progesterone and the formation of a viable egg less likely. The diminished levels of progesterone and the increased levels of prolactin, in turn, disrupt the normal maturation of the uterine wall. Thus, if an egg is fertilized against these considerable odds, it is less likely that proper implantation into the uterine wall will occur. And if that is not enough, certain stressors disrupt reproduction in another way. Females of numerous species secrete androgens (male sex hormones) from their adrenal glands. Although the amounts are small, they would normally be enough to impair reproduction. However, they are typically converted to estrogen by enzymes in fat cells. When stressors involve loss of body fat in females (from famine, wasting illnesses, extreme degrees of exercise, or anorexia nervosa), this conversion step is diminished. The result is a smaller amount of circulating estrogen and a buildup of circulating androgens, which can be disruptive to reproduction.

Among males, the regulatory steps are nearly as numerous. As with the female, CRH and β-endorphin inhibit GnRH release. As with the female, prolactin inhibits pituitary sensitivity to GnRH, and glucocorticoids inhibit testicular sensitivity to LH. The net result is decreased testosterone secretion and, under more extreme circumstances, decreased sperm production. Cell biologists have uncovered some of the ways in which β-endorphin, prolactin, and glucocorticoids exert their inhibitory effects in both sexes. In some cases, they decrease the numbers of LH receptors; in others, they have postreceptor effects, and in still others, they sensitize the brain to the inhibitory effects of other hormones. The body is creative and varied in its means of suppressing reproduction during stress.

Another aspect of male reproduction can be maddeningly vulnerable to stressors: attaining and maintaining an erection. The initial erection requires parasympathetic tone. With continued stimulation and arousal, breathing and heart rate increase, and the physiologic profile becomes more sympathetic rather than parasympathetic in tone. Ejaculation consists of a sudden and major inhibition of parasympathetic tone and stimulation of sympathetic tone. With the inhibition of parasympathetic tone during stress, it becomes difficult to have an erection—resulting in impotency. And if the erection has already occurred, the tendency of a stressor to shift autonomic tone from parasympathetic to sympathetic accelerates the normal transition—resulting in premature ejaculation.

Why are there so many mechanisms by which stressors can suppress reproduction? Another way to frame this question is to ask how effective these numerous collective mechanisms are. Surprisingly, the answer is, not very. Humans continue to reproduce under dreadful circumstances; for example, in one frequently cited study, nearly 50% of the women in a Nazi concentration camp were continuing to ovulate despite starvation, slave labor, and unspeakable psychological stressors. I suspect that so many mechanisms are needed to suppress reproduction during a stressor because the basic reproductive physiology is so robust.

The Consequences of a Prolonged Stress-Response on Growth

If the stress-response involves postponing anabolism, then stressors should be particularly disruptive in young, growing animals, in whom anabolism is nearly continuous. Indeed, in rats, stressors promptly inhibit circulating growth hormone (GH) concentrations. Secretion of GH is under bidirectional control from the hypothalamus, which contains a GH-releasing hormone (GHRH) and a GH-inhibiting hormone (known as somatostatin). GH secretion can thus be inhibited during stress either because a metaphorical foot is pressed on the brake (more somatostatin) or because a foot is taken off the accelerator (less GHRH). The inhibition in fact appears to be due to increased somatostatin, since stress-induced suppression of GH release is blocked with antibodies against somatostatin.[842, 867]

In humans, the picture is more complicated. Initially, stressors increase GH release. With chronic stress, however, GH secretion declines to below basal levels. The neural mechanisms underlying the initial increase or the delayed decrease are not known.

If GH secretion is inhibited long enough in a young organism, growth is disrupted profoundly. For example, maternal deprivation in rat pups inhibits growth; the same thing occurs in human children living in a war zone. These examples, however, are difficult to interpret. A rat pup deprived of its mother undergoes nutritional as well as emotional deprivation. A child in a war zone is psychologically stressed but is also likely to suffer from poor nutrition and inadequate medical care. Thus, impaired growth may not be due to the non-specific stressfulness of the situation but instead to poor nutrition or parasitic infestation. However, syndromes of growth inhibition do occur in children with no obvious organic cause (such as starvation, chronic wasting illness, and so on); instead, there is a history of major emotional disturbance and deprivation. In such cases of "psychosocial dwarfism" (also known as "stress dwarfism"), children average half the expected height for their age and secrete little GH, even after stimuli that normally elicit GH secretion. They may even be unresponsive to exogenous GH. Typically, within a few months of being placed in a less stressful environment, GH concentrations and rates of growth become normal, and if the child has not yet reached puberty, there can be sufficient "catch-up" growth for the child to eventually attain normal stature. It should be emphasized that stress dwarfism is a rare disorder seen only in tragically stressful (and often psychopathologic) circumstances.

Adults, obviously, no longer grow. In such cases, the "growth" that is inhibited during stress is the repair of existing tissues. For example, calcium is normally removed from bone and replaced with new calcium. Glucocorticoids inhibit this anabolic housekeeping. Thus, with glucocorticoid overexposure, bones become decalcified, thin, and prone to fractures. The glucocorticoid hypersecretion seen with chronic stress is rarely sufficient for this sort of pathology; rather, it arises in patients given large doses of glucocorticoids to control an autoimmune or asthmatic disorder.[842]

The Stress-Response and Analgesia

It has long been recognized that pain perception can be blunted during extreme stress and emotional arousal.[165] Such stress-induced analgesia (pain reduction) was often thought to be purely psychological. However, an understanding of the neurochemical nature of the phenomenon came from an explosion of discoveries in the early 1970s. Considerable interest had focused on opiates such as morphine, heroin, and opium, which had similar chemical structures and were analgesic. It was during that period that opiate receptors were discovered in the brain. This discovery carried a vital implication: The brain could not have evolved receptors for a plant compound. Instead, there must be "endogenous opiates" (or "opioids") somewhere in the body that normally bound to these receptors. This triggered a fevered search for opioids. Soon, three types were discovered: the endorphins, the enkephalins, and the dynorphins. They occur in the pituitary, brain, and a number of peripheral organs and serve endocrine, paracrine, and neuromodulatory roles.

Previous lesion, stimulation, and electrical recording studies had already mapped the neuroanatomy of pain pathways. These included relay sites in the dorsal horn of the spinal cord and, within the brain, the periaqueductal gray area and the raphe complex. These regions were shown to contain opiate receptors, opioids caused analgesia when microinjected at these sites, and opiate receptor antagonists blocked such analgesia.

It was soon shown that foot-shock stress caused secretion of β-endorphin from the pituitary. Other stressors were soon shown to stimulate secretion as well. Atheletes began to call the analgesia that comes about 30 minutes into exercise the "β-endorphin high," and the subject appeared solved. Two complications have emerged, however. First, it is not clear whether circulating β-endorphins, derived from the pituitary, actually cause analgesia. Variations in circulating levels of the hormone do not predict analgesia very well. Moreover, it is not clear how the peptide normally gets past the blood-brain barrier from the circulation in order to bind to these neural opiate receptors. Instead, it is probably the release of opioids from neuron terminals within the brain and spinal cord that mediates the analgesia.

As a second complexity, some aspects of stress-induced analgesia occur independently of opioids. Such analgesia shows no cross-tolerance with exogenous opiates and cannot be blocked with opiate receptor blockers. Various neurotransmitters have been implicated, including serotonin and histamine. In general, early phases of stress-induced analgesia appear to be opioid-independent, while slower phases (approximately 30 minutes or more) are opioid-mediated.

Are there pathogenic consequences of analgesia following chronic stress? Seemingly not, because the analgesia wanes over the course of hours to days. This does not represent "exhaustion" of the stress-response as Selye conceptualized it (i.e., the system does not run out of opioids); rather, this represents habituation to the stressor. As proof, imposition of a new, painful stimulus at the point where the analgesia has waned will reinstate the analgesia.

The Effects of the Stress-Response on the Brain

The hormones of the stress-response have numerous effects on the brain; they can influence learning and memory, vulnerability to depression, feeding behavior and aggression, to name just a few of their effects. In recent years, data have emerged showing that chronic stress, acting through glucocorticoid hypersecretion, can directly damage the brain. These findings are discussed in chapter 11.

A Detailed Analysis: The Stress-Response and Immune Function

A Brief Introduction to the Immune System

The immune system, whose primary job is to defend the body against infectious challenges,[311] is frighteningly complex, and it is beyond the scope of this chapter to give anything other than a brief overview. The basic cell types that make up the circulating components of the immune system are **lymphocytes** and **monocytes**. There are two classes of lymphocytes: **T cells** and **B cells**. Both classes originate in the bone marrow, but the former migrate to and mature in the thymus (hence the T in T cells), whereas, the latter mature in the bone marrow. B cells principally produce antibodies, but there are several kinds of T cells (T helper and T suppressor cells, cytotoxic killer cells, and so on).

The T and B cells mediate very different forms of attack upon infectious agents. The former bring about **cell-mediated immunity** (figure 10.3). When an infectious pathogen invades the body, it is recognized by a type of monocyte called the **macrophage**, which presents the foreign particle to a T helper cell. A metaphorical alarm is now sounded, and T cells begin to proliferate in response to the invasion. This alarm system ultimately results in the activation and proliferation of the cytotoxic killer cells, which attack and destroy the pathogen.

B cells, in contrast, are central to **antibody** (or **humoral**) -**mediated immunity** (figure 10.4). Once the macrophage/T helper cell combination has become alarmed, the latter will also stimulate B-cell proliferation. The main task of the B cells is now to differentiate and generate antibodies, which are large proteins that will recognize and specifically bind to some feature of the invading pathogen (typically, a distinctive surface protein). The molecular biology of the ways in which the immune system can generate distinctive antibodies to recognize a very large (but not quite infinite) number of novel infectious pathogens is fascinating but is beyond the scope of this chapter. Once the antibodies against the pathogen are generated and secreted, they can bind to and immobilize the pathogen and target it for destruction.

For the immune system, a difficult part of this complex system of activation is that these cascades involve different cell types scattered throughout the circulation. In order to sound alarms throughout the far-flung immune system, there must be bloodborne chemical messengers that communicate between different cell types. A variety of such messengers exist, including cytokines, chemicals that trigger cell division. For example, when macrophages first recognize an infectious agent, they release the cytokine **interleukin-1**. This triggers the T helper cell to release **interleukin-2**, which stimulates T-cell proliferation. At present, at least four other interleukins have been identified, but these additional ones need not be detailed here. On the humoral front, T cells

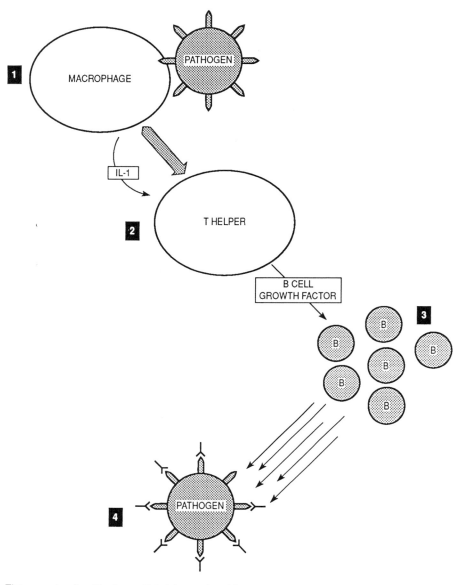

Figure 10.3 The cascade of antibody-mediated immunity. (1) A pathogen is encountered by a macrophage. (2) This encounter stimulates it to present the pathogen to a T helper cell and to release interleukin-1 (IL-1), which stimulates T helper cell activity. (3) The T helper cell then secretes B-cell growth factor, triggering differentiation and proliferation of another lymphocyte, B cells. (4) The B cells make and release specific antibodies that bind to surface proteins on the pathogen, targeting it for destruction by a large group of plasma proteins known as complement.

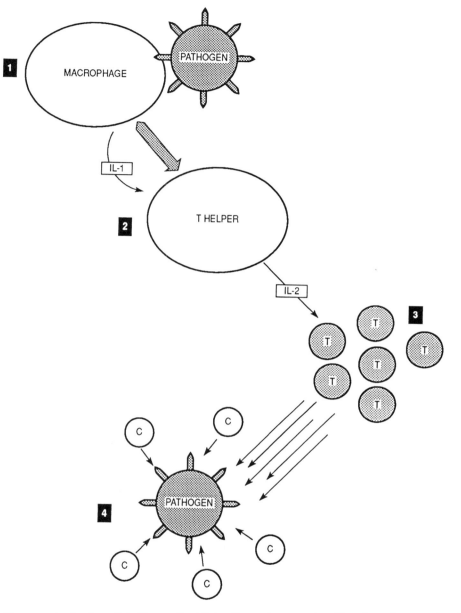

Figure 10.4 The cascade of cell-mediated immunity. (1) A pathogen is encountered by a type of monocyte called a macrophage. (2) This stimulates the macrophage to present the pathogen to a T helper cell (a type of lymphocyte) and to release interleukin-1 (IL-1), which stimulates T helper cell activity. (3) The T helper cell, as a result, releases interleukin-2 (IL-2), which triggers T-cell proliferation. (4) This eventually causes another type of lymphocyte, cytotoxic killer cells, to proliferate and destroy the pathogen.

also secrete **B-cell growth factor**, which stimulates B-cell differentiation and proliferation. An additional class of cytokines known as the **interferons** exists. These are secreted by T cells and fibroblasts, among other cells, and have broad activating effects on lymphocytes and monocytes. The critical point in this simplistic summary is to recognize the number of cell types involved in immunocompetence and the broad range of messengers needed to coordinate their function. It turns out that numerous points in these cascades are subject to the disruptive effects of stress.

The Mechanisms of Immunosuppression During Stress

If stress can influence immune function, then the brain must be able to influence the immune system, since stressors are first perceived in the brain. The recognition of neural regulation of immune function arose from two types of studies. First, lesioning or stimulating different brain regions could alter immune function. Second, organisms could be conditioned to change their immune function; such conditioned learning, of course, required the participation of the brain. These studies help found the field of **psychoneuro-immunology** and have paved the way for acceptance of the fact that neuro-endocrine systems can influence immune function during stress.[311, 768, 1058]

Glucocorticoids are by far the most important mediators of such regulation, and their general effects are inhibitory. They were also the first hormones to be recognized for that role, when Selye showed that adrenocortical extracts could involute (shrink) the thymus gland in the same way that stress did. What is most striking about glucocorticoid-induced immunosuppression is the breadth with which it is accomplished; some of the means are subtle, some extraordinarily crude.

On the subtle end, glucocorticoids inhibit release of most of the cytokines as well as the sensitivity of target cells to them. In some cases, glucocorticoids decrease sensitivity by decreasing the numbers of receptors for these cytokines; this occurs with IL-2, for example. In addition, glucocorticoids can inhibit the action of these cells once they are activated. By disrupting this network of signaling, glucocorticoids inhibit proliferative responses of the immune system. Glucocorticoids also inhibit B cell-mediated immunity by inhibiting IL-1 release. The steroids also inhibit production of certain components of complement, the system needed for antibody-mediated killing of target cells.

Other mechanisms of glucocorticoid-induced immunosuppression are anything but subtle. The steroids can block the maturation of developing lymphocytes; this accounts for the involution of immune tissue first observed by Selye. The steroids also can pull lymphocytes out of the bloodstream. This effect is far more pronounced in some species (for example, humans and guinea pigs) than in others (rats, mice). Finally, glucocorticoids can actually **destroy** some lymphocytes, causing them to burst. This "lysis" is due to a discrete, active process of programmed cell killing. Glucocorticoids induce the synthesis of a protein that appears to be an endonuclease, an enzyme that cleaves DNA. Not surprisingly, once its DNA is fragmented into little pieces, a cell does not last long.

The sympathetic nervous system (SNS) may also contribute to stress-induced immunosuppression. The SNS (and probably the parasympathetic nervous system as well) sends projections into immune tissues such as the spleen, thymus, and bone marrow. While the data are somewhat controversial, it appears that after destruction of these SNS projections, immune activity is enhanced, suggesting an inhibitory role for the SNS. Studies of opiates in vivo suggest that they mediate stress-induced immunosuppression. For example, following foot-shock stress, mice have reduced natural killer cell (a type of T lymphocyte) activity and reduced survival time from a tumor; this effect of stress can be blocked with the opiate receptor blocker naltrexone. Various cells of the immune system have opiate receptors, suggesting direct opiate effects upon these cells. Alternatively or additionally, injection of opiates into the periaqueductal gray area of the brain suppresses natural killer cell activity. Injection into other brain regions was not effective. Thus, opiate-induced immunosuppression may be relayed by the brain.

Why Suppress Immune Function During Stress?

There are many ways in which stress suppresses immune function.[311, 768] Why should this be desired? Earlier, I offered some pleasing teleology as an explanation. I noted that the job of the immune system is to search for tumors that will kill you in months or to raise antibodies to help you over weeks against an infectious agent. In that context, immunosuppression seems another logical example of suppressing costly anabolism. But this explanation actually makes very little sense. To suppress growth or reproduction during stress, growth hormone or gonadotropin secretion is merely inhibited. If the goal is merely to stop any new and costly immune responses, it should be enough to halt the formation of new lymphocytes and to stop the proliferation of preexisting ones. But the immunosuppression is more profound than that: Tumoricidal macrophages that are about to do their job are inhibited, lymphocytes are killed. The body actively **works** to disassemble the immune system. Few scientists, including myself, believe the easy explanation I gave earlier, that stress-induced immunosuppression exists merely to defer costly immunity.

Then why does immunosuppression occur? An early theory was that B lymphocytes burst during stress to release antibodies that they had made. In this scenario, cell killing would actually promote immunity. This idea, however, predated the discovery that a B lymphocyte need not be lysed to release antibodies. Another theory focused on the role of suppressor cells in the immune system, whose job it is to dampen immune activation. This theory held that stress preferentially destroys suppressor cells, thus promoting immune function. There is some evidence for this, e.g., moderate amounts of glucocorticoids can promote antibody production by inhibiting suppressor cells.

However, over the bulk of the glucocorticoid secretory range, the hormone inhibits not just suppressor cells, but *most* components of the immune system, thus compromising immune function.

In another theory, lymphocytes are destroyed during stress in order to scavenge their remnants for energy. This has generally been rejected as implausible. The energy gained would be small, and there are more likely cells to cannibalize if things are that bad. Another theory is that the anti-inflammatory effects of stress are quite logical, and it is not possible to obtain the anti-inflammatory effects without causing immunosuppression as well. Most of the cytokines are pro-inflammatory, supporting this idea.

In what is currently the dominant theory,[768] stressful emergencies are seen as times when the immune system is likely to be very active. This raises the danger that the system may become overactive, attacking the body's own tissues (i.e., an *auto*immune disorder). Stress hormones thus serve the role of reining in the immune system. In this scenario, the stress-response exists not so much to reduce normal immunity to abnormally low levels as to prevent normal functioning from becoming abnormally overactive.

Although this theory has gained some adherents, I am personally skeptical about it. The theory generates three predictions. (1) Shortly into the stress-response, before glucocorticoid concentrations have risen and have had time to affect the immune system (i.e.,, in the first 30 to 60 minutes), there should be a marked activation of the immune system. This should occur in response to all types of stressors. (2) Addison's disease is a disorder in which individuals cannot secrete glucocorticoids in adequate amounts. This theory predicts that the immune systems of these patients should be hyperactive during stress and that prolonged Addison's disease should be associated with autoimmune disorders. (3) If the goal during stress is merely to keep the immune system functioning normally (rather than suppressing it), prolonged stress should not be associated with pathogenic collapse of immune function. To my knowledge, none of these predictions are borne out in the literature.

It is not clear to me *why* the immune system should be suppressed during stress. But there must be a good reason: When the immune system is provoked with an infectious challenge, it stimulates the adrenocortical axis to secrete glucocorticoids. In other words, during immune activation, the immune system *asks* to be suppressed.

This is a very exciting topic in neuroimmunology. Everyone now accepts that neuroendocrine systems regulate immune function, but these data show that the immune system can also regulate neuroendocrine function in return (figure 10.5). Initially, it was found that immune activation after viral infection causes glucocorticoid secretion. Then it was shown that IL-1 is the immune factor responsible for stimulating glucocorticoid secretion. It is controversial how IL-1 does this, however. Two laboratories, including my own, were able to show that IL-1 directly stimulates CRF secretion from the hypothalamus. This was pleasing because IL-1 was already known to have effects upon the hypothalamus. The peptide, also known as "endogenous pyrogen factor,"

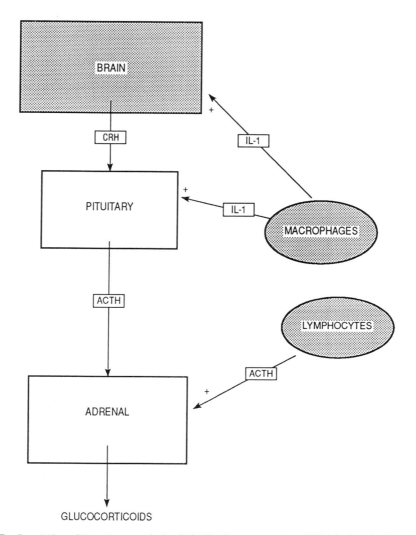

Figure 10.5 Regulation of the adrenocortical axis by the immune system. At left is the classic adrenocortical axis, with the brain releasing CRH (and related secretagogs), the pituitary releasing ACTH, and the adrenal cortex releasing glucocorticoids. Activated macrophages release IL-1; this cytokine stimulates CRH release directly from the brain and may directly stimulate pituitary ACTH release as well. Activated lymphocytes themselves secrete ACTH, which in theory can stimulate adrenal release of glucocorticoids. As discussed in the text, it remains unclear whether the amount of ACTH secretion from lymphocytes is enough to stimulate the adrenal to a physiologically relevant extent. The text also discusses other, less well documented routes by which the immune system stimulates this endocrine axis.

changes temperature regulation in the hypothalamus and promotes sleep (which explains why we run a fever and become sleepy during infectious illnesses). Others have reported that IL-1 directly releases ACTH from the pituitary, although others have failed to replicate this. Finally, supraphysiologic concentrations of IL-1 release glucocorticoids directly from the adrenal. Regardless of the mechanism, during immune activation the immune system uses IL-1 to stimulate the glucocorticoid secretion.

The immune system may accomplish this in additional ways. There are reports that activated lymphocytes may themselves secrete ACTH. This has not been replicated by all investigators, nor is it likely that the cells produce enough ACTH to stimulate the adrenals. Just to make life more complicated, other immune factors appear to stimulate the adrenocortical axis at either the brain, pituitary, or adrenal. These include IL-2 and IL-6 (a poorly characterized mixture of peptides from the thymus gland).

Clearly, the activated immune system works very hard to cause the adrenocortical axis to eventually inhibit it. In this case, immunosuppression makes sense, in that this is a time when an activated immune system may be teetering on the edge of generating inappropriate autoimmunity; glucocorticoids apparently evolved as the means to accomplish this self-policing. Perhaps glucocorticoid-induced inhibition of normal immune function during stress is the price paid in order to guarantee glucocortiocid-induced inhibition during immune activation. Obviously, a great deal more work is needed in this exciting area.

The Pathogenic Effects of Chronic Stress on the Immune System

These data allow one to construct a syllogism. First, chronic stress suppresses immune function. Second, immune systems whose functioning is suppressed cannot fight disease effectively—this has been proved by the AIDS epidemic. Thus, chronic stress should make a vast number of diseases more likely to occur and more damaging once they do occur. This syllogism is irresistible to psychoneuroimmunologists because it is the bottom line of the whole field—stress should have widespread effects on health.[134, 371, 380, 504, 939]

Unfortunately, it has been difficult to prove this syllogism, or to prove its importance. Probably the most work in the area has been done on whether stress causes or worsens cancer. Theoretically, this could occur in a number of ways: (1) By suppressing the immune system, and particularly natural killer cell activity, it is easier for tumors to become established. (2) Once established, a major task of a tumor is to obtain nutrients to fuel its wild growth rate. Thus, an early event after tumor formation is its stimulation of angiogensis, which is capilllary ingrowth. Glucocorticoid concentrations in the high stress range potentiate angiogenesis. (3) The glucose-mobilizing effects of stress might inadvertently divert glucose to the tumor and aid its growth.

Thus, there are many mechanisms by which chronic stress might promote cancer. A very large literature has tested whether this is so, and some broad conclusions can be made. (1) In animals, stressors can aid the establishment of tumors and speed their growth. The effects on tumor growth are generally stronger. (2) Nevertheless, many tumors are insensitive to the effects of stress, and some even have their growth inhibited by stress. (3) In humans, some studies have shown a relationship between life stressors and increased cancer risk. For example, an episode of a major depression seems to increase cancer risk for decades afterward, independent of age, diet, smoking, and other risk factors. (4) Nevertheless, the overall association between stressors and cancer in humans is quite weak.

A body of research has also examined the relationship between stressors and other diseases that are normally combated by the immune system, such as viral infections. Again, although there does seem to be a relationship, it is a quite weak one.

Given how seductive this syllogism seems, why has the link between stress and any of these diseases been so difficult to establish in humans? There are a number of possible reasons. (1) Endless studies have shown that stress (or glucocorticoids, for example) suppress immune function. But these have typically focused on only a few reductionistic pieces of the immune system (because it is so difficult to measure many things simultaneously), and the *overall* immune system may be capable of compensating for those small pieces of dysfunction. (2) Animal studies have usually shown stronger links between stress and disease than the human studies. But the animal studies typically involve more severe stressors and more severe (and artificial) disease exposure. (3) Many of the human studies are retrospective, requiring sick people or their families to recall histories of stressors accurately. Prospective studies (in which a population undergoing some pattern of stress is identified and followed for decades afterward) should be more reliable, but these are difficult and therefore more rare.

Few areas of the life sciences are considered more exciting these days than psychoimmunology because its potential impact on health and disease is so profound. Nevertheless, it is clearly a nascent discipline, and one should be cautious about overemphasizing its findings. Even more so than in most fields of science, more research is clearly needed.

Table 10.1 summarizes the effects of acute physical stressors upon physiology and the most common diseases that emerge from or are exacerbated by prolonged stressors. Amid this mountain of data, two conclusions seem clear: If you are that lion or zebra and you cannot appropriately initiate a stress-response, you are in deep trouble. But just as clearly, if you are unable to terminate a stress-response appropriately, there is a considerable pathologic price as well.

How Generalized Is the Stress-Response?

Figures 10.1 and 10.2 depict the hormones and neural systems thought to be turned on by *all* stressors and those inhibited by *all* stressors, respec-

Table 10.1 The Principal Components of the Stress-Response and the Most Common Pathologic Consequences of Prolonged Exposure to Stress

THE STRESS RESPONSE	ITS PATHOLOGIC CONSEQUENCES, WHEN PROLONGED
Mobilization of energy at the cost of energy storage	Fatigue, myopathy, steroid diabetes
Increased cardiovascular and cardiopulmonary tone	Hypertension
Suppression of digestion	Ulceration
Suppression of growth	Psychogenic dwarfism, bone decalcification
Suppression of reproduction	Anovulation, impotency, loss of libido
Suppression of immunity and the inflammatory response	Impaired disease resistance
Analgesia	
Neural responses, including altered cognition and sensory thresholds	Accelerated neural degeneration during aging

tively.[376, 669] For Selye, one of the cornerstones of the stress-response was this nonspecificity. This was the idea that whether you were too hot or too cold, the stress-response was essentially similar. It was no accident that Selye used the word "general" with "adaptation syndrome." He wrote:

It is difficult to see how such essentially different things as cold, heat, drugs, hormones, sorrow and joy could provoke an identical biochemical reaction in the organism. Yet this is the case; it can now be demonstrated by highly objective quantitative biochemical determinations that certain reactions of the body are totally nonspecific and common to all types of exposure.

This has turned out not to be the case, however; not all stressors provoke the identical package of responses. In Selye's view, any stressor would provoke norepinephrine release from all of the many branches of the system. Yet there is some specificity of response. For example, hypoxia stimulates renal and gastric sympathetic activity, while hypotension stimulates only the former. Furthermore, norepinephrine and epinephrine secretion during stress can dissociate. For example, hypotension affects both renal and adrenal sympathetic activity similarly, whereas hypoglycemia does not. Thus, the entire sympathetic nervous system is not necessarily turned on in a nonspecific way in response to any stressor. This specificity of coding is also observed when comparing different endocrine systems. Some stressors provoke adrenocortical activity far more than adrenomedullary activity, while others do the opposite. Some stressors also influence glucocorticoid secretion without affecting growth hormone secretion.

I predict that there is another way in which the stress-response will be shown to code for specific stressors. As discussed, CRH is not the sole hypothalamic hormone that triggers ACTH release. Instead, numerous "secretagog" hormones carry out that task. On the hypothalamic level, there appears to be a stressor-specific coding, in that different stressors cause a different profile of the secretagogues to be released. This appears to support Selye's view because all these different stressors produce increased ACTH secretion.

My expection, however, is that these secretagogs will be found to have additional and different roles at the pituitary. For example, CRH may be shown to inhibit FSH release also, while vasopressin might also stimulate prolactin release. This would be a mechanism for some degree of stressor-specific coding at the pituitary level.

Stressors of all sorts *tend* to provoke glucocorticoid and catecholamine secretion, *tend* to inhibit reproductive hormone release, and so on. Yet, there is clearly some stress-specific coding of the physiologic response.

Psychologic Stress

I have summarized the understanding of stress that would satisfy most physiologists. Much of the remainder of this chapter examines individual differences in the stress-response. By thinking purely in terms of the physiology presented in this chapter up until now, it would be easy to approach the question of why two organisms differ in some feature of their stress-response. One would first point out the obvious, that the two organisms might differ in the amount of stressors they are exposed to and then move on to the next and more interesting level of analysis—two organisms that are exposed to the same stressor but differ in the resulting stress-response. We can speculate about interesting mechanisms to explain the differences. Suppose two monkeys are both deprived of food to the point where metabolic homeostasis is disturbed and to an equal extent in both animals. Both should then secrete glucocorticoids; if there are marked differences in the amount of glucocorticoids secreted, the well-trained physiologist should immediately think of explanations such as differences in ACTH half-lives in the blood, differences in adrenal perfusion rates, numbers of glucocorticoid receptors, and so on. This would be the traditional approach of stress physiologists.[629, 724, 937, 1095]

One study suffices to show how much more complex the picture really is. In the study cited above, the two monkeys differed in one critical way. While both were deprived of any nutrition, the second was fed a non-nutritive, flavored placebo. That monkey did not secrete glucocorticoids, whereas the first one had a sizeable stress-response. Nothing in the world of Selye and the physiologists could have predicted this outcome because their homeostatic balance was equally disturbed (they were equally hypoglycemic). The second monkey did not **perceive** things to be as stressful as did the first one.

This study signaled a major change in the study of stress physiology. The prior view held that if you knew how physiologically disruptive the external insult was, you had a good chance of predicting the magnitude of the stress-response. Suddenly, there was a critical intermediary—psychological factors could modulate the stressfulness of a stressor. Psychological factors could even trigger a stress-response in the absence of homeostatic disruption: Animals and humans were shown to have classic stress-responses during bereavement, difficult cognitive tasks, conditioned fear, and so on.

How much can psychological variables modulate the stress-response? Clearly, a great deal. Numerous physical stressors are no longer stressful when the organism is counterconditioned to the situation and is thus accustomed to it. Yet it cannot be true that all physical stressors are stressful *only* to the extent that they cause emotional arousal. As evidence, an anesthetized person has a stress-response following a surgical incision.

Most scientists now accept the power of psychological variables to modulate stress physiology. The question, of course, is, What are these variables? What is stressful about psychological stress? Elegant studies have shown these to include a **lack of control, lack of predictability**, and **lack of outlets for frustration**. Other terms and constructs have been used in the field, but these encompass the important ideas.

Loss of control is critical. In one demonstration of this, rats were subjected to intermittent electric shocks. One rat could control the situation because it was able to press a lever to decrease the rate of shocks. The second rat received a shock whenever the first one did, but without control. The latter had far more glucocorticoid secretion and a greater chance of developing ulcers; this result occurred despite identical extents of physical perturbation. Similar findings have emerged with dogs and humans. In a subtle elaboration, if a rat is trained to press a lever to avoid a shock and is then prevented from performing that avoidance behavior when it expects a shock, there is glucocorticoid secretion even if no shock is actually delivered. Here, loss of control is a trigger, even in the absence of a physical stressor.

Loss of predictability is also critical. If rats are given a signal indicating the impending delivery of a shock, or when the shock period has ended, they have less glucocorticoid secretion than rats given identical shocks with no warning. In the former case, the signal allows the rat to predict when a shock is and is not about to occur and thus when it can relax its vigilance.

Some have noted that loss of control and of predictability share the trait of the outcome being **discrepant with expectations** (or, in other words, **novel**). Thus, the simple act of putting a rat in a novel environment—a new cage—activates the stress-response. In men learning to parachute jump, their first jump elicited a robust stress-response. With subsequent jumps, however, the response eventually habituated as the novelty of the situation lessened. Some have also emphasized that the common theme in loss of control and of predictability is the consequent **arousal** or **vigilance**, as the animal searches for the new rules of control and prediction.

A number of studies have emphasized the importance of **outlets for frustration**. For example, when rats are shocked, there is less glucocorticoid secretion and fewer ulcers if they can gnaw on a piece of wood or can attack another rat. Eating, drinking, or access to a running wheel can also serve as protective outlets.

One can ask some subtle questions. For example, does novelty stimulate the stress-response in a linear or all-or-none fashion? It appears to be linear. Thus, the more novel an environment for a rat (handled and returned to home cage, returned to a new but similar cage, to a new type of cage, to a new type of cage illuminated with bright lights . . .), the higher the level of glucocorticoid secretion. This question has the flavor of the questions that the bioengineering physiologists have asked about the system and shows the rigor of some psychoendocrine studies now being conducted.

Thus, the extent to which a physical insult is "stressful" is modulated dramatically by intervening psychological variables, and psychological factors can initiate a stress-response even in the absence of a physical insult. Clearly, one vital prerequisite for responding to psychological stressors is a certain level of intelligence. One needs to have a decent memory to perceive a novelty stressor—"I know what is normal, and what's happening now is not normal, and this makes me nervous," or a conditioned stressor—"Uh oh, I remember what occurred last time this happened and it wasn't good." Thus, only the more cognitively sophisticated species can have psychologic stressors. Humans excell at this, as will be discussed in the final section of this chapter.

Individual Differences in Stress Physiology

Why is it interesting to study individual differences? Most physiologists hate individual variability. Just when you think you have discovered something and can announce that "X causes Y," you have to qualify your observation by saying "X causes Y most of the time, but not in a subset of animals, and don't ask me why not." Individual variability makes data messy, makes it harder to know what is really going on. The emphasis in physiology on using inbred strains of animals with identical housing conditions is meant to eliminate individual variability. Why study it?

The answer must be because individual variability is a major chance to understand the prevention of stress-related disease. No one has to be convinced any longer that stress can make you sick. It sometimes seems miraculous that any of us manage to survive the lifetime of stressors that we are all subject to. Yet only some of us get stress-related diseases. To study individual differences in stress physiology is to study what some individuals are doing right, to study why some bodies and some psyches deal with stressors better than others.

I will review how individuals differ in their stress-response as a function of behavior and personality. In particular, I will concentrate on the effects of social rank in dominance hierarchies. I will then briefly review how some of these differences might arise. How do chronic stress, early experience, and genetics contribute to the workings of the stress-response? Rather than exhaustively cover every endocrine system relevant to stress, I will concentrate on individual differences in patterns of glucocorticoid secretion.

A Detailed Analysis: Social Status, Personality, and the Stress-Response

THE PHENOMENON OF SOCIAL DOMINANCE
Among social species dominance systems frequently emerge. Resources in the ecosystem are not infinite, competition occurs, and the resources are often

divided unevenly. Every contested resource could be fought for in a bloody showdown. Instead, systems of conventionalized gestures often evolve so that individuals need not fight it out. Two animals approach a desired food item, for example, and one of them makes a facial expression, gives a certain type of growl, releases a certain pheromone, which, in that species, means dominance. And the second individual usually relinquishes the food without an overt contest. Presumably, it can remember what happened the last time conflict with this individual came to a head.[906, 908, 909, 1110]

In some species, dominance systems are linear, in that a hierarchy of ranks emerge. Number one has a different quality of life from number five, who is different from number ten. Some dominance systems are nonlinear in which, for example, number one does all the mating. In this case, it is not meaningful to try to define a number five or a number ten. You are either a "number one" or a "not number one."

The quality of life of an animal depends tremendously on its social rank. Rank determines how hard it has to work for food and influences who it gets to mate with, or if it gets to mate at all. Social rank determines whether it gets a safe spot during a predator attack, a warm spot in the cold, an ideal spot to build a nest to ensure the survival of its offspring. It influences how often the individual is harassed in petty, irritating ways. Many studies have examined whether the physiology of the stress-response differs among animals of different ranks. Most studies examine social primates.

Initially, the results of these studies appear to be a mess. Sometimes, dominant animals have lower resting levels of glucocorticoids than do subordinates, sometimes higher. Sometimes their adrenals are bigger, sometimes smaller. Sometimes the speed of their stress-response is faster, sometimes sluggish. Other measures are just as confused. Researchers have come to recognize that not all dominance hierarchies are the same. A critical variable appears to be how **stable** the hierarchy is.

STABLE VERSUS UNSTABLE DOMINANCE HIERARCHIES
In a stable dominance hierarchy, the status quo is maintained, and ranks do not change. The contrasting situation of instability occurs in the wild when new animals migrate into a social group and destabilize the status quo, or when someone has died or been injured. In captivity, such instability is seen when social groups are first formed. And in both cases, the hierarchy restabilizes slowly, as everyone learns where they stand in relation to each other.

Psychologically, dominance is very different in stable versus unstable hierarchies. In the former, dominant individuals have tremendous amounts of predictability and control and numerous outlets for frustration. They can seize food from someone at will, need not fear harassment, can terrorize someone smaller when they are in a bad mood. But during instability, dominance is a very different experience. Typically, the rates of dominance interactions, of aggression, are elevated, and are focused on animals at the top. Ranks shift daily and unexpectedly, injuries are more common. This is a situation that has anything but control and predictability. Everyone, especially the top-ranked individuals, are experiencing stress. It is a very different experience to be the dictator of a country in which all dissent has been crushed than to be the same dictator when the palace is being stormed.

This explains a lot of the confusion seen in the physiologic studies. In stable hierarchies, dominant males have the lowest amounts of basal glucocorticoid secretion. During a stressor, they have as large a stress-response as subordinates because they turn on their system faster. This is ideal—less of the damaging hormones are around when they are not needed. They have other distinctive physiologic features as well. In a stable hierarchy, dominant individuals are probably less at risk for stress-related disease. This makes sense because they have far more control and predictability, and more outlets for frustration, than do subordinates.

During periods of social instability, the ideal adrenocortical profiles of dominant animals disappear. They no longer have low basal glucocorticoid concentrations or the largest stress-response. Moreover, their adrenals tend to be larger than those of subordinates. This makes sense, given the stressfulness of hanging on at the top of a shifting hierarchy.

Thus, there is no single physiologic profile that goes along with being dominant. What matters is not so much the rank as the **type** of society in which the rank is occurring. I now review a second variable that turns out to be even more important: whether you can **perceive** how stressful your situation is or not.

STYLES OF DOMINANCE

Social primates are too complex to be reduced to a mere rank. Two monkeys may have similar ranks yet differ in the **style** with which they go about that rank. They may differ in how likely they are to form cooperative coalitions or nonsexual friendships with the opposite sex, how reliable a coalitional partner they are, how often they play with infants, or whether they chase innocent bystanders after losing a fight. These highly individualistic animals have strong styles and personalities. Do dominant animals of differing styles all have the same distinctive physiology?

I have examined this issue in my studies of stress-related physiology, rank, and behavior among male wild baboons living in East Africa. I found that low basal glucocorticoid concentrations are not, in fact, a marker of high rank. Instead, low glucocorticoid levels are found only among dominant males with a certain personality. Dominant males without those personality traits secreted just as much glucocorticoids as did subordinates.

Low basal glucocorticoid concentrations occured in males with any of the following traits: an ability to differentiate (behaviorally) between neutral and threatening social situations; a tendency to initiate fights when those situations were indeed threatening; an ability to differentiate between winning and losing fights; a high likelihood of displacing aggression onto an innocent bystander after losing a fight; high rates of nonsexual "friendships" with females.

These traits reflect high degrees of social control and predictability. The animal can tell when things are threatening; if they are, it makes quick decisions when they come to a head. It can tell if the outcome was good or bad; if it was bad it has outlets for its frustration. If you were running stress management courses for baboons, these would be the traits you would encourage in your clients.

These "low glucocorticoid" males were high-ranking longer than males without these personality traits. This observation might immediately suggest that the personality and physiology are merely a *consequence* of a long dominance tenure—because males are in that position for a longer period, perhaps they learn how to predict social outcomes better and become more socially savvy, and their glucocorticoid concentrations drop. But that is not the case. The low glucocorticoid males had the endocrine and personality traits from the start of their dominance tenure. Where, then, did the distinctive personality and physiology come from?

These differences can appear at an extraordinarily early age. In studies of both humans and primates, infants (who in some cases may be only a few months old) are already different in personality traits reminiscent of some of those seen in adult baboons. They vary in how exploratory they are in novel or stressful circumstances, how emotionally reactive they are to novelty, how introverted or extroverted they are, and so on. Even at those young ages, the ones who are less emotionally reactive to mere novelty tend to have lower basal glucocorticoid concentrations. Moreover, these endocrine and behavioral traits persist into adulthood.

The studies of stable versus unstable hierarchies show that low glucocorticoid concentrations emerge among dominant animals only in the type of society where dominance carries with it certain psychological advantages. These studies of style show that low glucocorticoid levels are observed only in the animals that can perceive these advantages. A similar theme emerges from classic studies of humans under stress. Parents of children dying of cancer were studied and found to hypersecrete glucocorticoids. Whereas some parents had extremely elevated levels, some had only moderate elevations. It was found that a number of coping traits were associated with lower glucocorticoid secretion. These included having a religious structure that could rationalize the disease (i.e., parents who thought that they had been selected by God for some special test), an ability to ignore the facts of the disease, and an ability to lose themselves in the details of managing the disease.

Collectively, these studies of style among humans and baboons reiterate the lessons learned from the psychology of stress. Knowledge that an organism is undergoing something stressful (watching a child die of cancer, having a rank that is unsatisfying) allows us to make some predictions as to what that organism's physiologic profile will be. But the intervening variables of the psychological makeup of the individual, and its personality, and its capacity to rationalize, deny, look the other way, or look at the bright side are immensely powerful. We differ in whether we see the world consisting of glasses half empty or half full, and that difference seems to exert a profound effect on our physiology.

Chronic Stress and Glucocorticoid Profiles

Thus, two individuals may differ in their adrenocortical profiles because they differ in social rank or in personality. They may also differ because they have had differing histories of exposure to stressors. This variable interacts with social rank and personality in a complex manner.[915]

It is not really surprising that low-ranking animals secrete more glucocorticoids than high-ranking ones, or that animals with a personality who perceive everything as stressful secrete more than those who do not perceive things that way. If you are exposed to many stressors (or think you are), you will secrete more glucocorticoids. This is a "social/psychological" cause of this individual difference. But there is a more mechanistic cause as well. When stress causes an organism to secrete glucocorticoids repeatedly, the regulation of the system stops working as well, and the organism starts to hypersecrete glucocorticoids even under nonstressful circumstances. This occurs with animals or humans undergoing sustained stress (people suffering from major depression and medical interns during periods of stressful case presentations are two of the best-studied cases).

The reasons are complex. On a rather nontechnical level, one can use an automotive metaphor. During a stressor, a neural "accelerator" stimulates glucocorticoid secretion. At the end of stress and under basal conditions, a neural "brake" curtails secretion. When the system is stressed repeatedly, the brake stops working as well. The hippocampus is one such brake, and chronic stress impairs its ability to carry out that job. This need not be because hippocampal neurons are damaged. In milder cases, the neurons survive, but their functioning is altered transiently. At such times, organisms hypersecrete glucocorticoids basally and do not turn off the stress-response promptly at the end of stress.

Thus, at the beginning of a period of being stressed frequently (for example, shortly after dropping precipitously in rank), glucocorticoids are hypersecreted because frequent stressors are present; there are many peaks of stress-responses. But with time, as the regulation of the system is impaired, there is hypersecretion basally as well.

Early Experience and Glucocorticoid Profiles

Two adults may also differ in their glucocorticoid profiles because of differences in early experience. In rodents, a number of different developmental variables (separation from a mother, any of a number of other stressors, the extent of exploration, and so on) influence adult adrenocortical function. This endocrine system can "imprint," in that there is a developmental critical period in which experience alters functioning of the system for the rest of life. Probably the best-studied of these phenomena is neonatal "handling." Removing a pup from its mother and placing it in a new cage for 15 minutes a day for the first three weeks of life induces a more efficient adrenocortical stress-response in adulthood. These rats have smaller stress-responses and return to baseline faster after the end of stress. In old age, they have lower basal glucocorticoid concentrations. Handling after 3 weeks of age does not cause the effect.[628, 701]

Levine, in first describing this effect, called it "stress immunization," and this is an apt phrase. In medicine, infants are immunized with a mild version of a disease to stimulate the immune system into more efficient defenses against it thereafter. Similarly, handling represents stimulation of the stress-response with a mild stressor early, producing a more efficient response later.

Recent work has shown how handling causes these permanent changes. While the details are beyond the scope of this chapter, there is an increase in the sensitivity of the brain and pituitary to the signal of circulating glucocorticoids, causing more efficient regulation of glucocorticoid secretion. This is accomplished by the creation of lifelong changes in the pattern of receptors for the hormones.

Sex Differences and Glucocorticoid Profiles

In many species, including humans, females tend to have higher circulating concentrations of glucocorticoids than do males. When this was first observed, many investigators attributed this pattern to the greater "sensitivity" of females to stress. However, subsequent research has shown this sex difference to be more apparent than real and of little functional importance because of the way glucocorticoids are transported in the blood. Because they are steroids, glucocorticoids are hydrophobic and circulate best when bound to a protein. This role is mostly served by corticosteroid-binding globulin (CBG), also known as transcortin. Typically, 95% of circulating glucocorticoids are bound to CBG. It is the unbound 5%, in the process of entering a target tissue, that is biologically active.[193]

Importantly, estrogen induces the synthesis of CBG in the liver, producing higher circulating levels of this protein in females. Thus, in order to have the same glucocorticoid signal reach a target tissue (i.e., to have the same amount of hormone in an unbound state), more glucocorticoids must be secreted into the circulation. Therefore, while females typically have higher circulating glucocorticoid concentrations, the amount of hormone in the free, biologically active fraction does not usually differ by sex.

Do fluctuations in estrogen levels alter CBG concentrations and thus total glucocorticoid concentrations? This may account for changing glucocorticoid profiles over a lifetime because estrogen levels rise at puberty and decline post-reproductively. In general, the fluctuations in estrogen over the course of menstrual cycles is too small to alter CBG significantly. In the past, when oral contraceptives contained far more estrogen than they do now, their use led to higher CBG concentrations. But again, there is little reason to believe that under any of these circumstances in which total glucocorticoid concentrations might flucuate that this is of much functional importance.

One circumstance in which there is a sex difference in the amount of *free* glucocorticoids occurs during pregnancy. At such times there is a huge rise in CBG and, for reasons that are not well understood mechanistically, a rise in glucocorticoid secretion that more than compensates for the rise in CBG. Thus, the free fraction increases. This can produce some symptoms of glucocorticoid excess in pregnant women, including elevated blood pressure and mild glucose intolerance. The most plausible explanation for the purpose of this rise is that the female must provide glucocorticoids both for herself and for the fetus (before its own adrenal axis matures).

Genetics and Glucocorticoid Profiles

Two individuals may also differ in glucocorticoid profiles because of genetic differences. In rats, a few strains have been shown to be congenitally less capable of dealing with mild, novelty-related stressors. They do not learn as well, are less exploratory, and defecate more (a sensitive index of anxiety in rats). They also hypersecrete ACTH and glucocorticoids at such times. Importantly, these rats are normal under basal situations or in response to major, physical stressors. The genetic difference seems to be one of sensitivity to mild, psychological stressors.[395, 1010]

Little is known about the causes of these strain differences. Even less is known about the genetics of the stress-response in primates and humans. In one study, emotional reactivity, glucocorticoid secretion, and styles of mothering were characterized in rhesus monkeys in which cross-fostering experiments had been carried out—a child of a highly reactive high-cortisol female might be raised by an unreactive, low-cortisol female, and so on. A small amount of heritability of these traits was suggested.

Some Remaining Questions About These Models and Their Interactions

These previous sections suggest that two individuals may differ in their glucocorticoid profiles because of their social rank, the stability of the society in which they live, their personality, their immediate history of frequency of exposure to stressors, their perinatal experience, or their genetics. How do these different causes interact? This is an immensely complicated question. A few conclusions can be emphasized. The "good physiology" (for example, the low basal glucocorticoid concentrations) does not cause the dominance rank. First, dominant males do not always have that physiological profile (for example, those without the personality described, or those with that personality during the unstable season). Second, in studies of captive primates it is generally impossible to look at adrenocortical measures in animals when they are housed alone and predict who will be dominant in a social group. Finally, artificially lowering glucocorticoid concentrations does not make someone dominant. In contrast, I would suspect that personality traits involving social control and predictability contribute a great deal to the achievement (and maintenance) of high rank and to the physiology. One would then predict that males with the "low cortisol" personality had those distinctive personality traits even when they were younger and socially subordinate; this is now being studied. If that is the case, it implies that for some males the main point is that they are not in the lowest rank (whether they are number two or number nine in a hierarchy of ten) whereas for others, the point is that they are still not in the highest rank (whether they are number two or nine). The personality differences, in turn, seem to reflect both genetic and perinatal influences.

What neuroendocrine mechanisms underly these differences? The task is to take the complex endocrine cascades encompassing the brain, pituitary, and peripheral organs and then to determine what point in the cascade works differently, depending on rank, personality, history, genetics, so on. Some of these complex studies have been alluded to. As a broad conclusion, these mechanisms are extremely varied. You cannot conclude that, for example, the pituitary accounts for individual differences in all of these systems or that a decreased number of receptors is the main cellular mechanism mediating these differences, and so on. For example, dominant baboons have lower basal glucocorticoid concentrations in part because their *brains* are *more sensitive* to the inhibitory effects of circulating glucocorticoids. In contrast, these same animals have higher testosterone concentrations during stress in part because their *testes* are *less sensitive* to the inhibitory effects of circulating glucocorticoids. The individual differences occur at the brain, pituitary, or peripheral level and can involve enhanced or decreased tissue sensitivity to signals, involving, most likely, effects on numbers and functioning of receptors as well as postreceptor mechanisms.

Finally, do any of these individual differences matter? Do organisms with the lower basal glucocorticoid concentrations live longer and have fewer heart attacks and better immune systems to combat disease? These are difficult questions to answer. In the laboratory, animals are not exposed to the normal array of pathogens, so laboratory study requires rather artificial controlled exposure to disease. In the field, the difficulty is that the investigator must follow the same wild individuals over many decades of their lifetime, and it is difficult to be certain what diseases they might have. Moreover, because dominance rank among male Old World monkeys tends to change over time, there is more pressure to follow the animals over their whole lifetime—a subordinate male with elevated glucocorticoid concentrations this year may be a dominant terror in a few years, with lower glucocorticoid levels. Any given year's data are like single still photographs of a very dynamic, changing scene.

Nevertheless, there is evidence that these individual differences matter. For example, in stable social groups of primates, high-ranking monkeys are less prone to atherosclerotic plaque formation in their blood vessels than are subordinates. A fair amount is known about the long-term consequences of the neonatal handling in rats. As will be discussed in chapter 11, chronic stress does cause effects on the brain. Glucocorticoid exposure over the lifetime of a rat contributes to some aspects of hippocampal aging and degeneration. Thus, one would guess that handled rats, in their old age, should have less hippocampal degeneration and less of the cognitive deficits that arise from such degeneration; this is observed.

Summary and Conclusions

1. The stress-response involves changes in a tremendous array of endocrine and neural systems. These responses are somewhat (but not entirely) nonspecific to the type of stressor that triggers them.

2. When provoked for relatively brief periods in response to physical stressors, these responses seem fairly adaptive in helping an organism survive. Thus, an inability to initiate this stress-response appropriately can be highly deleterious.

3. These same responses, when provoked chronically or repeatedly, can cause or exacerbate numerous diseases. Stress-related disease can be considered to emerge most frequently from an overactivation of the stress-response rather than from a failure of that response. Thus, an inability to terminate the stress-response appropriately can be highly pathogenic.

4. The extent to which an external stressor provokes the stress-response can be modulated by intervening psychological variables. In the right psychological setting, a stress-response can be provoked even without an external stressor. Psychological stressors appear to be stressful to the extent that they contain elements of loss of control, loss of predictability, and absence of outlets for frustration.

5. Considerable individual variation exists in the workings of the stress-response. These differences can arise from differing genetic or developmental histories, and from more recent factors, such as social status and the stressfulness of life. These differences may reflect differing psychological makeup (i.e., organisms may differ in whether they perceive the same event as being stressful) and physiological makeup (i.e., once the event is perceived as stressful, organisms differ in how their various organ systems respond).

How are these findings most relevant to us? An inability to initiate a stress-response would obviously be catastrophic. In two human examples of that situation, Addison's disease (in which the glucocorticoid component of the stress-response is blunted because of adrenal insufficiency) and Shy-Drager syndrome (in which the sympathetic component is blunted), individuals are extremely fragile. But these are rare cases. Few of us will get sick because we have too small a stress-response. Our problem, overwhelmingly, is an overactivation.

This problem is compounded further by the circumstances under which our stress-response is overactivated. If we were to list the stressful things in our lives, the leading categories would probably be time and financial pressures, family conflicts, the tensions and disappointments of our social lives, job dissatisfaction. Few of us are likely to list droughts, locust infestations, malaria attacks during the rainy season, close calls with predators. In our ecologically buffered lives, we encounter few of the physical stressors that our ancestors did and that most mammals on earth still do. Instead, we have the luxury of making ourselves sick with psychological and social stressors. Given the pathogenicity of psychological stressors, we are more at risk for developing an ulcer at some point in our life than is a zebra.

Because of this, the studies concerning psychological modulation of the stress-response are profoundly important for us. Repeatedly, the lesson from such studies is that although external events may be stressful, the pathogenic impact of such events can be blunted considerably by psychological variables. If that is the case for a rat encountering something as unambiguously stressful as electric shocks, it should certainly be true for ourselves and our lives encompassing far more subtle, ambiguous stressors. We may have to rely on highly interventionist medical technology to repair us once we get sick with stress-related disorders. But my feeling is that by manipulating psychological variables concerning sense of control, predictability, and so on, we have a tremendous power within ourselves to control whether we get those stress-related disorders in the first place.

Acknowledgement

All the figures in this chapter were prepared by Becky A. Stein.

11 Hormonal Influences on Extrapyramidal Sensorimotor Function and Hippocampal Plasticity

Jill B. Becker

In this chapter we find that hormones can affect neuronal activity in areas of the brain that are important for the complex processing of cognitive and sensorimotor information. Several interesting models have taken advantage of pharmacological methods to reveal and measure effects of gonadal hormones on motor activity, sensory processing, and the integration of sensorimotor information. We also find evidence that both adrenal and gonadal hormones can affect cognitive functioning by affecting neuronal development and morphology in the hippocampus. Furthermore, as we saw in the previous chapter, prolonged stress can kill neurons and this impairs memory.

What are the effects of gonadal steroids on neurotransmitter activity and on neural activity and structure? How can we measure the behavioral consequences of such changes? How does long-term hormone exposure affect the neural substrates of these behaviors?

Introduction

Sexual behaviors, courtship behaviors, parenting behaviors, and aggressive behaviors are just a small sample of the many sexually dimorphic or hormonally modulated behaviors exhibited by animals. In this chapter, sex-related differences and hormonal influences on three brain regions, the **striatum**, the **cerebellum**, and the **hippocampus**, will be considered. These brain regions will be used as examples of the wide impact that hormones can have on the brain and the consequence on functions as diverse as motor activity, sensory perception, and neuronal plasticity.

The striatum and the cerebellum are components of the **extrapyramidal motor system**. Both of these brain regions receive direct or indirect input from all sensory systems and are implicated in the control of movement. The hippocampus has been shown to exhibit considerable neuronal plasticity and is implicated in learning and memory. At first, the relations among these three brain regions and their functions may not be apparent to the reader. But sex-related differences and hormonal influences on motor activity and sensory perception can affect one's performance in tasks of learning and memory. For example, if estrogen treatment increases general activity, a test that requires an animal to learn to keep still will be more difficult for an animal that has received estrogen than for one that has not. Hormonal modulation of sensory perception can also result in test bias by increasing or decreasing sensory thresholds that can directly influence performance. In other words, sex-related differences or hormonal influences on one behavior can result in behavioral biases that make a test easier for one group than for another. Therefore, it is important to take into consideration sex-related differences and hormonal influences on sensorimotor function when comparing behaviors thought to be mediated by the hippocampus in males and females or evaluating the effects of hormones on tests of learning and memory. For these reasons, these brain regions are discussed together in this chapter.

The chapter will begin with an overview of hormonal and sex-related influences on the striatum and cerebellum, followed by speculation about how this might affect more complex measures of activity and sensory perception. Then the evidence for sex-related differences and hormonal modulation of the hippocampus and hippocampal plasticity will be presented. How these differences affect hippocampal development and function as well as learning and memory performance will be discussed in light of the hormonal effects on sensorimotor function.

Hormonal Influences on the Striatum and Cerebellum Affect Sensorimotor Function

Sex Differences and Hormonal Influences on the Striatum

The striatum is composed of two nuclei, the caudate nucleus and the putamen. In conjunction with the globus pallidus, these nuclei are referred to as the basal ganglia. Anatomically the afferent and efferent connections of the striatum are organized into four feedback loops that process sensory information and produce motor output (figure 11.1).

THE NIGROSTRIATAL DOPAMINE SYSTEM
As illustrated in figure 11.1, cells in the substantia nigra project their axons to the striatum. These neurons use the neurotransmitter dopamine. Over 90% of the dopamine-containing neurons in the brain are found in this projection from the substantia nigra to the striatum, called the nigrostriatal dopamine projection. When dopamine activity increases, animals exhibit an exaggerated motor response to a sensory stimulus. For example, **amphetamine** is a drug that acts by stimulating dopamine release from dopamine terminals. Behaviorally, a rat that has received amphetamine is hypersensitive and hyperresponsive to sensory stimuli. For example, if you snap your fingers over a rat's head, normally no response or a small startle is seen. In a rat that has received amphetamine, however, snapping your fingers over its head will elicit an exaggerated startle response. A similar behavioral response is seen when the drug **apomorphine** is administered. Apomorphine is a dopamine receptor agonist (it mimics the effect of dopamine at its receptor), so the motor response to a given sensory input is greater when dopaminergic activity is increased. In contrast, the dopamine receptor antagonist, **haloperidol**, acts by blocking dopamine receptors.

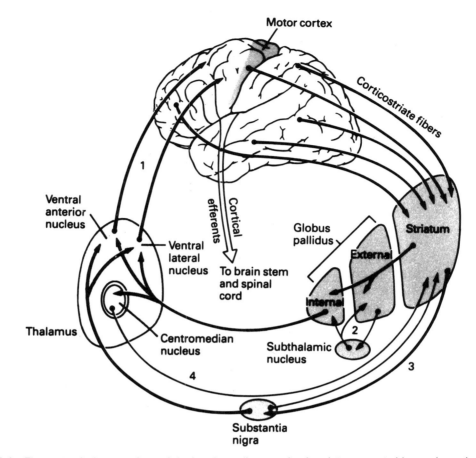

Figure 11.1   The anatomical connections of the basal ganglia comprise four interconnected loops. Loop 1: Corticostriate fibers to striatum, striatum to globus pallidus, globus pallidus to thalamus, and thalamus back to cortex. Loop 2: Globus pallidus to the subthalamic nucleus, subthalamic nucleus to globus pallidus. Loop 3: Striatum to substantia nigra, substantia nigra to striatum. Loop 4: Striatum to globus pallidus, globus pallidus to thalamus, and thalamus back to striatum. (From Kandel and Schwartz, 1985.[553])

When a rat receives haloperidol, it becomes hyporesponsive, lethargic, and sometimes even cataleptic or unresponsive to sensory input.

FUNCTIONS OF THE STRIATUM

Behaviors induced by activation with specific dopamine agonists (e.g., apomorphine) or antagonists (e.g., haloperidol) illustrate that the saliency of sensory stimuli and the consequent motor response produced seem to become greater when dopamine activity is increased (and vice versa), suggesting that dopamine enhances sensorimotor integration. However, since there are also dopamine neurons in other brain regions, these phenomena do not prove that the striatum mediates this integration of sensorimotor information. In fact, while a role for the striatum in the integration of sensorimotor information has been postulated for years, delineating the specific role that it plays is still quite difficult. We know quite a lot, however, about what happens when activity is abnormal or when damage to the striatum or its input occurs. This does not tell us what the striatum or basal ganglia are normally doing in animals without brain damage; nevertheless, clinical syndromes can tell us some things about the role of the striatum in sensorimotor function.

Two devastating disorders are caused by specific basal ganglia degeneration: **Parkinson's disease** and **Huntington's disease**. In Parkinson's disease the dopamine neurons of the substantia nigra degenerate. This leaves the striatum without dopaminergic input. The consistent and prevalent symptom of Parkinson's disease is *bradykinesia*, a reduction in the speed of movements. This occurs even though there is no evidence of paralysis. During the final stages of the disease, patients can be so bradykinetic that it may appear that they cannot move at all. In fact, these patients behave very much like animals or patients who have taken high doses of a neuroleptic drug (e.g., the dopamine receptor antagonist haloperidol). Another symptom of Parkinson's disease is *resting tremor*. Resting tremor is frequently one of the first symptoms of the disease. This appears as a regular involuntary, oscillatory movement of a body part. The hands and extremities are usually affected first, but the entire body may also be subjected to persistent resting tremor.

Huntington's disease is a hereditary disease of the basal ganglia. Onset of symptoms occurs late in life (usually in the third to fourth decade). It is characterized neurologically by cell loss in the basal ganglia. In many ways Huntington's disease is the opposite of Parkinson's disease. In Parkinsonism there is excessive inhibition of motor systems causing the bradykinesia. In contrast, in Huntington's disease there is a **loss** of inhibition causing *chorea* as well as cognitive deficits. Chorea means dance in Latin, and it is characterized by the presence of rapid flick-like movements of the limbs and facial muscles. At advanced stages of the disease patients are no longer able to care for themselves because of the pervasive cognitive deficits and motor dysfunction.

Summary of the Functions of the Striatum   The clinical symptoms of basal ganglia damage and the results obtained from animal research have given us some ideas about the functions of the striatum and basal ganglia. Unfortunately, we still don't know the complete story. Marsden has suggested "that the basal ganglia...are required to set up the correct motor programmes to execute complex simultaneous and sequential movements." He goes on to suggest that these functions are performed in the basal ganglia. The basal ganglia integrates information after it has been received by the sensorimotor cortex. The integrated or processed information from the basal ganglia is then transmitted to the premotor cortex for subsequent motor action.[661]

GONADAL STEROID MODULATION OF STRIATAL ACTIVITY
In order to determine whether the gonadal steroid hormones influence the functional activity of the striatum and in particular the nigrostriatal dopamine

system (the neural system that degenerates in Parkinson's disease), a number of behavioral tests have been used. By far the most widely used behavioral tests are behaviors induced by dopamine agonists. When dopaminergic mimetics such as apomorphine or amphetamine are administered to the rat, a wide variety of behaviors are induced. Shortly after administration of a high dose of apomorphine or amphetamine an animal shows increased locomotor and exploratory behavior and this is followed by a stereotypic phase. Stereotyped behaviors in the rodent are repetitive movements of the head, mouth, snout, whiskers, and forelimbs. Behaviors included are chewing movements, excessive sniffing (directed at nothing), up and down movements of the head, and jerky movements of the forelimbs. These stereotyped behaviors are thought to be due to activation of the striatal dopamine system in conjunction with increased dopamine activity in the nucleus accumbens and olfactory tubercle.

Another behavioral test used to assess dopamine activity in the striatum is drug-induced rotational behavior. When the nigrostriatal dopamine system is selectively damaged unilaterally (i.e., only on one side) by the catecholamine neurotoxin 6-hydroxydopamine (6-OHDA), rats and mice exhibit persistent circling toward the side of the lesion. A large number of studies have established that animals typically turn in the direction contralateral to the nigrostriatal dopamine system having the greatest activity (figure 11.2). Thus, after a unilateral 6-OHDA lesion of the substantia nigra, the dopamine terminals in the striatum on that side degenerate, and amphetamine can release dopamine only on the intact side. Activity in the intact striatum induces turning toward the damaged side. However, dopamine receptors in both striata are intact following a unilateral substantia nigra lesion. Apomorphine, acting on dopamine receptors, elicits turning in the other direction. This is thought to reflect the unilateral increase in the number of dopamine receptors on the denervated side. Apomorphine activates more receptors on the side of the lesion, so the animal rotates away from the lesioned side toward its intact side.

Studies of stereotyped behaviors, rotational behavior, and postural asymmetries have found that female rats exhibit a greater behavioral response to dopaminergic drugs when the dopamine system is stimulated during late proestrus or early estrus than in diestrus.[98, 100, 543] During the estrous cycle of the rat, estrogen peaks on the afternoon of proestrus. The onset of behavioral receptivity (behavioral estrus) occurs 8 to 12 hours after the estrogen peak in association with ovulation, usually after the onset of the dark phase of the light-dark cycle (see chapter 3). Neurochemical measures suggest that changes in both presynaptic and postsynaptic dopamine activity occur during the estrous cycle. On the presynaptic side, striatal dopamine release, dopamine synthesis, and dopamine turnover all are greatest during estrus. Postsynaptically, the number of striatal dopamine receptors increases when presynaptic activity decreases, during diestrus. There are at least two types of dopamine receptors (called D_1 and D_2 dopamine receptors), and similar changes are found with both receptor types.

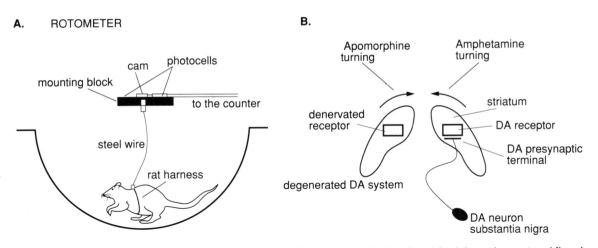

A. ROTOMETER

B.

Figure 11.2 The behavioral apparatus used for assessing asymmetry in the nigrostriatal dopamine system (*A*) and a schematic model for mechanisms of dopaminergic drug-induced rotational behavior (*B*). *A*, The behavioral apparatus employed is called a rotometer. As illustrated, during testing the rat wears a nonconfining elastic harness around its chest. The harness is attached to a rigid steel wire that turns with the animal. The steel wire is attached to an assembly that can turn freely, opening and closing photocells as the animal turns. Output from the photocells is sent to a computer-controlled counter that records the number of 360-degree turns the animal makes during the test session. *B*, Following unilateral dopamine (DA) degeneration induced by injection of the neurotoxin 6-hydroxydopamine into the substantia nigra, rotational behavior is induced when drugs that stimulate the dopaminergic system are administered. The direction of turning is indicated by the arrows at the top of the figure. There has been considerable research to demonstrate that animals turn in circles away from the striatum that is most active. Since striatal DA receptors become supersensitivie after DA denervation, administration of the DA receptor agonist apomorphine induces a greater postsynaptic response in the denervated striatum than in the intact striatum, and animals turn away from the side of the lesion. On the other hand, amphetamine induces DA release from intact DA nerve endings. So, following amphetamine administration there is greater DA release in the intact striatum, and animals turn away from the intact striatum.

Results from studies investigating estrous cycle–dependent variation in neurochemical and behavioral indices of striatal dopamine activity are summarized in table 11.1. In general, spontaneous activity and behavior induced by drugs or treatments that stimulate presynaptic activity are increased when estrogen secretion is elevated, during late proestrus and early estrus. Estrous cycle–dependent variations in the response to drugs that act on dopamine receptors are not as evident and have been seen in only a few of the studies reported. When an effect is seen, the results agree with the variations reported in striatal dopamine receptors during the estrous cycle.

What hormones are mediating these estrous cycle–dependent changes in striatal dopamine activity? Experiments that have manipulated ovarian hormones using physiological doses indicate that estrogen or estrogen plus progesterone can mimic the estrous cycle–dependent effects. Following ovariectomy, decreased rotational behavior is induced by drugs or treatments that stimulate dopamine release. Decreased presynaptic striatal dopamine release is also induced by amphetamine. Treatment of ovariectomized rats with estro-

Table 11.1 Estrous Cycle-Dependent Variation in Striatal Activity

WHAT WAS MEASURED	RESULTS	REFERENCE
Behavioral Indices		
Sensorimotor performance on balance beam task	Performance better on estrus than on other days of the cycle	Becker et al. (1987)[101]
Amphetamine-induced rotational behavior	Females in estrus turned more than those in diestrus	Becker et al. (1982)[100]
Amphetamine-induced stereotypyed behaviors	Females in estrus exhibited greater stereotypy than did those in diestrus	Becker and Cha (1989)[98]
Haloperidol-induced catalepsy	No effect of estrous cycle	Kazandjian et al. (1988)[558]
Rotational behavior elicited by electrical stimulation of ascending dopamine fibers	Females turned more during estrus than they did on other days of the cycle	Robinson et al. (1982)[863]
Apomorphine-induced stereotyped behaviors	No effect of estrous cycle	Steiner et al. (1980)[984a] Hruska et al. (1982)[506]
Apomorphine-induced stereotyped behaviors	Decreased stereotypy on afternoon of proestrus compared with estrus or diestrus	Kazandjian et al. (1987)[559] Miller (1983)[273a]
Neurochemical Indices		
Dopamine turnover in striatum	Greater dopamine turnover on estrus than on other days of the cycle	Kazandjian et al. (1988)[558]
Amphetamine-stimulated striatal dopamine release in vitro	Greater amphetamine-stimulated striatal dopamine release on estrus than diestrus	Becker and Ramirez (1980)[99]
Spontaneous striatal dopamine release in vitro	Estrous cycle–dependent variation in profile of striatal dopamine release over time	Dluzen and Ramirez (1985)[297a]
Amphetamine-stimulated dopamine release from striatum of freely moving rats determined using in vivo microdialysis	Greater amphetamine-stimulated striatal dopamine release on estrus than on diestrus	Becker and Cha (1989)[98]
D_1 striatal dopamine receptors	There is an increase in the number of D_1 dopamine receptors on diestrus compared to proestrus	Levesque et al. (1989)[624]
D_2 striatal dopamine receptors	No change in the number of D_2 striatal dopamine receptors, increased agonist binding during late diestrus	DiPaolo et al. (1988)[284]

gen reinstates the behavioral response to amphetamine, enhances striatal dopamine turnover, and increases amphetamine-induced dopamine release.[96, 97, 286]

Sex differences are seen in behaviors mediated by the striatum. Male rats exhibit lower rates of rotational behavior, locomotor activity, and stereotypy in response to amphetamine than do female rats in estrus, even when brain concentrations of the drug are demonstrated to be equivalent. In addition, behavior induced by stimulation of the nigrostriatal dopamine system in female rats decreases dramatically following ovariectomy. Castration of male rats, by contrast, has no effect on rotational behavior or on striatal dopamine release induced by amphetamine.[99, 180, 862]

The dose and regimen of hormone administration are important factors mediating the effects of estrogen in the striatum. In both males and females treatment with estrogen in high doses (e.g., 50 to 125 μg of estradiol benzoate or estradiol valerate) or even low doses for prolonged periods (e.g., 0.1 μg of estradiol twice a day for 10 days) results in an increase in amphetamine- and apomorphine-induced behaviors. These treatments also produce an *increase* in the density of striatal dopamine receptors and *decreased* presynaptic dopamine activity. This is in contrast to the effects of acute treatment with physiological doses of estrogen, which causes *decreased* postsynaptic activity and *increased* presynaptic dopamine activity.[283, 285, 507, 625] What causes this dose-dependent effect of estrogen on striatal dopamine systems? Most likely, this effect is caused by the sensitive feedback system between the striatum and substantia nigra. Heightened activity in dopamine neurons activates a negative feedback loop that eventually shuts down dopamine activity at the cell body.

Therefore, the effects of the estrous cycle and of physiological doses of estrogen are quite different from the effects of high doses or prolonged estrogen treatment. Different effects of estrogen doses and treatment schedules are also seen in the reproductive system. Physiological variation in estrogen regulates the reproductive and gestational systems beautifully. In contrast, prolonged estrogen treatment can produce a very different effect—mammary and uterine cancer.

The effects of gonadal steroids on striatal activity are also seen in spontaneous behaviors. In one study, experiments conducted in my laboratory looked at a naturally occurring sensorimotor behavior.[101] Female rats were trained to walk across a narrow beam suspended about 3 feet above the floor. The rats quickly learned to walk across the beam and would do so without being deprived of food. Sensorimotor function was assessed by examing the accuracy of foot placement on the beam. If the foot was placed on top of the narrow beam, that was considered correct. When the foot slipped off the top or grabbed onto the side, that was called a footfault. We found that female rats made fewer footfaults on estrus than on diestrus 1 or proestrus (figure 11.3).

Is this estrous cycle-dependent effect on foot placement mediated by the action of estrogen in the striatum? To address this question, we next trained ovariectomized female rats to walk across the suspended beam. After 2 or 3 weeks of training, their performance had stabilized. These rats then received

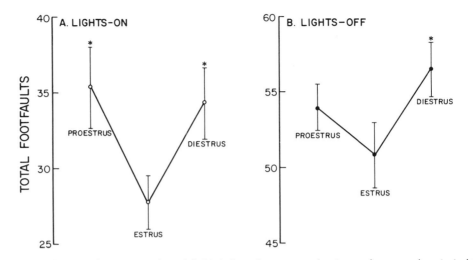

Figure 11.3 The influence of estrous cycle and light-dark cycle on sensorimotor performance in rats trained to walk across a narrow suspended beam. Female rats were repeatedly tested 2 hours after lights on (*A*) or 2 hours after lights off (*B*). The mean number of footfaults made during 3 consecutive days during the estrous cycle is depicted. The bars indicate the standard error of the mean (SEM). Note the different ranges in the scales for *A* and *B*, suggesting that the task was more difficult when animals were tested in the dark (under red-light conditions so that the experimenter could see, but the albino rats could not). The asterisk indicates performance significantly different from estrus (p < .05). (From Becker et al., 1987.[101])

implants of 17β-estradiol or a control substance (cholesterol or the biologically inactive estrogen 17α-estradiol). The implants were inserted bilaterally into the striatum for 6 hours. Within 4 hours there was a dramatic improvement in sensorimotor performance: Rats with cannulae that contained 17β-estradiol were making fewer footfaults! Animals continued to show improvement for 24 hours, and then behavior returned to baseline levels (figure 11.4). Importantly, control implants were ineffective, as were implants that contained 17β-estradiol that missed the striatum. This suggests that estrogen can act directly on the striatum to improve sensorimotor performance. Other work from my laboratory has confirmed neurochemically that estrogen can act directly on the striatum to affect dopamine release in isolated tissue.[96]

How does estrogen induce effects on the striatum? Autoradiography is usually used to identify neurons with estrogen receptors. Studies of this type have shown that the striatum in the adult rodent contains very few neurons that concentrate estrogen in their nucleus. However, as the earlier discussion indicates, there is both behavioral and neurochemical evidence that estrogen can act directly on the striatum to modulate basal ganglial activity.[96, 101, 544, 1068, 1069]

The striatum may not be the only site where hormonal or sex-related differences produce some of the behavioral effects observed. The frontal cortex has extensive input to the striatum, and recent evidence indicates that sex-related differences and hormonal influences also exist in the morphology of neurons in the frontal cortex.[596] Importantly, both the cortex and the striatum,

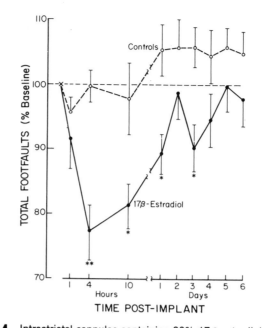

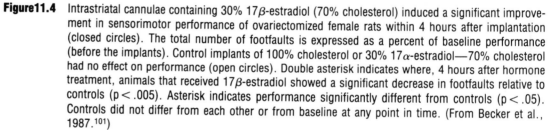

Figure 11.4 Intrastriatal cannulae containing 30% 17β-estradiol (70% cholesterol) induced a significant improvement in sensorimotor performance of ovariectomized female rats within 4 hours after implantation (closed circles). The total number of footfaults is expressed as a percent of baseline performance (before the implants). Control implants of 100% cholesterol or 30% 17α-estradiol—70% cholesterol had no effect on performance (open circles). Double asterisk indicates where, 4 hours after hormone treatment, animals that received 17β-estradiol showed a significant decrease in footfaults relative to controls (p < .005). Asterisk indicates performance significantly different from controls (p < .05). Controls did not differ from each other or from baseline at any point in time. (From Becker et al., 1987.[101])

brain regions previously thought to be devoid of gonadal steroid receptors, have recently been found to contain receptors for estrogen during early postnatal development.[946, 1039] Thus, it seems that our understanding of where, how, and when gonadal steroid hormones act may soon need to be revised. Additional research is needed to determine the specific mechanism(s) through which sensorimotor function and striatal activity are modulated by estrogen and progesterone.

HORMONAL INFLUENCES ON THE STRIATUM:
CLINICAL IMPLICATIONS

One of the rarest complications of pregnancy is the development of chorea. In an analysis that was published in 1950, it was estimated that the incidence of this disorder, known as chorea graviderum, was between 0.015% and 0.035% in the British Isles.[112] In the 1960s and 1970s the association between choreiform movement disorders and ovarian hormones became apparent when it was found that some patients taking oral contraceptives developed chorea.[53, 772] The symptoms of chorea were transient and subsided within 1 to 2 months after oral contraceptive treatment was terminated. In one case study, chorea movements associated with oral contraceptives ceased after the patient stopped taking the medication. Symptoms returned a short time later when the patient became pregnant.[854] Further evidence that ovarian hormones induced behavioral effects symptomatic of basal ganglial disorders came from clinical observations of schizophrenic patients. Chronic estrogen treatment has been reported to precipitate Parkinsonian symptoms in patients receiving neuroleptic drugs.[102]

Hormonal Influences on the Cerebellum

The cerebellum contains complete motor and sensory representations of the body, and its anatomical microstructure has been well characterized. As illustrated in figure 11.5, the cerebellum is a layered structure having five different intrinsic types of neurons. The largest neurons in the cerebellum are known as Purkinje cells. The Purkinje cells send their axons to deep cerebellar neurons to modulate output from the cerebellum to the motor system.

FUNCTIONS OF THE CEREBELLUM
The cerebellum controls the timing and the pattern of muscles activated during movement, postural support, and the integration of vestibular and kinesthetic input with the maintenance of muscle tone. Lesions of the cerebellum produce neither muscle weakness nor disorders of perception, but there is a loss of ability to perform some movements automatically. This occurs because the cerebellum is involved in the control of very rapid or "preprogrammed" movements. In many ways, the functions of the cerebellum are complementary to those of the basal ganglia.

Disorders of the cerebellum result in distinctive symptoms. These include *decomposition of movement* or a failure of synergistic muscles to produce smooth, well-controlled movements. This can result in movements that either overshoot the mark or underestimate a distance as well as *ataxia* (ataxia means loss or lack of muscle coordination). Other symptoms of cerebellar damage include *hypotonia* or loss of muscle tone, and *tremor* during movement. As mentioned earlier, the tremor associated with basal ganglia *damage* occurs during rest. Finally, slurred speech can be a symptom of cerebellar damage.

If electrical activity from a Purkinje cell is recorded in a freely moving rat, Purkinje cell firing is found to be correlated with movement. To conduct these studies, a rat is positioned on a treadmill. When the treadmill is turned on, the animal begins to walk. Activity in a given Purkinje cell is correlated with the movement of one of the limbs. As the rat walks, every time one of its feet reaches a particular place in the step cycle, the Purkinje cell being recorded will fire. The phase of the step cycle that is associated with firing varies from Purkinje cell to Purkinje cell, but all Purkinje cells show this relationship with the step cycle. Complex recording studies in monkeys have shown that movement-correlated firing of cerebellar Purkinje cells precedes changes in

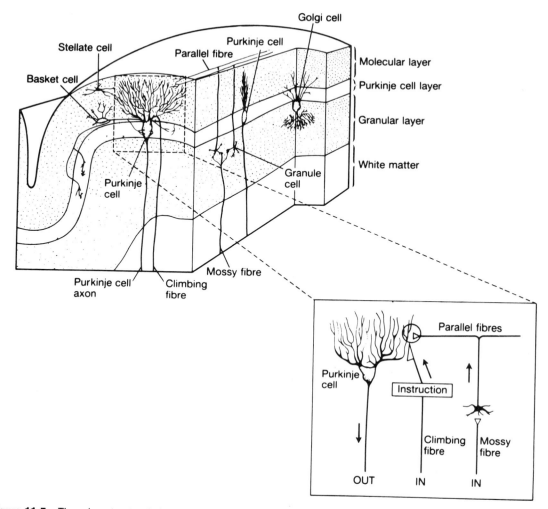

Figure 11.5 The microstructural simplicity and regularity of the cerebellar cortex is illustrated in this figure. Only five types of neurons—Purkinje cells, granule cells, Golgi cells, stellate cells, and basket cells—are organized into three layers of the cerebellar cortex. The sole output from the cerebellar cortex is provided by the Purkinje cells. Input to the cerebellum arrives through the climbing fibers, which synapse on the Purkinje cells, and through the mossy fibers, which synapse on the granule cells. The inset shows a simplified schematic neuronal circuit, illustrating the convergence of the two major cerebellar inputs on the Purkinje cell. (From Dudai, 1989.[309a])

motor cortex neuronal activity. This suggests that the cerebellum may be integrating sensorimotor functions and then activating the appropriate motor output.

HORMONAL INFLUENCES ON CEREBELLAR PURKINJE CELL ACTIVITY

S. S. Smith and colleagues[973] have recorded electrophysiologically from cerebellar Purkinje cells in animals trained to walk on a treadmill. She has shown that both estrogen and progesterone modulate the firing of Purkinje cells during this step cycle-correlated activity. Estrogen augments the movement-correlated increase in Purkinje cell discharge. Progesterone has an opposite or suppressant effect. These two effects are additive. If both hormones are administered together, they counteract one another.

Therefore, in this neuronal system during the proestrous increase in estrogen, the Purkinje cells fire more vigorously during the step cycle. When progesterone begins to increase during the late afternoon of proestrus, the previous effect of estrogen is counteracted. A decrease in the response of Purkinje cells correlated with movement occurs.[973] From these studies one would predict that cerebellum-mediated sensorimotor function would be augmented maximally during the proestrous increase in estrogen. As progesterone increases, this function would be attenuated.

The effects of progesterone on cerebellar Purkinje cell activity are thought to be caused by the binding of progesterone (or one of its metabolites) to receptors for the inhibitory neurotransmitter gamma-aminobutyric acid (GABA). One particular class of GABA receptors, called the $GABA_A$ receptors, has a very high affinity for progesterone and its metabolites.[928] When progesterone is administered to a rat, the response to GABA is potentiated within 30 seconds. This enhanced response to inhibition by GABA is thought to mediate the decrease in movement-associated Purkinje cell activation following progesterone administration.

Possible Implications: Sex-Related Differences and Hormonal Influences on Motor Activity and Sensory Perception

Specific sex-related differences and hormonal effects on striatal and cerebellar function have been demonstrated only recently. It has been known for many years, however, that there are sex-related differences and hormonal influences on many different measures of motor activity and sensory perception. Therefore, the behavioral impact of hormonal modulation of the basal ganglia and cerebellum probably extends beyond those few behaviors and functions described earlier. A survey of some of the other sex-related differences and hormonal influences on motor activity and sensory perception follows to give the student a grasp of how widespread these effects may be. It is possible that the effects of hormones on the striatum or cerebellum are important factors in these behaviors. However, these are complex behaviors, so there may be multiple sites of hormone action that result in the behavioral effects to be discussed.

Determining the neural substrate of the hormonal effects to be discussed will be important for advancing our understanding of these hormone-behavior relations.

MOTOR ACTIVITY

Motor activity depends on the cerebellum for control of gate and posture and on the striatum for components of exploratory motor behavior, including rearing and sniffing. Other brain regions, the nucleus accumbens in particular, are also involved in locomotor activity.

Open-Field Activity When rats are placed in a large open testing arena (about 90×90 cm), females tend to walk around (ambulate) more than males; they also rear more than males, but defecate less. The effect of gonadectomy on open-field activity is sex dependent. Castration of males has no effect, but ovariectomy causes a decrease in ambulation and rearing. The effect of ovariectomy is not consistent, however, because some authors report no effect on open-field behavior.[94, 964, 989, 990]

The administration of either estrogen or androgen to females during the perinatal period of sexual differentiation suppresses open-field behavior in the adult female rat. The absence of androgens and estrogens during the perinatal period is necessary for feminization of this behavior. In addition, exposure of female rats to estrogen during later postnatal development may also be necessary to produce high levels of open-field activity in the adult.[990] In a study by Stewart and Cygan,[990] female and male rats were gonadectomized on day 1; then animals were treated with estrogen for 10 days, either from 10 to 20 days of age or from 30 to 40 days. Either treatment was effective in increasing ambulation and rearing in adults of both sexes. The presence of high concentrations of testosterone or estrogen during the perinatal period suppressed open-field activity. The additional presence of estrogen later in life was apparently necessary to complete the sexual differentiation process that resulted in open-field activity comparable to that seen in normal females.

Locomotor Activity There are species differences in the organizational effects of gonadal hormones on activity. For example, some species of rodents show sex differences in activity but not always under the same conditions as those seen in rats. Mice frequently do not show sex differences in open-field activity. However, if locomotor activity is tested in the home cage, an organizational effect of perinatal hormones on general locomotor activity is seen in mice. Intact females are more active than intact male mice. If male mice are castrated on day 1 of life, then they are more active as adults than males that were castrated after the critical perinatal period. Conversely, if females are given androgens on day 1, they are less active than normal females.

Females that are located in utero between two male fetuses (and therefore exposed in utero to the adjacent males' androgens) exhibit less locomotor activity as adults than females located between two females in utero. Interestingly, male mice are also influenced by intrauterine position. Males located in utero between two females are more active as adults than males located between two males. Therefore, in mice there is a graded effect of perinatal hormones on adult activity. The hormones secreted by an individual mouse as well as those of its adjacent siblings contribute to the animals' activity level as an adult, presumably through sexual differentiation of the brain. Whether there is an additional requirement for estrogen during adolescent development (as was true for rats) has not been investigated.[32, 155, 582]

Sex differences in general activity are probably also prevalent in other species, but few species have been studied as extensively as rats and mice. For example, sex differences in activity have been reported in the African clawed frog *Xenopus laevis*. As was true in rodents, female frogs are more active than males. The organizational or activational role(s) of hormones on activity in *Xenopus* have not yet been investigated.[708]

Running Wheel Activity   The activity of rodents in a running wheel is a curious phenomenon. Anyone who has had a pet hamster or gerbil with an activity wheel in the cage has observed this phenomenon. During the night, hamsters, rats, or gerbils step into the wheel and run the equivalent of miles! In female rodents this behavior is hormonally modulated. There is a dramatic increase in running wheel activity on the evening of behavioral estrus.

Running wheel behavior has been shown to be activated by estrogen in both males and females, and progesterone inhibits the effect of estrogen in activating running wheel activity, although not completely. The preoptic area (POA) of the anterior hypothalamus has been implicated in the mediation of the effects of estrogen on running wheel behavior. Implants of crystalline estradiol into the POA activate running wheel behavior.[1084] It is not clear that this effect is specific to the hypothalamus, however, because implants of estradiol into the striatum also activate running wheel activity.[884]

Other hormones may also modulate wheel running behavior in rodents. For example, in adult rats running wheel behavior decreases when growth hormone secretion increases and vice versa.[42, 568] However, further research is needed to demonstrate cause-and-effect relations between growth hormone and running wheel behavior.

SENSORY PERCEPTION

Tests of sensory perception usually require that an animal make a motor response to indicate its detection of a stimulus. Because of this, hormonal influences in these tests could be due to a direct effect of the hormone on the sensory system, to an effect of the hormone on the brain areas that receive sensory information, or to hormonal influences on the brain regions that transduce the input into the motor output: the striatum and cerebellum.

Chemical Sensation   In many species of mammals, chemical signals originating from other animals of the same species (i.e., pheromones) are detected by a specialized organ in the nasal cavity called the vomeronasal organ. As discussed in chapter 4, the vomeronasal organ is important for activation of male sexual behavior in the rat and for the induction of estrus in the vole. In addition, there are sexual dimorphisms in the detection of pheromones that are mediated by the vomeronasal system.

Hormonal modulation of the vomeronasal system can be demonstrated behaviorally in preference tests. In these tests, male and female rats choose between various odors. Both males and females show a preference for odors from gonadally intact members of the same species (conspecifics). This preference for conspecifics is abolished by gonadectomy and restored by testosterone administration in males or estrogen in females.[957]

Conversely, there is pheromonal modulation of hormonal systems in rodents. As summarized by Simerly,[957] "removal of olfactory bulbs exerts profound effects on copulatory behavior in hamsters and rats, and exposure of female mice that are in various reproductive states to urine from intact male mice can result in the suppression of estrus (Lee-Boot effect), the induction of estrus (Whitten effect), the blockage of pregnancy (Bruce effect), and the acceleration of puberty (van den Bergh effect)." These effects on reproductive functions in mice and other animals are thought to be induced by pheromones and to be mediated by the sexually dimorphic vomeronasal pathway. Other effects of pheromonal activation of the vomeronasal system on sexual behavior will be discussed in chapter 13.

Taste Female rats exhibit a greater preference for sweet tastes (either glucose or saccharin) than do males. The ovarian hormones, estrogen and progesterone, are apparently involved in *establishing* taste preference in adult females. Once the sweet taste preference has been established in the intact female rat, the preference is retained in the absence of the hormones. Ovariectomy has no effect on the behavior. Adult female rats also develop a greater taste preference for salt solutions than do males. Neonatal hormone manipulations can reverse the development of salt taste preferences in adults.[94]

Perhaps related to the hormonal influences on taste preferences, male rats, mice, and guinea pigs eat more than do females of their respective species. This results in sex differences in body weight that are hormone dependent. The effect of hormones on body weight is partly due to activational mechanisms. Estrogen reduces body weight and testosterone increases it in both castrated males and ovariectomized females. However, there are also organizational effects that influence the magnitude of body weight changes induced by estrogen and testosterone in guinea pigs. Male guinea pigs show greater body weight increases in response to testosterone and a smaller decrease in body weight induced by estrogen than do females.[241] It should be noted that in some species (e.g., hamsters and spotted hyenas) females are bigger than males. In these species, one does not find the same relations between hormones and body weight described above for rats, mice, and guinea pigs.

Pain Sensitivity and Analgesia Female rats tend to be more responsive than males to stimulation with electric shock to the feet. This response is indicated by both lower pain thresholds and shorter escape latencies. This sensitivity to shock is modulated by perinatal androgenization and by gonadectomy in the adult. However, it is not always clear in these studies to what extent central mechanisms are involved, since hormonal influences on secondary sex characteristics may also change sensory sensitivity.

For example, estrogen increases fatty deposits whereas testosterone increases muscle mass. Both of these hormonal effects may alter the sensitivity of an animal to tactile stimuli. By measuring both threshold and response latencies (when pain thresholds are being measured, this is called nociceptive reactivity), it is possible to determine whether secondary sex characteristics are interacting with an animal's sensitivity to stimulation. Subsequent studies of sex-related differences in response to pain and analgesia (i.e., relief from pain) have demonstrated that sex differences persist even when nociceptive reactivity is comparable for males and females.[894] Thus, sex-related differences in the central processing of pain and its alleviation (analgesia) may exist.

The endogenous opioids (β-endorphin, enkephalin, and dynorphin) may be involved in sex differences in analgesia. Analgesia induced by either the administration of morphine or intermittent stress (animals are forced to swim in cold water at various time intervals) have been shown to be mediated by opioid systems. The analgesia induced by stress or morphine is greater in males than in females. Administration of morphine into the cerebroventricle also produces a sex difference in analgesia, suggesting that the greater analgesia seen in males is mediated by neural mechanisms.[128]

There are also small but significant effects of gonadal hormones on the analgesic response. Castration of male rats produces a slight reduction in the analgesia induced by intracerebroventricular morphine. In addition, in females there is estrous cycle–dependent variation in both morphine and stress-induced analgesia. Thus, there are activational effects of gonadal hormones on analgesia. The magnitude of the sex difference in the sensitivity to opioid analgesia is much greater than the effect of either castration or the estrous cycle, suggesting that there may also be organizational hormone effects on this system. This question is currently under investigation.[128, 894]

Summary

1. The gonadal hormones can modulate motor function and sensory responsiveness by producing direct effects on both the striatum and the cerebellum. Hormonal modulation of sensorimotor function in the striatum and cerebellum normally occurs during the estrous cycle in female rats and can be mimicked by physiological concentrations of gonadal steroid hormones. In both brain regions, estrogen potentiates neuronal responsiveness. In the cerebellum, but not the striatum, progesterone attenuates the effects of estrogen.

2. Hormones can influence both motor activity and sensory perception in rodents and other species. Sex-related differences in sensation may be mediated by hormonal influences on peripheral components of sensation as well as

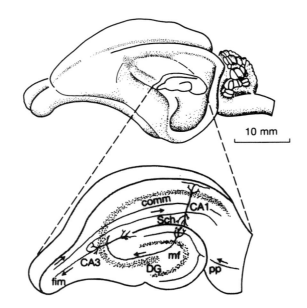

Figure 11.6 The hippocampus in the rat brain. The top illustration shows the position of the C-shaped hippocampus as it is located in the rat brain. A cross-section of the hippocampus is enlarged to illustrate the cell fields of the hippocampus known as CA1 and CA3, and the dentate gyrus (DG). Field CA2 is located between CA1 and CA3, CA4 is found between CA3 and the DG. The perforant pathway (pp) arrives from the overlying region of cortex referred to as the entorhinal cortex and perforates the DG. Axons arriving from the contralateral hemisphere, referred to as the commissural projection (comm), and collaterals from neurons within the hippocampus (Schaffer collaterals, Sch) sprout in response to perforant pathway deafferentation. Other abbreviations: fim, fimbria; mf, mossy fibers. (From Dudai, 1989.[309a])

through sex-related differences in the effect of hormones on the striatum, cerebellum, and other regions of the brain.

In the next section of this chapter, we will see how these hormonal influences and sex-related differences on motor activity and sensory perception may influence our assessment of other functions. In particular, we will examine how assessment of learning and memory, thought to be mediated by the hippocampus, can be affected indirectly by hormones and sex-related differences.

Hormonal Influences on Hippocampal Plasticity

Early neuroanatomists thought that the hippocampus looked like a seahorse, which is how it got its name (hippocampus is Greek for seahorse). In cross-section (figure 11.6) it is a C-shaped structure that looks like a jelly roll, with the dentate gyrus folding around the the cells of the CA3 and CA4 regions of the hippocamus. As can be seen in figure 11.6, input to the hippocampus comes predominantly from the entorhinal cortex through the perforant pathway, from the hippocampal commissure, and from the septal nucleus.

The hippocampus has received considerable attention because of its role in the processes of learning and memory. The importance of the hippocampus in learning and memory became apparent from clinical reports of a patient known as H. M.[729] As a young man, H. M. suffered from severe intractable epilepsy. To stop his epileptic seizures, his hippocampus was removed bilaterally. The neurosurgical procedure also resulted in the bilateral removal of the amygdala and some of the parahippocampal cortex (the temporal cortex was left intact). After the surgery, the epilepsy ceased, and H. M. could remember everything leading up to the surgery except for the last few days before the operation (a phenomenon referred to as retrograde amnesia). What was surprising was that H. M. could no longer form new memories (this is called anterograde amnesia). After these memory deficits were reported, no surgeon ever again intentionally removed the hippocampus bilaterally in human patients. However, in a few cases in which one hippocampus was removed (usually for epilepsy), it was subsequently discovered that the contralateral hippocampus was already damaged. These patients also suffered mild retrograde amnesia and profound anterograde amnesia. The finding that specific memory deficits were associated with lesions of the hippocampus led to considerable research on the role of the hippocampus in learning and memory in other vertebrate species.

No one has established conclusively how the brain forms new memories. But we do know that in response to a learning experience, neurons may change their pattern of synaptic connections to store the memory, and this process, referred to as **neuronal plasticity**, is thought to be reflected in the dendritic arbor of neurons. This is important because the dendrites of a neuron represent about 95% of the available receptor surface and are capable of rapid changes in their shape and their synaptic connections. Changes in specific parts of the dendritic tree are thought to represent specific changes in input to the cell. Furthermore, changes in dendritic morphology of neurons in the cortex, cerebellum, and hippocampus are correlated with learning or experience. For example, an increase in the complexity of dendritic branching in the visual cortex and cerebellum occurs with training in adult rats, and changes in hippocampal morphology occur as a result of experience during development. Also important in the context of this chapter, widespread hormonal effects and sex-related differences in hippocampal function exist that may underlie sex-related differences in learning and memory.

There are at least three different ways that hormones have been shown to affect the hippocampus in rodents. (1) Hormones can affect dendritic outgrowth during development of the hippocampus, after injury, and during the estrous cycle. Hormonal influences on the hippocampus are reflected in sex-related differences in the effect of early rearing conditions on the development of the hippocampus, hormonal modulation of compensatory sprouting that occurs following neuronal injury, and the response of hippocampal neurons to circulating hormones. (2) There are sex-related differences in some learning and memory tasks that suggest that hormones may produce organizational effects on the hippocampus. The impact of hormonal influences on motor activity and sensory perception on behavioral assessment of hippocampal function is an important factor in this regard. (3) Chronic stress hormone secre-

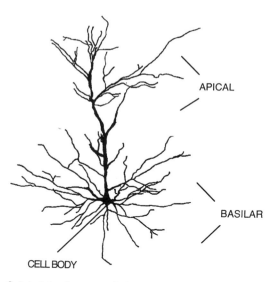

Figure 11.7   Golgi-stained neuron. Apical dendrites are those oriented on the side of the cell body closest to the cortical surface at the top of the figure; basilar dendrites are those farthest from cortex at the bottom of the figure. (Courtesy of Dr. Bryan Kolb.)

tion may result in hippocampal damage and deficits in learning and memory. Each of these hormonal effects on the hippocampus will be discussed in turn.

Sex Differences in the Hippocampus

Sex differences and hormonal sex-related influences on neuronal morphology are found in the hippocampus.[427, 546] The gonadal steroids and glucocorticoids are known to act on specific populations of neurons in the hippocampus. In both males and females estradiol receptors are found only in the CA1 region of the hippocampus. No estradiol receptors are found in other regions of the hippocampus or in the dentate gyrus, and no testosterone receptors are found in the hippocampus.[643] In the CA1 region of the hippocampus, either estrogen or progesterone administration will increase the number of spines and the complexity of branching in apical dendrites (figure 11.7). This suggests that estrogen can affect the synaptic connections that are made between neurons in the hippocampus. The effect of estrogen and progesterone is also seen following ovariectomy, when a decrease in spine density occurs in CA1 pyramidal cells. Estrogen or estrogen plus progesterone can prevent this decrease.[427]

In contrast to gonadal steroid receptors, which are not sexually dimorphic, there are sex-related differences in hippocampal glucocorticoid receptors. Female rats have a larger number of glucocorticoid receptors than males, and ovariectomy increases the number of glucocorticoid receptors even more, whereas castration in the male has no effect on glucocorticoid binding.[1055] The importance of receptors for steroid hormones will become apparent as we see how these hormones can modulate the hippocampal response to experience or injury.

SEX DIFFERENCES IN THE HIPPOCAMPUS AND THE EFFECTS OF EARLY EXPERIENCE

Similar changes are seen in the cortex, cerebellum, and hippocampus when animals are raised in enriched environments where there are other animals and many objects with which to interact. It is thought that these animals have richer experiences than animals raised under normal laboratory conditions and so form more complex memories.[439, 546] As a result of rearing in an enriched environment, male and female rats have larger brains and a thicker cortex.

More subtle effects of rearing in an enriched environment are seen in the hippocampus. Sex differences in the apical dendrites in the CA3 region of the hippocampus and the dentate gyrus have been reported. These sex differences are differently modulated by environmental influences during development. The dendrites of females raised in enriched environments are more concentrated in the apical tree proximal (close) to the soma than are those of males. This sex difference was most prominent in the neurons of females raised in the enriched environment. The direction of sex differences was reversed in the apical dendrites distal to the cell body. Males had a greater proportion of apical distal dendrites than females. As in the proximal dendritic tree, this pattern of sex differences was primarily found in neurons of rats from the enriched environment. There were no sex differences in the basilar dendritic tree of CA3 neurons.[547, 548]

In the dentate gyrus, sex differences were also modulated by environmental influences during rearing. Rearing conditions had very little effect on dentate granule cell morphology in males. By contrast, dentate granule cells of females reared in an enriched environment had increased dendritic length compared with those in females reared in normal laboratory conditions. In comparisons between the sexes, males reared in enriched conditions had a smaller dendritic tree than that of females raised under the same conditions. In contrast, with normal laboratory rearing male rats had a more complex dendritic tree than females.[547, 548]

Thus, as a function of the environment during development the morphology of neurons in the hippocampus is profoundly changed. Because we believe that the morphology of a neuron reflects the synaptic connections it receives from other neurons, the enriched environment is thought to have altered these connections. Learning and memory are thought to be represented by similar changes in neuronal morphology. This effect of the environment on dendritic morphology occurs in different regions of the hippocampus and in different regions of a neuron's dendritic tree depending on the sex of the animal and presumably on the hormones to which the neurons are exposed during development. Since the dentate gyrus and CA3 regions of hippocampus do not have estrogen receptors, but sex differences in glucocorticoid receptors exist in these regions, it is possible that environment-dependent sex differences are mediated by the effects of rearing conditions on adrenal hormone secretions.

HORMONAL MODULATION OF NEURONAL SPROUTING

The effects of steroid hormones are also seen in the hippocampus following damage. When the hippocampus is deafferented by lesions of the entorhinal cortex, rapid growth of new branches from surviving neurons occurs, called sprouting. Sprouting is a form of neuronal plasticity because adult neurons make new synaptic connections as a function of the partial loss of input to the hippocampus. Since it is generally believed that learning requires the formation of new synaptic connections and that memory requires using these new connections, sprouting is considered a simple model of the neuronal changes that occur during learning and memory.

There are sex differences in the sprouting responses that occur following damage to hippocampal input. In addition, sprouting responses are modulated by gonadal steroids and by glucocorticoids. In females, sprouting is decreased by ovariectomy, and estrogen restores sprouting to intact levels. In contrast, adrenalectomy increases the sprouting response to some extent. Females subjected to both adrenal and gonadal removal exhibit a sprouting response that is no different from that in the intact animal. In females, therefore, there is an interaction between the hormones of the adrenals and gonads that modulates the sprouting response.[922, 923]

In males, the effect of adrenal and gonadal hormones is quite different. Castration in males does not affect sprouting, suggesting that testosterone does not play a comparable role to that of estrogen in females. Adrenalectomy also does not affect sprouting in males. However, if males are both adrenalectomized and gonadectomized, sprouting decreases. In the male, the hormones of the gonads and adrenal may serve complementary functions (the adrenal gland also produces androgens) which maintain the sprouting response.[920–923]

If hormonal modulation of sprouting is mediated by the same mechanisms that are acting during normal development, perhaps in females both adrenal and gonadal hormones promote enhanced dendritic branching. In males, gonadal and adrenal hormones seem to produce less effect on neuronal sprouting, and this seems to be reflected during development in neural outgrowth that is influenced less by environmental effects on endocrine systems. How these hormonal influences on hippocampal morphology and plasticity may affect learning and memory will be discussed next.

Sex-Related Differences in Learning and Memory

The study of sex differences in cognitive functions has been a source of controversy for over a century. While a great deal has been written about sex differences in behavior, the amount of tightly controlled research is still quite small. This problem is confounded by the tendency of scientists to avoid the complications associated with ovarian cycles and use only male subjects. However, the existence of sex differences continues to be raised as a phenomenon. As Beatty pointed out in his excellent review of the question,[94] "Despite the long tradition of designing experiments in a manner that precludes discovery of sex

differences in behavior, differences on several behaviors have been described."
I rely heavily on Beatty's review in the discussion that follows.

We will examine the evidence for and against sex differences in various learning paradigms in which sex differences have been evaluated in rodents. The possible underlying mechanisms mediating any sex differences in learning behavior will be discussed. This will include possible sex differences in peripheral effects, or sex differences in sensorimotor function that might contribute to the results reported. Sex differences and hormonal influences on cognitive functions in humans will be discussed in chapter 12.

It should be pointed out that there is also an extensive literature on the acute influence of pituitary and adrenal hormone effects on learning and memory. This topic is quite complex and therefore, unfortunately, is beyond the scope of this chapter. The interested reader is referred to reviews by McGaugh[691] and Martinez.[666]

PASSIVE AVOIDANCE LEARNING

In passive avoidance learning an animal is placed on a platform, and when it steps off the platform it receives a mild shock on its feet. If the next time the animal is placed on the platform it remains passive and does not step down, this is called response suppression, and the animal is said to have retained the memory of the previous training experience. Male rats and gerbils show greater response suppression than do females on this task. This has been interpreted by many to indicate that males learn passive avoidance tasks better than female rats or gerbils.[94]

Do gonadal hormones activate this behavior? The results are not clear. Ovariectomy is reported to have no effect on passive avoidance behavior in female rats. In contrast, castration of male rats has been reported to decrease response suppression. In a conflicting report, no effect of castration has also been reported.[94, 107]

The sex difference in response suppression on this task appears to depend on a number of factors. First, the interval between training and subsequent retest is a factor. If passive avoidance is tested immediately after training, there is no sex difference. Only when testing is delayed does the sex difference emerge. A number of investigators have attempted to dissociate the variables contributing to this sex difference. Factors that have been eliminated include age, weight, shock intensity, and an active adrenal gland. This means that sex differences can be dissociated from differences in age and weight. It can't be just that males and females sense different shock intensities because sex differences persist with a variety of shock intensities. Finally, the sex difference persists when adrenal steroid release is suppressed pharmacologically, so sex differences in adrenal steroid secretion cannot be responsible for mediating this effect.[307, 480, 1073]

Interestingly, if females are given a choice between entering a compartment where they have never been shocked in or entering the one where they received the shock, females do not enter the shock-paired compartment, indicating that they have retained the memory of what happened in the shock-paired compartment.[1066]

So why is it that females show less response suppression on passive avoidance tasks than males? As discussed earlier, female rats tend to be more active than males. One possibility is that shock reduces activity to a greater extent in males than in females. Heinsbroek and colleagues (1988) have shown that passive avoidance training suppresses open-field activity to a greater extent in males than in females. Since male rats are already less active than females, the additional suppression by the presentation of shock in males may tend to exaggerate sex differences in activity. The sex difference in passive avoidance "learning" may simply be a reflection of the sex difference in activity. In other words, after receiving shock, males are less active. The response suppression may reflect simply the decreased activity rather than a superior cognitive representation of the learned behavior.[477, 478]

ACTIVE AVOIDANCE LEARNING

In active avoidance learning, animals learn that in response to a cue (e.g., a light or a tone) they must quickly move to another part of the test chamber to avoid being shocked. As summarized by Beatty,[94] female rats learn to respond appropriately more rapidly than do males. The magnitude of the effect varies with the strain of rat and with the specific avoidance task. No sex difference is reported in gerbils or hamsters.

Work from Beatty's laboratory and others indicates that organizational influences of androgens during the prenatal period in the rat may mediate some of the sex differences seen in active avoidance learning. Castration of male rat pups at birth or treatment with an antiandrogen increases the rate of acquisition of avoidance learning in males to a rate comparable to that seen in females. Conversely, treatment of female rat pups with testosterone perinatally, usually combined with testosterone treatment in the adult, impairs acquisition of avoidance behavior. When adrenal cortex activity is depressed by repeated treatments with dexamethasone, sex differences in acquisition of active avoidance behavior persist. This indicates that sex differences in the release of adrenal cortex hormones do not underlie the sex difference in acquisition of an active avoidance response.[481]

As was the case with passive avoidance learning, it is likely that sex differences in activity underlie the sex difference in acquisition of active avoidance learning. Females are generally more active, and they are less likely than males to show suppression of activity following shock. Therefore, a task that requires an animal to walk actively into another compartment to avoid a shock is probably biased in favor of females.

While females acquire active avoidance responses more rapidly, extinction of avoidance behavior occurs more rapidly in males than in females. When adrenal cortex activity is depressed, the rate of extinction is the same for females as for males. The rate of extinction in males is not affected by depression of adrenal cortex activity.[481] This suggests that sex differences in the rate of extinction may be mediated by sex differences in the pituitary-adrenal axis. Estrogen, progesterone, and testosterone have also been reported to influence extinction of avoidance behavior, but the direction of the effect varies. More research is needed before a cohesive picture of the influence of gonadal steroids on extinction of active avoidance behaviors can emerge.

DIFFERENTIAL REINFORCEMENT OF LOW RATE RESPONDING (DRL)
Training an animal to push a lever at a very low rate (e.g., once per minute), is called DRL. Female rats learn to perform a DRL task more efficiently than males. This means that females make fewer unreinforced responses than do males during acquisition of the behavior. This sex difference is due at least in part to the sex difference in general activity. Between responses, female rats tend to engage in other activities, whereas males do not. If males are provided with an alternative response in which to engage during DRL training, their rates of acquisition of the behavior are comparable to those of females.[94, 1070]

TASTE AVERSION
When a treatment that makes an animal feel sick is paired with a novel taste, animals will develop an aversion for the taste. For example, if an animal drinks saccharine and then receives lithium chloride, the animal will feel sick for a while and learns to associate the sick feeling with the saccharine. Male rats acquire taste aversions at lower concentrations of saccharine than those required for females.[244] The sex difference in the acquisition of taste aversions may be related to the sex difference in taste preference. Since females tend to have a greater preference for saccharine than do males, it is possible that this preference interacts with the aversive association. To develop a taste aversion for saccharine, females must overcome an initial greater preference for the taste of saccharine. The possible interaction between sex differences in taste preferences and taste aversions has not been studied experimentally.

The acquisition of a taste aversion does not appear to be hormonally dependent. However, male rats are slower to extinguish a taste aversion after it has been developed. The slow rate of extinction is determined by the hormonal state of the animal during the extinction procedure. Administration of testosterone to either males or females can produce the male-like, slow pattern of taste aversion extinction. Estrogen ameliorates this effect, speeding the rate of extinction.[195, 196]

COMPLEX MAZE LEARNING
Maze tasks are frequently used to assess more complex problem-solving abilities. Mazes vary in difficulty, the most simple being the **T-maze**, in which a rat must run down an alley and choose whether to turn right or left to obtain a goal. A more complex maze has multiple choice points. Much more complex tests include the **radial-arm maze**, in which an animal has to choose whether to enter arms (usually 8 to 17 different arms) that project off a center island in a radial fashion, or the **Morris water maze**, in which a rat must find a hidden

platform while swimming in a large pool. Maze tasks, especially the radial arm maze and the Morris water maze, are considered tests of **spatial abilities** in rodents because animals usually solve these maze tasks by using cues from the surroundings outside of the maze. Each of these tasks can be modified to become nonspatial tests by placing cues within the maze (proximal cues) for the animal to use.

The hippocampus in rats is thought to be essential for solving tasks that require the animal to use its spatial abilities. In other words, animals without a hippocampus have a difficult time solving mazes like the Morris water maze or the radial-arm maze when only spatial cues are available. If the task is changed so that it can be solved with landmarks or proximal cues, the same animals have no problem with the task.

Studies that have found sex differences in maze learning in rats, have most often reported that males learn to solve a maze with fewer errors than females. There are probably two components to the errors made in a complex maze— inappropriate exploratory behavior and inappropriate general activity. Beatty[94] argues that most of these mazes are just open fields, with many additional walls. Females make more errors on such a task because they are more active. The argument is that the greater activity of females translates into "errors" in the maze.

T-Maze Learning: Spatial Alternation Spatial alternation in a T-maze requires animals to alternate the direction in which they turn at the choice point in each trial. It has been reported that male rats are superior to females on spatial response alternation in a T-maze. Since this task is less like an open field than most complex mazes, it is more difficult to make the case that this sex difference is mediated by sex differences in activity levels. However, sex differences in exploratory activity may still underlie this effect.[1111]

Variation in Sex Differences on Performance of Complex Maze Learning In studies of sex-related differences in complex maze performance in the vole (a small field mouse), two species of vole that differ in spontaneous activity levels were compared. These investigators found that meadow voles were more active than prairie voles but that errors on complex maze tasks (seven different mazes were used) did not vary with activity level. Furthermore, the two vole species showed different sex-related differences in maze performance. In the prairie vole, females were more active than males, but females made fewer errors than males on the mazes.[394] In the meadow vole (the more active species), females were less active than males but made more errors than males on the mazes. When the hippocampus of the meadow vole was examined, the hippocampus of the male was found to be 11% larger than that of the female.[394, 527] By contrast, in a third species of vole, the pine vole, there was no sex-related difference in maze performance or in the size of the hippocampus.[527] Thus, the effect of activity on complex maze performance can be dissociated from sex differences in spatial tasks in the vole. It should also be pointed out that the presence and even the direction of the sex-bias may vary with the species.

Radial-Arm Maze Learning   An alternative strategy in trying to distinguish sex differences in maze learning from differences in exploration or activity is to look at behavior in a maze where performance is less influenced by general activity. Three studies have investigated sex differences in performance in the radial-arm maze. In two studies, male and female rats were found to solve the maze task in the same amount of time and with the same number of trials.[545, 1067] In one report, sex differences in the number of errors were found. In this study, males were more likely to adopt a successful strategy of visiting adjacent arms than were females.[321]

The difference in response strategy may provide interesting information about sex differences in spatial learning. Drawing from this idea, Williams and associates[1102] have looked at sex differences and the effects of perinatal hormone manipulations (estrogen treatment on days 1, 3, 5, 7, and 9 to masculinize females, castration on day 1 to feminize males) in a version of the radial-arm maze that allows the investigator to address questions of response strategy more directly. These investigators used a 12-arm maze in which the food cup at the end of eight of the arms always contained food (baited), while four of the arms never contained food (unbaited). The errors made by the animal provide information about both reference or long-term memory (remembering not to go into the unbaited arms) and working or short-term memory (remembering the baited arms that have already been visited during the trial). They found that males, or masculinized females, showed faster acquisition of the radial-arm maze task and increased working memory capacity during acquisition than did females or feminized males. Following acquisition of the radial-arm maze task, there were no sex differences.

Further tests, manipulating cues within the maze (landmarks) and outside the maze (geometry), demonstrated that males or masculinized females used fewer cues (geometry only) than did females or feminized males, who used both landmarks and geometry to solve the maze task. The idea presented by these investigators is that spatial abilities (the ability to use only geometry to solve the maze) are promoted by perinatal exposure to gonadal steroids, perhaps through an effect of estrogen on the hippocampus.[1102]

Morris Water Maze Learning   Of all maze tasks, the one thought to have the fewest sexual biases is the Morris water maze (when water temperature is controlled). In the Morris water maze animals must swim to a submerged platform using cues from the environment external to the maze (i.e., spatial cues) to find the platform. In one experiment that looked at performance of males and females on this task, no sex differences were found. Males and females learned where the hidden platform was in the same number of trials. Swim time (the amount of time it took to find the platform) and directional accuracy (the direction in which the animals headed when first placed in the maze) were comparable for both sexes.[1025, 1026] Whether sex differences would be found if the task were made more difficult has not been investigated.

Interestingly, Therrien found that there were sex differences after removal of the hippocampus. Male rats showed severe deficits in performance after unilateral removal of the hippocampus (either left or right side). After removal of the right hippocampus, females were not as impaired in the Morris water maze task as were male rats. But they were just as impaired as males after removal of the left hippocampus. Female rats had greater behavioral deficits after bilateral hippocampus removal than did males. Thus, it seems that there are sex differences in hippocampal function mediating performance on the Morris water maze that are revealed when the hippocampus is damaged. Further research is needed to determine the contribution of this factor to sex differences in morphology and function of the hippocampus.

The gonadal hormones are not the only steroid hormones that may be important for hippocampal function and the modulation of learning and memory. The glucocorticoids, produced and released by the adrenal cortex in response to stress, may also affect the hippocampus and learning and memory.

Effects of Chronic Stress Hormones on the Hippocampus and Learning and Memory

As summarized by McEwen and Brinton recently,[688] "the pituitary-adrenal axis has two principal modes of operation: diurnal variations in secretion and a stimulus-coupled mode which occurs during stress-induced activity." There is a daily rhythm of glucocorticoid secretion that is thought to be important for behavioral activation during the appropriate phase of the light-dark cycle. There are also stress-associated changes in adrenal secretions that are superimposed on the diurnal rhythm. These two effects of glucocorticoids may be mediated by two different receptor populations in the brain. The response to diurnal variation of low concentrations of glucocorticoids is thought to be mediated by the corticosteroid receptors. These are high-affinity receptors that are found in specific brain regions, including the hippocampus, septum, and amygdala. The response to stress is thought to be be mediated by the second type of receptor, the glucocorticoid receptor. These receptors are found more uniformly throughout the brain and the periphery (i.e., kidney, liver, and so on). Thus, the glucocorticoids can affect the brain through two different mechanisms: acute diurnal modifications of hippocampal activity and long-term adaptive responses to stress mediated by changes in activity throughout the brain and body.[688]

As animals get older, there is a tendency for individuals to begin to show memory deficits. A loss of cells in the hippocampus is implicated in the onset of age-associated memory loss. It seems that in addition to the effects of glucocorticoids on neuronal development and plasticity discussed above, the glucocorticoids might influence how many neurons the hippocampus loses during aging.[902–904, 911, 914]

Many changes in the body and brain are associated with aging in addition to the loss of neurons in the hippocampus. For example, with aging there is an elevation in the level of serum glucocorticoids. There is also a failure to terminate glucocorticoid secretion after a stressful incident. To find out if these two events are related, Landefeld and colleagues[611] removed the adrenal gland in middle-aged rats (12 months old). Low levels of glucocorticoids were then given to the animals. This combination of treatments prevented the rise in serum glucocorticoids that typically accompanies aging. When these animals were examined in old age (1 year later), their hippocampi had *not* lost neurons. Perhaps more important, these rats also did not have the memory problems that usually plague aged rats.

Sapolsky asked whether elevated glucocorticoid levels could accelerate aging in two related studies. In one study, animals received treatments that produced high levels of circulating glucocorticoid concentrations for 3 months. The amount of glucocorticoids the animal received was comparable to the levels seen after major stressors. The hippocampi of these young rats were found to have lost neurons and to have degenerated to the extent seen in aged rats. Sex differences in the effects of glucocorticoids on hippocampal function have not been investigated, but since there are sex differences in glucocorticoid receptors in the hippocampus it would be an interesting topic.

Sapolsky points out that the glucocorticoid-induced degeneration of hippocampal neurons has an insidious implication. You will recall from the last chapter that in addition to its role in learning and memory, the hippocampus inhibits CRH release. Recall also that in response to stress, a large number of hormones are secreted, and feedback then occurs to terminate these secretions. The hippocampus serves as an additional "brake" to terminate CRH secretion, thereby inhibiting secretion of the adrenal steroids. When the CA3 region of the hippocampus is damaged, there is increased secretion of CRH and consequently an increase in the secretion of ACTH and the hormones of the adrenal cortex. This creates a vicious circle. With damage to the hippocampus there is increased secretion of glucocorticoids. The increased glucocorticoids produce additional hippocampal damage, and so on. It seems, therefore, that glucocorticoid levels may be elevated in aged rats because of prior damage to the hippocampus caused by glucocorticoids.[702, 910, 912]

Does this mean that hippocampal damage and memory loss are an inevitable consequence of aging? Some recent research suggests that there still is hope. An animal's early experience has a dramatic influence on the development of its brain and endocrine systems. For example, rats that are handled as infants have lower resting levels of glucocorticoids as adults. Sapolsky and colleagues reasoned that these animals should be exposed to lower cumulative glucocorticoid levels over their lifetimes, and have less hippocampal degeneration. This is what they found. Rats that had been handled once a day for 2 weeks as infants, in old age had not lost hippocampal neurons. These animals also did not have the memory problems typical of aged rats, and their hippocampal brake still functioned as in young rats.

How do glucocorticoids damage the hippocampus? These hormones seem to endanger hippocampal neurons in some way. You will recall from chapter 10 that the effect of glucocorticoids in the periphery is to mobilize energy stores. They do this by blocking glucose transport into cells. At first, during times of acute stress, for example, this may benefit neuronal function by providing more glucose to neurons and facilitating learning and memory. However, the glucocorticoids can also block glucose transport into neurons. The effect is not large. There is only a 20% to 30% inhibition of glucose uptake by glucocorticoids in neurons. But this may be enough to put hippocampal neurons at risk during periods of chronic stress when the increase in available glucose can no longer compensate for the decrease in glucose uptake.

This damage occurs because neurons are already very susceptible to demands on energy and oxygen supply. Neurons are some of the most metabolically active cells in the body. Furthermore, neurons use glucose as their primary energy source. They depend upon the rest of the body to provide them with a continuous supply of glucose and, of course, oxygen. If there is a significant drop in neuronal glucose uptake due to a glucocorticoid-mediated stress response, the neurons in the hippocampus may be among the first neurons to be damaged if there is some additional trauma, such as loss of oxygen. In fact, it has been demonstrated that glucocorticoids exacerbate damage to the hippocampus induced by seizure, hypoxia-ischemia, or hypoglycemia.[902–904]

If glucocorticoids or stressors cause comparable damage in the human hippocampus, this has important implications for the treatment of clinical symptoms of brain damage. Neurologists frequently administer glucocorticoids to control brain swelling when treating victims with neurological injuries. This might not be the best treatment because they might be increasing hippocampal damage. Alternatives to glucocorticoids to control the swelling should probably be considered.

Many of us undergo stressful lives. Are we all producing irreparable damage to a vital part of our brain that is going to result in senescence later in life? Hundreds of thousands of people each year receive high doses of glucocorticoids to control autoimmune disorders (to take advantage of the immunosuppressive actions of the hormones). Is this producing brain damage? We don't yet know the answers to these questions.

Some rather frightening data have emerged recently, however, from studies of nonhuman primates. In one study, fetal monkeys were exposed to high concentrations of the synthetic glucocorticoid dexamethasone. In another study, adult monkeys had glucocorticoid-secreting pellets implanted into the hippocampus for 1 year. In the third study, the brains of monkeys who were under a great deal of social stress and had died of peptic ulcers were examined. In all three studies, damage occurred preferentially in the hippocampus. The pattern of damage in the hippocampus was very similar to that seen in the rodent studies described above.[916, 1060] These results suggest that when careful studies are carried out on chronically stressed humans or those who have received glucocorticoids for long periods of time, the news will not be good. Prolonged stress may come to be viewed as neurodegenerative.

On the other hand, I wouldn't recommend that you have your adrenal glands removed to ensure preservation of your hippocampus in old age. A recent report by Sloviter and associates[965] indicates that complete removal of the adrenal gland of rats also produces selective loss of cells in the dentate gyrus region of the hippocampus 3 to 4 months later. Animals that received low amounts of corticosterone in their drinking water had hippocampi that were preserved. In other words, a small amount of glucocorticoids seems to preserve some hippocampal cells. Too little or too much results in neuronal degeneration of others.[965]

Summary

1. Hormonal modulation of hippocampal neuron morphology and hormonal influences on plasticity occur in response to experiences during development or to injury. The dendritic morphology of the hippocampus in females is influenced to a greater extent by experience than is that of males. This suggests that no one single typical pattern of female brain exists, but that there is greater plasticity in the hippocampus (and other brain regions) of females. Some of the variation noted between species in sex-related differences in learning and memory may be due in part to species differences in rearing or living environment.

2. Many standard tests of learning and memory require that an animal either remain still, exhibit a specific pattern of locomotor activity, or become active when a cue is presented. Sex differences in sensorimotor function, and in particular sex differences in motor activity and sensory perception, may bias the results of such tests in favor of males or females. When tests of learning and memory that do not have this bias are used, sex differences are present but are minimal. In spite of the small sex differences noted in acquisition of spatial tasks, it is important to remember that criterion performance is no different for males and females in any of the tests of learning and memory. Both males and females are capable of performing the tasks with equal facility, but different cognitive strategies seem to be employed.

3. Stress hormones produce long-term effects on the hippocampus. Specifically, the glucocorticoids can endanger hippocampal neurons. This damage results in the eventual degeneration of these neurons and is correlated with deficits in learning and memory. The effects of stress hormones on the hippocampus are not all bad. Low concentrations of glucocorticoids are required to sustain granule cells in the dentate gyrus. The chronic presence of stress hormones in high concentrations, however, is detrimental to the hippocampus and endangers these neurons, leading to memory deficits. It is possible that these effects of stress hormones contribute to the memory deficits found in aging animals and humans.

General Summary

Are there any common themes to guide the student? The effects of hormones on the brain and behavior discussed in this chapter were chosen to illustrate both the variety and the inter-relatedness of hormone-brain-behavior relations. All of the neural systems mediating sex-related differences and hormonal modulation of motor activity, sensory perception, learning, and memory remain to be elucidated, but the striatum, cerebellum, and hippocampus are certainly involved, and the impact of hormones on these functions is closely related.

1. We have seen that there are sex-related differences in the activational effects of gonadal steroid hormones. In females, removal of gonadal steroids attenuates whereas estrogen treatment enhances striatal dopamine activity, cerebellar Purkinje cell activity, and hippocampal spine density and dendritic sprouting. By contrast, in males castration does not alter striatal dopamine activity or hippocampal sprouting. The effects of castration on Purkinje cell activity have not been investigated. Thus, one common component of the sex-related differences in the functions of these three brain regions is that in the female there is variation in activity during the estrous cycle, whereas in the male endogenous gonadal steroid hormones do not modulate neural activity.

2. The striatum, cerebellum, and hippocampus mediate complex behaviors. Therefore, making the leap from anatomical, electrophysiological, and chemical indices of neuronal function to spontaneous behaviors is not easy. However, many behaviors that are used as indices of activity in the cerebellum, striatum, or hippocampus show patterns of hormonal modulation that reflect those of the mediating brain region. For example, if estrogen has an activational effect on behavior, sensory perception and motor activity are enhanced. By contrast, testosterone has less effect on motor activity or sensory perception found in adult animals. In regard to learning and memory, the developmental influences of gonadal and adrenal hormones on the hippocampus may have a greater effect on the expression of sex-related differences than the activational effects of these hormones, although estrous cycle influences on spatial abilities have not been investigated.

3. Finally, in both the hippocampus and the striatum, chronic hormone exposure can have very different effects than acute hormone treatment. Chronic glucocorticoids put hippocampal neurons at risk and can lead to neuronal death. Chronic estrogen in the striatum has an effect opposite to that of acute estrogen. Striatal dopamine function is suppressed with chronic estrogen exposure and enhanced with acute estrogen. Similar dose-response characteristics may be important in other endocrine relations as well.

Acknowledgments

My thanks to William Beatty, Marc Breedlove, David Crews, Janice Juraska, Bryan Kolb, Bruce McEwen, Terry Robinson, and Ed Roy for their comments on earlier versions of this manuscript. The section of this chapter on chronic glucocorticoids was adapted from a summary written by Robert Sapolsky. Supported by USPHS grants NS22157 and NS25662 (RCDA) to JBB.

12 Sex Differences and Hormonal Influences on Cognitive Function in Humans

Elizabeth Hampson and Doreen Kimura

This may be one of the more controversial and challenging chapters in this book. There is one species that, because it has an excellent brain and will attempt even very difficult tasks, allows us to examine higher cognitive function. That species is Homo sapiens, *of course. But these are very complicated creatures that have a social history stretching back long before they came to the laboratory, a history over which we have no control. Perhaps, then, it is not too surprising that there are great individual differences in cognitive function that make it difficult to detect possible differences between populations (say men versus women, or women during the luteal phase versus the follicular phase of the ovulatory cycle). As you will see, there are small but reliable sex differences in cognitive function. There is even evidence that adult hormones contribute to these subtle differences in humans. Furthermore, contrary to popular notions, one sex does not have superiority in all cognitive functions in which there are sex differences. Sometimes males are better, sometimes females are better.*

How does one measure cognitive function in humans, and which of these measures reveal sex differences? Are such differences the result of hormonal or experiential differences? How do changes in gonadal hormone levels affect cognition and the lateralization of function?

Introduction

In the past 25 or 30 years, behavioral endocrinology has become a burgeoning science. By far the bulk of the research in this area has focused on nonhuman species, in which it is possible to manipulate hormones experimentally and study the resultant effects on the brain and behavior. Much of this research has focused on the steroid hormones secreted by the gonads, specifically, androgens, estrogens, and progestins. The influence of these hormones has been shown to extend far beyond the reproductive organs; they are essential to the normal sexual differentiation of the brain during development and to the production and maintenance of sexually dimorphic behaviors throughout life. Much less research attention has been devoted to the study of hormonal modulation of *human* behavior, in part because of the methodological difficulties inherent in such research. As a result, very little can be said definitively about how, in conjunction with cultural and psychosocial factors, hormonal factors may influence human behavior. Nevertheless, a small but growing body of evidence suggests that human behavior also may be influenced by the hormonal milieu, presumably through its myriad actions on brain structure and function. In this chapter, we will review some of the evidence showing that gonadal steroids can affect human behavior, conceptualizing the effects according to the traditional organizational versus activational distinction observed in nonhuman species, and focusing mainly on specific cognitive (or intellectual) abilities and motor skills.

Sex Differences in Cognitive Abilities

In nonhuman species, the behaviors that have been shown to be influenced either by sex hormones present during some critical developmental period or by hormones present in the mature organism tend to be sexually dimorphic. That is, they show qualitative or quantitative differences between the two sexes. This is not to say that behaviors that do not show sex differences are immune to the effects of hormones necessarily, merely that the effect of the gonadal hormones may be most evident among sexually dimorphic behaviors. Therefore, in humans, we might expect the influence of gonadal hormones to be most evident in behaviors that show consistent sex differences. We must, however, be careful in making any inferences about hormonal effects simply on the basis of sex differences. Some differences, such as how men and women dress, are clearly under cultural or environmental control, and it would be far-fetched to hypothesize a hormonal effect on these behaviors. The role of nature seems predominant in other differences, such as sex differences in muscular strength or voice frequency. There are many other sexually dimorphic behaviors in which the relative roles of nature versus nurture are more difficult to delineate, including sex differences in a number of cognitive or intellectual abilities.

On standardized tests of intelligence, there are no sex differences in the general IQ. But men, on average, differ from women, on average, in a number of more specific abilities. For some abilities, the difference favors males, for others the difference favors females. We say "on average" because it is not possible to predict, merely on the basis of sex, whether a particular man or a particular woman will be good or bad at a particular task. Figure 12.1 shows a hypothetical situation in which ability A is measured by the same paper-and-pencil test in adult men and women. The frequency distribution of scores is plotted separately for each sex. In a typical situation, the frequency distributions overlap considerably, and the means are only slightly different for the two sexes. Assuming equal variances in the two distributions, this means that the number of individuals scoring above a given point will be different for the two sexes. In our hypothetical example, the mean for females is higher than the mean for males by about half a standard deviation, which means that only about 25% to 30% of males score above the female mean. Although this is a hypothetical situation, and actual sex differences do not always favor

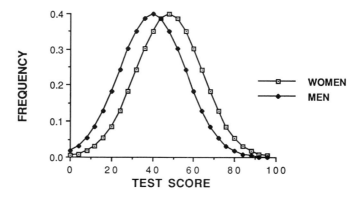

Figure 12.1 Scores for men and women on a test measuring hypothetical cognitive ability, plotted separately for each sex. The vertical axis shows the probability of obtaining any particular test score.

Table 12.1 Abilities That Typically Show Sex Differences in Humans

MALE ADVANTAGE	FEMALE ADVANTAGE
Spatial abilities	Verbal abilities
Quantitative abilities	Perceptual speed and accuracy
Strength	Fine motor skills

women, several cognitive abilities do in fact show sex differences of approximately this size. Sex differences in specific cognitive or motor abilities are often of this type: relatively small in size compared to the more striking sex differences in behavior usually studied in nonhuman species.

Many sex differences in cognitive and motor abilities have been reported, and there is a very extensive literature on the topic (for reviews see Halpern,[453] Hyde et al.,[516] Jarvik,[530] Linn and Petersen,[637] Maccoby and Jacklin,[647] Tyler[1056]). Among the more widely recognized sex differences in ability are those listed in table 12.1. We will be referring to several of these abilities throughout this chapter.

Spatial ability is measured by tests that require the subject to imagine the rotation of a depicted object, or what an object would look like when folded together or seen from a different perspective, without these physical changes actually occurring. Other spatial tests require the subject to imagine changes in the relative positions of objects, to recognize specified shapes that are embedded in a more complex visual array, to read a map, or to solve a maze problem. Although we will be referring to these collectively as tests of spatial ability, factor analytic studies in fact have shown that there are at least three different subtypes of spatial ability, all showing a sex difference in favor of males. These subabilities are referred to as spatial orientation, spatial visualization, and flexibility of closure. Sample items from tests known to load on each of the three spatial factors are shown in figure 12.2. The sex difference varies in size depending on the test and subability being measured, with the

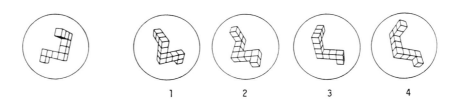

SPATIAL ORIENTATION

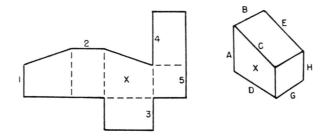

SPATIAL VISUALIZATION

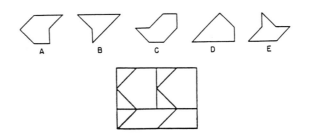

FLEXIBILITY OF CLOSURE

Figure 12.2 Sample items from tests measuring three different aspects of spatial ability. Many tests of *spatial orientation* require the subject to rotate a configuration mentally in space (top). In this example, which of the figures on the right correspond to the target figure on the left? (Choices 1 and 3 are correct). Tests of *spatial visualization* often require stimulus transformations or dynamic serial operations (middle). In this example, the lettered edges on the object are to be matched with the corresponding numbers on the unfolded pattern. *Flexibility of closure* refers to the ability to disembed a target configuration from a more complex pattern or design (bottom). In this example, which one of the simple figures A to E is embedded within the complex pattern shown? (Choice A is correct). (From Vandenberg, S. G. [1976][1061]; *Mental Rotations Test*, In R. B. Ekstrom, J. W. French, and H. H. Harmon (Eds.), *Manual for Kit of Factor-Referenced Cognitive Tests*, Educational Testing Service, Princeton, N.J. Reprinted by permission.)

largest differences typically being reported on the more difficult tests requiring the imagination of three-dimensional rotations in space (e.g., see figure 12.2, top), where differences as large as almost one standard deviation have been reported.[898] On less difficult but still demanding spatial tasks, the average sex difference is usually around 0.5 standard deviation in size. Spatial ability is important for competent performance in a number of occupations, such as architecture, engineering, carpentry, mechanics, or any other occupation requiring large amounts of visualization in the absence of real-world stimuli.

Sex differences in spatial ability have been demonstrated in adults across a number of Western and non-Western cultures,[1108] and may also occur in nonhuman species, at least insofar as comparable tasks can be devised.[393, 1102] Much of the existing literature on hormonal effects on human cognitive abilities has focused on spatial ability because the sex difference is relatively large and is found very consistently. Also, the sex difference in spatial ability has been reported not to appear in full force until puberty, raising the possibility that hormonal changes occurring at that time may play some role in its ontogenesis.

It is often assumed that all sex differences favor men, but this is definitely not the case. Sex differences that favor women have been reported in a variety of verbal skills, including spelling, grammar, rate of acquisition of speech in childhood, and ability to comprehend or decode language. Also, boys more often than girls show language impairments, such as stuttering or dyslexia (inability to read). An aspect of language production that often shows sex differences is verbal fluency, which is defined as a facility in thinking rapidly of appropriate words, phrases, or sentences. In the laboratory, fluency can be assessed by having subjects write down or orally report, within a specified time limit, as many words as possible that meet a particular phonetic or semantic criterion. For example, subjects may be asked to report all the words they can think of beginning with the letter J within 1 minute, or all the words they can think of that belong to some category, such as birds.

Sex differences in verbal abilities are often on the order of 0.25 standard deviation units but vary tremendously in size depending on the specific verbal skill being measured. For example, Hines[490] reported a large sex difference in some preliminary data on a difficult associational fluency task (a task requiring subjects to generate words similar in meaning to a given word). The task showed sex differences of approximately 1 standard deviation in size. Sex differences in vocabulary, as assessed by tests sampling knowledge of word meanings, are occasionally reported, and more often than not these differences favor females. However, maybe because vocabulary tests are highly related to general intelligence, which does not show sex differences, and to educational or socioeconomic level, sex differences in vocabulary tend to be very small and are not reported consistently. In a recent review article, Hyde and Linn[517] reported that sex differences in verbal abilities are actually decreasing in size over time. But their review emphasized verbal tests, such as vocabulary and reading comprehension, which are not known to show reliable sex differences in adults. It should also be noted that many current verbal tests have been standardized to help eliminate the sex differences favoring females that appeared on earlier versions of the tests, e.g., the SAT-Verbal.

Women typically also outperform men in certain nonverbal abilities such as some tests of short-term memory that use either verbal or pictorial stimuli. For example, Galea and Kimura[386] gave men and women 1 minute to view a display consisting of 40 pictures of animals and common objects, randomly arrayed. After a 20-minute delay, women were able to recall significantly more of the items than men, even though there was no sex difference in recall when subjects were tested immediately following the stimulus presentation. A similar sex difference was reported by Wilson and Vandenberg[1104] in a very large-scale study of cognitive abilities conducted in Hawaii. This difference may seem paradoxical given the sex difference in spatial ability, but it is important to recognize that no dynamic transformations are required to memorize designs or other pictorial stimuli. There has been relatively little research in this area, however.

Women also have the advantage in tests of perceptual speed and accuracy. This is defined as the ability to perceive quickly and accurately the details of a visual array. The sex difference in this ability favors women regardless of whether the visual material to be scanned is verbal or nonverbal in nature. Figure 12.3 shows sample items from tests assessing perceptual speed and accuracy. On paper-and-pencil tests, this ability can be assessed by having subjects make rapid comparisons of figures or symbols, or by rapid scanning to find a particular visual configuration. In published studies demonstrating a sex difference in perceptual speed, the size of the difference is typically on the order of half a standard deviation.[1056] This makes it roughly comparable in size to the sex difference seen in spatial ability, although in favor of women rather than men.

Obviously, sex differences in cognitive abilities are quite specific. One cannot always tell simply from the face validity of a test (that is, what it appears at first glance to be measuring) whether it actually measures a particular ability or whether it will show a particular sex difference. However, sex differences in abilities other than spatial and verbal abilities have received relatively little direct study, and their hormonal contributors even less.

Sex Differences in Motor Skills

Sex differences in certain motor skills are widely recognized. Although males dramatically excel in strength, especially after the early teenage years,[539] women typically show greater speed and agility at fine motor skills, both manual and articulatory. The latter sex difference can be demonstrated in the laboratory in tasks such as speeded syllable repetition or the test of speeded manual coordination shown in figure 12.4. This sex difference is also apparent in many other tests of manual dexterity, including some tests used for voca-

(A)

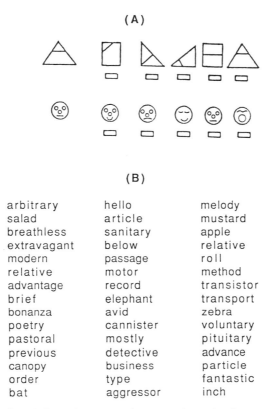

(B)

arbitrary	hello	melody
salad	article	mustard
breathless	sanitary	apple
extravagant	below	relative
modern	passage	roll
relative	motor	method
advantage	record	transistor
brief	elephant	transport
bonanza	avid	zebra
poetry	cannister	voluntary
pastoral	mostly	pituitary
previous	detective	advance
canopy	business	particle
order	type	fantastic
bat	aggressor	inch

Figure 12.3 Sample items from tests of perceptual speed and accuracy. *A*, On the identical pictures test, each item requires the subject to select the figure on the right that matches the target figure shown on the left. (From *Manual for Kit of Factor-Referenced Cognitive Tests.* Copyright © 1962, 1976 by Educational Testing Service. Reprinted by permission.) *B*, The subject must find all the words containing a designated letter of the alphabet as quickly as possible.[1061]

tional screening. For example, subjects may be asked to place pegs quickly into holes or to assemble metal components in a specified order under time constraints. In many tests, the sex difference is large enough to warrant separate norms for men and women. Although the female advantage in such tasks may be at least partly related to their smaller finger size,[805] central nervous system factors probably also contribute to the sex difference in performance.

Studies of patients with localized brain damage have revealed that there is a common neural system that contributes to motor programming of both manual and articulatory movements.[575] Patients with stroke or other sudden brain damage affecting the specialized regions of the left hemisphere where these motor control areas are located show a fascinating phenomenon. Although they are able to move their limbs freely, they display great difficulty in organizing sequences of movements, and so make errors in movement selection and movement ordering, a disorder called manual apraxia. These patients also have an analogous difficulty with movements of the mouth and oral musculature (oral apraxia). When speaking, these patients typically display a form of speech

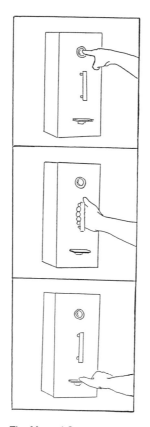

Figure 12.4 The Manual Sequence Box. Subjects must learn to produce the simple sequence of three movements shown here.

disturbance called aphasia, in which syllables or even larger parts of speech are omitted, misarranged, or substituted. Although aphasia is often conceptualized as a pure language deficit, detailed analysis of the types of speech errors produced has suggested that the same underlying motor programming problem is at least partly responsible for the disturbance in spontaneous speech as well.

Neuropsychological tests are a special class of tests that sample sensory, perceptual, cognitive, or motor skills for which the integrity of a particular region of the brain is known to be essential. A neuropsychological test that samples the type of manual skills that are dependent on this complex motor control region of the left cerebral hemisphere is the Manual Sequence Box, shown in figure 12.4. Patients with left hemispheric damage in the critical motor-programming regions have great difficulty in mastering the simple sequence of three movements shown in the figure, despite adequate limb strength and mobility. Most of these patients also have aphasia, as mentioned earlier. The fact that there appears to be a common region of the brain that is involved in complex motor control of both the oral musculature and the upper limbs may well be important to our understanding of the basis for the sex differences noted in manual and articulatory speed and accuracy. This is particularly true because, as we shall see later, there appears to be a sex difference in the exact cortical localization of these specialized motor control regions.

Sex Differences in Brain Organization in Humans

Why do sex differences in abilities exist? The underlying reasons are hotly disputed. One hypothesis is that there may be sex differences in the physical structure of the human brain. Structural differences could lead to cognitive differences through differences in processing efficiency, capacity, or preferred strategy for task solution. The types of structural differences that might exist range from macroscopic differences that are evident on casual inspection to microscopic differences in synaptic termination pattern; regional cell size, density, or number; dendritic arborization patterns; or the interconnectivity of particular brain regions. From the animal literature, we also know that similar-appearing macroscopic brain structures can be built from sexually dimorphic neurotransmitter systems. In chapter 2, some sex differences in the structure of the human brain were described, and these are reviewed briefly below. The existence of such sex differences raises a strong possibility that the human brain is subject to the organizational effects of gonadal steroid hormones during sensitive periods in gestation or early postnatal life.

Sex Differences in the Functional Organization of the Cortex

In most humans, the left side of the brain is the one primarily responsible for the control of speech and certain types of manual movements, as mentioned earlier. This is an example of cerebral specialization, or lateralization of function. However, there is some variability in the degree to which this is true. For example, in many left-handed people, the right side of the brain also controls speech to some degree. In extreme cases, the situation may be completely reversed, with the right rather than the left side of the brain predominant for speech control. Sex differences in the cerebral lateralization of speech as well as certain nonverbal functions have been hypothesized by many researchers. Typically, it has been argued that in adults the two sides of the brain may be more differentiated or specialized in men than in women, not only for language but also for nonverbal functions. In other words, men may show a greater degree of cerebral lateralization than women, whereas women may tend to show a more bilateral representation of function.[166, 468, 695] This generalization is based largely on two types of evidence.

First, some studies of the degree of intellectual or behavioral deficits observed following brain injury have shown that damage restricted to one side of the brain (i.e., unilateral damage) may have more devastating consequences in males than in females. For example, investigators such as McGlone[694] and Inglis[523] have independently investigated the effects of unilateral brain damage on IQ. Sample findings are shown in figure 12.5. Notice that, in this example, left hemispheric damage impaired verbally weighted aspects of IQ more than

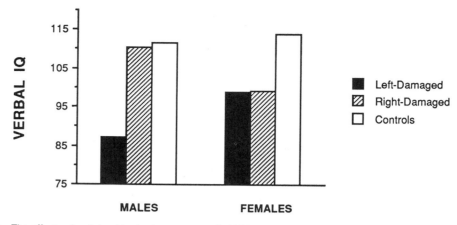

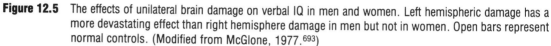

Figure 12.5 The effects of unilateral brain damage on verbal IQ in men and women. Left hemispheric damage has a more devastating effect than right hemisphere damage in men but not in women. Open bars represent normal controls. (Modified from McGlone, 1977.[693])

right hemispheric damage, as one would expect if the left hemisphere is responsible for language functions. But this was true only for males, not for females. One interpretation of this finding is that females with left hemispheric damage could rely on the language capabilities of their intact right hemisphere in performing the verbal tasks. As another example, Lansdell[612] administered a verbal proverbs test to 55 patients before and after various neurosurgical procedures. Among his results was the finding that left temporal lesions were disruptive to performance on this task only in males. Again, this finding is compatible with a greater degree of involvement of the right hemisphere in complex verbal functions in females.

The second source of evidence of sex differences in cerebral lateralization is the finding that there are sex differences in the size of certain perceptual asymmetries usually seen in normal adults when they are tested in the laboratory using standard **dichotic listening** or **tachistoscopic** tests. In these tests, simple auditory or visual stimuli are presented to a subject for extremely short durations. When the stimuli are of a verbal nature (e.g., words or nonsense syllables), a typical subject accurately reports more of the stimuli being presented to the right ear or the right visual field. Because of the way the visual and auditory pathways project to the brain, this is presumed to reflect left hemispheric lateralization of verbal functions. Conversely, a left ear or a left visual field advantage typically is seen when briefly presented stimuli tap the specialized processing capacities of the right hemisphere (e.g., melodies or dot arrays). As with the evidence from patients with brain damage, women often tend to show smaller perceptual asymmetries than men, which may in turn reflect a lesser degree of underlying cerebral lateralization of function (see McGlone[695] for a review of the literature).

Although these arguments seem straightforward, more recent evidence suggests that the picture may not be as simple as this. Specifically, it is unlikely that *all* functions are less lateralized in the female brain. In a more detailed analysis of performance on the subtests of the Wechsler Adult Intelligence Scale and several other neuropsychological tests, Kimura and Harshman[578] found that not all verbal abilities showed the same pattern of sex differences following left or right hemispheric brain damage. Although certain aspects of the results were consistent with earlier suggestions of more bilateral representation of verbal functions in women, other aspects were more compatible with sex differences in *intra*hemispheric organization.

In at least two studies, detailed analysis of language disturbances following brain damage has suggested that basic speech functions may indeed be organized along an anterior-posterior gradient within the left hemisphere, with the anterior region being relatively more important for the production and decoding of speech in females than the posterior region.[576, 1078] Kimura,[576] for example, studied 81 right-handed patients with restricted anterior or posterior damage, and found that aphasia and manual apraxia resulted significantly more often in women from damage to the anterior part of the left hemisphere than from damage to the posterior part of the left hemisphere. This was not true for men. Also in that study, of 169 patients with restricted right hemispheric damage, only a tiny fraction showed speech disorders, and the incidence of these did not differentiate the sexes, contrary to what would be expected if these basic speech capacities showed increased dependence on the right cerebral hemisphere in females.

Evidence from cortical stimulation also supports the notion of anterior-posterior sex differences in the cerebral organization of speech.[673] Cortical stimulation is used to determine clinically safe boundaries for resection in patients about to undergo neurosurgery to remove an epileptic focus, so that they will not be left with a lasting speech deficit. The cortex is exposed and stimulated with a mild electrical current to map out areas of the cortex that are involved in speech. In Mateer's study, electrical stimulation of the left neocortex evoked naming deficits from many more sites in males than in females, and stimulation of the posterior parietal cortex evoked naming errors in almost 60% of men but affected none of the women.

Thus, sex differences in at least two planes have been suggested, and there is some evidence in favor of both types of sex difference (see figure 12.6). Although this may seem contradictory, the secret to reconciling these studies may lie in the fact that different investigators have sampled very different verbal functions. It is possible, for example, that basic motor or acoustic functions related to speech show one type of sex difference in the brain, while more abstract or complex verbal functions show another type of sex difference. A lesson to be learned from all this is that researchers who are interested in studying sex differences in cerebral organization from indirect behavioral data must delineate both the neuroanatomical locus and the behavioral function to be examined as precisely as possible. We are still very much in the early stages of understanding how behavioral functions relate to sex differences in cerebral organization.

ANTERIOR----POSTERIOR   RIGHT----LEFT

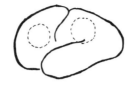   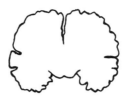

Kimura (1983)[576]   Lansdell (1961)[612]
Mateer et al. (1982)[673]   McGlone (1978)[694]
Vignolo et al. (1986)[1078]   Inglis & Lawson (1981)[522]

Figure 12.6 Clinical studies have suggested sex differences in cerebral language representation within both the anterior-posterior and the left-right planes.

Table 12.2 Anatomical Studies Showing Sex Differences in the Human Brain

Crichton-Browne (1880)[238a]	Weight differences between L and R hemispheres less marked in females than in males
Wada, Clarke and Hamm (1975)[1083]	Planum temporale larger on R more often in females than in males (but usually larger on L in both sexes)
Wada (1976)[1082a]	Cuneate area of occipital lobe larger on R in females, larger on L in males
deLacoste and Horvath (1985)[270]	Entire R cortex more developed in males, L perfrontal cortex in females, at 13 weeks gestation
Lewis et al. (1988)[632]	Volume of caudate nucleus larger on R in males, larger on L in females
Rabl (1958)[834a], Morel (1948)[748], Davie and Baldwin (1967)[262a]	Agenesis of massa intermedia more frequent in males than in females
deLacoste-Utamsing and Holloway (1982)[272]	Maximum splenial width larger in females; area of splenium larger in females than in males ($p < .08$)
Allen and Gorski (1986)[17]	Anterior commissure at the midsagittal plane larger in females
Swaab and Fliers (1985),[1014] Allen et al. (1989)[18]	Nuclei of the preoptic-anterior hypothalamic area larger in males than in females

Other Sex Differences in Brain Organization

Direct anatomical studies have contributed to our understanding of more visible structural sex differences, although until recently surprisingly few researchers analyzed their data according to sex. Some of the studies that have done so are summarized in table 12.2. Wada and colleagues[1083] reported that brains in more females than males showed a larger planum temporale on the right side than the left, an area on the superior surface of the temporal lobe believed to be involved in auditory speech functions. This is a reversal of the typical pattern of asymmetry, in that the planum temporale is usually larger on the left in both sexes. This particular morphological asymmetry was already apparent by the twenty-ninth week of gestation, the youngest brains available in Wada's study. In the fetus, deLacoste and Horvath[270] showed that as early as 13 weeks' gestational age, the entire right cortex in males and the left prefrontal cortex in females are more developed relative to other brain regions (see also deLacoste et al.,[271]). Interestingly, it is around this time that testicular androgens reach peak concentrations in the human male fetus. In the rat, perinatal androgens have been hypothesized to exert a suppressant effect on the growth of the left hemisphere.[991] At present, there is no published evidence of persisting differences in the adult human brain that would suggest that such a phenomenon occurs in humans. However, Lewis and associates[632] reported an asymmetry in the volume of the human caudate nucleus, as judged from magnetic resonance imaging (MRI) scans. The caudate nucleus in males tended to be larger on the right than on the left, whereas in females it tended to be larger on the left than on the right ($p < .055$).

Sex differences in the interhemispheric commissures have also been reported. In the human brain, five major fiber pathways interconnect the two cerebral hemispheres: the corpus callosum, the anterior commissure, the posterior commissure, the massa intermedia, and the hippocampal commissure. Several investigators have reported that the massa intermedia (MI), a band of neural tissue that connects the two halves of the thalamus across the third ventricle, is more frequently absent in men than in women. Lansdell and Davie[613] noted a trend in which males without the massa intermedia tended to have higher nonverbal factor scores on a test of general ability than those in whom the MI was present. More recently, deLacoste-Utamsing and Holloway[272] reported that the splenium of the corpus callosum, the most posterior portion of this structure, is larger and more bulbous in women. This finding is disputed, in light of failures by several other investigators to replicate the original finding.[1107] However, deLacoste and her associates have replicated their results in a new sample of adult brain specimens[496] as well as in fetal brains as young as 26 weeks of age.[269] It is not clear whether methodological differences, such as differences in procedures used to estimate callosal size, the method of correction for overall brain size, or uncontrolled subject variables might account for the discrepancies among studies. Even more recently, Allen and Gorski[17] calculated the midsagittal area of the anterior commissure in 30 human brains ranging in age from 4 to 78 years. Although the weight of the male brain was larger, the anterior commissure was larger in the absolute sense in females than in males, and even more so after correction for brain weight. It is not known whether the commissural differences that have been reported so far represent a greater number of fibers traversing the cerebral commissures in women or simply a greater diameter of fibers.

Within the past few years sex differences in hypothalamic nuclei have also been reported in humans. Swaab and Fliers[1014] reported a sex difference in the preoptic area of the hypothalamus such that the volume and cell number are approximately 2.5 times greater in males than in females. Allen and colleagues[18] confirmed the presence of two sexually dimorphic cell groups in the preoptic-anterior hypothalamic area. They reported that both brain regions are more than twice as large in the male as in the female brain, and one was 3.7

times larger in women of reproductive age compared with a small group of prepubertal and postmenopausal women. These hypothalamic findings are particularly exciting and noteworthy because the preoptic area has been shown to be sexually dimorphic in several nonhuman species and more important, to be sensitive to prenatal or perinatal hormonal influences (see chapter 2). The critical period for sexual differentiation of the human hypothalamus is unknown but most probably occurs during gestation or the first few months of postnatal life.

To summarize, a variety of sex differences in brain organization have been reported in humans. These sex differences in brain organization may provide the neuroanatomical substrate for sex differences observed in behavior and cognitive abilities.* It is not known, however, how these neural sex differences arise. In particular, it is not known whether or not they are a direct result of organizational influences of sex hormones in the human brain.

Evidence of Organizational Effects of Prenatal Hormones on Cognition and Lateralization

If we were to look for evidence that gonadal hormones early in life can permanently influence human cognition and behavior, where would we look? Theoretically, we could measure testosterone or other hormones in amniotic fluid obtained from at-risk pregnancies or in umbilical cord blood obtained at the time of birth and see how these correlate with behavioral or cognitive measures obtained later in development or at maturity. Although such studies are being done, they are very time consuming because of their longitudinal nature and are extremely rare.[351, 526] A more common source of information about the possible organizational effects of sex hormones in humans comes from the study of individuals exposed to unusual hormone environments prenatally. This exposure typically results from genetically based abnormalities in the synthesis, metabolism, or sensitivity to particular hormones or more rarely, from the ingestion of synthetic hormones by the mother during pregnancy. The latter hormones typically have been synthetic estrogens or progestins that were administered to prevent miscarriage.

Because we cannot experimentally manipulate hormones in humans and observe the resultant effects on brain and behavior, we must try to infer possible effects from such "experiments of nature," hoping that they will shed light on the role of sex hormones in *normal* development. A number of methodological and inferential problems plague such clinical research, however. (1) Double-blind studies are often impossible, since affected individuals and their

---

*An interesting question is how sex differences in brain organization might interact with the handedness differences alluded to earlier. Do left- and right-handed men and women differ in their brain organization and consequently in their patterns of cognitive abilities? The answer may be yes. Harshman and co-workers[467] reported some evidence in favor of consistent variations in spatial ability as a function of sex, handedness, and reasoning level. Dichotic listening scores showed somewhat parallel interactions in the same groups of subjects. Studies such as this emphasize that sex of subject may be only one of the factors contributing to subtle interindividual variations in brain organization and cognitive abilities.

parents are typically aware of their condition. (2) Because many of these syndromes are extremely rare, it is difficult to obtain large enough sample sizes to provide an adequate test of hypotheses of interest. (3) Childhood upbringing may be atypical due to the need for chronic hormone replacement or, in some instances, to genital ambiguity or other physical stigmata that can result in parental ambivalence or gender identity problems in the offspring. Although individuals exposed to exogenous hormones in utero provide a population that circumvents some of these difficulties, other problems are unique to these populations: (4) The timing and type of synthetic hormone exposure varies markedly from one individual to another, and, since the timing of any possible critical period for CNS development in humans is unknown and the exact nature and strength of different synthetic compounds may vary enormously, it can be difficult to know whether a given individual provides an adequate test of one's hypothesis or not. (5) Possible effects on the nervous system of the factors that necessitated hormonal intervention in the first place must also be taken into account. (6) The influence of socioeconomic or other selection factors, which may be operative in determining who receives prenatal therapy, must be considered.

However imperfect these clinical data may be, they have provided most of the information we have at present on the role of prenatal hormones in human behavioral development. There is suggestive evidence that hormones may influence our brains and behavior in a manner similar to that seen in other species. To the extent that a variety of different syndromes support an influence of hormonal factors, we are on stronger ground in attributing developmental differences to abnormal hormone exposure. This is particularly true when possible confounding factors differ across syndromes.

Effects on Noncognitive Behaviors

GENDER IDENTITY
Gender identity is defined as a person's primary identification with one or the other sex—in other words, whether we view ourselves as male or female. In a review of the literature, Ehrhardt and Meyer-Bahlburg[318] concluded that the prenatal hormonal environment exerts little influence on gender identity. This conclusion was based mainly on case histories showing that gender identity appears to depend largely on sex of rearing, even when this is in contrast to some of the biological indicators of sex[736] (but see also Diamond[290]). For example, children born with ambiguous genitals reportedly develop a gender identity that agrees with their assigned sex, provided steps are taken early in life to correct the physical ambiguity and there is no ambiguity in parental upbringing. Proponents of this view argue that sex of rearing is the major factor in determining gender identity, which is thought to be established irrevocably by about 3 to 4 years of age.

Other studies draw the strict social learning view into question, at least in its strongest form. Imperato-McGinley and associates[519, 520] described a group of genetic males in the Dominican Republic called *guevedoces* by the locals, literally, "penis at 12 (years of age)." Although genetically male, these individuals were raised as girls because they were born with female-appearing external genitalia owing to an inherited enzyme deficiency (5α-reductase deficiency). These males had deficient dihydrotestosterone production but normal synthesis of and sensitivity to testosterone. As a result, they suddenly became masculinized or **virilized** at puberty as their testosterone levels rose toward adult concentrations. They experienced penile growth, descent of the testes into the scrotum, and deepening of the voice. Imperato-McGinley and colleagues reported that, despite being raised unambiguously as girls, 17 of 18 males made a relatively effortless change in gender identity at puberty in response to the physical changes. This would not be expected from a strict social learning perspective and has been interpreted by some researchers as favoring the supremacy of hormonal factors over rearing practices. It at least seems to question the immutability of gender identity despite contradictory physical evidence. The studies remain controversial, however, because in our culture, other reports of sudden virilization at puberty have suggested that a change in gender identity, when it occurs at all, requires a very long and difficult period of readjustment.[318] Further research is needed to resolve the controversy.

SEXUAL ORIENTATION

The prenatal hormonal environment has been hypothesized to exert a predisposing influence on adult sexual orientation, although again, postnatal socialization also makes a very important contribution.[735] Theoretically, the presence of androgens in prenatal life should contribute to the development of a sexual orientation toward females, while a deficiency in prenatal androgens or tissue insensitivity to androgens should contribute to a sexual orientation toward males, regardless of genetic sex. Ehrhardt and co-workers[317] examined a sample of women exposed to excessive levels of adrenal androgens both prenatally and well into adolescence or adulthood. Despite many years of severe virilization, homosexuals did not predominate in their sample, although there did appear to be an increase in bisexuality as judged from fantasy and sexual experience. An increased incidence of bisexuality in imagery or sexual experience was confirmed in a recent controlled study of such women exposed only to virilizing effects in utero.[739] In that study, 37% of the women rated themselves as bisexual or homosexual. In contrast, only 5% of a similar group of women reported bisexual or homosexual activity in a recent study by Mulaikal and colleagues.[766] However, this difference may reflect the narrower focus in the latter study on overt behavior per se rather than on other recognized indices of sexual orientation such as sexual imagery, arousing stimuli, and attractions. Exposure prenatally to diethylstilbestrol (DES), a synthetic estrogen known to exert masculinizing or defeminizing effects in the central nervous system of other species, has also been reported to increase the incidence of bisexuality or homosexuality in women,[319] although in this study the majority of DES-exposed women (75%) nevertheless reported a heterosexual orientation. You may recall that it is not clear whether estrogen is important for the differentiation of sexual preferences in primates. Taken together, these studies suggest that fetal androgens might exert a predisposing influence on sexual orientation in humans but appear to rule out a rigidly deterministic effect.

Genetic males who are exposed to an androgen-deficient prenatal environment through an inherited insensitivity to androgens typically are female in appearance, are reared as females, and as adults tend to be sexually attracted to men.[712] Unfortunately, in this syndrome, the effects of rearing and hormones are confounded. What about genetically normal homosexual men? In normal homosexuals, an androgen deficiency during some critical period in fetal development has been suggested but has not been confirmed to date. Tentative support for the notion of a prenatal androgen deficiency comes from reports that homosexual men show a pattern of luteinizing hormone (LH) release in response to an injection of estrogen that is intermediate between that of heterosexual males and heterosexual females.[305, 406] A similar positive feedback response has been demonstrated in male rats deprived of androgens perinatally. This line of research in humans has been criticized on several grounds, however. First, there have been failures to replicate the proposed homosexual versus heterosexual distinction in LH responsiveness.[419, 483] Second, you may recall that in contrast to rodents, it is not clear that the capacity for a positive feedback response to estrogen is a sexually dimorphic characteristic in primates.[779] Under some circumstances, human males apparently also show a positive feedback response to an estrogen stimulus.[409, 410, 420] Thus, the absence of a positive estrogen feedback effect may not be a permanent feature of the hypothalamic-pituitary axis in heterosexual men. Finally, there is also the possibility that the LH effect, even if it did reliably distinguish between homosexual and heterosexual men, is somehow secondary to the homosexual lifestyle rather than a marker of differences in the prenatal hormone environment.

GENDER ROLE BEHAVIOR

Other aspects of behavior, including certain sexually differentiated social behaviors, also may be subtly influenced by prenatal hormone exposure. Genetic females with a disorder called congenital adrenal hyperplasia (CAH) are masculinized genitally to varying degrees by prenatal exposure to excessive androgens, a disorder arising from an adrenal enzyme deficiency. The genital masculinization can be surgically corrected, and these girls typically are raised as females and develop a female gender identity. Nevertheless, several studies have found evidence of behavioral masculinization in females with CAH. Girls with CAH have been reported to show a more masculine pattern of toy preference than their unaffected sisters[111, 315] as well as more rough-and-tumble play, a preference for male rather than female playmates, greater tomboyism, reduced rehearsal through childhood play of adult female roles as wife and mother, reduced interest in infant care, and reduced interest in physical appearance or attractiveness compared with female controls.[315, 316] Boys with

CAH are reported to differ from their unaffected male siblings in higher levels of intense energy expenditure in rough outdoor play and sports. They also show a nonsignificant increase in a propensity to initiate fighting.[315] With the exception of the Berenbaum and Hines study, this research has unfortunately tended to rely almost exclusively on self or parental reports rather than direct behavioral observation.

Interestingly, results similar to those reported in CAH females have also been reported in females whose mothers were treated during pregnancy with masculinizing progestins to prevent miscarriage.[320] In some cases, the female offspring of these pregnancies were born with partially masculinized genitalia, sometimes necessitating surgical correction. Based on interview data, Ehrhardt and Money[320] reported that a group of girls with evidence of genital masculinization at birth showed high levels of tomboyish energy expenditure in childhood and a strong interest in boys' toys, such as guns and trucks, rather than dolls and other toys generally preferred by girls. They typically were characterized as "tomboys" by their parents and themselves. In addition, progestin-exposed individuals purportedly show a heightened potential for physical aggression compared to sibling controls, as judged by a paper-and-pencil questionnaire.[843] This was true despite the fact that none of the female subjects in Reinisch's study had been genitally virilized. As in CAH, gender identity and sex of rearing in the progestin-exposed girls typically are female.

Thus it seems that there may be some behavioral changes in individuals with CAH and in women exposed to masculinizing progestins during gestation that are consistent with the virilizing prenatal environment to which they were exposed. This suggests that hormones present in the normal uterine environment may be capable of exerting a lasting but subtle influence on certain aspects of gender role behavior in humans.

Effects on General Intelligence

The effect of the prenatal hormone environment on cognitive abilities has been assessed by studying both general intelligence and, more rarely, sexually dimorphic abilities. The results so far have been somewhat difficult to interpret.

In 1967, Ehrhardt and Money[320] reported that females whose mothers were treated with androgenic progestins during pregnancy to prevent miscarriage had significantly increased IQ scores relative to population norms. Their sample was very small, consisting of only ten girls, nine of whom had some degree of genital masculinization. The mean IQ in their sample was 125, and 60% of the subjects had IQs over 130, compared with the expected 2% in a random population sample. Similarly, above average intelligence has repeatedly been found in samples of male and female patients with CAH.[696, 737, 804] For example, Money and Lewis[737] found that 60% of a group of 70 patients with CAH had IQs above 110, compared with the expected population frequency of 25%, and fully one-third of the group had IQ scores over 120.

Other studies examining the role of sex steroids in intellectual development have come from England, where Dalton[248] examined the school performance of children exposed to *natural* progesterone in utero. This hormone had been administered as a supplement to their mothers during pregnancy for relief of toxemic symptoms. Natural progesterone does not have the virilizing effects associated with some of the synthetic progestins. At age 9 to 10 such children were rated by teachers, who were unaware of their hormonal history, as significantly superior in verbal reasoning, English, and mathematics compared to normal children or children from untreated toxemic pregnancies, who were matched for age, geographical area, social class, and other variables. At age 17 to 20, treated children exceeded the educational attainments of controls on a variety of measures.[250] Unfortunately, direct IQ testing was not carried out in Dalton's studies. There has been one attempt to use standardized tests to examine IQ in natural progesterone-treated children, but unfortunately this study failed to provide conclusive results due to methodological problems.[645]

Results such as these have been interpreted by some investigators as indicating a potentially favorable effect of prenatal hormones, possibly progestins, on intelligence. Studies using siblings or other family members as controls have brought this conclusion into serious question, however. In several studies, family members who were *not* exposed to an abnormal prenatal environment were tested and also found to show superior intellectual performance.[45, 696, 844] For example, no significant difference in IQ was found between a group of women exposed in utero to one or more of 23 different progestins and their unexposed siblings.[844] Similarly, Baker and Ehrhardt[45] found no IQ differences between a group of people with CAH and their unaffected sibling and parent controls, who also showed superior intelligence. These findings seem to rule out the unusual fetal hormone exposure as the explanation for the high IQ scores. Instead, it has been suggested that sampling bias, not abnormal hormone exposure, may be the true explanation for the apparent IQ elevation reported in hormone-exposed subjects.

It is possible, for example, that the clinics where these studies are conducted may attract families with higher than average intelligence, or that these families may agree to participate in research projects in disproportionate numbers. Whatever bias may be present, it is not directly related to socioeconomic status (SES). In the Baker and Ehrhardt study,[45] for example, CAH patients and controls showed higher than average IQ scores but did not have high SES. Also, the Dalton studies controlled for social class and therefore presumably for SES as well. Differences between the progesterone-treated and untreated groups were nevertheless significant. One might expect a selection bias in families attending specialty clinics in the United States in favor of higher SES families. But in a summary of IQ findings in patients with various endocrine abnormalities seen at the Johns Hopkins clinic, Money and associates[738] reported that the only endocrine syndromes associated with IQ elevation were CAH and idiopathic precocious puberty. Patients attending the same clinic who had genetic syndromes that did not involve abnormal exposure to androgens or progestins, or an accelerated rate of physical maturation, were not found to show increased IQ scores. Patients with most other syndromes did not differ from the norm in intellectual functioning, although a few showed selective deficits. We must be cautious in interpreting these findings, however, because no information on other family members was provided in Money and colleagues' report. It is possible that average intelligence in the clinic patients may nevertheless represent an IQ depression relative to other family members.

Other factors also complicate interpretation of these studies. In the initial Ehrhardt and Money[320] sample of females exposed to androgenic progestins, nine of ten girls had been genitally masculinized by the prenatal hormone exposure. In the Reinisch and Karow[844] study, none of the subjects were so affected. If a facilitative effect of exogenous progestins on IQ does exist, it may be more obvious in more virilized cases, perhaps reflecting differences in dose, type, timing, or sensitivity to hormone exposure. As a possible indication that timing may be an important factor, Dalton found in her studies that academic achievement was positively related to high dosage and early administration of natural progesterone during gestation.[248, 250]

To summarize, sampling bias currently is regarded as the most likely explanation for the IQ elevation reported in some hormone-exposed patients and their families. CAH or exposure to exogenous progestins themselves has not been demonstrated to contribute directly to high IQ scores. In particular, it is generally believed that prenatal androgens do not have any enhancing effect on intelligence. This makes sense when one considers that sex differences in general intelligence are not found in the population at large. On the other hand, it is not always clear what type of selection bias may be operating in published studies in this area, and a more subtle hormonal influence of some kind cannot be totally discounted.

Effects on Specific Cognitive Abilities

Only rarely have studies examined the effects of prenatal hormones on more specific cognitive abilities. If the prenatal hormone environment normally does contribute to cognitive sex differences, we might expect females exposed to an unusually masculinizing environment to show an enhancement of cognitive abilities that normally favor males. In particular, enhanced visuospatial ability might be expected.

Studies testing this hypothesis using visuospatial tests have produced mixed results to date. The inconsistent findings may partly reflect methodological factors such as the lack of statistical power associated with small sample sizes and the bias in many subject samples toward younger, prepubertal subjects in whom sex differences in spatial ability are usually less pronounced. McGuire and colleagues,[697] for example, did not detect significant differences between females with CAH and matched controls using the Embedded Figures Test, a test sampling the subtype of spatial ability we have called flexibility of closure (see figure 12.2). Baker and Ehrhardt[45] examined performance on the verbal and spatial subtests of the Primary Mental Abilities battery. As expected, females with CAH showed slightly lower verbal scores and slightly higher spatial scores than their sisters, but the differences were not significant in this study. Perlman[804] reported that females with CAH performed significantly better on a pictorial test that was not clearly spatial in nature but that did show a sex difference in favor of males in Perlman's normal sample. The females with CAH performed significantly better than a group of matched female controls. Interestingly, a group of androgen-deficient males showed the reverse pattern, with significantly lower performance on the test compared to normal male controls.[804] Finally, a recent and methodologically very sound study by Resnick and associates[847] succeeded in demonstrating significantly enhanced performance by females with CAH compared with unaffected female relatives on three separate tests of spatial ability. This study is therefore the strongest evidence to date in favor of an enhancing effect of prenatal androgens on visuospatial ability in females with CAH.

Two studies have reported decreased performance on arithmetic tests in females with CAH compared to siblings[45] and nonfamilial matched controls.[804] However, the study by Resnick and colleagues,[847] using a simple test of speeded calculations, failed to confirm this finding. Such a deficit in females with CAH may seem paradoxical at first glance, since mathematical reasoning is a skill at which males normally excel. But if anything, females normally have the advantage at performing simple arithmetic operations and computations.[531] This result may perhaps reflect the perceptual speed component implicit in such tasks. The two studies reporting a numerical deficit in CAH used simple arithmetic tests that do not tap the kind of mathematical problem-solving ability at which males typically excel. Further studies are needed to clarify whether the nature of the problem in CAH is really one of mathematical aptitude, perceptual speed and accuracy, or something else. Since perceptual speed is a skill that generally favors females in normal populations, we might expect it to be adversely affected by the excessive androgen exposure in CAH.

Finally, a few studies have examined cognitive performance in individuals exposed in utero to the synthetic estrogen DES. Recall that DES is known to have masculinizing effects in rodents. Although the role of estrogens in differentiation of the primate brain is less certain, the possible involvement of estrogen in cortical differentiation is suggested by the fact that aromatase complex activity has been noted in the association cortex of the perinatal rhesus monkey brain.[649] With regard to behavioral studies, Yalom and associates[1121] found that boys exposed prenatally to DES and small amounts of a synthetic progestin were less aggressive, less athletic, and showed poorer performance on the Embedded Figures Test compared with two comparison groups. Reinisch and Sanders,[845] in a preliminary analysis of 13 pairs of brothers, one of whom was DES-exposed, found that the exposed brothers resembled females more than males in their performance on a test of nonverbal cerebral lateralization. No further details of this study have been published. In contrast, Hines and Shipley[491] found that DES-exposed women showed a more *masculine* pattern of lateralization than their sisters on a verbal dichotic listening task. However, an unconventional measure was employed, and no significant differences in two other sexually dimorphic tasks were found. Thus, the few studies involving DES exposure that have been conducted to date have produced seemingly contradictory results. These may be partly explicable on the basis of sex of subject, since some animal studies suggest that excessive levels of androgens or estrogens may have a *de*masculinizing effect on behavior.[83, 292]

Most of the studies that we've been describing in this section share a common underlying assumption: They assume that if the human CNS is sensitive to the organizing influence of gonadal steroids, the critical period for sexual differentiation of the brain and behavior most likely occurs during prenatal development. Although this is a reasonable working hypothesis, we should not be blind to other possibilities. Hier and Crowley,[487] for example, reported an impairment in spatial ability in men with severely low androgen levels due to a lifelong deficiency in gonadotropin-releasing factor. This disorder typically becomes manifest as a failure to undergo puberty. However, these males are believed to undergo normal masculinization in utero, thanks to the presence of maternal gonadotropins. In Hier and Crowley's study, administration of androgens to a small group of these men as adults did not appear to improve their spatial ability. Interestingly, men with a similar disorder, which was acquired after a normal puberty as a result of a brain tumor or other cause, did not show any spatial deficit despite having severely low androgen levels. These data suggest a possible postnatal organizing influence of androgens on spatial ability, exerted at or before the time of puberty.

To summarize, studies of the effects of prenatal hormone exposure on human cognitive abilities have produced suggestive but hardly definitive results to date. A prenatal sex hormone influence on cognitive abilities would not be surprising considering that other behavioral sequelae of hormone exposure have been detected in humans. These indicate that sex hormones can exert lasting effects on the neural template. However, such an influence seems to be more likely on specific, sexually differentiated abilities than on general IQ. This conclusion is consistent with the fact that there is no sex difference in the general population in global IQ. Unfortunately, detection of hormonal influences has been hampered by many factors, including the relative scarcity of suitable subjects, methodological shortcomings inherent in many previous studies (some of them unavoidable), and the possibility of alternative interpretations. Surprisingly, most researchers have not focused specifically on skills that are sexually dimorphic, although one would expect that this subset of abilities would be most influenced by gonadal hormones.

Evidence of Activational Effects of Gonadal Hormones on Cognition and Lateralization in Adults

Very few studies have been explicitly designed to test the hypothesis that sex hormones might exert an activational influence on the brain and behavior in humans. But fortunately, some studies designed for other purposes are relevant

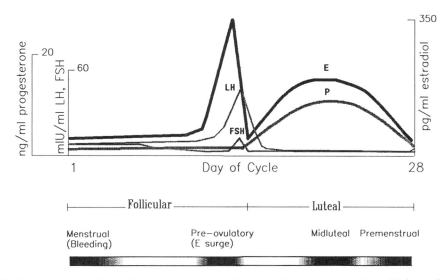

Figure 12.7 Patterns of variation during the menstrual cycle in the plasma concentration of E (estradiol), P (progesterone), LH (luteinizing hormone), and FSH (follicle-stimulating hormone). Note the terms used to denote different subphases of the cycle.

to this question. Once again, because our ability to experimentally manipulate hormone levels in humans is very limited, we typically must rely on naturally occurring biorhythms or medical conditions and their interventions for relevant data. The menstrual cycle provides one convenient, nonintrusive method for studying how fluctuations in hormone levels might influence cognitive functions in women. Some findings from the menstrual cycle literature are summarized below. We will also summarize some nonmenstrual findings. However, nonmenstrual cognitive studies have been very rare to date. One consequence of this is that very little is known about the possible activational effects of testosterone or other androgens in humans.

Evidence from the Menstrual Cycle

Plasma concentrations of several hormones vary systematically during the menstrual cycle. The nature and timing of the major variations are shown in figure 12.7, for 17β-estradiol, progesterone, luteinizing hormone (LH) and follicle-stimulating hormone (FSH). By convention, the first day of menstrual bleeding is denoted day 1 of the cycle, and other days are numbered consecutively from this point. As figure 12.7 shows, secretion of the hormones estradiol and progesterone is lowest during menstruation (menses). Then estrogen gradually rises to a high peak just before ovulation. If the egg is not fertilized, both estrogen and progesterone levels rise more gradually in the week following ovulation and then drop off again just prior to menses. The onset of menstruation marks the beginning of the next cycle. On average, this whole process recurs every 28 to 29 days. But there are substantial inter- and intra-individual variations in the length of the cycle. Absolute concentrations of the various hormones present at each stage also vary considerably. Figure 12.7 shows the terms we will be using in this chapter to identify the various phases of the menstrual cycle. You will need to be familiar with these to understand the following discussion.

The menstrual cycle literature is broad, complex, and often very poor methodologically. Methodological problems that have plagued many studies include (1) small sample sizes, which are inadequate to detect the small fluctuations in cognitive performance that might be expected to occur as a result of changes in steroid levels in women; (2) failure to verify that women were actually tested at the targeted phases of their menstrual cycles through the use of radio-immunoassays (RIAs) or indirect measures; (3) use of cognitive tests that are inappropriate for detecting changes in performance; (4) interpretation of non-significant findings as if they were statistically significant; (5) use of idiosyncratic terminology for identifying phases of the cycle; and, in some cases, (6) selection of inappropriate phases of the cycle for testing hypotheses of interest. The studies described below were selected because they shed some light on hormone-behavior relationships and because they have managed to avoid the worst of these methodological pitfalls.

FLUCTUATIONS IN AFFECT DURING THE MENSTRUAL CYCLE

The majority of menstrual cycle studies to date have been devoted to studying variations in mood during the menstrual cycle. Most of these studies have focused on negative changes in affect reported premenstrually, either in ordinary women or in women with "premenstrual syndrome." Typically, self-reported depression, anxiety, and hostility peak in the premenstrual or early menstrual phases of the cycle.[525, 674] But not all women consistently experience emotional changes at this time, and the reported severity of such changes can vary markedly from woman to woman and from cycle to cycle. The term premenstrual syndrome (PMS) has been used to decribe the most severe premenstrual affective and physical changes. However, the literature on PMS is complex and difficult to integrate owing to methodological problems in many existing studies and definitional problems with the concept itself.

Partly because research has tended to focus on the premenstrual phase and partly because most instruments designed to assess mood are heavily weighted toward negative items, increased feelings of well-being around the time of ovulation have been less thoroughly documented but apparently do occur, at least in some women.[1, 877, 900] In our own research, we confirmed enhancement in vigor and positive affect during the preovulatory surge in estrogen in a sample of university undergraduates and young working women.[456] Interestingly, Sherwin and Gelfand,[943] in a double-blind cross-over study, reported an amelioration of depression in surgically menopausal women during periods when they were on hormone replacement therapy. This seems to confirm that the mood changes are somehow tied to the hormones per se, rather than arising through some independent biorhythm that just happens to be correlated with the menstrual cycle.

In the menstrual cycle literature, cognitive changes often have been assumed to be a secondary result of affective changes. But the affective changes themselves presumably result from transient hormone-induced variations in neurochemistry, perhaps within catecholamine or serotonin-containing neuro-transmitter systems. Clinical studies have suggested a role for these particular neurotransmitters in depression. If affective changes during the menstrual cycle do indeed arise from neurochemical variations induced by sex hormones, it is not clear why cognitive changes could not arise independently through similar mechanisms.

SPATIAL ABILITY

The possibility of cognitive variations occurring during the menstrual cycle has been considered in a number of studies. Most of the research carried out in the 1970s and early 1980s was stimulated by a controversial and highly spec-ulative theory proposed by Broverman and colleagues.[161] This suggested that sex differences in cognitive functioning arise because estrogens and androgens influence the balance of neural activity in subcortical areas controlling the sympathetic and parasympathetic branches of the autonomic nervous system. Depending on the balance of activity in these areas, individuals were thought to be more or less adept at simple perceptual-motor tasks as opposed to com-plex "perceptual-restructuring" tasks. The latter were defined as tasks requir-ing a response to stimulus characteristics that are not immediately apparent and that require mental effort to extract the relevant information. Broverman and colleagues' theory was heavily criticized on theoretical grounds and re-ceived only limited empirical support. Nevertheless, some of the research it generated remains of interest because in many cases the cognitive tasks chosen for study were tasks known to show sex differences in performance.

A number of studies designed to test the Broverman theory compared perfor-mance during phases of the menstrual cycle on tasks that we would consider spatial, such as disembedding tasks, or the Rod-and-Frame test. Disembed-ding tasks involve finding a simple figure hidden within a more complex design or pattern, or what we have termed flexibility of closure. The Rod-and-Frame task requires subjects to determine the true vertical and set a rod to that position when they are able to view only a tilted, and therefore spatially con-fusing, visual background. Unfortunately, either by accident or design, many of these early studies ended up making comparisons between phases of the menstrual cycle that are not hormonally distinct. Not surprisingly, mixed and often nonsignificant results were obtained.

However, a few studies looking at more tightly defined stages of the men-strual cycle suggested that spatial performance may indeed vary as a function of the hormonal state. The size of the changes observed is quite small. But theoretically, these findings are very important. Komnenich and associates[597] found that women performed significantly more poorly during the estrogen

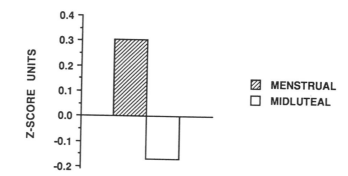

Figure 12.8 In our study, normally cycling young women showed better performance on a combined measure of spatial ability at the menstrual phase (when plasma levels of estradiol (E) and progesterone (P) are low) than at the midluteal phase of the menstrual cycle (when E and P are high).

surge just prior to ovulation than at other points in the cycle on the Embedded Figures Test, a test of disembedding. The sample size in this study was tiny, but phase of cycle was verified directly using plasma radioimmunoassays. Broverman and colleagues[162] predicted that performance on the Embedded Figures Test and on a task that involved copying designs made out of blocks would be worse during the estrogen surge just prior to ovulation than during the luteal phase of the cycle. (Although estrogen levels are also high during the luteal phase, Broverman believed that progesterone might somehow counteract the effects of high estrogen at that time.) Phase of cycle was estimated indirectly from basal body temperature records. Due to variations in cycle length, only 19 of 87 subjects provided adequate data with which to test the hypothesis. But in this subgroup, as predicted, performance on the Embedded Figures Test was significantly poorer on day 10 than on day 20 of the cycle. No significant differences occurred on the block design test.

Little information on spatial ability is available from studies predating the Broverman hypothesis. Wickham[1100] studied aptitude test performance in a very large sample of women in the British armed forces. She reported better performance during menses, when estrogen and progesterone levels are lowest, on a test that involved assembling parts into a model with the aid of diagrams. While performance on this test probably depended on several abilities, spatial ability was probably the single most important contributing factor.

Our own recent data also suggest that spatial ability may vary systematically with the phase of the menstrual cycle. As shown in figure 12.8, a composite measure of spatial ability was significantly higher in a group of undergraduate women tested during menses than in a group of women tested during the midluteal peak in estrogen and progesterone.[455] This confirmed the pattern we had seen in an earlier study using the Rod-and-Frame Test.[457] In that study, too, women performed significantly better during menses than they did during the midluteal phase of their cycles. More recently, Hampson[456] reported similar results on a composite spatial measure derived from tests sampling the three subtypes of spatial ability described earlier in this chapter. Women were tested during the estrogen surge just prior to ovulation and also during the menstrual phase of their cycles. Once again, higher estrogen levels were associated with poorer performance on tests of spatial ability. RIAs were used in this study to verify the phase of testing.

VERBAL ABILITY AND PERCEPTUAL SPEED
If higher levels of gonadal steroids tend to be associated with poorer spatial performance, as several studies now seem to suggest, do other cognitive skills show the same pattern of variation during the menstrual cycle? The answer seems to be no. Fewer studies have looked at possible variations in abilities that favor females, but the data that are available so far suggest that if there are variations in these abilities, the pattern may be quite different from that seen for spatial ability.

Snyder[974] reported faster performance on days 17 to 22 of the cycle than during the premenstrual and early menstrual days on the Matching Familiar Figures Test. This task requires making fine visual discriminations as quickly as possible among similar appearing visual stimuli and therefore might be assumed to have a strong perceptual speed component. Similarly, Anderson[27] reported better performance on a measure of perceptual speed during the luteal phase of the cycle compared to the early follicular days. However, in this study almost all of the tests included in Anderson's battery tended to show better luteal phase performance, including two spatial tasks, the Rod-and-Frame and the Embedded Figures Tests.

Several studies have found faster luteal phase performance on simple verbal-articulatory tasks, such as reading words aloud, naming colors, counting, or repeating syllables (e.g., Anderson[27]). Broverman and associates[162] reported that performance on one such task was faster during the presumed estrogen surge just prior to ovulation than during the luteal phase of the cycle, while a second similar task failed to show a significant difference.

Variations in performance on more complex verbal tasks have seldom been examined. Wickham[1100], using an extremely large sample, found slightly poorer performance during the menstrual phase on a test involving comprehension of complex instructions compared to other days of the cycle. Further details about the nature of the task were not supplied. Hampson[455] reported very small variations during the menstrual cycle in verbal fluency, as assessed by tasks requiring subjects to think of either single words or whole sentences fitting particular phonetic criteria. Women's performance was slightly better during the midluteal estrogen and progesterone surge than during the menstrual phase of the cycle, when gonadal hormones are at low levels. This effect needs replication. In another study, we failed to find a similar facilitation during the high estrogen levels just prior to ovulation.[456] Both studies, however, did reveal a strikingly significant enhancement at higher estrogen levels of the types of simpler verbal-articulatory skills mentioned above (e.g. syllable repetition, speeded counting, and so on). These findings are shown diagrammatically in figure 12.9.

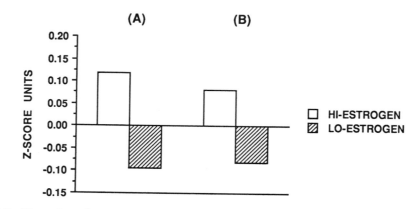

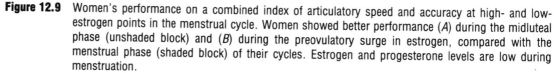

Figure 12.9 Women's performance on a combined index of articulatory speed and accuracy at high- and low-estrogen points in the menstrual cycle. Women showed better performance (*A*) during the midluteal phase (unshaded block) and (*B*) during the preovulatory surge in estrogen, compared with the menstrual phase (shaded block) of their cycles. Estrogen and progesterone levels are low during menstruation.

A different measure of verbal output was examined by Silverman and associates who observed in a small sample of women stutterers (N = 4) that more speech dysfluencies were produced premenstrually than at midcycle.[956] In a later study with nonstutterers, Silverman and Zimmer[955] counted speech dysfluencies during spontaneous speaking on designated topics. Though ovulation was not always targeted successfully, 9 of 12 women produced more speech dysfluencies premenstrually than at midcycle. In both studies, the premenstrual and periovulatory phases of the cycle were selected for study to maximize differences in anxiety, which was thought to underlie the observed changes. However, in light of our own findings, it is possible that the articulatory changes reflected variations in gonadal steroids per se rather than anxiety.

To summarize, to date there have been few studies of verbal and perceptual speed abilities during the menstrual cycle. The data that are available suggest that simple verbal output tasks, such as speed and accuracy of articulatory performance, may be facilitated during phases of the menstrual cycle characterized by higher serum concentrations of estrogen. The picture for more complex verbal abilities and for perceptual speed remains unclear.

BASIC SENSORY PROCESSES
Other studies have examined changes in perceptual or motor functions during the menstrual cycle. Parlee[797] reviewed the evidence showing changes in basic sensory processes. Visual sensitivity appears to increase around the time of ovulation,[291, 381, 1112] as does olfactory sensitivity to certain volatile compounds.[306] Generalizations about other sensory modalities are more difficult to make owing to insufficient study or inconsistencies among studies. One methodological shortcoming that has plagued much of the research in this area is imprecise or inaccurate identification of cycle phase, a shortcoming shared by many of the cognitive studies as well, as noted earlier.

MOTOR PERFORMANCE

A number of studies have looked for objective evidence of changes in motor performance during the menstrual cycle. One impetus for this line of research has been self-reports by some Olympic woman athletes[1131] and other sportswomen[328] of a menstrual or premenstrual decline in athletic performance. Furthermore, Dalton[247] reported that among women, more than half of all accidents requiring hospitalization orimmediate medical attention occurred during menstruation or the 4 days preceding menstruation, a finding she suggested may be related to slowed reaction time.

Prior to our own studies in this area, several studies seeking objective evidence of changes in motor performance had been conducted, and although not definitive, several showed nonsignificant trends in support of a menstrual or premenstrual decline.[992, 1091] Zimmerman and Parlee[1137] reported that arm-hand steadiness was greater during the early luteal phase than premenstrually, and probably menstrually as well. In a sample of seven women, Becker and colleagues[95] found that during menses the total time needed to trace a line was significantly longer and the preferred tapping frequency was slower than during the follicular phase. Two studies have looked at the frequency of spontaneous limb movement during the menstrual cycle.[759, 985] Both studies reported significant variations in activity, although certain aspects of the methodology employed leave any conclusions open to question. Stenn and Klinge[985] found that two of seven women examined during several cycles showed variations in spontaneous arm movement activity, with peak activity most likely to occur in the late luteal phase and least likely to occur in the menstrual phase. Morris and Udry[759] obtained a midcycle peak in pedometer-recorded physical activity, with two lesser peaks menstrually and premenstrually. However, this pattern was apparent only when several cycles were averaged together, and only when data were artificially standardized to a 28-day cycle, a questionable procedure. The validity of the data are brought into further question by the fact that a subgroup of women on oral contraceptives showed a similar cyclic pattern. This should not occur, given that the contraceptives had suppressed their hormonal cyclicity.

Our own menstrual cycle studies have revealed significant changes in manual motor performance during the cycle. Hampson and Kimura[457] reported significantly better midluteal than menstrual performance on several measures of manual speed and coordination, including the Manual Sequence Box described earlier in this chapter (see figure 12.4). In another study, we found better performance on the same motor tasks in women tested during the preovulatory surge in estrogen compared with their performance during menstruation. These findings suggest that higher levels of sex hormones may be associated with improved manual performance in women, at least on the sorts of small-amplitude motor tasks used in these studies.

With respect to reaction times, many studies have failed to find significant cyclic variations in either simple or choice reaction time.[515, 532, 818, 1137] This result is contrary to Dalton's[247] speculation that reaction times may be slower around the time of menstrual onset, thus contributing to accidents, and contrary to the predictions made by Broverman and associates'[161] theory. A West German group of investigators, however, has reported that reaction time to a 30-Hz light flicker is shortest during the luteal phase.[227, 1117, 1118] In other research, the same group of investigators studied a variety of simple and choice reaction time measures administered as part of a larger battery. No significant results were reported for the reaction time measures except for an increased number of errors during menses in reaction to a specified tone.[95] It is not clear what factors account for the discrepancies among reaction time studies.

OVERALL ABILITY AND WORK PERFORMANCE

Finally, many menstrual cycle studies have looked for potential deficits in women's everyday work performance during the menstrual and premenstrual phases of the cycle, on the assumption that affective or physical factors may cause performance to be poorer at that time. Some of this literature has been reviewed by Gamberale.[387] Dalton[249] found slightly lower examination marks among British schoolgirls when the examinations were taken during menses or premenses. But other researchers studying college students' performance on course examinations have failed to find any significant fluctuations with the menstrual cycle.[40, 114, 977] Smith[966, 967] studied the work performance of women employees in an aircraft factory and two garment factories. Menstrual data were collected separately. Supervisor's blind ratings of daily activity levels showed a trend toward lower activity during the menstrual and premenstrual phases, but the magnitude of the difference was small and did not reach statistical significance.[966] In a companion study, Smith also reported that the quality of the work produced, as indicated by female factory workers' production of defective units, did not change during the cycle, and, in particular, there was no decrement during the menstrual phase.[967]

It should be stressed that if activational effects of gonadal hormones contribute directly to cognitive performance, the effects on most types of activity can be expected to be very small and, for most women, are probably unnoticed in everyday life. Morever, in evaluating actual work performance, such factors as familiarity and previous practice on that or related tasks, the absence of sex differences in most complex tasks (i.e., tasks requiring many different abilities), and motivational or other psychological factors, may also mitigate against finding significant differences.

VARIATION IN TESTS OF CEREBRAL LATERALIZATION
DURING THE MENSTRUAL CYCLE

Variations in regional brain activity are assumed to underlie the activational effects of hormones on cognition. But direct evidence of hormone-related changes in the brain in humans is scarce. This scarcity is due partly to lack of study and partly to the limitations of the technology that is currently available for detecting these sorts of changes in living human beings. One indication that this might be a fruitful area for future research comes from recent studies

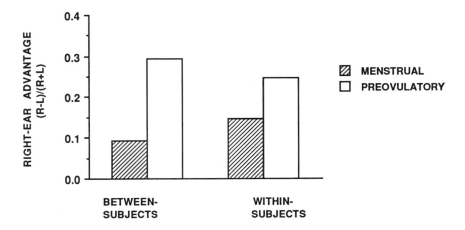

Figure 12.10 On a verbal dichotic listening task, we found that the degree of right-ear advantage changed significantly during the menstrual cycle. The disparity between ears was reduced during the menstrual phase, when plasma concentrations of estrogen and progesterone are low. This was true in both between-subject and withinsubject types of comparisons.

showing variations in performance on tests of cerebral lateralization during the menstrual cycle. Recall that these are perceptual tests that yield visual field or ear asymmetries in speed or accuracy of response that are believed to reflect underlying cerebral asymmetry of function. Although it is difficult to imagine how there could be changes in the degree of hard-wired cerebral asymmetry during the menstrual cycle, there may be changes in the degree to which this hard-wiring is functional or operative and therefore apparent on perceptual or other tests.

Hampson,[456] for example, found significant variation during the menstrual cycle in the degree of right ear advantage on a verbal dichotic listening test (figure 12.10). In a group of young women, the degree of asymmetry was greater at high estrogen levels just prior to ovulation than during the menstrual phase of the cycle. A trend toward greater asymmetry during the midluteal estrogen and progesterone peaks had been seen in an earlier study.[455] Similarly, Altemus and colleagues[23] recently reported a premenstrual decrease in the size of the right ear advantage on a verbal dichotic listening task compared with that seen on days 6 to 12 of the cycle. Using a visual face perception task, Heister and colleagues[482] found a significant left field advantage during menstruation, which was reduced during other phases of the cycle. Finally, Chiarello and associates[203] did not detect any interaction between phase of cycle and visual field on two tachistoscopic tasks presented by means of a computer.

Except for the Chiarello study, these results are consistent in suggesting a shift in relative hemispheric activity during the higher estrogen phases of the menstrual cycle, such that the left hemisphere is somehow facilitated relative to the right. This relative change could reflect true facilitation of underlying left hemispheric areas, suppression of right hemispheric areas, or both. The mechanisms causing this result are unknown.

Summary of Menstrual Cycle Results

Although a number of studies, not described here, have failed to find significant variations in cognitive test performance during the menstrual cycle, many of the nonsignificant results can be explained by the particular research methodology employed. To date, the studies that have reported significant variations during the menstrual cycle suggest that higher levels of estrogen and perhaps progesterone may have a detrimental effect on spatial ability, an ability at which males typically excel. Conversely, higher levels of these hormones may simultaneously be associated with better performance on certain tasks at which women typically excel, particularly tasks requiring abilities involving speech and speeded motor performance. Can these findings be explained on the basis of variations in mood, as older studies sometimes suggested?

The fact that reciprocal changes in different abilities seem to occur at the same point in the cycle makes this sort of explanation less likely. Moreover, in the studies by Hampson and Kimura, variations in cognitive and motor performance were seen in women who did not report significant variations in mood at the points in the cycle at which they were tested.[455, 457] In another study,[456] poorer spatial ability was found in women during a phase of the cycle when enhanced feelings of vigor and well-being were reported, which seems contrary to expectation. Statistically, variations in mood did not appear to explain any of the cognitive or motor changes reported. These sorts of findings suggest that cognitive and affective variations during the menstrual cycle may be separable effects.

Another question that naturally arises from these studies is whether, if these cognitive and motor variations during the menstrual cycle are real, they can be attributed to the effects of sex hormones per se, or might both the variations in cognition and the variations in hormone output appear linked because they are both a function of some central pacemaker mechanism in the CNS? There are a number of arguments against this possibility, but perhaps the strongest comes from preliminary evidence involving the administration of exogenous hormones, which in the majority of women would not be in synchrony with any internal pacemaker. This situation exists in postmenopausal women taking hormone replacement therapy, whose regimen typically starts on the first day of the calendar month and involves the administration of conjugated estrogens for about 25 days. At the end of the month there is typically a 4 to 6 day break from hormone treatment, during which steroid levels decline.

In a study conducted by Kimura,[577] postmenopausal women were tested while undergoing their estrogen therapy and, in a separate session, when they had been off their medications for at least 4 days. The abilities tested in these women were the same as those described previously for younger women in the menstrual cycle studies. However, a slightly different set of tests was used. Table 12.3 shows a comparison, made during the first session, of a group of women tested while on estrogen therapy and a group of women tested while temporarily off therapy. Performance on both the Manual Sequence Box and

Table 12.3 Performance on Fine Motor and Spatial Tasks in Postmenopausal Women Who Take Estrogen Replacement Therapy (ERT)

	OFF ERT (N = 17)	ON ERT (N = 16)
Fine Motor Tasks		
Manual sequence box		
Time to acquisition (sec)	14.0	10.9
Speeded trials (sec)	8.1	6.5
Tongue twister (sec)	16.5	14.5
Spatial Tasks		
Card rotations (% corr)	44.0	41.5
Hidden patterns (% corr)	38.7	39.5

a speeded articulation test involving the recitation of tongue twisters tended to be faster and more accurate during the estrogen treatment compared with the off-treatment phase of the cycle. The same pattern was apparent in within-subject comparisons. In this study, spatial tasks did not show a significant decrement during hormone replacement therapy, contrary to expectations. However, for the motor tests at least, these preliminary results tended to bear out the patterns of variation seen during the menstrual cycle in younger, spontaneously cycling women. These results suggest that the activity of an internal pacemaker, working independently of hormonal influences, is unlikely to explain the patterns of correlations observed.

Correlates of Hormonal Variation in Men

In the studies we have been discussing, women were chosen as a population of convenience, since variations in estrogen and progesterone concentrations during the menstrual cycle are quite marked compared to hormonal variations in men. Nonetheless, men are unlikely to be immune to the effects of gonadal steroids on cognition.

In several studies involving men, Broverman and his colleagues[161, 586, 648] reported results that are compatible with a curvilinear relationship between testosterone levels and cognitive function. Men with higher testosterone production and clearance rates were cognitively **more** similar to women than their lower testosterone male peers, in that they tended to display relatively better performance on simple perceptual-motor tasks, such as color-naming, than on perceptual-restructuring tasks, such as the Embedded Figures Test. This pattern was described as being more "automatized." Diurnal variations in performance also were reported in men.[648] Mean morning performance on a color-naming task was slightly but significantly faster than afternoon performance, whereas the reverse pattern was seen on an Embedded Figures Task. This pattern was attributed to the diurnal variation in plasma testosterone levels (approximately 20% higher at 9 A.M. than at 4 P.M.). Since adrenocortical hormones show a similar cyclicity in diurnally active humans, and since female controls were not included in these studies, this conclusion is tentative at best. However, the afternoon decline in "automatization" ability was reported to be partially but significantly reversed by the infusion of intravenous testosterone.[586]

Recently, Gouchie and Kimura[425] reexamined the possibility of diurnal variations in male cognitive performance, using a different battery of cognitive tests. Testosterone concentrations were verified through salivary assays. Using normal university students as subjects, no statistically significant diurnal variations in spatial performance were detected. It may be true that the types of changes reported by Mackenberg are small and select or, alternatively, that the diurnal variation in blood levels of testosterone is simply too minor to exert any major effect on men's cognitive functioning. Of course, it is also possible that there is a time lag between the period of maximal testosterone concentration in the circulation and its behavioral consequences, and if so, it is difficult to know exactly when any behavioral "assay" should be performed.

A more interesting outcome of the Gouchie and Kimura study was their finding of a stable, nonlinear relationship between testosterone levels and certain cognitive abilities.[426] The results are in some ways similar to those reported previously by Shute and colleagues[947] for performance on the Minnesota Paper Form Board Test (MPFB), a well-known test of spatial ability. In the study by Shute and colleagues, individual differences in spatial tasks in a group of male and female university students proved to be related in a nonlinear fashion to free androgen levels as determined by plasma radioimmunoassay.[947] On the MPFB, low-androgen level males performed better than high-androgen males, whereas high-androgen females performed better than low-androgen females. The study generated some controversy about whether the responsible hormone was actually testosterone or some other androgen because the assay technique used by Shute and associates was apparently not specific to testosterone. McKeever and associates,[699] using a more specific antibody, failed to find significant correlations between testosterone and performance on the MPFB, but they used a less sensitive statistical analysis. Others have questioned whether the relationship between testosterone and ability is truly nonlinear. In a large sample of young men, for example, Christiansen and Knussman[207] reported small negative correlations between testosterone and verbal test scores and small positive correlations between testosterone and spatial test scores. However, the statistical technique used in this study may have obscured nonlinear relationships that were originally present.

Figure 12.11 shows that in the Gouchie and Kimura study,[426] females with higher levels of free testosterone showed better performance on a test of spatial ability than females with lower testosterone levels, whereas the reverse was true for males—i.e., higher levels of free testosterone were associated with poorer spatial performance. In contrast, measures of perceptual speed and articulation did not show this pattern. Naturally, testosterone levels were considerably different in the two sexes (approximately 175 pg/ml for males versus

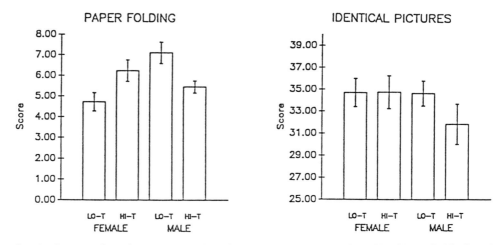

Figure 12.11 Results from the Gouchie and Kimura (1991) study on a test of spatial ability (Paper Folding) and a test of perceptual speed and accuracy (Identical Pictures Test). Subjects within each sex were subdivided into low- and high-testosterone groups according testosterone (T) levels measured in saliva.

50 pg/ml for females). This study not only confirms and extends Shute and colleagues' results, it also demonstrates a definite relation between testosterone specifically and spatial performance. Thus, although diurnal variations in testosterone levels may not be correlated with noticeable cognitive variations in males, males do not appear to be immune to hormonal variations correlated with cognitive ability. It should be noted, however, that the nondiurnal Gouchie and Kimura results are not necessarily activational in nature. Until other studies in men are available, the evidence for activational effects of hormones will be based mainly on evidence obtained from spontaneous or exogenously induced variations in hormone levels in women.

Nonmenstrual Studies

Nonmenstrual cognitive studies in adults have been extremely rare to date. Aside from the studies on males just described, very few such studies exist. Memory decline is a common complaint among postmenopausal women, and there have been several attempts to show that improvement in memory occurs in postmenopausal women taking estrogen replacement therapy.[451] Results have been inconclusive. Hackman and Galbraith,[451] for example, reported a significant improvement in memory in a double-blind pilot study of a small group of women on estrogen replacement therapy compared to controls receiving a placebo. But the results varied considerably from woman to woman in the treated group, and there appeared to be some initial disparity between the treated and nontreated groups in their pretreatment memory performance. Recently, memory also has been studied in *surgically* menopausal women receiving hormone replacement therapy following hysterectomy with bilateral removal of the ovaries.[942, 944] Results have suggested that administration of exogenous estrogen may reverse some of the mild memory impairments seen in untreated women. Further studies are needed, which should include measures to rule out affective changes as the mechanism for this improvement in light of the apparent buoyant effect of estrogen on mood.

Finally, results consistent with an activational effect of steroids on adult cognitive abilities were obtained in a recent nonmenstrual study by Woodfield.[1113] In this study, performance on the Embedded Figures Test was examined in women before and after childbirth. The predicted deficit in performance was seen in women tested during the thirty-eighth to fortieth weeks of pregnancy compared with their performance 6 weeks after delivery, when gonadal hormone levels had declined. Performance on a control task, a vocabulary test, did not change as a function of hormone state. The observed changes in Embedded Figures Test performance were above and beyond the effects of practice, which were assessed using two hormonally stable control groups.

Several recent studies have first quantified hormone concentrations directly through the use of radioimmunoassay techniques and then examined the correlations between these measurements and scores on cognitive tests. Although some significant relationships between gonadal hormones[436, 456] or gonadotropins[421] and cognitive performance have been obtained, the interpretation of these findings is very difficult. Do these relationships reflect the activational effects of the hormones? And if so, which hormones? The answers are not clear-cut. Given the dearth of information in this area, we are unable to draw any conclusions from these studies at present.

At the beginning of this section, we set out to describe some evidence that gonadal hormones may have activational effects on certain cognitive and motor skills in humans. There is a long history of menstrual cycle research, culminating in our own studies, that is relevant to this question, although the studies as a rule were not explicitly designed to test this particular hypothesis. We have seen that despite many nonsignificant and inconsistent results, the pattern that emerges from recent studies, as well as from some of the past studies that employed more precise methodology, is that the ambient hormone state may indeed affect cognitive functioning. Morever, this relationship may not be a simple one. It is not the same, for example, for all cognitive abilities, and for some it may be nonlinear or in other ways highly complex.

Discussion and Summary

Two major questions arise from all of the data that we've presented here. If there are in fact organizational or activational effects of sex steroids on human behavior, particularly on human cognitive and motor skills, (1) what are the mechanisms responsible for these effects, and (2) what implications do these effects have for research and for our everyday lives?

A Question of Mechanism

The very existence of sex steroid effects on human cognitive and motor behavior is still disputed, so it is not surprising that the possible neural bases for these effects are largely unexplored. Furthermore, in humans, technical and ethical considerations place stringent limits on the types of research that might shed light on possible hormonal interactions with the brain. Therefore, at present there are few empirical data in the human literature that pertain to questions of mechanism, and we must rely on the animal literature for clues to the possible bases for these effects, on the assumption that similar mechanisms operate in humans as well.

In earlier chapters we saw how prenatal or perinatal exposure to androgens or androgen metabolites in other species can produce lasting structural changes or changes in hormone sensitivity in specific regions of the brain. The SDN-POA and songbird nuclei are examples of such effects. Although sex differences in human brain organization have been reported, as we outlined earlier in the chapter, there is so far no direct evidence that any of these result from the actions of sex hormones on neural tissue. However, given that such effects do occur during sexual differentiation in other species, it would be surprising if analogous effects did *not* occur in the human brain.

Perhaps the strongest evidence that this may be the case are reports of sex differences in the preoptic area of the human hypothalamus,[18, 1014] since this area is known to be hormone sensitive in other mammalian species. If predictable differences in this area were to be found in individuals with recognized endocrine abnormalities, such as in females with CAH for example, we would have grounds for believing that sex hormones may contribute to this particular sex difference. Unfortunately, there has been almost no attempt to study the possibility of variations in brain organization in individuals with endocrine abnormalities, even by indirect means. An exception is the Hines report of differences between DES-exposed women and controls in certain aspects of their dichotic listening performance.[491] Although this finding raises the possibility of the presence of a hormonal influence on cerebral language lateralization, the effect noted in that study was weak and needs confirmation. If fetal exposure to gonadal steroids does influence neural differentiation at specific brain sites, it would be easy to see how this might provide a possible basis for organizational effects on behavior, both in normal individuals and in those with endocrine disorders.

There are several possible mechanisms by which gonadal steroids may exert more transient effects on the central nervous system as well. In nonhuman species, many of the effects of steroids are believed to be mediated through the actions of the hormone on the genome as described in chapter 1. Specifically, steroids are thought to induce selective gene activation, which results in the synthesis of specific proteins. Estradiol, as well as other gonadal hormones, has been shown to regulate the concentrations of specific enzymes involved in neurotransmitter synthesis and breakdown. Variations in a number of such enzymes as a result of exposure to estradiol have been documented (for reviews see McEwen,[685] McEwen et al.,[687] McEwen et al.,[689]), including reductions in monoamine oxidase (MAO), an enzyme involved in the degradation of catecholamines. That this enzyme may be similarly hormone dependent in humans is suggested by the fact that MAO activity in plasma varies as a function of estrogen state.[585, 587] (MAO is normally present in blood to metabolize catecholamines and serotonin released peripherally.) The ability to influence differentially the synthesis, reuptake, and degradation of various neurotransmitters provides a means by which a single hormone may simultaneously exert different effects on different behavioral systems.

Other effects of estrogens and progestins on the central nervous system that do not require the presence of cytosolic receptors are also possible. For example, changes in neuronal firing rates, with onset latencies on the order of milliseconds to seconds, can be produced by local application of gonadal steroids.[567, 811, 972, 1122] These effects occur too rapidly to be mediated by genomic interactions, and it has been hypothesized that such direct steroid effects involve some kind of membrane receptor sites.[686] Morever, it is likely that steroids evoke secondary effects on neural activity in brain areas that are connected synaptically with regions that are more directly sensitive to gonadal steroids. Finally, estrogens can be hydroxylated in the brain, thus conferring a catechol structure on the steroid molecule. There is some evidence that these so-called catecholestrogens are biologically active, and so the interaction of catecholestrogens with enzymes involved in catecholamine metabolism, and possibly even with catecholamine receptors themselves (i.e., norepineprine, dopamine) must be considered.[432, 689]

Thus, there are multiple possible mechanisms by which the activational effects of estrogens and progestins may be mediated. However, *where* in the human brain such effects may occur is unknown. The results of studies in our own laboratory[457] suggest that areas involved in manual and oral motor control may be among the areas directly or indirectly sensitive to gonadal steroids, estradiol in particular. Cortical areas known to be involved in manual and oral movement programming have been reported to be sexually differentiated in humans,[576] as we saw earlier in this chapter. Women as a group show greater dependence on the anterior left hemisphere for these functions. It is possible that these areas are sensitive to the influence of gonadal steroids during adult life. Since androgen receptors have been detected in the neocortex of the human temporal lobe in brain specimens obtained from adult males,[917] it is possible that estrogen receptors may exist in other cortical locations. In the rat, Becker and associates[101] also have reported a modulatory influence of 17β-estradiol on motor functions thought to be dependent on the striatum, raising the possibility that other areas involved in motor control, even those containing few if any genomic estrogen receptors, may also be estrogen sensitive (see chapter 11).

In the Hampson and Kimura studies, visuospatial ability also appeared to be hormone sensitive. The right hemisphere is generally acknowledged to be specialized for perceptual and spatial analysis in humans,[110] and in females the right anterior region in particular has been reported to be important, at least for visuoconstructional functions.[576] One could speculate on the basis of the changes in spatial performance displayed during the menstrual cycle that certain regions of the right hemisphere may be transiently suppressed by high levels of estradiol. It is possible that these areas may include sexually dimorphic regions of the right frontal lobe. Interestingly, there is some evidence that depressed moods may be accompanied by asymmetrical electroencephalographic (EEG) activation over the frontal lobes, with greater activity in the right frontal region.[919, 1053] Consistent with the hypothesized release of suppression or inhibition at lower blood estrogen levels, women report greater depression and other types of negative affect during the menstrual than during the preovulatory phase of the menstrual cycle.[456]

One very interesting observation arising from the menstrual cycle studies is that dichotic listening performance appears to vary during the menstrual cycle. Women consistently showed greater ear asymmetry scores during the preovulatory phase, when estradiol levels were high, compared with menses, when estradiol levels were low (figure 12.10). Similar trends were apparent when the dichotic performance of menstruating versus midluteal phase women was compared, and also in a study by Altemus and colleagues,[23] comparing the late follicular and premenstrual phases of the cycle. In our study, when the two ears were examined separately, left ear accuracy was found to be significantly poorer with higher levels of estrogen, whereas the right ear if anything, did better at that time. Again, this is consistent with the notion of reduced effective right hemispheric engagement at higher blood estrogen concentrations. Further studies are needed to determine whether this finding can be generalized to other types of dichotic stimuli.

Although a differential effect of hormones on the two hemispheres may sound very unlikely, the animal literature shows that the neural effects of gonadal steroids may be highly localized within discrete regions of the brain.[687] In fact, there is some suggestive evidence that the two cerebral hemispheres may at some points in development actually differ in their sensitivity to hormones (also, for the hypothalamus, see Nordeen and Yahr[778]). In the adult rat, for example, the right cerebral cortex is reported to be thicker than the left in males but not in females.[293] This asymmetry may be due to a suppressant effect of testicular androgens on cortical enlargement, especially in the left hemisphere, during perinatal development.[991] In the neonatal male rat, estrogen receptor density has been shown to be significantly greater in the left cortex, while in the female the right cortex contains a greater density of estrogen receptors.[273, 901] A difference in receptor concentrations may underlie the differential effects of perinatal hormones on the growth of the two hemispheres.

Similarly, in humans, Geschwind and Galaburda[397] have speculated that the presence of testosterone during fetal development may slow the growth of the left hemisphere, permitting relatively greater growth in the right hemisphere. There is so far no direct evidence for this hypothesis. However, deLacoste and

Horvath[270] have reported that in humans as early as 13 weeks of gestational age, the entire right hemisphere is larger than the left in the male fetus, whereas in females the left prerolandic cortex is larger and more developed than the right. (Secretion of testosterone in the fetus peaks at around 13 to 15 weeks of gestation.[535]) It is not known whether the two hemispheres are different in sensitivity to the effects of gonadal steroids in adults.

It should be remembered that any activational effects on the two cerebral hemispheres may represent either direct or indirect effects of steroids. It is possible, for example, that certain regions of the left hemisphere are facilitated by high levels of estrogen but that suppressant effects on right hemispheric functions are indirect, acting through steroid-induced variations in inhibition of the right hemisphere by the left. The fact that high levels of estrogen and progesterone appear to facilitate finger-tapping speed on the left as well as the right hand argues for some regional specificity, however, in that not all regions of the right hemisphere appear to be similarly affected by high levels of steroids. Another possible mode of indirect action might involve the hypothalamus, an area known to contain high densities of estrogen and progestin receptors in all species examined to date.[556, 808] An asymmetry in the gonadotropin-releasing hormone (GnRH) content of the two sides of the hypothalamus has been reported in the adult female rat, favoring the right side,[396] but whether this results from different sensitivities to the feedback effects of estrogen is unknown. Hypothalamic efferents project to numerous limbic and brainstem areas and through these indirectly to the cerebral cortex.[154]

To summarize, at present we can only speculate about possible mechanisms that might mediate the effects of estrogen and progesterone on cognition, mood, and motor performance. The variations in these abilities noted during the menstrual cycle suggest that it may be profitable to explore the adult human brain to determine the locations of estrogen, progestin, and androgen receptors, and especially to determine whether these are present in sexually dimorphic regions of the cerebral cortex.

Implications

The study of hormone-brain-behavior relations in humans is difficult and controversial among both scientists and laymen. Therefore, it is very important to keep the influence of hormonal factors in perspective and to recognize that they represent only one among a complex multitude of biological and environmental influences on human abilities and behavior. The demonstration of hormonal contributions to performance does *not* imply that our abilities are "determined" solely by our biology, nor that environmental factors are unimportant. Moreover, the size of the hormonal effects on cognition and motor abilities demonstrated to date has tended to be small, and in fact this small magnitude has contributed substantially to the difficulty of isolating and distinguishing these effects experimentally.

So why study such small effects? There are important theoretical benefits to this area of research. The study of endocrine abnormalities, for example, may provide valuable new insights into the role of fetal hormones in normal cognitive development, including the types of intellectual functions that may be affected by hormones and the extent, direction, and timing of any influence. Discovery of statistically significant hormone effects on cognition may lead to exciting new hypotheses about the sites and mechanisms involved in hormonal actions in the human brain. The results of these studies may greatly enhance our understanding of the biological factors underlying individual differences in behavior and, more specifically, may shed light on one of the factors contributing to widely recognized sex differences in abilities. Finally, if prenatal hormones are shown to influence later intellectual abilities significantly, even if the influence is minor, this may have important implications for the medical control of hormonal deficiencies or excesses in *utero*, for the administration of exogenous hormones to prevent miscarriage, and for the detection of these abnormalities through neonatal or even prenatal screening programs. Any underlying sex differences in normal brain organization may be of potential significance to neurologists and others who need to understand the different behavioral and cognitive effects of brain damage in men and women.

The menstrual cycle literature has been particularly controversial, but in the menstrual cycle studies conducted to date, no phase of the menstrual cycle has been identified that is characterized by either a generalized decrement or a generalized facilitation in women's performance. If anything, the picture is one of complex minor trade-offs among different abilities. There are some women for whom the observed variations in performance are sufficiently large to be of practical importance, but this is the exception rather than the rule. The fact that the effects vary considerably in direction and degree among individual women emphasizes the inappropriateness of judging any *particular* woman on the basis of these group results. The same can be said of the cognitive correlates of variations in testosterone levels in men. The tests used in these studies were specifically selected to be sensitive to hormonal effects, and in everyday life it seldom happens that we engage in activities that require a single "pure" ability such as these. Our everyday activities typically require a complex interplay of different abilities that may be differently affected by hormones, resulting in little net change in efficiency from one hormone state or one individual to another. Furthermore, the effects of practice might mitigate against these effects in some instances. As mentioned earlier, many studies have failed to detect significant variations during the menstrual cycle in women's performance on complex intellectual tasks (such as course examinations in college), suggesting that one should not be too hasty in generalizing these laboratory findings to everyday life. Therefore, these results are of value not so much for their practical significance as for their theoretical implications.

IMPLICATIONS FOR SEX DIFFERENCES
Sex differences in human cognitive and motor skills are widely acknowledged, but the basis for these differences remains controversial. In some of the men-

strual cycle studies, variations were observed during the cycle in several abilities known to be sexually dimorphic in humans. The direction of hormone effects on specific cognitive and motor skills appeared to be dissociated and to some extent predictable from the direction of known sex differences in population performance. High levels of estrogen and progesterone facilitated certain abilities known to favor females but were detrimental to certain abilities known to favor males. Assuming that males do not show the same pattern of cyclic fluctuations as females, an assumption that is supported by other research,[597] these results suggest that sex differences in specific abilities may fluctuate in magnitude as a function of ambient hormone levels. For example, the sex difference in spatial ability may be somewhat smaller during menses than at higher estrogen points in the female menstrual cycle. Of course, future studies including both men and women as subjects are needed to verify this. In the Hampson[455] study, on first exposure to the tests the difference between women at the menstrual and women at the midluteal phase amounted to a 5% to 15% difference between the means on most sexually dimorphic tests. Most reported sex differences in cognitive abilities are of a similar magnitude. It is therefore possible that hormonal variations may account for a relatively large proportion of the observed sex difference on specific tests despite the relatively small magnitude of these effects in absolute terms. Future studies should include both male and female subjects to clarify more directly the extent to which transient variations in hormone levels contribute to sex differences in abilities.

Acknowledgments

We would like to thank Jill Becker and Jo-Anne Finegan for their valuable comments on earlier versions of this manuscript. The research by E. Hampson and D. Kimura reported here was funded by grants from the Medical Research Council and the Natural Sciences and Engineering Research Council of Canada. Elizabeth Hampson was the recipient of an NSERC post-doctoral fellowship during preparation of this chapter.

We begin now to consider how hormones and behaviors travel a two-way street. Changing an animal's hormonal levels can affect its subsequent behavior, as we have seen in previous chapters. But if they are to survive, organisms must be very sensitive to environmental cues such as those that help predict food availability, coming bad weather, and the presence of potential mates. The individual must also attend to internal cues such as whether there are sufficient body stores of food, water, and other nutrients. These are just a few of the hundreds of stimuli to which animals must attend. All of these cues, plus hundreds of others, affect hormone secretion to prepare the body physiologically for the future. In other words, experience can alter hormone secretion, and, because the animal's behavior often determines whether it will be exposed to stimuli such as daylight, odors, tastes, and so on, changes in behavior can cause changes in hormone secretions.

This reciprocal relationship between hormones and behavior has come up in previous chapters. For example, in chapter 9 we saw how androgens can increase aggression, but aggressive encounters can also change androgen levels. In chapter 10 we learned how the perception of danger, whether real or imagined, can maintain the secretion of "stress hormones." However, for the most part, we have spoken as though hormones alter behavior but not vice versa. This is a convenient manner of thinking that allows us to understand a great many of the relationships between hormones and behavior, but it is clearly an oversimplification. Therefore, in this final portion of the text we dwell futher upon this additional complication to our study of behavioral endocrinology.

Why have hormones and behavior come to affect each other in this reciprocal fashion? Evolution has not conspired to confuse would-be students. Rather, as we suggested above, it is absolutely crucial that organisms carefully respond to external and internal cues so that they can survive. Often the optimal response to such cues is to alter hormonal secretions to prepare the body and the brain for what lies ahead. In chapter 13 we will see that sensory input (sight, taste, touch, smell) provides important cues for the reproductive future of mammals and therefore can have powerful effects on reproductive hormones and behavior. Chapter 14 reviews work with invertebrates showing how hormone release affects behavior, which then affects subsequent hormone release, and so on, resulting in the metamorphosis of the caterpillar to the moth. Chapter 15 covers the relations between the substances ingested and the internal levels of water, salt, and calories. Hormones play a role in maintaining a balance in these elements both in response to behavior (food intake, for example) and in response to the nutrients ingested. Finally, chapter 16 reviews the importance of biological rhythms for virtually all physiological and behavioral processes, and how hormones are an integral part of those rhythms. The rhythms are usually coordinated by external events or regularly occurring behaviors.

13 Environmental Factors Influencing Hormone Secretion

Rae Silver

The sensory input that an animal receives can affect hormonal systems and, in so doing, affect reproductive function. Visual, tactile, olfactory, and auditory cues are all used in this regard, as is illustrated in this chapter. Many mammals are nocturnal, however, and rely heavily on the sense of smell to find food, to avoid danger, even to find and select mates. Furthermore, odorants have powerful influences on reproductive physiology, including the maintenance of pregnancy and the acceleration of puberty. Many of the environmental cues that can affect hormonal secretion and consequently change the physiology or behavior of an individual will also be discussed.

How can environmental stimuli affect hormore secretion and reproductive status, and why might such responses be advantageous? What is the evidence that each of the senses can mediate such influences, and are these effects seen in humans?

Introduction

The reader by now should be familiar with the idea that chemicals produced by our bodies influence how we feel, how we behave, and how we respond to our surroundings. This idea is not new. In ancient times personality traits were attributed to the body's chemical composition; people were thought to be sanguine, phlegmatic, bilious, or splenic according to the proportions of blood, mucus, bile, and spleen produced by their bodies. In modern times, theories about the ways in which hormones influence behavior have evolved to a more refined state, as has been illustrated in the first 12 chapters of this book. There is no doubting the basic concept that body chemistry alters mood, behavior, and perception. We are much less familiar with the idea that our moods, behavior, and perceptions can also alter our body chemistry. The aim of this chapter is to provide an overview of some of the remarkable ways in which the operations of our senses of sight, sound, smell, and touch can change endocrine function. To illustrate this concept we will focus on the chemical changes mediated by the reproductive system.

The plan of the chapter is to describe first the variety of environmental conditions under which hormonal secretions can be altered in humans. The second part of the chapter focuses on similar effects in animals and demonstrates how experiments with animals allow us to isolate specific sensations involved in particular hormonal effects. In the final section we show how environmental stimuli and hormonal responses are integrated during the life cycle of a single animal species. Here we emphasize the ways in which the various sensory and endocrine systems act in unison or in sequence in animals to ensure the coordination between sex partners, and between parents and offspring, that is necessary if reproduction is to be successful.

Environmental Factors that Influence Hormones in Humans

The Pubertal Stage

The first example of an environmental factor that alters hormonal response involves the onset of puberty, the time at which an individual becomes capable of reproduction. In the last 120 years there has been a dramatic decline in the age at which girls reach puberty.[1021] In the mid-1840s, the average Norwegian girl began menstruating at 17 years of age. Today the average age at onset of menses is 13 years (figure 13.1). A similar decrease in the age of puberty has occurred in many other European countries and in the United States. The trend seems to have leveled off in the past 30 years, suggesting that girls may now be reaching sexual maturity at the maximum possible rate.

It is difficult to isolate the environmental factors involved in this interesting shift in the age of puberty because the lives of people today differ in many ways from those of people living 100 years ago. One obvious difference is the increase in the percentage of people living in urban rather than rural settings. If urbanization has a role in the advancement of human puberty, one might expect to see a difference in the average age of puberty between girls living in urban centers and those living in rural communities. There is some evidence for this. For example, during the last century the average age of puberty in girls living in Warsaw has been earlier by almost 2 years than that in girls living in rural parts of Poland.[1021] However, this demographic approach to the question of accelerated puberty is only marginally helpful in the search to isolate the particular environmental factors involved in this acceleration. After all, urban and rural people may differ in the amount and type of work they do, in the nutritional content of their food, and in the sights, sounds, smells, and temperatures to which they are exposed.

There is some evidence that the senses are involved in the onset of puberty in girls. Blind girls with some perception of light reach puberty earlier than normally sighted girls.[1130] Totally blind girls with no light perception reach puberty even earlier than minimally sighted girls. Furthermore, in the springtime, when daylight is present for more than 12 hours of each 24-hour period (and the proportion of light is increasing), fewer girls start to menstruate than during seasons of reduced or decreasing amounts of daylight.[130] Increasing day length, or light, appears to inhibit gonadal development in human beings. However, without direct evidence, we cannot be certain that photic information is the critical seasonal factor that influences the onset of puberty.

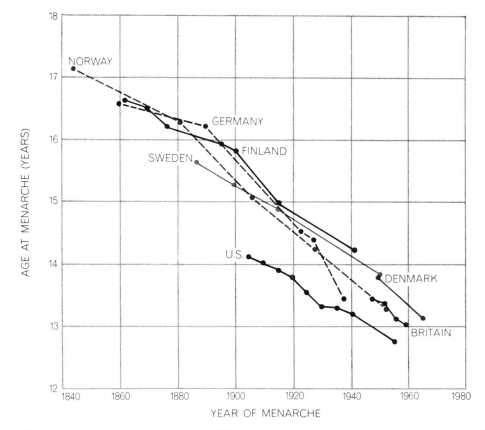

Figure 13.1 The age at menarche has declined in the U.S. and Europe. On the average, girls begin menstruation 2.3 to 3.3 years earlier than they did a century ago. (From Tanner, J. M., 1976[1021] *Earlier Maturation in Man.* © Scientific American, Inc. All rights reserved.)

It might be that the changes of temperature characteristic of the seasons influence the onset of puberty more than the amount of sunlight. However, this seems unlikely. Eskimo and Nigerian girls reach puberty at the same age. Although this suggests that the influence of climate on puberty is a small one, a strong statement to this effect cannot be made based on available correlational data. We do not know the effects (if any) on puberty caused by the increase in mean world temperature that occurred between 1850 and 1940. In fact, we have no data on puberty in equally nourished groups of people living in environments that differ only in climate.

The Adult Stage

MENSTRUAL CYCLES

Stimuli from the environment affect the reproductive functions of the adult as well as the immature individual. Olfactory stimuli can affect women's menstrual cycles. Timing of menstruation was studied in a group of women students living together in a college dormitory[682] (see also chapters 3 and 5). If each woman's menstrual cycle were determined strictly by internal factors, then one would expect that living together would not change the timing of menstruation. However, as the semester proceeded, the scatter in the timing of the menstruation periods decreased in roommates and close friends. That is, the menstrual cycles of women who had spent a lot of time together became synchronized. Of course, people who spend a lot of time together have many shared experiences. They probably keep similar hours, engage in the same activity cycles, eat similar foods, and experience the stresses of exams and other problems at about the same times. Nevertheless, it is reasonable to conclude that the synchronization of menstrual cycles in these college women was at least partially due to olfactory stimuli.

To evaluate whether perspiration smells could synchronize menstrual cycles, perspiration from a donor was mixed with alcohol and applied to the upper lip of experimental subjects.[889] Alcohol alone was applied to the upper lips of control subjects. At the beginning of the study the menstrual periods of the experimental subjects started about 9 days away from the donor's. Four months later, the difference had been reduced to about 3 days. The control group showed no such shift. These results demonstrate that odors can change the menstrual cycle. Of course, this result does not preclude environmental factors such as light, temperature, sound, nutrition, and stress as additional influences on menstrual cycle. In fact, some of these other environmental factors may have altered the chemical quality of the sweat of the donors!

The ability to detect odors has also been associated with reproductive function. In one study olfactory acuity was measured in 96 women with menstrual irregularities and in 500 women with normal menstrual cycles.[662] A high percentage (83%) of the women with menstrual abnormalities had subnormal olfactory acuity. Many of the subjects were not aware of this lack of sensitivity to smells, but a substantial percentage (20%) of those with irregular menses were virtually unresponsive to odors.

A similar effect arises in Kallman's syndrome in men (see also chapter 5), in which small testicular size is accompanied by an inability to smell (anosomia). For a long while the relationship between olfaction and gonadal condition was hard to understand. While the data might indicate that a poor sense of smell results in hormone levels that are too low to ensure normal testicular development and regular menses, they could just as well be taken to suggest that a low hormone level causes a poor sense of smell or that there is no causative but only a correlative relationship between hormone levels and acuteness of the sense of smell. Very recently, however, an explanation for the association between olfactory and gonadal function has emerged, first from studies in mice[930, 1116] and later in related work in humans.[931] In ontogeny, gonadotropin-releasing hormone (GnRH)-expressing cells migrate from the epithelium of the olfactory placode to the hypothalamus (figure 13.2). The principal endocrine deficit in Kallman's syndrome is a failure of secretion of GnRH. In patients with Kallman's syndrome, the agenesis of the olfactory bulbs early in development results in a failure of GnRH neuronal migration

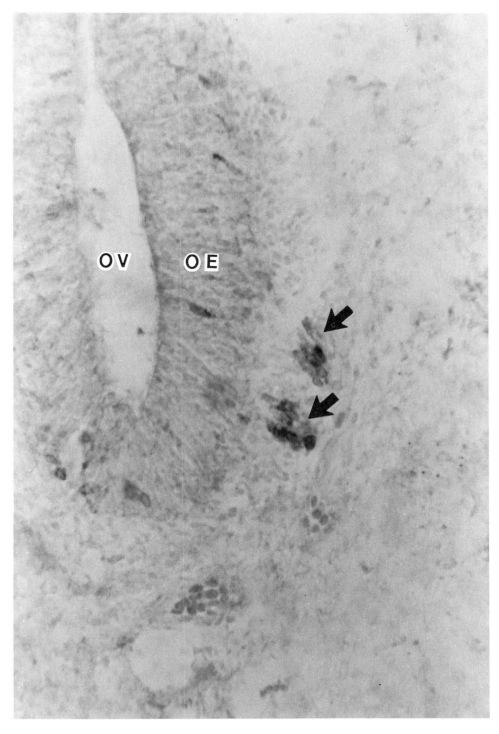

Figure 13.2 GnRH-immunoreactive neurons in the 4-day-old embryonic chick. A cluster of embryonic GnRH cells (arrow) are seen near their origin in the epithelium. OV, olfactory ventricle; OE, olfactory epithelium. (Courtesy of K. A. Sullivan and A. J. Silverman; supported by HD 10665.)

from the olfactory region to the hypothalamus. That is, abnormal olfactory bulb development results in a failure of normal development or migration of GnRH-expressing neurons, resulting in small testes in men and irregular menses in women.

COITUS AND PREGNANCY

Hormonal changes associated with copulation occur in both men and women. In one study the relationship between hormone levels and sexual activity was determined.[372] Serum testosterone concentrations were higher in men during and immediately after intercourse than under resting conditions. In contrast to the changes that accompanied coitus, testosterone levels either increased slightly or not at all after masturbation, indicating that stimuli associated with sexual arousal by a partner are more reliably correlated with changes in testosterone than is ejaculation.

The idea that ejaculation need not precede an increase in male hormone production seems to be supported by an amusing and widely cited letter to the editor of *Nature* magazine.[29] An anonymous author claimed that his beard growth was greater when he anticipated (and when he actually engaged in) sexual activity with his girlfriend than when he was isolated on a remote island. Anonymous suggested that the enhanced beard growth can be explained by an increase in the production of testicular hormones, which are known to influence the rate of beard growth. Needless to say, this report elicited several critical letters to the editor noting that a number of factors, including water content of the skin, thickness of the skin (which changes 2 to 3 hours after awakening), degree of tension exerted by the muscles of the hair follicles, and so on, all influence beard growth. It was suggested that Anonymous could do a better controlled study if he enticed his friend to drop in on him unexpectedly or if she unexpectedly withheld her favors during randomly selected visits.

In a review of annual cycles of human reproduction, Roenneberg and Aschoff[864] integrated data on climatic and photoperiod information for 380 geographical locations. They showed that on a global scale, photoperiod influences the physiology of human reproduction (see figure 6.2). Thus, conception rates are highest during the vernal equinox at high latitudes, where changes in day lengths are pronounced. Temperature also appears to be a major influencing factor. Conception rates are above the annual mean when temperatures are between 5°C and 20°C, and conception rates fall when temperatures lie beyond these extreme values. Roenneberg and Aschoff note that the influence of environmental factors is decreasing in recent decades as people become increasingly shielded from photoperiodic cues (by indoor work) and from temperature (by heating and air conditioning).

Finally, the frequency of birth of fraternal (or dizygotic—from two separate eggs) twins has been reported to be higher in northern countries than in tropical countries. Also, the rate of twinning in the southern parts of France and Japan is lower than in the northern parts of these countries.[551] In this work it has not been determined whether the relevant climatic cue is day length or some other correlated factor such as temperature.

NURSING

One of the most important and easily demonstrable contexts in which external stimuli are known to affect the production of hormones involved in human reproduction occurs during nursing. Milk production begins 2 to 3 days after childbirth. When the baby suckles at the nipple, tactile information from the nipple is transmitted from nerves in the breast to the brain, causing the release of oxytocin and prolactin, which circulate in the blood and ultimately reach the breast to promote milk production and release (see chapter 8). If the baby does not suckle, the mother becomes unable to produce milk. On the other hand, if suckling continues, the mother can continue to produce milk for her own child (or for other children) for many years.

Although relatively rare, milk production and milk release, which together constitute lactation, can occur in women without pregnancy and without a suckling infant, or in men. Lactation can occur after manual stimulation or suckling of the breast of either virgin women or of men. Poorly fitting clothes about the chest can produce lactation. In each of these instances, stimulation of the nerves of the breast releases hormones that produce lactation. Visual or auditory stimuli acting alone can also cause milk release in lactating mothers when they see or hear their baby crying. This response can become conditioned to other cues such as the sound of a nurse opening the door to bring the baby into the mother's room.

In studies of humans we often cannot identify the stimuli that result in changes in hormone secretion. In other cases we can identify the stimuli but cannot always tell precisely how they work. Only in rare instances are we able to control fully a stimulus and to measure precisely a neural and hormonal response.

In the ensuing sections of this chapter animal research that has permitted the isolation and quantification of environmental stimuli that affect hormone production will be explored. Four major sensory modalities (sight, smell, touch, and hearing) will be examined in turn. The effectiveness of stimuli from each modality on seasonal breeding, puberty, cycles of ovulation, pregnancy, and lactation in animals will be discussed.

Environmental Factors that Influence Hormones in Animals

The Visual System

The first experimental demonstration that external stimuli affect the development of reproductive glands was reported by William Rowan in 1925.[881] Rowan kept two groups of migratory birds called juncos in outdoor cages during the cold winter in Edmonton, Alberta. One group was exposed to extra periods of artificial light while the other group experienced only the normal periods of sunlight and darkness of a Canadian winter. At regular intervals after Christmas, Rowan performed autopsies on the birds. He found that the ovaries or the testes of the birds exposed to additional periods of light were enlarged. This remarkable effect was caused by the extra light despite temperatures that dropped to −45°C. In later experiments, Rowan released birds and watched the direction they took as they flew away from the aviary. Juncos that had been exposed to the extra artificial light traveled north as though it were summer, while those kept in normal winter light headed south. Somehow the additional light produced gonadal growth and determined the direction in which the birds migrated.

In recent years the analysis of effects of light on the gonads of birds has reached a very sophisticated level. Substantial evidence indicates that birds (as well as many other animals) are able to measure time, using a "biological clock" in their brain (see chapter 16). These "clocks" allow animals to be awake and alert when they should be—during the daytime for such animals as seed-eating pigeons, and at night for such nocturnal predators as rodents. Interestingly enough, the clock control mechanism in birds receives information through light-sensitive receptors in the brain itself and not exclusively through the eyes or the pineal gland.[1103] If the eyes of a bird such as the white-crowned sparrow are covered by a light-proof shield, the growth of the gonads in response to the light proceeds normally, as if the shield were not present. On the other hand, shielding the brain from light (by injecting an opaque substance such as India ink under the skin overlying the skull) prevents normal gonadal growth even when the eyes are exposed to light.[706] The brain's clock responds to light only during a certain phase of the animal's day, and not to the total amount of light.[367] Animals exposed to short day lengths (e.g., 6 hours of light and 18 hours of darkness) have regressed gonads. Exposure to an additional 15-minute period of light each day is sufficient to produce full growth of the testes if the light exposure is correctly timed. If the 15-minute period does not occur during the clock's sensitive period, no testicular growth occurs (figure 13.3). By shining light of different wavelengths directly on the skull and measuring plasma luteinizing hormone (LH), Foster and colleagues[370] were able to show that the spectral sensitivity of the brain photoreceptor is like that of rhodopsin with a peak sensitivity around 492 nm.

Light has also been shown to affect the onset of puberty in animals. When a female rat reaches puberty, the membrane covering the vagina ruptures. The age at which the vaginal membrane ruptures is therefore a convenient measure of the onset of puberty. Female laboratory rats exposed to normal seasonal fluctuations of light and dark demonstrate an influence of light upon attainment of puberty. Females born in April show vaginal membrane rupture at an average of 40 days, whereas those born in November do not show rupture until they are 47 days of age. Further evidence of an effect of light on puberty in rats comes from experiments in which females are raised under conditions of constant artificial light from the day of birth. Their vaginal membranes rupture

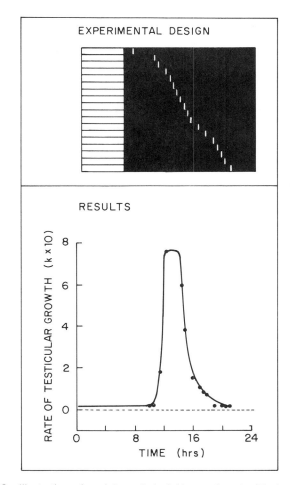

Figure 13.3 Illustration of an interrupted night experiment with Japanese quail. The effect of 15-minute light administered at various phases of the day on the rate of testicular growth in birds maintained under a photoperiod of 6 hours light and 18 hours of darkness. The upper panel shows the experimental design. Each row describes a different experimental group. The white bars represents periods of light, while the black represents periods of darkness. In the lower panel the ordinate shows the rate of testicular growth. (From Follett and Sharp, 1969.[367])

4 to 7 days earlier than the membranes in females housed in conditions of alternating periods of artificial light and dark each day. It is interesting that the effects of light on puberty in rats, which are nocturnal are opposite to those seen in humans, who are diurnal. In diurnal birds such as white-crowned sparrows, light has a delaying effect on puberty, as it does in humans.[1128]

The influence of light on the age of puberty, as measured by testicular descent, has also been studied in male rats. At the time of birth the testes of rats lie in the abdominal cavity. Sometime before puberty, the testes descend from the abdominal cavity into the scrotum. The time of descent of the testes was advanced by several days in rats housed in constant light compared to control males housed in an environment of alternating periods of light and dark.

Visual stimuli more complex than light also affect hormone production in animals. A very good example is provided by the factors affecting ovarian development in certain adult female lizards, *Anolis carolinensis*. As discussed in chapter 6, the male lizard courts the female by bobbing his body up and down in a manner resembling push-up exercises and by extending his dewlap, a semi-circular flap of tissue under his throat. In one experiment, the dewlaps of some males were painted with blue India ink, thereby masking the normal red color. In other males, the dewlap was surgically prevented from extending from the throat. This surgery did not interfere with the lizard's ability to perform the bobbing movements. If a female were courted by a male that could not extend his dewlap, her ovaries did not grow. The color of the male's dewlap did not influence the female's ovarian response. Clearly, ovarian development in a female lizard of this particular species is not induced merely by seeing a male but by seeing it court by bobbing and extending its dewlap. As Crews points out (chapter 6) while courtship by the male promotes ovarian development, aggressive displays are inhibitory.

A final example of the effects of visual stimuli on reproductive hormones involves the effect of light on pregnancy.[730] The total length of pregnancy and the timing of delivery were measured in rats kept on one of three schedules of artificial light: short (2 hours of light per day), long (22 hours per day) or intermediate (14 hours per day). The results showed that the duration of pregnancy was 12 hours longer in animals exposed to long periods of light each day than in animals exposed to short or intermediate light length schedules. The time of delivery (parturition) was also influenced by light in that all three groups of animals tended to give birth during the time of day in which the lights were turned on.

From all these accounts of animal research it is obvious that visual stimuli are capable of affecting reproductive processes such as the onset of puberty, growth of the gonads in adulthood, and duration of pregnancy. We will see that the senses of smell, touch, and hearing also affect these processes.

Olfaction and Chemical Cues

Chemical substances released by one animal that affect the behavior or physiology of another animal are called pheromones (see Vandenbergh[1063] for review). Dogs deposit chemical cues when they urinate on tree trunks and fire hydrants. Other dogs are very interested in these deposits and spend substantial amounts of time sniffing them. Male moths of a certain species fly from considerable distances to approach the source of an odorous substance released by a conspecific female.

The term **signaling pheromone** was coined by Bronson[156] to distinguish complex mammalian responses to chemical cues from the term **releasing pheromone**, used to describe the more rigid, stereotyped responses of insects to chemical cues. Signaling (or releasing) pheromones affect the behavior of the recipient. In contrast, **priming pheromones** can induce physiological changes in the recipient. Priming pheromones are less rapid and less direct in their effects.

One of the best known signaling pheromone systems involves the behavioral responses of the hamster to odor cues. If the olfactory system is destroyed, the male hamster will neither court a female nor show sexual behavior (see Johnston[537] for review). Male hamsters that are sexually experienced prefer the odor of estrous females to that of pregnant or lactating females. This is an adaptive response because lactating and pregnant hamsters are very aggressive toward males.

It has been established that the vaginal discharge from the female hamster contains chemosignals that attract and stimulate the sexual behavior of the male.[769] If the hamster vaginal discharge is applied to the hindquarters of a male hamster, either anesthetized or alert, it is sexually attractive to other males. In addition to eliciting male sexual behavior and related responses such as approaching and sniffing at the odor, hamster vaginal discharge produces a short-latency rise in testosterone and a lowering of aggressive tendencies. This response may involve learning because responses to hamster vaginal discharge can be conditioned.[538] Finally, early androgen exposure influences responses to hamster vaginal discharge. Females that receive testosterone neonatally have a significant preference for hamster vaginal discharge following gonadectomy.[442]

Priming pheromones are capable of acting at all stages of the reproductive life of an animal. They have been shown to affect the timing of puberty (Vandenbergh effect), the suppression of ovulation (the Lee-Boot effect), the induction of ovulation (Whitten effect), and the maintenance of pregnancy (Bruce effect) in a number of rodent species, particularly mice.

ONSET OF PUBERTY

Female mice attain puberty earlier when they are exposed to a pheromone in adult male urine than when they are not (Vandenbergh effect). If a small quantity of urine from adult males is dabbed between the nose and mouth of immature mice, these mice reach puberty sooner than females dabbed with a control substance such as water.[219] Additional research indicates that the pheromones are produced only by animals that have androgen in adequate quantities in their circulation.

Social factors that presumably cause decreases in production of androgen also cause decreases in the production of the pheromone. Among these social factors are subordination by other males and the presence of pregnant or lactating females. Isolation of the puberty-accelerating pheromone from male urine has not yet been achieved. The pheromone itself is not an androgen; column chromatography of male urine suggests that it is a factor with a molecular weight of 860 daltons.[1064] Also, it is not volatile and therefore is not carried by the air from the male to the female. Rather, the female must directly contact the urinary pheromone by touching, tasting, or ingesting it.

A pheromone produced by adult female mice may inhibit the onset of puberty in young females. The first indication that this might be so came from a study showing that isolated female mice reach puberty earlier than female mice kept in groups. By itself, this finding does not necessarily mean that a pheromone is involved. The effect could be due to crowding, to tactile contact among females, to auditory stimuli, or to visual stimuli. Proof of the involvement of a pheromone was shown by brushing a small amount of urine taken from grouped female mice on the noses of isolated immature females. When this procedure was followed for 7 consecutive days, puberty occurred later than in control females that had water brushed on their noses.[698] Further studies showed that this puberty-retarding pheromone is produced by adult as well as juvenile female mice that are in physical contact with one another.

It has been suggested that the male pheromone (that favors onset of puberty) and female pheromone (that inhibits onset of puberty) help to regulate population density. Thus, the total amount of male pheromone released will be low when *many* males are present because production of male hormones is stifled in males that become subordinate during intense male-male aggressive interactions. The total amount of female pheromone present should theoretically increase with increasing population density, and this should increase the likelihood that immature individuals will reach puberty later when population density is high and earlier when population density is low. Puberty-accelerating pheromone appears to be less stable than puberty-inhibiting pheromone, suggesting that they are not identical.[1064]

ONSET OF ESTRUS

As in immature female mice, grouping of adult females seems to inhibit the ovaries. To test whether the inhibitory effect of grouping females is due to a pheromone, several experimental strategies have been used. Grouped female mice, in the absence of a male, show a suppression of ovarian function even if they are blinded, deafened, or prevented from having direct body contact with one another. By the process of elimination, this indicates that a pheromone is involved. More direct evidence for this supposition comes from an experiment in which isolated female mice stopped showing regular ovulatory cycles when they were exposed to sawdust soiled by a group of females. It is not yet certain whether the pheromone that inhibits reproductive activity in adult female mice is identical to the pheromone that inhibits the onset of puberty in mice.

PREGNANCY

The best known experiments on the effects of pheromones on reproductive hormones were carried out by H. M. Bruce.[164] She noticed that pregnancy failed in mice that were exposed to a male other than the inseminator (termed the Bruce effect). If the new male belonged to the same strain ("strange male") as the inseminator, pregnancy failed in 30% of cases, but if the new male belonged to a different strain ("alien male"), pregnancy failed in 80% of the cases. If the strange or alien male was not introduced within 4 days after the insemination by the first male, pregnancy did not fail. A role of pheromones in this phenomenon is shown by several type of experiments. When the sense of smell is eliminated in females before mating, the presence of alien males did not result in pregnancy failure. Furthermore, pregnancy failure did occur in female mice with an intact sense of smell when they were exposed to bedding material that had been soiled by alien males. The pheromone is contained in the urine of animals that have adequate quantities of androgen. The primary way in which the pheromone disrupts pregnancy appears to involve a decrease in prolactin.[654] Pheromonal stimuli from an alien male decrease prolactin release, preventing formation of corpora lutea. The consequent decrease of progesterone prevents implantation. Administration of exogenous progesterone prevents the male-induced pregnancy block. Finally, column chromatography indicates that the active fraction of the pregnancy-blocking pheromone is approximately the same as the puberty-accelerating pheromone, suggesting that they may be the same agent.[1064]

The Sense of Touch

The sense of touch or pressure has been shown to be involved in the alteration of hormone levels at all stages of reproductive life in nonprimate mammals. The effect of tactile stimulation on hormones involved in ovulation in adult animals of certain species is very well documented (see chapter 3). For example, cats, rabbits, and ferrets generally do not ovulate unless they are mounted and the male achieves intromission. If the female's ovaries are adequately developed and in a state of readiness to ovulate, this tactile contact during copulation provides the neuroendocrine signal that causes a surge of LH from the pituitary. Ovulation then occurs within a few hours. How do we know that such "reflex ovulation" is caused by tactile cues from the male rather than visual, olfactory, or auditory cues? There are several ways of establishing this. For example, the nerves leading from the genital area of the female can be severed or anesthetized so that the nerve impulses caused by tactile stimulation of the genitals do not reach the brain. When this is done, intromission by the male fails to cause reflex ovulation. Another approach is for the experimenter to stimulate the cervix of a cat, rabbit, or ferret with a glass rod. This tactile stimulation causes ovulation even though the male of the species cannot be seen, smelled, or heard by the female.

Of course, females of many species do not require contact by other members of their species to ovulate. These species, of which humans are one, are known as "spontaneous ovulators." In some instances we can change a spontaneous ovulator into a reflex ovulator by experimental manipulation. For example, female rats kept in continuous light fail to ovulate spontaneously, as rats normally do. When a male copulates with a continuous light-exposed female rat, she ovulates reflexively. Glass rod stimulation of the female's cervix produces the same result.

When a male mouse copulates with a female mouse who is about to ovulate "spontaneously," the female usually becomes pregnant. If the male is vasectomized before he copulates, the tactile stimulation provided to the female's cervix by the male's penis causes changes in the female's hormonal condition that are quite similar to the hormonal conditions that prevail early in pregnancy. This condition, induced by the vasectomized male, is called pseudopregnancy. These findings suggest that hormonal changes characteristic of the start of pregnancy or pseudopregnancy arise as the result of tactile stimulation of the female's cervix at about the same time as she is spontaneously ovulating. If this is so, an experimenter should be able to stimulate the cervix of a mouse with a glass rod or mechanical vibrator and induce a state of pseudopregnancy. However, many attempts to do this have failed.

Diamond[288] sought to understand the basis of these pregnancy failures. He observed that when male mice copulate they intromit into the female about 5 to 13 times before they ejaculate, and there are intervals of 90 to 215 seconds between intromissions. Diamond reasoned that this pattern of repeated intromissions with characteristic intervals between them constitute a kind of "vaginal code" of tactile stimulation. He then imitated this code with mechanical stimulation of the female's cervix. When this code was imitated, pseudopregnancy was induced, but when the vaginal code was not imitated (i.e., too few insertions of the mechanical vibrator or inappropriate intervals between insertions), pseudopregnancy was not induced. Apparently, not only the amount but also the pattern of tactile stimulation of the cervix is important for starting the changes in hormone secretion that accompany the early stages of pregnancy in mice. Similar findings have been made in rats and hamsters, each species of rodent having a different vaginal code. A further description of the function of pacing intromissions is provided in chapter 3.

The importance of tactile cues from the cervix in initiating the hormonal changes of pregnancy has been shown in other ways. For example, the nerves leading from the cervix to the brain were severed in female rats. The females were then allowed to mate with male rats. Even though mating and spontaneous ovulation occurred, no pregnancy or pseudopregnancy ensued in the female rats. Further experimentation showed that a deficit in prolactin secretion caused by the severance of the nerves first become apparent about 8 hours after mating. If nerve-severed female rats were given an injection of prolactin 8 hours after mating, pregnancy occurred. Prolactin seems to potentiate the release of progesterone from the corpus luteum, thereby facilitating pregnancy. Note the parallels between this effect and the mechanism whereby pheromones disrupt pregnancy, described earlier. From these experiments one can conclude that tactile stimulation of the cervix of rats somehow signals the brain to cause the release of prolactin from the pituitary gland. Without this tactile signal, prolactin is not released in adequate quantities to ensure sufficient progesterone release, and pregnancy does not ensue in the rat.

Not only does tactile stimulation of the cervix serve an important role in starting the production of hormones in early pregnancy, it also seems to influence the later stages of pregnancy in at least some rodents. In hamsters, artificial insemination fails to produce pregnancy.[289] If a hamster is artificially inseminated and is then given an injection of progesterone, pregnancy results, but only 25% of the offspring are born alive. If a hamster is artificially insemi-nated and her cervix is mechanically stimulated at the same time, pregnancy ensues, and all the offspring are born alive. In some unknown way, tactile stimulation of the cervix (perhaps by causing the release of prolactin, which maintains the production of progesterone) ensures the well-being of the fetuses. It seems truly remarkable that the information provided by tactile stimulation of the vaginal cervix during copulation of the hamster should be translated and stored in such a way as to influence the viability of the offspring.

We have now seen that tactile stimuli influence the onset of puberty, the occurrence of ovulation, and the start and maintenance of pregnancy. The sense of touch has an influence on hormones at yet another stage of the repro-ductive process, the nursing phase. The sense of touch is important for the initiation of adequate mammary growth for nursing. This has been shown in experiments with rats. Pregnant rats that had a kind of Elizabethan ruffle collar placed around their necks had much smaller mammary glands than rats with-out such a collar. Apparently, this result occurred because collared females could not lick their own bellies, and failure to self-lick the teats resulted in a failure to produce hormones that encourage mammary gland growth. When collared pregnant female rats had their teats mechanically stimulated, mam-mary growth was similar to that seen in normal rats. In fact, mechanical stimulation or massage of the teats induced mammary gland growth even in virgin rats (see chapter 8).

The Sense of Hearing

Although auditory signals are important during courtship and sexual behavior, their effects on reproduction have not been examined as intensively as the effects of other environmental factors such as light, odor, and touch. For this reason we will have to depart from our usual form of discussing, in order, the effects of sensation on hormones involved in puberty, ovulation, start of preg-nancy, maintenance of pregnancy, and lactation.

In some species, sounds produced by one member affect the production of hormones by a reproductive partner. Some interesting examples of the way these intraspecific (within species) sounds function as a normal component of reproductive cycles have been reported in birds. For example, Kroodsma[605] tape-recorded the songs of male canaries. One group of female canaries heard a large repertoire of songs while another group heard a smaller song repertoire. Females that heard the larger repertoire built nests sooner and laid more eggs than females that heard only a small variety of songs. Evidently, female repro-ductive hormone production and female reproductive behavior are stimulated by the content of the song of the male canary. A similar conclusion can be drawn from Brockway's[152] work with an Australian parrot, the budgerigar. Female budgerigar vocalizations were recorded on tape and played daily to the females in 2-hour sequences for a total of 6 hours or in one continuous 3-hour sequence. When the tape consisted of males singing a "soft warble," the females' ovaries grew and ovulation resulted. When the tape consisted of other male vocalizations such as "squacks," "chedelees," "whedelees," "tuks," and "loud warbles," the ovaries were not stimulated. Later work with budgerigars showed that females reach a higher degree of reproductive development when exposed to male song during the first half of the day than when exposed during the second half.

Not only does the male budgerigar stimulate the ovaries of females by his song, his song may also cause stimulation of his own testes. Brockway[153] "devocalized" male budgerigars by cutting the nerves and muscles involved in song production. The devocalized males had smaller testes and a lower sperm count than unoperated males. This difference was apparent even when the devocalized males were allowed to hear the songs of normal males. Thus, the male budgerigar seems to stimulate his own gonads by singing. The component of the song that seems to be involved is the long warble.

A few studies on the effects of intraspecific audible sounds on hormone production by mammals also have been performed. In one such study, a lactating female (female A) rat, exposed to the stimuli emanating from another lactating rat (female B) with her litter, ejected more milk in response to suckling than a control lactator (female C) that was not exposed to these stimuli. However, if female A was surgically deafened, no difference in ejection of milk occurred between female A and female C. From this, one would suppose that auditory stimuli from female B and her litter somehow increased release of the hormone that regulates the ejection of milk in female A.

Ultrasounds (i.e., sounds of too high a frequency to be heard by humans) have been shown to form part of the intraspecific communication mechanism in several mammals, but so far no reports of the effects of ultrasonics emitted by one member of a species on the hormone production of another member of the same species have appeared.

The Behavior of Ring Doves: How Environmental Factors Coordinate Hormones and Behavior

In the preceding sections, hormonal responses of the reproductive system after activation of the visual, auditory, tactile, or olfactory system in several different species were described. Although these examples give us a feel for the variety of ways in which the senses can affect the chemical constitution of the body, they do not illustrate how the senses operate together or in sequence to produce hormonal changes that are required for successful cycles of reproduction in a particular animal. To illustrate how the various senses come into play during the reproductive cycle of a particular animal, I will describe reproduction in an intensively studied laboratory species of bird, the ring dove. The story of the breeding cycle of the ring dove, first told by the late D.S. Lehrman,[618] provides an incomparable example of the delicate relationships among external stimuli, hormones, and behaviors required for successful reproduction (reviewed in Buntin,[171] Cheng,[199] Silver,[951] see chapter 8).

Male and female ring doves look alike: they weigh the same, and they have the same porcelain-like creamy color and semicircle of black feathers around the back of the neck (figure 13.4). The female and male court each other, build a nest together, share in incubating their eggs, and feed their young squab. When the young are able to eat by themselves, the adults begin a new cycle of courtship, incubation, and rearing of young.

How are the senses involved in cyclic occurrence of these hormone-dependent reproductive activities? In the first phase of the reproductive cycle, the perception of light is important for gonadal growth. Courtship behavior by the male depends on adequate gonadal development. If laboratory doves are housed in artificial lighting conditions that resemble those of winter (short days and long nights), the testes of the male remain small. If the doves are then placed in artificial light conditions that resemble summer (long days and short nights), the testes begin to grow. But light is not the only factor in the external environment that affects the growth of the male's gonads. If a male dove is placed by himself in a short day length environment, his testes grow less than those of a male housed with a sexually active female under identical conditions of short day length. These results indicate that two visual factors are important for testicular growth in males: photoperiodic stimulation by light and the presence of a sexually active female.

How do we know that it is sight rather than touch, sound, or smell that induces increased testicular development in the male? Furthermore, how do we know that the sight of another male or the sight of a sexually *inactive* female would not be as effective as the sight of a sexually active female? To obtain definitive answers, we performed the following series of experiments. On one side of a cage, we placed individual male ring doves, and on the other side, separated by a clear glass partition, we placed either another male, a sexually inactive female, or a sexually active female.[785, 786] We then measured the amount of hormone produced by testes of the experimental males. The sight of a sexually active female (but not of a sexually inactive female or of a male) on the other side of the glass partition caused as much production of male hormone as that resulting from placing a male and a sexually active female in the same cage. By placing a glass partition between the male and the sexually active female we prevented them from touching one another. Thus, physical contact between the male and female is not required for increased testicular activity in the male. The transparent glass barrier still permits the males to hear (and possibly to smell) as well as to see the sexually active female. Further experiments will have to be done (e.g., using an opaque barrier, blocking the sense of smell of the males) to rule out the senses of hearing and smell as important contributors to the activation of testicular hormone production in doves.

Nevertheless, it is clear that the female influences the production of hormones in males during the period of courtship. Does the perception of the male by the female influence the production of hormones by females during courtship? If a female is kept by herself under conditions of long day length,

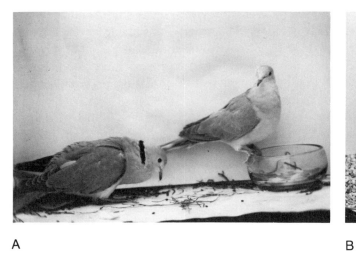

A

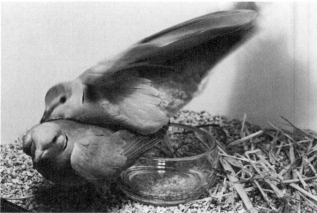

B

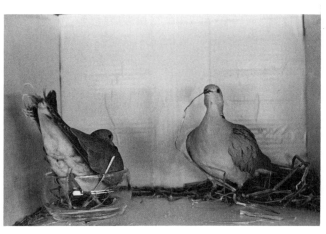

C

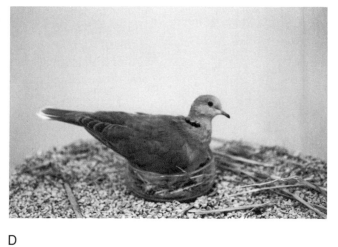

D

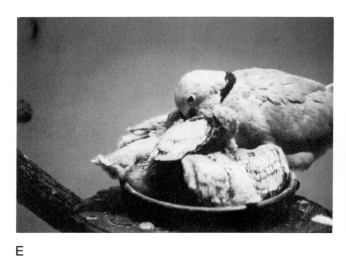

E

F

her ovaries will grow, and she will ovulate about every 6 months or so. However, if females are placed with males, and the long day length conditions are maintained, most (80%) of the females will ovulate and lay eggs in about 8 days.[952] If a female is placed with a male *and* with straw suitable for building a nest, most females (95%) will ovulate and lay eggs about 6 days after pairing. One can show that tactile stimulation is not necessary for egg-laying to occur by separating the female from the male with a transparent glass plate. In this situation, most females will lay (infertile) eggs within about 8 days, just as when they are not separated by a glass barrier. Both the sound and the sight of a courting male are effective in producing ovarian growth. Female birds kept alone in sound-proofed cages show little ovarian growth, but if the sounds from a breeding colony are piped into the cage, significant ovarian growth occurs. If, in addition, the female can see a courting male, and if he responds to her behavior, then ovarian growth is even greater.[382]

Does the sight of any other bird result in ovarian growth, or is there something especially stimulating to the female ring dove about the sight or sound of a courting male? Male ring doves that are castrated do not exhibit courtship behaviors when introduced to a sexually active female, and sexually active females do not ovulate when they are exposed to such noncourting males. Therefore, it seems likely that the sights or sounds of male courtship itself are important for full ovarian development in female ring doves.

While it has long been assumed that the mate's displays induce endocrine changes in its partner, it is also possible that endocrine changes occur in response to an animal's own behavior subsequent to seeing the mate. Females prevented from nest cooing show little or no follicular development in response to active courtship by the male. This suggests that nest cooing stimulates the female's own ovarian system through audio or proprioceptive feedback.[200]

To summarize the events of the courtship part of the reproductive cycle, long day length is important for gonadal growth in both sexes. Males show courtship behavior if they have adequate quantities of testicular hormone in their blood. Perception of the male's courtship behavior increases production of ovarian hormones (estrogen and progesterone) in his female partner. Production of these hormones by the female causes her to act in a sexually active

Figure 13.4 The reproductive cycle begins when the female and male ring doves start to court each other. The male bow-coos at the female (A) and initially, she usually turns away from him. After several days, mating occurs (B), and the pair start to build a nest together, with the female sitting in the nest and the male carrying straw to her (C). The pair take turns incubating their nest (D), with the male sitting for a block of time in the middle of the day and the female sitting the rest of the time. The eggs hatch after about 15 days, and both parents brood their offspring by sitting on them, and feed the young by regurgitation (E). The young grow up very quickly (F). At hatching the young are featherless, they cannot regulate their body temperature, and their eyes are closed. By the time they are 21 days of age, they are weaned and resemble adults, except that they lack the black neck ring. (Photos by Rae Silver.)

manner, and the perception of the female's behavior by the male causes an increased production of testicular hormone (testosterone). This mutual stimulation of hormone secretion ends when the female lays eggs. This marks the end of the courtship and the beginning of the second phase of the breeding cycle, incubation.

Soon after the female lays eggs, the parents take turns incubating to keep the eggs warm. In all pairs, the male sits on the eggs for 6 to 8 hours during the middle of the day, while the female sits on the eggs the rest of the time. The eggs are thus continually covered by one or the other parent. How do ring doves know when to court and when to incubate? If a pair of birds is introduced into a cage already containing a nest with eggs laid by another female, the pair will begin incubation only after several days of courtship and after having built their *own* nest and laid their own eggs over those that had been provided.[619] Why do the birds not incubate immediately, and why do they incubate later? The answer to this question is different for each sex.

Before the female will build a nest or incubate, she must produce the hormones estrogen and progesterone. Proof for this statement comes from a series of experiments in which the ovaries were removed, and the female's behavior was observed after she received various hormone treatments.[201] If the ovariectomized females were given both estrogen and progesterone, both nest building and incubating behaviors were restored. These experiments suggest that in order for the female to show the transition from courtship to incubation behavior, she must produce adequate quantities of estrogen and progesterone in the ovary. As we have already seen, these hormones are produced in response to the sight and sound of a courting male.

The story is quite different for the male, as shown by the following experiment. Shortly after castration, male ring doves were paired with females.[953] Most of the castrated males showed very little courtship behavior, and their mates laid eggs only after a very long interval. Nevertheless, when the females finally laid their (infertile) eggs, the castrated males helped to incubate, even though they received no androgen replacement. Thus, the presence of the male's gonadal hormones is not necessary for the transition from courtship to incubation behavior. Nevertheless, it should be noted that castrated males must reside with female partners for a while before they will incubate. The incubation-encouraging sensory cues that the female provides to the castrated male during this period of cohabitation are not known.

So far we have described how the doves court each other and share in incubating their eggs. Sitting on the eggs has hormonal consequences for both mates. The incubation period (from the time of egg-laying to the time of squab hatch) lasts about 15 days in doves. During this time, the crop gland in the neck of each parent dove grows, and a milky substance, called crop milk, is produced. When the young hatch, the parents feed them crop milk. It is well known that the pituitary hormone prolactin is the most important hormone for the induction of crop growth. We can now ask, which perceived stimuli initiate the secretion of prolactin?

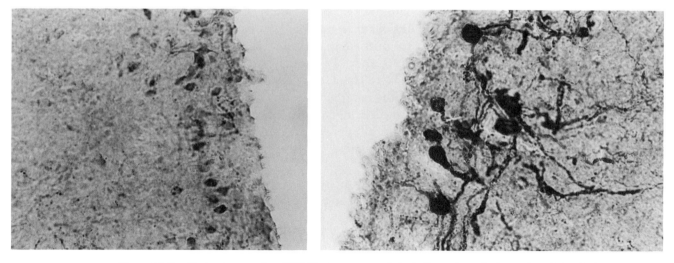

Figure 13.5 Photomicrographs of VIP-like immunoreactivity in the periventricular region of the third ventricle. The left panel shows VIP-like immunoreactive cells in a bird housed in isolation; the right panel shows the same brain region during late incubation. The diameter of VIP-expressing cells increases from about 9 to about 19 microns during incubation. (From Cloues, Ramas, and Silver, 1990.[215])

When female and male doves sit on their eggs, the tactile stimulation provided by the nest and eggs to the breast region of the sitting bird induces prolactin secretion. If birds are removed from the breeding cage after the eggs are laid, thereby depriving them of the opportunity to sit on the nest and eggs, they do not produce prolactin and do not show crop growth. Remarkably, visual stimuli are also effective in promoting prolactin production. If a male is separated from his incubating female mate by a transparent glass plate, his crop gland will still grow, just as though he was sitting. It seems that the visual stimuli provided by the sitting female are sufficient to support prolactin production in the male.

Stimuli associated with incubation influence prolactin secretion through an action on the brain neuropeptide, vasoactive intestinal polypeptide (VIP). VIP is known to release prolactin in birds. In both sexes, an increase in the diameter of VIP-like immunoreactive cells in a highly localized site in the ventral infundibular region is detectable during courtship and early incubation, anticipating the increase in plasma prolactin levels[215] (figure 13.5). VIP cell diameter remains enlarged during late incubation until about the time the squab start feeding themselves. Parents rearing one squab have a less prolonged period of enlarged VIP-like immunoreactivity cells than do parents rearing two squab.

Once the eggs hatch, external stimuli from the squab are very important for maintaining and furthering crop development. If the parent's contact with the young is restricted by a transparent glass plate placed over the nest, crop growth is reduced, indicating decreased prolactin production. The presence of young also acts to delay the start of a new cycle of courtship and egg-laying in the parents. Thus, if two eggs hatch, the parents do not start to court anew until the young reach about 21 days of age. If only one squab hatches, the parents start to court when the squab is about 15 days old. Finally, if the squab are removed altogether, the parents start to court very soon, and new eggs are laid in about 7 days. The data clearly show the coordination of the behaviors of the adult male, the adult female, and the developing young and involve visual, auditory, and tactile cues that elicit changes in adult hormone production. The hormones in turn alter the behaviors of the parents and ensure that correct behavioral responses are shown at appropriate times in the reproductive cycle.

Summary

This chapter has demonstrated that the operation of cues from the internal and external environment act on the senses and have important influences on neuroendocrine systems. Each of the five senses has been shown to exert such effects, often after altering reproductive hormones. These phenomena help to coordinate reproductive function with the animal's environmental conditions, including changes in day length and temperature, food availability, and social context. In the ring dove, such sensory cues are crucial for the chain of behaviors and physiological events required for successful reproduction.

14 *Hormonal Regulation of Behavior: Insights From Invertebrate Systems*

James W. Truman

Invertebrates account for far and away the majority of animal species on this planet. Although built according to diverse body plans, invertebrates have sophisticated endocrine systems that play a major role in coordinating behavior with changing physiological or developmental states. Besides being of interest in their own right, these animals also provide convenient models in which to study general mechanisms by which hormones alter nervous system development or function.

What organs control the neuroendocrine systems of invertebrates, how do hormones coordinate behavior with the physiology of reproduction and metamorphosis? What are motor programs and how do hormones activate them?

Introduction

Although invertebrates have relatively simple nervous systems, their behaviors are rich and diverse. This diversity is orchestrated through a heavy reliance on chemical signals for triggering and shifting behaviors. Internal chemical signals, in the form of circulating hormones or locally released neuromodulators, act on the central nervous system (CNS) to adjust behavior to meet changing developmental and physiological needs. A hallmark of these hormonal agents is that their actions are not rapid in the manner of neurotransmitters, which act in the span of milliseconds to seconds. Rather, their effects may take minutes or hours to become manifest and then may persist for hours or days. Also, the responses to these agents are typically coordinated pieces of behavior rather than simple twitches or isolated movements.

This chapter is not intended to be a comprehensive review of the involvement of hormones in the behavior of invertebrates. Considering that these animals constitute well over 90% of all known species, such an attempt would be futile and superficial given the space available. Also, other chapters in this book include material about invertebrates where appropriate. One advantage in the study of invertebrates is their relatively simple nervous systems. This simplicity allows a level of analysis that is rarely attained in vertebrate systems, and such analyses have commonly produced basic insights into the neural mechanisms that underlie behavior. While focusing on a number of specific examples, this chapter will emphasize mechanistic principles that arise from

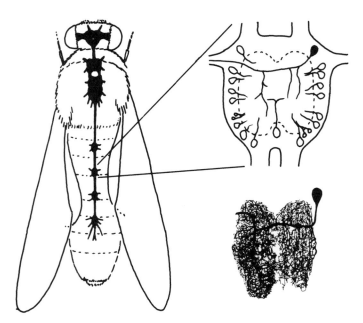

Figure 14.1 The organization of the invertebrate central nervous system (CNS) as illustrated by that of a moth. In this insect, the CNS is composed of the brain and a series of ventral ganglia linked through the paired longitudinal connectives. The organization of one of the segmental ganglia is given at the right. The neuronal cell bodies are situated in the "rind" that surrounds a central neuropil (dashed line). Neuronal processes such as dendrites extend into the neuropil, which is the area of synaptic interaction. A complete reconstruction of the central processes of the neuron depicted with the black cell body is shown at lower right.

the study of invertebrate systems and that are probably relevant to these issues in animals with more complex nervous systems. The student is also referred to some recent reviews[119, 601, 1046,] that deal with the role of hormones in regulating nervous system development and behavior in invertebrates.

Overview of the Invertebrate Central Nervous System

The nervous systems of invertebrates possess a number of attributes that facilitate studies of the neural basis of behavior. With the notable exception of cephalopod molluscs (e.g., octopus and squid), in which the complexity of the CNS rivals that of their fish competitors, the numbers of neurons found in the CNS of invertebrates range up to hundreds of thousands of cells[169] rather than the tens of billions that are estimated for the brains of some mammals. These neurons are typically grouped into discrete aggregations of neurons called **ganglia** (figure 14.1). Many of the cells in a ganglia are always found in the same place and can be reliably identified from one animal to the next. In invertebrates such as the arthropods and the molluscs, many neurons are quite large, making intracellular microelectrode recording relatively easy, even under conditions in which the animal is only partially restrained and able to perform somewhat normal behavior. Thus, it has been possible to examine neurons on a cell-by-cell basis to determine their roles in particular behaviors. In the context of the actions of neuromodulators and neurohormones, such analyses are aimed at linking cellular actions with the accompanying changes in overt behavior.

Invertebrate Endocrine Systems

In the coelenterates, such as *Hydra*, the nervous system is arranged as a diffuse nerve net with concentrations of neurons in the tentacles and around the mouth. The neurons in *Hydra* seem to lack the classic transmitters such as acetylcholine, the catecholamines, and serotonin, but they contain a rich store of neuropeptides.[443] In *Hydra*, of course, there is no circulatory system, and hence these peptides are not strictly speaking hormones. Nevertheless, when released from synaptic terminals to affect post-synaptic cells, these peptides probably also diffuse through tissues to act on distant targets. This arrangement undoubtedly provided the basis from which the neuroendocrine system in vertebrates eventually evolved.

In more complex invertebrates, a circulatory system is present to transport peptides that are released from the CNS to distant target sites. As discussed in chapter 1 on vertebrates, neurons that release their peptide products directly into the blood are termed neurosecretory cells. The same terminology applies to invertebrates. Many of the hormones that are released into the circulation from specialized endocrine or neuroendocrine cells are also found in other neurons within the invertebrate CNS, from which they are released in a local, neurotransmitter-like fashion. This scheme is analogous to the dual use of oxytocin and vasopressin in vertebrates. Because of the organization of the invertebrate CNS into multiple ganglia with free access to the circulatory system (i.e., no blood-brain barrier as in vertebrates), target neurons may encounter a given neuropeptide as a hormone arriving through the circulation or as a neuromodulator released from a neighboring neuron.

Biogenic amines such as serotonin, octopamine, and dopamine are also found throughout the invertebrate species. As with the peptides, the amines are released both locally and systemically and have profound effects on behavior.[119, 601]

Advanced invertebrates, such as the arthropods and molluscs, have both neuroendocrine and endocrine components. For example, figure 14.2 shows that larvae of the tobacco hornworm moth have an extensive neurosecretory system as well as two well-defined endocrine glands, the **corpora allata** and the **prothoracic glands**. The corpora allata synthesize and release **juvenile hormones**, a family of sesquiterpenoid hormones that regulate **metamorphosis**[852] and, in some insects, also regulate adult reproduction.[595] The prothoracic glands produce a family of steroid hormones, the **ecdysteroids**,[492] which are involved in **molting** and may also have a role in reproduction. Other organs such as the gut and the gonads may also have an endocrine role. Since hormones from these glands arise outside of the CNS, their only access to the nervous system is through the circulation.

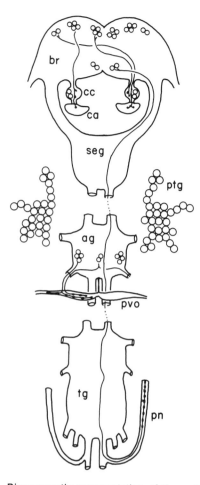

Figure 14.2 Diagrammatic representation of the endocrine system of an insect such as the tobacco hornworm caterpillar. A prominent feature is a diverse group of neurosecretory cells whose locations are indicated by the small circles. The major groups of brain (br) neurosecretory cells extend their axons to the corpora cardiaca (cc), the main neurohemal release site associated with the brain. The cc also contain intrinsic neurosecretory cells that release peptides that regulate lipid and carbohydrate metabolism. Some of the brain axons also extend to the corpora allata (ca), an endocrine gland that produces juvenile hormone. Another set of brain neurosecretory cells sends their axons the length of the ventral CNS to release sites on the proctodeal nerve (pn). Insects also possess segmentally arranged neurosecretory cells such as those shown in an abdominal ganglion (ag); these cells project to the segmental perivisceral organs (pvo). The prothoracic gland (ptg) is a diffuse gland situated in the anterior thorax that synthesizes and secretes the ecdysteroids. seg, subesophageal ganglion; tg, terminal ganglia).

Types of Actions of Hormones on Behavior

Biogenic amines, peptides, and steroids all have pronounced behavioral actions in invertebrates. Most commonly, these effects are of a "modifier" character, i.e., the hormone does not directly cause a particular behavior pattern but, rather adjusts the gain of the nervous system such that a particular stimulus now produces an altered response. A good example of this type of action is seen in the development of sexual behavior in female crickets.[996] Sexually receptive females have high concentrations of juvenile hormone and respond to the calling song of males by showing a positive phonotaxis—they approach calling males. Females that are not yet sexually mature either ignore the song or require a much greater intensity of stimulus before they respond. When the corpora allata (the sole source of juvenile hormone) were removed from immature females, they failed to become responsive to the song. Responsive behavior could be induced in these females, however, by implantation of glands or by application of juvenile hormone. Thus, juvenile hormone appears to act on the CNS of these females to alter their response to the stimulus of a calling male.

Besides changing the behavioral gain, hormones may directly trigger specific behavioral responses. A well-documented example involves the stereotyped behaviors that insects show at the end of each molt. Because of their rigid **exoskeleton**, insects must periodically molt. During the molt they form a new exoskeleton and shed the old one (a process termed **ecdysis**, which literally means to strip off). The specialized **ecdysis behaviors** are very stereotyped and are triggered by a neuropeptide, **eclosion hormone**.[1045] **Eclosion** is the technical term that refers to a larva hatching from its egg or an adult insect coming forth from the pupal case, but eclosion hormone activates ecdysis behavior after every molt. Injections of eclosion hormone are followed by the onset of ecdysis behavior, and studies on isolated CNS preparations show that exposure to the peptide is both necessary and sufficient to induce the ecdysis motor programs (see later).

Hormones also serve a priming function to prepare the CNS to respond to subsequent hormone signals. For example, eclosion hormone triggers ecdysis behavior only if given to animals during a narrow window of time late in each molt. The onset of responsiveness requires that the insect first be exposed to **ecdysteroids**, the steroid hormones that initiate the molting process.[1052] Such a relationship between steroid and peptide hormones is a common theme in the vertebrates as well.

Organizational effects of hormones are permanent changes in the nervous system that are generally brought about by actions relatively early in development. The behavioral results of these actions, however, may not be evident for months or years. In vertebrates, the most common examples of organizational effects occur in the context of sexual differentiation of the hypothalamus and spinal cord (see chapter 2). In invertebrates, by contrast, mechanisms for controlling sexual differentiation are extremely diverse, and many groups, such as the insects, do not use hormones for this task. However, insects show other types of **polymorphisms** as seen in social insects, in which the various castes (worker, soldier, queen) are characterized by morphological and behavioral specializations. In these cases, the determination of caste (and the resultant behavioral modifications) results from different regimens of hormonal exposures when these insects were larvae.[462,773]

Selected Invertebrate Systems

Regulation of Egg-Laying Behavior in *Aplysia*

The sea hare, *Aplysia californica*, shows a complex sequence of behaviors associated with egg deposition (see Mayeri and Rothman[678] for a review). In the appropriate season, bouts of egg-laying occur at approximately 7-day intervals. The animal typically climbs a vertical surface and then becomes stationary. An egg string is extruded from the genital pore and extends along the genital groove to the mouth. Back and forth motions of the head weave the egg string into a sticky mass that is pressed to the substrate. An entire egg string can be many centimeters long and requires several hours to be deposited. An inhibition of feeding behavior and changes in cardiac output and respiratory movements are also seen in association with this behavior.

The bag cells, a paired cluster of several hundred neurosecretory cells located along the abdominal connectives, are involved in controlling egg-laying behavior.[609] These cells are electrically coupled and typically fire a sustained burst that lasts for 15 to 20 minutes. Studies on intact animals showed that a burst discharge of the bag cells preceded a bout of egg-laying.[819] When extracts of the bag cells were injected into intact animals, egg-laying behavior promptly commenced,[609] suggesting that a hormonal signal from the bag cells triggers the behavior.

When examined at the level of responses of specific neurons, the bag cell extracts were found to elicit a wide variety of electrophysiological effects (e.g., Mayeri and Rothman[678]; figure 14.3). These included *transient* or *prolonged*

Figure 14.3 The bag cell system of *Aplysia*. *Top left*: Schematic diagram of the dorsal and ventral surfaces of the abdominal ganglion showing the locations of the two bag cell clusters and identified target neurons and neuronal clusters that respond to bag cell activity. The texturing of the target cells indicates their responses to a bag cell discharge. *Bottom left*: Schematic diagram of the precursor protein for egg-laying hormone (ELH) that is produced in the bag cells. ELH, α-, β-, and γ-bag cell peptide (BCP), four candidate transmitters for various bag-cell–induced responses, are represented on the ELH/BCP precursor protein along with an acidic peptide. The signal sequence for the precursor begins with a methionine residue followed by a hydrophobic region (horizontal lines); arrows show peptide cleavage sites. *Right panel*: Intracellular recordings of a bag cell burst discharge and the types of responses it produces in identified neurons of the abdominal ganglion. The traces are aligned as if they were recorded simultaneously, although they were taken from several preparations. The neurons provide examples of the types of responses to a burst discharge of the bag cells that was triggered by a brief electrical stimulation (arrow) and lasted 20 minutes. There is burst augmentation (cell R15), prolonged excitation (LC cell), prolonged inhibition (cell L6), and transient excitation (cell R1). The peptide transmitter candidate for each response is shown at the right. Impulses in individual neurons are often seen fused together. (Adapted from Mayeri and Rothman, 1985.[678])

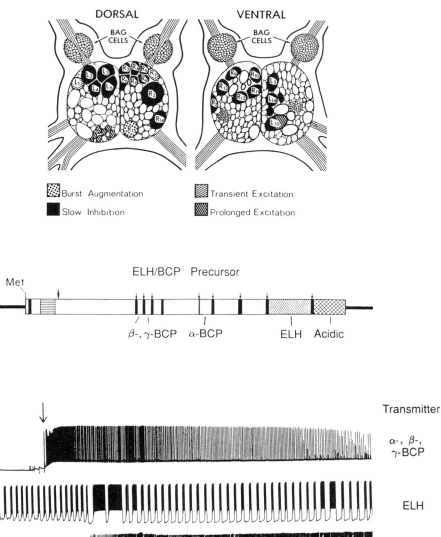

DORSAL   VENTRAL

BAG CELLS   BAG CELLS

▨ Burst Augmentation   ▨ Transient Excitation
■ Slow Inhibition   ▨ Prolonged Excitation

ELH/BCP Precursor

Met

β-, γ-BCP α-BCP   ELH   Acidic

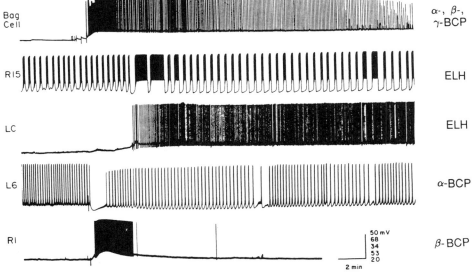

Transmitter

Bag Cell α-, β-, γ-BCP

R15   ELH

LC   ELH

L6 α-BCP

R1 β-BCP

50 mV
68
34
53
20

2 min

excitation, burst augmentation, and slow inhibition, depending on which target neuron was examined. The roles of many of these abdominal neurons in egg-laying behavior itself are unknown, although some of the neurons are important in regulating respiratory or circulatory physiology and hence may be responsible for some of the physiological changes that occur during egg-laying.

The hormone primarily responsible for egg-laying behavior is a 36-amino acid peptide dubbed egg-laying hormone.[204] Synthetic egg-laying hormone induces egg-laying behavior, but it does not reproduce in detail all of the neural effects evoked by either bag cell discharge or by injections of bag cell extracts. The reason for this discrepency became apparent when the gene that codes for egg-laying hormone was cloned and sequenced.[924] As seen in figure 14.3, egg-laying hormone is produced from a large precursor that includes a number of small peptides, α-, β-, and γ-bag cell peptides. During bag cell activity these small peptides are co-released along with egg-laying hormone. The various products of the egg-laying hormone precursor then have distinct actions in the CNS.[678] For example, as seen in figure 14.3, the prolonged excitation of the bag cells can be caused by all three of the bag cell peptides, the inhibition of L6 is caused by α-bag cell peptides, and burst augmentation in R15 and prolonged excitation of LC are caused by egg-laying hormone itself. Thus, the egg-laying hormone gene is responsible for the variety of changes that occur during egg-laying but not through the action of a single peptide. Rather, the gene codes for a precursor that is then processed to produce a mixture of discrete peptides, each having its own distinct action. The coordinated actions of these peptides then result in the full spectrum of changes seen during egg-laying.

Hormonal Activation of Premetamorphic Behaviors

In insects that undergo complete metamorphosis, the behaviors of the larva are directed toward feeding and growth. At the end of larval life, however, feeding ceases and a new set of behaviors appear that prepare the insect for metamorphosis. Species that spin cocoons show the most complex of these premetamorphic behaviors. In the Cecropia silkmoth, for example, the larva invests almost a mile of silk in an elaborate cocoon that takes over a day to complete and that consists of outer and inner envelopes, each containing a one-way valve for the future emergence of the adult moth.[1065] Such **premetamorphic** behaviors are triggered by the steroid hormones, the ecdysteroids.[641]

THE WANDERING BEHAVIOR OF THE TOBACCO HORNWORM
Unlike the giant silkmoths, the tobacco hornworm does not spin a cocoon but shows a simpler set of behaviors termed the **wandering behavior.** Figure 14.4 summarizes some of the behavioral changes that occur as hornworm larvae switch from the feeding to the wandering states.[300] Wandering larvae become positively geotactic (i.e., they move down off the food plant) and show intense activity involving three primary behaviors: crawling, burrowing, and cell

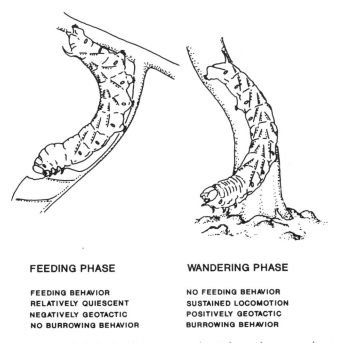

FEEDING PHASE

FEEDING BEHAVIOR
RELATIVELY QUIESCENT
NEGATIVELY GEOTACTIC
NO BURROWING BEHAVIOR

WANDERING PHASE

NO FEEDING BEHAVIOR
SUSTAINED LOCOMOTION
POSITIVELY GEOTACTIC
BURROWING BEHAVIOR

Figure 14.4 The changes in behavior that are seen when tobacco hornworm larvae shift from the feeding phase to the wandering phase.

building. Crawling movements involve anterior waves of segmental lifting and promotion. Although larvae can crawl at essentially any time during larval life, the intensity and sustained nature of this behavior is unique to wandering. Wandering larvae may crawl for hundreds of feet but if given an appropriate substrate, they immediately initiate burrowing behavior. This type of behavior is shown only by wandering larvae and involves repeated dorsal thrusts and flexions of the head and thorax while the abdomen remains rigid. After a series of these shoveling movements, the larva takes a small step into the cleared space and then repeats the cycle, thereby gradually forming a tunnel. Cell-building behavior occurs within the soil and involves tunneling in tight circles to excavate the chamber and compact its walls. During the course of the wandering behavior, the larva may switch between the various behavior patterns depending on external conditions.

Wandering behavior generally lasts about 20 hours.[300] Importantly, this duration is seen whether the animal is placed in the soil where it can burrow and prepare a normal chamber or simply placed in a plastic Petri dish where only crawling behavior is possible. Thus, the duration of the behavior appears to be set internally rather than being dependent on external stimuli. Indeed, when newly wandering larvae were placed in preformed cells, they tunneled out through the wall of those cells and later prepared cells of their own.

External stimuli cannot shorten the duration of wandering activity, but they can prolong it. For example, when larvae were removed from their cells soon after they had ceased activity, they resumed crawling and burrowing behavior

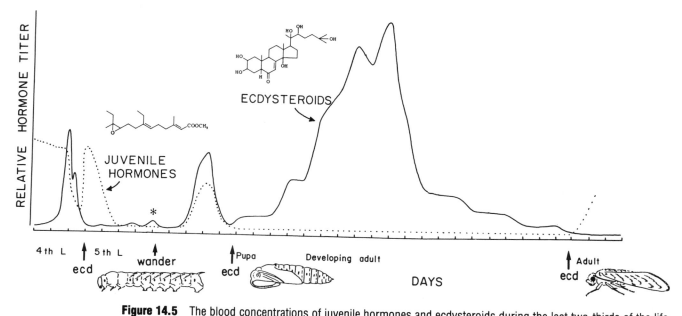

Figure 14.5 The blood concentrations of juvenile hormones and ecdysteroids during the last two-thirds of the life history of the tobacco hornworm. Each of the large peaks of ecdysteroids brings about a molt, which is ended with the ecdysis (ecd) of the new stage. The presence of juvenile hormones during the ecdysteroid peak ensures that the fourth stage larva (4th L) will molt into the fifth larval stage (5th L). The subsequent decline in juvenile hormones permits a small release of ecdysteroids (*, the commit- ment peak) to induce wandering behavior (wander) and also to set the animal irreversibly on the way to metamorphosis. Subsequent ecdysteroid releases bring about the formation of the pupal and adult stages, respectively. The chemical structures are of juvenile hormone I and of 20-OH ecdysone. (Titer data from Bollenbacher et al., 1981,[131] and from many sources as summarized in Riddiford and Hiruma, 1990.[853])

and attempted to construct a new cell. Typically, the cell was incomplete as if the animal had run out of time.

ENDOCRINE REGULATION OF WANDERING BEHAVIOR
The onset of premetamorphic behaviors such as wandering behavior needs to be viewed in the context of the endocrine signals that control molting and metamorphosis. As seen in figure 14.5, the periodic molts that occur through larval life are caused by surges of ecdysteroids. During larval life, ecdysteriods act while the levels of juvenile hormone are high and the insect molts into another larval stage. Due to mechanisms that are still unknown, juvenile hormone titers decline during the last larval stage, and this decline allows meta- morphosis to commence. The transition from the feeding to the wandering stage occurs after a small steroid peak, the **commitment peak**, occurs, which is the first time the insect is exposed to ecdysteroids in the absence of juvenile hormone. This steroid peak "commits" the insect to metamorphosis, but it is not until 2 days later that a larger surge of ecdysteroids causes the molt to the pupal stage. Ecdysteroids then reappear after pupal ecdysis to cause the trans- formation of the pupa into the adult.

Evidence that the ecdysteroids released during the commitment peak induce wandering behavior came from experiments in which the prothoracic glands, which secrete the steroids, were surgically removed prior to the commitment peak.[301] These larvae lived for up to a month but never showed wandering behavior. Infusion of ecdysteroids into such glandless larvae then evoked the switch from feeding to wandering behavior. Moreover, intact animals were made to show precocious wandering behavior by infusing ecdysteroids after the juvenile hormone decline but prior to the animal's own commitment peak.

The ability to induce premature wandering by steroid treatment allowed an examination of the hormonal requirements for induction of the behavior.[301] A single injection of ecdysteroids was ineffective at inducing wandering. The steroid had to be infused over at least 3 hours to initiate the behavior. Total dosage was also important, and the response showed a clear dosage optimum. Response latencies were long, with intense locomotor activity generally starting about 10 to 12 hours after the initiation of the infusion.

THE NEURAL BASIS OF WANDERING BEHAVIOR

Wandering behavior is a very robust behavior. Larvae continued to show sustained crawling movements even when the middle abdominal segments were restrained and partially dissected. The experimenter could then transect the lateral nerves leading from the respective ganglia and place electrodes on the proximal nerve stumps to monitor motor activity.[302] As these larvae attempted to crawl, the arrival of the locomotor wave in the denervated area elicited strong motor bursts from the appropriate ganglia, but the patterning of each burst was highly variable. Presumably, this lack of stereotyped patterning in the denervated segments reflects the importance of sensory feedback in shaping the motor output necessary for crawling.

In insects as well as many other invertebrates, parts or all of the CNS can be removed and maintained in vitro in a normal physiological state for hours or days. When the CNS was removed from hornworm larvae and placed in isolation, the pattern of spontaneous motor activity reflected the behavior of the donor larva.[302] Nervous systems from feeding larvae showed variable levels of tonic activity but only occasional motor bursts. By contrast, those from wandering larvae showed sustained rhythmic motor bursts that continued for hours. The patterning of the bursts was extremely variable, a situation similar to that noted in relation to the bursts in deafferented segments of wandering animals. The duration of this intense bursting in the isolated CNS was similar to the duration of the behavior noted in intact animals. Thus, this high level of motor activity appears to be a central manifestation of the wandering state.

Are hormones responsible for the hyperactivity seen in the CNS of wandering larvae? The CNS from feeding larvae could be induced to display the wandering type of activity by bathing them in either the blood from a wandering larva or in saline containing ecdysteroids.[302] In both cases, the change in motor activity occurred about 10 to 12 hours after the start of the treatment. This latency was similar to that seen for the induction of the behavior by ecdysteroids in the intact animal. Thus, ecdysteroids act directly on the CNS to switch it from the feeding to the wandering state.

The use of isolated CNS preparations also permitted identification of the primary target site for ecdysteroid action. Diffusion barriers made of silicone grease were placed between various regions of the CNS, allowing treatment of restricted regions with ecdysteroids.[302] When such barriers were placed between the brain and the rest of the CNS (without severing axonal connections), treatment of the brain was sufficient to evoke sustained bursting from the remainder of the CNS. However, the opposite experiment, in which all of the CNS except for the brain was exposed, proved ineffective. Thus, the primary site for steroid action in evoking wandering behavior appears to be the brain.

Hormonal Regulation of Ecdysis Behaviors in Insects

The cuticular exoskeleton of insects provides a lightweight, rigid covering that is an effective barrier to water loss. While the cuticle has allowed insects to invade successfully most terrestrial habitats, it also has imposed the requirement that a new cuticle must be made periodically to accommodate growth and changes in morphology. The production of the new cuticle, a process termed molting, is under endocrine control (figure 14.5). Each molt is typically concluded by ecdysis (the shedding of the old cuticle) and the expansion and hardening of the new cuticle. Ecdysis behaviors are highly specialized and are seen only at the end of a molt. In some instances, their timing is also controlled by a circadian clock. This feature is especially striking in short-lived adults such as mayflies in which emergence synchrony is essential for an animal that has only a few hours to mate and lay eggs before it dies. The behaviors that occur around the time of ecdysis can be divided into three phases: (1) the preparatory phase, (2) the ecdysis phase, and (3) the postecdysial phase.

Preparatory phase behaviors are generally quite flexible and serve to bring the animal into a microhabitat appropriate for shedding the cuticle. In grasshoppers, for example, a successful ecdysis requires a perch from which the insect can hang as it is escaping from the old cuticle.[513] Shortly before ecdysis, the insect becomes restless and searches for such a site, and ecdysis may be delayed for hours until an appropriate location is found. In nonmobile stages, such as the pupal stage of moths, the preparatory behavior is reduced to a set of abdominal movements that loosen the connections between the old and new cuticles.[1044] The preparatory phase ends with the initiation of the behaviors that immediately precede ecdysis.

Behaviors of the ecdysis phase are very stereotyped and include behaviors responsible for the rupture and shedding of the old cuticle. The most detailed descriptions of this behavior have been made for crickets.[183] The initial behaviors involve anchoring the old cuticle to the substrate and swallowing air. This causes the body to swell and aids in rupturing the old cuticle. The ecdysis movements then involve a complex series of motor patterns, the major one consisting of rhythmic bouts of peristaltic contractions that move the abdo-

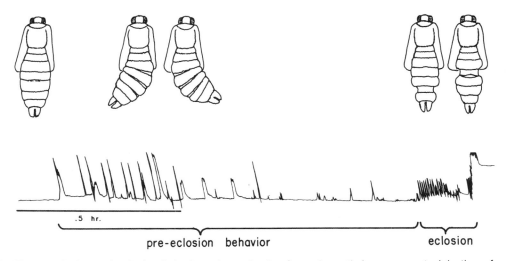

Figure 14.6 The preeclosion and eclosion behaviors shown by the Cecropia moth in response to injection of eclosion hormone. The bottom record is a trace of the abdominal movements of a preemergence moth starting about 5 minutes after injection of eclosion hormone. The record was obtained by running a thread from the abdominal tip of the surrounding pupal cuticle to a lever that wrote on a revolving drum. The large excursions on the left were due to abdominal rotations; the smaller ones at the right were produced by eclosion movements. At the end of the record the moth escaped from the pupal cuticle. The drawings are dorsal views of the moth after manual removal of the surrounding pupal cuticle, showing the major features of the abdominal movements during both behaviors.

men up and propel the old cuticle backwards along the body. Coordinated with these abdominal movements are specific motor subroutines that extract each appendage (legs, antennae) from its sheath of old cuticle. There are additional behavioral subroutines that are not displayed during a normal ecdysis. If certain aspects of the behavior go awry, such as when an appendage becomes stuck, these behaviors are then called into play. The segmental peristaltic waves are commonly observed during the ecdyses of most insects but other components vary widely depending on the size and shape of the appendages involved, and so on.

The postecdysial phase is devoted to expansion and hardening of the new cuticle. Some degree of expansion usually occurs during ecdysis, but many species show specialized behaviors after the cuticle is shed to inflate the new body structures. The most dramatic of these behaviors appear in adult stages that have new wings that must be expanded and hardened after the emergence.

ECDYSIS BEHAVIORS OF MOTHS

Studies of the endocrine regulation of ecdysis were first performed on **adult ecdysis** (also called eclosion) of moths. The Cecropia silkmoth (*Hyalophora cecropia*) shows a two-part behavior (figure 14.6).[1041] The first part, termed the **preeclosion behavior**, lasts for approximately 60 minutes. There is a 30-minute active period when the animal shows frequent rotary movements of the abdomen. This is followed by a quiescent period of equal length. Eclosion is accomplished primarily by cycles of abdominal retraction and extension. The retraction phase involves a rapid peristaltic wave of contraction that progresses up the abdomen and ends in the thorax with vigorous shrugging movements of the wing bases. This shrugging is accompanied by an extension of the abdomen, followed by initiation of the next retraction phase. After emergence, the moth searches for a suitable site from which to hang and inflate its wings. The wing inflation behavior includes a series of stereotyped wing movements and tonic abdominal contractions that force blood into the expanding wings.

The details of these behaviors vary even between closely related species.[1041] For example, in the giant silkmoths, the emerging moth must not only escape from the old pupal cuticle but also from the cocoon that it had spun as a larva weeks or months before. In the Cecropia moth, the ecdysing moth pauses for about 5 minutes after it has emerged part way out of its pupal cuticle. This pause is accompanied by the secretion of labial gland fluid, which is applied to the front end of the cocoon. This fluid moistens the threads around the escape valve, thereby making it easier for the moth to push through the opening. This pause is internally programmed and is seen even in animals that have been removed from their cocoon. The Polyphemus moth (*Antheraea polyphemus*) also shows a programmed pause, but in this case it lasts for about an hour. The cocoon of this species has a uniformly thick wall without an escape hatch, and the emerging moth uses an enzyme, cocoonase,[549] to digest through the wall. The long pause provides sufficient time for the enzyme to work. The Chinese oak silkmoth (*A. pernyi*) spins a cocoon similar to that of Polyphemus, but this insect, if taken out of its cocoon, shows no programmed pause during ecdysis. It immediately leaves the old cuticle unless it encounters a barrier while still partially encased. In the latter instance, it immediately stops, releases copious amounts of cocoonase and waits for about an hour for a hole to be digested in the cocoon before resuming its activity. Thus, the latter two species of silkmoths deal with the problem of a thick-walled, valveless cocoon in two different ways. One stops for a programmed period of time, the other has a reflexively induced pause. All of these silkmoths, if they are prevented from escaping from their cocoon in a timely manner, nevertheless begin wing expansion behavior but with disastrous results.

In contrast to the giant silkmoths, the tobacco hornworm does not have a cocoon and pupates underground. The animal shows no pause during ecdysis. The appearance of a barrier immediately elicits vigorous digging movements, and wing expansion is delayed as long as the moth is confined.[1049] Indeed, even after 24 hours of digging, most insects will commence the wing expansion behavior if they are then provided with an appropriate site.

Endocrine Regulation of Ecdysis-Related Behaviors

Many of the behaviors seen during ecdysis are highly specialized and dedicated only to this process. They occur in the context of molting, which is orchestrated by a series of hormonal cues. The relevant hormones are the ecdysteroids and the peptide hormone, eclosion hormone. The ecdysteroids have some behavioral actions on their own and also prime the CNS to make it responsive to eclosion hormone. The latter hormone then triggers the behaviors involved in the ecdysis phase itself.

THE ROLE OF ECLOSION HORMONE IN TRIGGERING ECDYSIS BEHAVIORS
A series of experiments in which the silkmoth brain was removed and then reimplanted elsewhere in the body provided the first evidence that ecdysis was hormonally triggered.[1051] The brain was found to control the timing of the behavior, but the form of the behavior was regulated by centers in the ventral ganglia. The brain was effective even when transplanted into the abdomen, suggesting that it acted through the release of a bloodborne factor. This factor, which was called eclosion hormone, was eventually purified from the tobacco hornworm and found to be a 62-amino acid peptide.[663] It is found widely throughout the insects, but it has no structural similarity to any other known peptide hormone in either vertebrates or invertebrates. Its sole known role is to cause ecdysis and its associated physiological changes.

The neural basis of ecdysis behavior was first studied in the Cecropia moth.[1041] Injection of preemergent adults with eclosion hormone was followed within 10 to 15 minutes by initiation of the preeclosion behavior, followed by ecdysis and then by wing expansion behavior. The system was experimentally simplified with the discovery that hormone treatment could evoke the first two behaviors from abdomens that had been separated from the rest of the insect.[1041] The behavior of isolated abdomens differed from that seen in intact animals in two respects: (1) Eclosion movements involved only the peristaltic retraction phase rather than the retraction-extension cycles, and (2) the abdomens did not show the brief pause in ecdysis associated with escape from the cocoon. These results indicated that the abdomen contained centers that could respond to eclosion hormone and could generate a respectable rendition of the two behaviors.

As illustrated in figure 14.7, studies on isolated abdomens were later extended to the isolated abdominal CNS.[1042] Without the addition of eclosion hormone, the isolated CNS showed low levels of tonic motor output with occasional motor bursts at 30 to 60-minute intervals. Addition of eclosion hormone, by contrast, resulted in a complex program of spontaneous, patterned motor output. Approximately 20 to 30 minutes after the addition of the peptide to the surrounding bath, the CNS started generating motor bursts with a rotary pattern. These occurred at a high frequency for 30 to 40 minutes, and then the CNS spontaneously became quiet. This quiet phase lasted for a similar period of time and then was terminated by the abrupt resumption of spontaneous bursting. The new bursts had a new pattern that generated peristaltic waves moving up the abdomen. Thus, the CNS contains not only the information for the patterning of the various movements seen during the preeclosion and eclosion behaviors but also the temporal information dictating how long

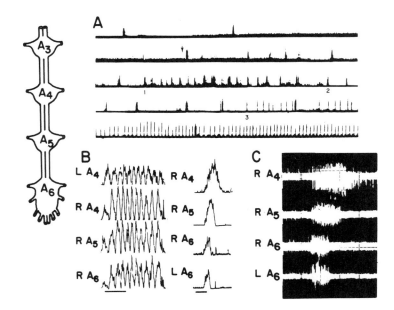

Figure 14.7 Response of the isolated nervous system (*left*) of a preemergence Cecropia moth to addition of eclosion hormone to the bathing medium. *A*, Continuous 5-hour integrated record of the spontaneous motor activity from an isolated CNS. Record from the right nerve of A4. Arrow, time of addition of eclosion hormone. 1, Start of preeclosion phase; 2, start of quiescent phase; 3, beginning of eclosion bursts. *B*, Simultaneous records from various nerve roots showing the integrated motor activity during a burst of the preeclosion active phase (*left*) and the eclosion phase (*right*). R and L refer to the right and left nerves from the various ganglia. Bar is 10 seconds (*left*) and 4 seconds (*right*). *C*, Example of unprocessed spike data recorded during an eclosion burst. (*A* and *B* from Truman, 1978.[1042])

each movement should be performed and the sequence of progression from one phase to the next. This is a striking example of a central "motor tape"[505] that can play out a set of behaviors without recourse to sensory feedback.

The motor programs are released through the direct action of eclosion hormone on the CNS. Exposure of the CNS to the peptide for as little as 5 minutes was sufficient to trigger the complete rendition of the preeclosion and ecdysis behaviors, which lasted for over $1\frac{1}{2}$ hours. Thus, the peptide serves only as a phasic signal to start the playing of the motor tape.

BEHAVIORAL ACTIONS OF THE ECDYSTEROIDS
The ecdysteroid titers increase during the early phases of a molt and then decline as the molt nears completion. Insects are vulnerable during the time of the molt, so they typically stay hidden and quiescent. Experiments performed on grasshoppers about 30 years ago[472] suggested that this quiescence was imposed by the direct action of ecdysteroids on the CNS.

The decline in ecdysteroids as the molt nears completion then brings about the behaviors of the preparatory phase. These were best demonstrated in the tobacco hornworm,[1044] in which the preparatory behavior, prior to adult ecdysis, consists of a 2-hour period of abdominal movements that loosen connections between the old and the new cuticles. This behavior occurs at its appropriate time even in debrained animals, showing that the behavior is not caused by eclosion hormone. Delay in the normal ecdysteroid decline by injection of exogeneous steroid results in a dose-dependent delay in the behavior. Thus, the declining steroid titer at the end of the molt appear to induce the behaviors that prepare the insect for ecdysis.

The declining ecdysteroid titer is also necessary both to release eclosion hormone and to prime the CNS to respond to eclosion hormone.[1052] Interestingly, during most of its life an insect is insensitive to eclosion hormone. In the case of the hornworm, for example, the animals become responsive to eclosion hormone only during a narrow window of about 8 hours duration near the end of each molt. These windows are set by the declining ecdysteroid titer. Injection or infusion of steroid to delay the decline results in a comparable delay in the onset of responsiveness to eclosion hormone. Thus during its life history, the insect shifts back and forth between times during which it is sensitive to eclosion hormone and times when it is not. Once eclosion hormone acts to trigger ecdysis behavior, it renders the CNS refractory to a further exposure to eclosion hormone, and the animal must undergo a cycle of steroid exposure and withdrawal before sensitivity is reestablished. Some of the events that are behind this steroid priming will be dealt with below.

General Features of Hormone-CNS Interactions

Hormones are often secreted in a pulsatile fashion, and, once in the circulation, they potentially have access to the entire CNS. The ways by which these features of hormone release have been exploited by the nervous system for organizing behavior will be examined in this section.

Hormones and the Duration of Motor Programs

The behavioral responses evoked by hormones may last for hours or even days. Both the wandering behavior of the tobacco hornworm and the preeclosion behavior of the Cecropia moth are characterized by relatively fixed durations—the wandering behavior lasts for about 20 hours, whereas the duration of the preeclosion behavior is 60 minutes. These behaviors illustrate, however, two different ways in which a hormone can control the timing of behavior.

As described in the previous section, studies on isolated CNS preparations have shown that in both cases the duration of the behavior is not set by external stimuli but is a property of an internal CNS program. Eclosion hormone initiates the preeclosion motor program in an all-or-none fashion. Once initiated, the program then runs to completion regardless of the continued presence or absence of the peptide. Thus, eclosion hormone appears to provide a phasic signal to trigger a motor program that is otherwise hormone independent.

With wandering behavior, by contrast, the endocrine system controls not only the onset of the behavior but also its duration.[301] As described previously, ecdysteroids had to be infused for a minimum of 3 hours to initiate the behavior. The behavior then began about 10 hours after the start of infusion, but it lasted only a few hours rather than the expected 20. When the length of the infusion was extended, the latency of onset remained the same, but the duration of wandering activity was extended accordingly. Infusions of 10 hours resulted in behaviors of essentially normal duration.

A similar quantitative relationship was seen after experimentally supplying juvenile hormone agonists.[301] The induction of wandering behavior requires that ecdysteroids act in the absence of juvenile hormone. Consequently, when juvenile hormone agonists were applied immediately prior to the start of the relevant ecdysteroid pulse, wandering behavior was blocked. When juvenile hormone agonist treatment was delayed until after the start of steroid secretion (so that larvae experienced an initial exposure to ecdysteroids alone before the addition of juvenile hormone), wandering behavior began at its appropriate time, but its duration varied as a function of the length of the juvenile hormone-free period of ecdysteroid exposure. Once wandering behavior was underway, the duration of the behavior was set, and treatment with juvenile hormone agonists was no longer effective.

Thus, both the infusion of ecdysteroids and the application of juvenile hormone agonists identify a critical period during the 10 to12 hours preceding the onset of wandering behavior. The action of ecdysteroids during this period produces a cumulative effect in the CNS. These effects summate in a linear manner to program the CNS to generate a behavior of the given duration. It is as though the CNS "remembers" how much hormone it has been exposed to during this time and acts accordingly. After the system has been "programmed" and the behavior begun, neither ecdysteroids nor juvenile hormone can influence the subsequent performance.

Hormones and the Coordination of Behavioral Sequences

Complex behaviors often involve a series of motor patterns arranged in a stereotyped temporal order. Hormones can play a number of roles in organizing such sequences. One way in which such sequences are organized results when different hormones each trigger a different behavior, and the sequential release of these hormones then results in the sequential display of the behavioral responses. For example, the end of a molt in insects is characterized by a decline in ecdysteroids followed by the release of eclosion hormone. In the tobacco hornworm, the ecdysteroids cause the abdominal movements of the preparatory behavior,[1044] whereas eclosion hormone then triggers ecdysis itself.[1051] The proper sequencing of the two behaviors is ensured because the decline of ecdysteroids is a prerequisite for eclosion hormone release.[1052]

The relationship between the decline in ecdysteroids and the preparatory phase behaviors has not been explored in insects with very complex behaviors such as grasshoppers and crickets. In these cases, though, the successful completion of the preparatory behavior (i.e., the acquisition of a suitable ecdysis perch) is apparently an additional component that acts in concert with a steroid decline to cause eclosion hormone release. Once the the peptide has been released, however, the insect is apparently irreversibly committed to the stereotyped ecdysis response.

Another example of successive hormonal signals triggering successive phases of a behavior is seen in cocoon spinning in the moth *Ephestic kuniella*.[401] In this case, however, instead of different hormones, the cue involves two pulses of the same hormone. The cocoon of this insect has an outer and an inner envelope. The construction of the outer envelope is caused by the commitment peak of ecdysteroids. Spinning of the inner envelope is caused by the following prepupal ecdysteroid peak that precipitates the larval-pupal transition. Importantly, the stimulus provided by an outer envelope is required to induce the prepupal ecdysteroid peak, resulting in completion of the cocoon.

A different relationship between a hormone and a behavioral sequence is seen in the action of eclosion hormone in triggering the preeclosion, eclosion, and wing expansion behaviors. The most detailed analyses have been carried out for the first two behaviors of the sequence. Studies of isolated CNS preparations showed that a single pulse of the peptide elicits the two motor programs in their appropriate temporal arrangement.[1042] Hence, sensory feedback is not necessary for either the timing or the transition from one pattern to the next (see figure 14.7), and this temporal sequence is an inherent property of the CNS response. A number of lines of evidence suggest that this sequencing occurs because of different response latencies of the respective motor programs.[1043] For example, in triggering adult ecdysis in the Cecropia moth, a low dose of eclosion hormone occasionally triggered only the preeclosion behavior. After the former was completed the animals then lapsed into random background movements instead of showing the next behavior (eclosion). When such animals were later challenged with a second and larger dose of eclosion hormone, they did not replay the preeclosion behavior but responded with only the eclosion behavior. Importantly, however, the behavior did not start until about 90 minutes after the second injection, the time of its usual appearance in the normal sequence.

A similar set of observations was made for eclosion and the wing expansion behavior except that the latency for the latter was about 120 minutes. These and similar observations suggest that the three behavioral programs involved in the sequence are each acted on separately by the peptide, and each has its own characteristic response latency—15, 90, and 120 minutes for the preeclosion, eclosion, and wing-expansion behaviors, respectively. These latencies ensure the appropriate ordering of the behaviors. They also provide an internal template of how long a particular behavior should take. Importantly, if the animal gets hung up in one phase, as when it has difficulties in escaping from part of the old cuticle, there appear to be neural mechanisms to suppress at least temporarily the performance of the next behavior until the conditions become appropriate.[1042] The mechanism by which these long latencies are established is not known. Nor has the role of different response latencies in the organization of other complex behaviors been explored.

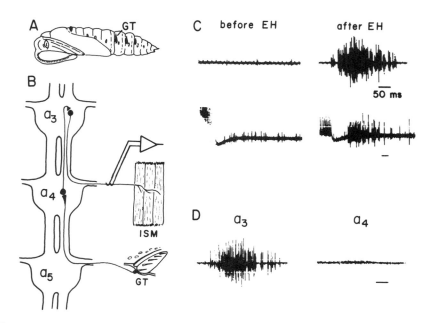

Figure 14.8   The gin-trap reflex and its activation by eclosion hormone (EH). *A*, Pupal stage of the tobacco horn-worm showing the location of a lateral gin-trap (GT). *B*, Schematic representation of the proposed circuitry underlying the gin-trap reflex and the location of the extracellular electrodes recording motoneuron activity. a_n, abdominal ganglion n; ISM, intersegmental muscles. *C*, Response of the intersegmental muscle motoneurons to tactile stimulation of the gin-trap receptors (*top*) or electrical stimulation of the gin-trap nerve (*bottom*). Before exposure to EH (*left*) neither stimulus evokes a response. One hour after exposure to EH (*right*) both stimuli evoke the characteristic reflex responses of the motoneurons. Tactile stimulation occurred at the start of the top records; stimulation artifacts are evident in the bottom traces. *D*, Results of selective exposure of individual ganglia to EH. Record-ings are from the lateral nerve of a_4 as shown in *B*. *Left*, Exposure of a_3 to EH activates the entire reflex pathway as shown by the motoneuron response to tactile stimulation of the gin-trap receptors approx-imately 1 hour after EH treatment. *Right*, Exposure of a_4 in another preparation to EH does not activate the reflex pathway. Bar equals 50 milliseconds. (Data from Levine and Truman, 1983.[627])

Spatial Actions of Hormones on the Invertebrate CNS

The example of behaviors in the emergence sequence given earlier suggests that the hormone does not act on a single "master" neuron that then orches-trates the various aspects of the behavioral response. Rather, there appear to be distinct hormone-sensitive components associated with each behavior, and these components may be distributed throughout the CNS. Physiological evi-dence of discrete hormone targets associated with discrete behaviors is seen with ecdysis of the pupal stage of the tobacco hornworm. Eclosion hormone triggers both pupal ecdysis and the permanent activation of a set of abdominal reflexes, the gin-trap reflexes,[627] which are specific to the pupal stage. The gin-traps are a set of sharp-sided pits located on the lateral margins of abdomi-nal segments 5 to 7 (figure 14.8). Stimulation of the sensory hairs in the pit results in reflexive contraction of the longitudinal muscles in the next anterior segment, thereby pulling the trap under a shelf of cuticle and crushing whatever may have entered it. This reflex serves to protect the otherwise helpless pupa from small soil arthropods such as ants and mites. Each reflex involves a set of sensory neurons, an interganglionic interneuron, and a defined population of motoneurons[69,70,627] (figure 14.8). This circuitry is repeated for each of the three segments that bear gin-traps.

Although global exposure of the CNS to eclosion hormone resulted in pupal ecdysis and the activation of all of the reflex circuits, the application of eclosion hormone to a single abdominal ganglion in the intact chain did not trigger the ecdysis motor pattern.[627] This selective exposure, however, did turn on a gin-trap reflex circuit but only for a single segmental unit—the one whose interneuron-motoneuron synapses were located in the treated ganglion (figure 14.8). Thus, the normal coactivation of all of the segmental reflexes and their coordination with ecdysis is mediated through a chemical linkage rather than through neural means. The broadspread action of eclosion hormone on a number of ganglia is essential for the coordinated behavioral changes seen at ecdysis.

Not all responses require the same type of broadspread action seen with eclosion hormone. A good counterexample is wandering behavior, in which the target appears to be much more restricted. The wandering type of bursting activity displayed by the isolated CNS is evident only if the brain is exposed to ecdysteroids.[302] The presence or absence of steroid exposure for the rest of the CNS appears to be irrelevant.

Even for a single circuit that generates a particular behavior, there may be multiple sites of hormone action. The best example of this sort comes from study of the effects of various neuromodulators on a simple invertebrate ganglion, the stomatogastric ganglion of the lobster. This ganglion, which is located over the stomach, contains only about 30 neurons and controls the striated muscles that move the various regions of the stomach—the pyloris, the cardiac sac, and the gastric mill. The ganglion produces various patterns of rhythmic motor output that control the patterns of contractions in the three areas. These patterns of motoneuron discharge are evident whether the recording is made in situ or from the isolated ganglion. Consequently, the ganglion has been an object of intense study for over 25 years, and the connections between the various neurons are known in detail. This circuitry includes both electrical and chemical synapses, the latter being predominantly inhibitory in nature.[723]

This simple set of only 30 neurons can generate a rich repetoire of rhythmic motor outputs. This plasticity is due to a wide variety of neurohormones and neuromodulators that act on this network and modify its pattern of rhythmic motor output. Importantly, the actions of a given neuromodulator are not confined to a single neuron but are distributed throughout the network.[557,655] The effects include changes in the strengths of specific synapses and in the bursting properties of particular neurons. The result is a new stable pattern of rhythmicity, characterized by altered phase relationships and altered frequencies, thereby resulting in new patterns of rhythmic movement. The important point is

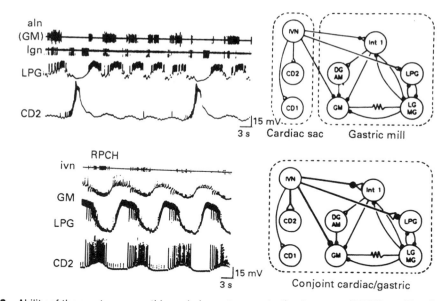

Figure 14.9 Ability of the crustacean peptide, red pigment concentrating hormone (RPCH), to "fuse" two pattern-generating circuits in the lobster stomatogastric ganglion. *Top*, Control preparations. *Left*, Extracellular and intracellular records showing the rhythmic motor activity controlling movements of the gastric mill and the cardiac sac regions of the lobster stomach. Upper three traces are gastric mill units, whereas the lower trace (CD2) is involved in the cardiac sac rhythm. The two rhythms run at different frequencies and interact only weakly. *Right*, Diagrammatic representation of the synaptic interactions that are involved in the two circuits. The IVN cells make weak synapses on various neurons in the gastric mill circuit. *Bottom*, Response to application of RPCH to the stomatogastric ganglion. *Left*, Cells in both patterns become active in a single rhythm. (GM and LPG are normally gastric, and IVN and CD2 are cardiac sac.) *Right*, Changes in the strength of the synaptic interactions caused by RPCH that allow the fusion of the circuits into one functional circuit.

Other abbreviations and symbols: open triangles, inhibitory synapses; closed circles, excitatory synapses; "spiked" line indicates electrical synapses; aln, anterior lateral nerve; AM, anterior median neuron; CD1, cardiac dilator neuron 1; DG, dorsal gastric neuron; int 1, interneuron 1; GM, gastric mill neuron; LPG, lateral posterior gastric neuron; LG, lateral gastric neuron; MG, medial gastric neuron; IVN, inferior ventricular neurons. (From Dickinson et al., 1990.[295])

that the neurons within the ganglion show a high degree of interconnectivity that can be described as a "wiring diagram" showing the anatomical connections. The hormones and modulators then act on this network to adjust synaptic strengths and neuronal bursting properties. These modifications cause a subset of the cells to form a functional circuit to generate a particular rhythmic pattern. A different hormone or modulator configures the same set of cells in a functionally different manner. Thus, the motor output is very fluid and is a function of the cocktail of neurohormones and neuromodulators that are acting on the ganglion at any given time.

A particularly striking example is shown in figure 14.9.[295] The rhythmic activity in the cardiac sac and the gastric mill are controlled by different sets of neurons in the stomatogastric ganglion. The neurons in one subset are synaptically connected to those of the other, but the synaptic connections are weak.

Consequently, under normal conditions the rhythms in the two regions are largely independent. However, when the crustacean neurohormone "red pigment-concentrating hormone" is added to the bath, the relationship between the two sets of neurons dramatically changes: Both subsets of neurons synaptically fuse together to produce a unified motor output. As seen in figure 14.9, this change comes about through the strengthening of the synaptic connections between a driving cell involved in the cardiac sac rhythm (IVN) and various neurons in the gastric mill set. This functional fusion of the systems persists only for the duration of action of the red pigment-concentrating hormone.

Priming Actions of Hormones on the Invertebrate CNS

Occasionally the physiological or developmental state of an animal prevents it from exhibiting a behavioral response to hormone treatment. This occurs because an animal may respond to a given hormone only during specific times in its life or after exposure to other hormones. The response to eclosion hormone provides a striking example of such restricted periods of sensitivity. During the life of the tobacco hornworm, the insect goes through long periods of nonresponsiveness punctuated by brief "windows" of sensitivity. The window is closed by eclosion hormone itself acting to evoke ecdysis behavior. Once ecdysis behavior has been induced, the CNS will not respond to eclosion hormone again until it is exposed to ecdysteroids.[1052] Hence, among their many actions, these steroids have an essential function of priming the CNS so that it can then respond to eclosion hormone.

The changes evoked by ecdysteroids are not evident at the anatomical level. There are, however, steroid-induced changes in the biochemical cascade that mediates eclosion hormone action. Eclosion hormone stimulates guanylate cyclase, resulting in a rise in intracellular cyclic 5'-guanine monophosphate (cyclic-GMP),[760,1050] which inturn activates a cyclic GMP-dependent protein kinase. This kinase then phosphorylates two membrane-associated proteins.[761] The nature of these membrane associated proteins and the manner by which their phosphorylation results in the activation of the ecdysis motor programs are not yet known.

Intermolt larvae are not sensitive to eclosion hormone, and they are also missing two components of the cascade. At this stage, treatment with eclosion hormone did not stimulate an increase in cyclic-GMP titers despite the fact that the CNS had normal levels of guanylate cyclase.[760] Consequently, either eclosion hormone receptors or some component that couples the receptor binding to activation of the guanylate cyclase appeared to be lacking. A second element that was lacking was the membrane-associated proteins that were normally phosphorylated in response to eclosion hormone.[761] With exposure to ecdysteroids, the CNS became able to respond to eclosion hormone with an increase in cyclic-GMP, indicating that the first block had been removed. Importantly, however, although the CNS showed a biochemical response to eclosion hormone, it did not show a neural response until after the ecdysteroids were then withdrawn. The removal of the steroid then caused the appearance of the membrane-associated proteins, and with them the constitution of the fully responsive system.[762] Thus, the priming effects of ecdysteroids appears to reside in the induction of the biochemical components needed for the response cascade.

Organizational Effects of Hormones in Invertebrates

Organizational effects occur within the invertebrates, but the cellular mechanisms are not well understood. Some of the most dramatic effects are seen in the case of caste determination in the social insects. In the honeybee, for example, there are striking differences between the brains of workers and the brains of queens.[541] This polymorphism is controlled by the pattern of juvenile hormone exposure in the larval stage (see Hardie and Lees[462] for a review). The details of the mechanisms by which the hormonal conditions cause these neural differences are lacking.

A more widespread type of organizational change in insects occurs during metamorphosis and is due to the reorganization of the nervous system caused by ecdysteroids acting in the absence of juvenile hormone. For example, in the tobacco hornworm, behaviors vary dramatically between the caterpillar, pupa, and moth stages. Some of the changes that underlie these differences are best seen by examining ecdysis behavior, one of the few behaviors that is shown by all three stages. In all stages, ecdysis is triggered in the same manner, i.e., by the action of eclosion hormone on an ecdysteroid primed-nervous system.

The form of ecdysis behavior differs in the caterpillar (larval), pupal, and moth (adult) stages because the movements needed for a successful ecdysis depend both on the character of the old cuticle and on the new morphology of the animal that is trying to shed this cuticle (figure 14.10). In the case of larval ecdysis, the old larval cuticle is shed through anterior-directed peristaltic waves that are coordinated with the transient retraction of the ventral abdominal prolegs. At pupal ecdysis, by contrast, the animal must still shed a larval cuticle, but pupae lack abdominal prolegs. Consequently, the proleg retraction component is lost, and the behavior is reduced to primarily the peristaltic movements. The adult stage is then faced with escape from a rigid shell of pupal cuticle rather than from a thin, flexible sleeve of larval cuticle. Its ecdysis movements involve the two-phase abdominal retraction-extension cycles accompanied by shrugging movements of the wing bases. These movements propel the cuticle backward and continue to be used as the newly emerged moth digs to the surface of the soil.

Both the transformation of the larva to the pupa and the pupa to the adult occur in response to ecdysteroids acting in the absence of juvenile hormone. We do not have a complete understanding of how ecdysteroids alter the neural substrates for ecdysis behavior, yet a few pieces of information are known. One of the major differences between the larval and pupal ecdysis behaviors is the lack of proleg movements in the pupa (figure 14.10). Electrophysiological

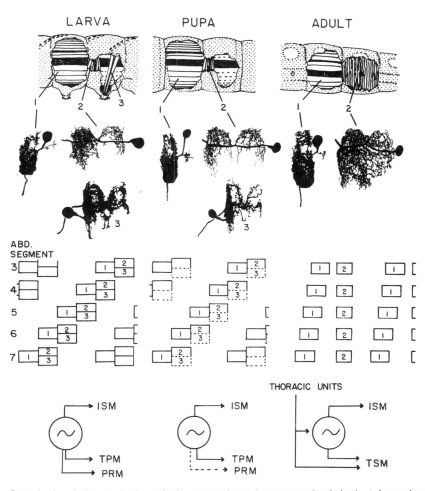

Figure 14.10 Organizational changes in the ecdysis system through metamorphosis in the tobacco hornworm. *Top*, Some of the musculature and motoneurons involved in ecdysis: 1, the intersegmental muscles (ISM) and one of its motoneurons; 2, motoneuron MN-3, which innervates the tergopleural muscles (TPM) in the larva and pupa. These muscles die and are replaced by the adult tergosternal muscles (TSM), and MN-3 shows a drastically remodeled dendritic arbor in the adult; 3, the proleg retractor muscles (PRM) and their motoneuron PPR; the muscle dies before pupal ecdysis and PPR shows loss of some dendrites at that time but then degenerates soon thereafter. *Middle*, Temporal organization of abdominal (ABD) muscle contractions during the respective ecdyses. The numbers refer to the muscle groups above and show the progression of the ecdysis wave with time. The dashed box at pupal ecdysis shows the timing of firing of the proleg retractor motoneurons despite the loss of their muscles. *Bottom*, Schematic representation showing the changing relationship of the larval ecdysis pattern generator (circle) through metamorphosis. In the larva, the oscillator causes the ISMs to contract out of phase with the TPMs and the PRMs. At pupal ecdysis the same phase relationship is seen, but the PRM motor output is weakened and the muscle itself is gone. The larval pattern generator persists into the adult, but its output is highly modified by descending inputs from the thorax. (From Truman, 1989.[1047])

recordings of the motor activity occuring during pupal ecdysis, however, revealed that the proleg motoneurons were still present and fired at their appropriate phase in the ecdysis cycle, despite the loss of their muscles.[1092,1093] They were not driven as strongly as they were during larval ecdysis, a finding correlated with a reduction in their dendritic branching in the pupa (figure 14.10).[1094] Thus, the main difference between the larval and pupal behaviors is not at the level of the ecdysis central pattern generator. Instead, it is due primarily to changes in the periphery: the loss of the prolegs and their musculature.

The ecdysis behavior used during adult ecdysis bears little resemblance to the behaviors used by earlier stages.[709] However, when neural communication between the thorax and abdomen was experimentally blocked, the abdominal movements immediately lapsed into the pupal-like, slow peristaltic waves rather than the rapid two-phase adult movements. These findings suggest that the central pattern generator for larval ecdysis persists through adult differentiation, but during this transition it becomes associated with thoracic units that strongly alter its output (figure 14.10). Thus, the sequential reorganization of the ecdysis behavior conserves the original pattern generator that was used throughout the larval stages. Peripheral (pupal ecdysis) or central (adult ecdysis) modifications are then used to modify the behavioral output to ensure that the behavior is appropriate for the present stage.

Role of Local Versus Systemically Released Hormone in the Alteration of Behavior

In the case of hormones that are secreted only by endocrine glands, it is clear that the only avenue by which they can gain access to the CNS is through the circulation. With peptides and biogenic amines, however, the situation is not so clear-cut because these substances can potentially be released locally into the CNS as well as into the circulation. In *Aplysia*, for example, egg-laying hormone will trigger egg-laying behavior when injected into a gravid animal. Also, large amounts of egg-laying hormone are released into the circulation prior to normal bouts of oviposition. However, as described earlier, there is also a small network of central neurons that contains egg-laying hormone and related peptides and that extends throughout the CNS. Egg-laying hormone released locally from this network is probably the normal pathway by which the behavior is triggered. This hormone released into the circulation is required for peripheral targets such as the ovo-testes.[880]

A similar relationship appears to hold for eclosion hormone and pupal ecdysis in the tobacco hornworm. At the pupal stage only four neurons produce eclosion hormone. Their cell bodies reside in the brain, but their axons descend through the length of the ventral CNS and exit from the terminal nerve where they form a neurohemal release site.[1048] Under conditions in which peripheral release from the terminal nerve site is abolished, the stimulation of these cells still results in the prompt triggering of ecdysis behavior.[486] Thus, sufficient peptide appears to be released from the descending axons into the ganglia through which they pass to evoke the ecdysis motor program. By contrast, changes in peripheral targets, such as the activation of secretion by dermal glands, are not seen in the absence of circulating eclosion hormone.[486]

A third example relates to the role of the biogenic amine serotonin in lobsters.[601] Injection of this amine caused animals to stand tall on the tips of their walking legs with their claws open. This posture mimics that shown by dominant animals during intraspecific interactions. Stimulation of a key set of neurons that contain serotonin resulted in both central and systemic release of the amine. The former selectively adjusted the central programs for postural output, whereas the latter enhanced the response of the muscles, the peripheral effectors for this output.

Thus, in these three cases, the release of a bioactive compound into the circulation is coupled with a similar release locally within the CNS. This arrangement thereby gives the CNS a chemical "copy" of the hormonal conditions found in the circulation.

Summary

This chapter has focused on three systems that illustrate different aspects of hormonal effects on invertebrate behavior—premetamorphic behavior of the tobacco hornworm, ecdysis behavior of several insects, and egg-laying behavior of *Aplysia*. One important characteristic of hormones is their broad action throughout the nervous system. This action usually comes about because the compounds are present in the circulation and hence are generally available. However, as seen in the last section, a similar situation can be accomplished through a dispersed set of neurons or processes within the CNS, which supplements the effects of the circulating material. The widespread access of hormones has been exploited by the CNS in accomplishing the temporal and spatial coordination of behavioral responses.

In some cases, the expression of the various elements of a behavioral response may be held together simply because they are all responding to a common chemical cue. Even within a given circuit or motor pattern, the action of a hormone is likely to be diffuse. We can contrast this with external chemical cues, of which the signal is intercepted at the body surface by a specialized set of cells that transduce the sensory information and convey it to particular parts of the nervous system. In this case, there is a logical chain of command that can be followed from its source. Such an orderly system is not operative for internal chemical cues; hormones appear to act at many levels in a given neural network. The studies on the stomatogastric system provide an elegant example of such dispersed actions. The studies of wandering behavior, though, caution that diffuse action may not be a universal property of hormonally driven systems in invertebrates.

Hormones also play a crucial role in the temporal organization of behavior. Sensory information is undoubtedly essential for the modification of behavioral outputs. Experiments on isolated nervous systems, however, show that the CNS carries a "template" that estimates how long a particular behavior should last and the order of sequential behaviors. The mechanisms by which this temporal information is stored in the nervous system will be an area of interest in the future.

Acknowledgments

I am grateful to Dr. Earl Mayeri for supplying me with the revised version of figure 14.3.

15 Hormones and Ingestive Behaviors

Edward M. Stricker and Joseph G. Verbalis

The thousands of chemical processes that take place in our bodies every day rely on the careful maintenance of internal chemisty and the continuous flow of nutrients and energy to sustain that chemistry. The brain provides the control center that monitors internal conditions and directs the activity of major organs such as the heart, liver, and kidneys as well as the ingestive behavior of the animal to maintain the internal milieu. Hormones act as messengers that direct information from various organs to the brain and deliver the brain's orders back to those organs to conserve needed nutrients. Furthermore, there is at least one instance in which hormones may act directly on the brain to affect ingestive behaviors.

Which hormones help maintain energy and fluid balance? What happens to that balance when there is loss of these hormones? How do changes in these hormones indirectly affect ingestive behavior? What is the evidence that hormones can also act directly on the nervous system to affect ingestive behavior?

Introduction

Ingestive behaviors provide the various nutrients that animals need for normal growth and development. These nutrients can be subdivided into three broad categories based on how quickly they are expended and need to be replaced. One such category consists of **oxygen** alone. Its rate of expenditure is uniquely high, and our ability to survive without it is uniquely low. Although evolution has not provided the capacity for long-term storage of oxygen within the human body, we satisfy our continuous demand for this vital nutrient readily because we live on a planet where it can be obtained rapidly by normal breathing. Deliberate behavior, involving a strong and willful motivation to obtain oxygen, analogous to intense hunger or thirst, usually is unnecessary but may develop suddenly whenever oxygen is not readily available or carbon dioxide accumulates in the blood.

Nutrients at the opposite end of the continuum from oxygen include **vitamins**, **essential amino acids**, and **trace minerals**. Their turnover is so slow that even when they are absent from the diet, animals can function normally for weeks or months at a stretch. There are no automatic physiological mechanisms akin to breathing that provide for the ingestion of these nutrients, nor are there taste mechanisms that permit each of them to be distinguished among other foodstuffs. Instead, animals obtain the relatively small amounts of needed nutrients incidentally, while they eat primarily for calories. They learn to avoid diets deficient in these nutrients, as they would shun a diet containing a toxic substance, and systematically expand the range of foods they eat until they meet their specific nutrient needs. Then the symptoms of nutrient deficiency disappear and intake of that diet is reinforced.[885]

Water, sodium, and **glucose** represent nutrients in a third category midway between these two extremes. Each is expended in large amounts very rapidly, though not as rapidly as oxygen. Each is available to a considerable extent in body stores, so their dietary absence does not provoke a crisis within minutes, as when the intake of oxygen is prevented, but in days or weeks, depending on the environmental conditions and the initial size of the stores. Gustatory mechanisms, using chemical sensors in the mouth, permit each of these three nutrients to be located readily by their distinctive tastes. The familiar tastes of salty and sweet are common among animals, and gustatory water receptors have been found in several species (but not in primates[60]). Finally, and of most relevance to this chapter, separate hormones help animals to conserve these nutrients and thereby limit their loss when body supplies are low.

In considering the various roles of hormones in ingestive behavior, it is appropriate to acknowledge at the outset the substantial influence of **vasopressin**, **aldosterone**, and **insulin** on the metabolism of water, sodium, and glucose, respectively. The critical contribution of these three hormones to the health and well-being of animals may be best appreciated by considering the consequences that result when any of them is absent or ineffective. For example, arginine vasopressin (AVP; also known as antidiuretic hormone or ADH) is a peptide hormone synthesized in the hypothalamus and secreted into blood from the posterior portion of the pituitary gland. AVP is normally secreted when animals are dehydrated and directly affects the tubules in the kidneys to increase the reabsorption of water from formed urine. Animals lacking AVP have a persistent and uncontrolled loss of water in urine. Consequently, they must drink large amounts of water to survive. For example, unless human patients with this disorder of continual thirst and excessive urinary water loss (called **diabetes insipidus**) are given synthetic AVP as a replacement therapy, they may drink and excrete as much as 15 to 20 quarts of water each day; that amounts to almost 1 quart per hour, every hour of the day, every day of their lives. AVP normally liberates us from the task of irrigating ourselves repeatedly, by promoting the maintenance of water balance with relatively little deliberate effort.[324]

Similarly, aldosterone helps animals to conserve sodium in urine. This steroid hormone is secreted from the adrenal cortex and acts upon tubules in the kidneys to promote sodium reabsorption from urine. Thus, animals lacking aldosterone have an uncontrolled loss of sodium in urine, and in compensation they must ingest sodium in amounts comparable to their sodium excretion. For example, adrenalectomized rats will consume (and excrete) sodium each day in amounts equal to their total extracellular sodium content. A similar phenomenon of adaptive sodium appetite, though of lesser magnitude, can occur in humans with adrenocortical dysfunction (e.g., Addison's disease[850]).

Finally, insulin has a similar influence on glucose metabolism. Glucose is a sugar molecule that is an important source of calories, providing metabolic fuel for basic cell function. Insulin is a peptide hormone secreted from the pancreas that enables glucose to be transported into muscle for use and into liver and adipose (fat) tissue for storage. Consequently, when insulin is not present, glucose is stranded in the blood, where its levels increase so much that the kidneys cannot reabsorb it all and glucose begins to appear in urine. Such pronounced increases in the sugar content of blood and urine are two of the cardinal symptoms of **diabetes mellitus** (not to be confused with diabetes insipidus, described previously). An appropriate compensatory response to the decreased transport of glucose into cells and the increased loss of glucose in urine is to eat more. It is therefore not surprising that rats eat three to four times their normal daily amounts of food after extensive damage has occurred to insulin-secreting cells in the pancreas, but they do not gain weight because they cannot store the caloric nutrients.[850] Similar overeating is a common symptom in human patients with uncontrolled diabetes mellitus.

In short, these three hormones help to maintain **homeostasis**—that is, they keep the circulating supply of water and sodium from getting too low and that of glucose from getting too high. By doing that, they also affect ingestive behavior indirectly by influencing the physiological processes by which these three vital nutrients are conserved and utilized. This chapter will not further dwell on these important matters but instead will address the question of whether these and other hormones also have more direct effects on the nervous system to influence food and fluid intake behaviors. During the past 20 years many hormones have been proposed to affect ingestive behavior by such direct action on the nervous system. A current list of the most likely candidates includes the three hormones mentioned above plus three others: cholecystokinin, angiotensin, and oxytocin (table 15. 1). In this chapter we will review the evidence suggesting that these six hormones directly influence ingestive behaviors.

Basic Concepts

Please note that in some cases these areas of research are marked by controversies and unresolved issues and thus are the focus of active research efforts and continuing debates. For that reason, we describe some of the experiments by which ingestive behaviors have been studied and emphasize the underlying principles by which results have been interpreted, so that readers can consider both the currently available evidence and future studies with some perspective and insight. First, however, we will briefly review the basic physiological processes of caloric and body fluid homeostasis, to provide an appropriate context in which to consider the possible direct role of hormones to influence ingestive behavior.

Table 15.1 Hormones Proposed to Directly Affect Ingestive Behavior

HORMONE	PROPOSED ROLE
Vasopressin	Stimulation of thirst
Aldosterone	Stimulation of sodium appetite
Insulin	Food satiety
Cholecystokinin	Food satiety
Angiotensin	Stimulation of thirst
	Stimulation of sodium appetite
Oxytocin	Food satiety
	Inhibition of sodium appetite

Note that this list is not comprehensive and that other hormones not discussed in this chapter have also been suggested as possibly inhibiting food intake (e.g., bombesin, glucagon) and salt intake (e.g., atrial natriuretic peptide, tachykinins).

Caloric Homeostasis

Animals continuously need metabolic fuels and oxygen to support cellular metabolism. However, they cannot depend on food consumption to provide fuels immediately upon need, as breathing provides oxygen, because the digestive process introduces a considerable delay between the ingestion of food and the availability of small-molecule nutrients to body cells. Consequently, the cells use nutrients, consumed some time ago and sequestered in body stores, which are readily made available.[177]

There are two phases of caloric homeostasis, involving the storage and mobilization of metabolic fuels. After a large meal, digested nutrients from the gastrointestinal tract flood into the circulation in far greater amounts than are immediately needed by the cells to support ongoing metabolism. Excess caloric nutrients are not excreted but efficiently stored in fat and the liver for later use (figure 15.1). Insulin is critical for this storage, altering enzyme activity in the liver and adipose tissue to promote the formation (from glucose) of glycogen and triglycerides, respectively, the two complex molecules that provide the bulk of energy reserves. For this conversion to occur, insulin must be secreted in appropriate amounts while the blood supply of caloric nutrients is abundant.

There are three principal controls of insulin secretion, each dominant during one of the successive, overlapping phases by which caloric nutrients move through the animal. The first control involves a conditioned release of insulin that accompanies the sight, smell, and taste of food. This preingestive, "cephalic phase" response is mediated largely by parasympathetic neural innervation of the pancreas. The second control is a "digestive phase," when food in the stomach and intestines stimulates secretion of various gastrointestinal hormones, which, among other actions, in turn stimulate further secretion of insulin. The third control occurs during the "absorptive phase," when glucose enters the circulation and acts directly on the pancreas to stimulate insulin secretion. These three stimuli for insulin secretion can act additively, thereby

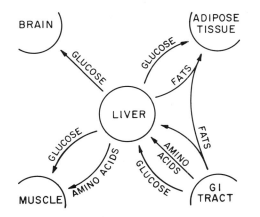

Figure 15.1   Disposal of caloric nutrients after a meal. Food consumption usually delivers nutrients in amounts that far exceed the animal's immediate caloric requirements. Because of the large capacity of the gastrointestinal tract to accommodate food and the relatively slow absorption of nutrients, feeding provides metabolic fuels long after the meal itself. During this time, ingested nutrients either are utilized directly or are stored for later use. Carbohydrates are broken down into utilizable sugars, such as glucose, and are absorbed from the small intestine into capillaries going directly to the liver; there they are oxidized to provide energy, stored in limited quantities as glycogen, or converted to fats, which enter the circulation and join adipose tissue for storage. The circulating glucose not removed by the liver is used for energy production in brain, muscle, and other tissues or else is stored in adipose tissue as triglycerides. Protein from the food is degraded to amino acids, which, after absorption into the bloodstream, are either reincorporated into new protein, used for energy production, or metabolized in the liver to carbohydrate or lipid. Dietary fat, mainly as triglycerides, is hydrolyzed in the capillary beds to liberate glycerol and free fatty acids. The glycerol is converted in the liver to glucose, which is handled as described above, whereas the free fatty acids usually reform triglycerides within adipose tissue and are stored there. The storage capacity of adipose tissue is quite large. (Adapted from Friedman and Stricker, 1976.[384])

ensuring that the levels of insulin in blood are adequate for the disposal of caloric nutrients from the time eating is anticipated until all the eaten food has been absorbed and assimilated.[341,1114]

Larger meals provide caloric nutrients for longer periods of time than smaller meals of similar composition. No matter how much food is consumed in a meal, ultimately its absorption is complete, yet the need for fuels to support cellular metabolism continues. Until the next bout of food ingestion occurs, the body obtains the needed metabolic fuels from body stores (figure 15.2). The mobilization of nutrients from liver, adipose tissue, and muscle is influenced largely by the absence of insulin, which results when all stimuli for its secretion have disappeared: The animal has stopped eating, the stomach and intestines have emptied, and the flow of nutrients into the blood has ceased as well. The mobilization of metabolic fuels from glycogen, lipid, and protein stores is controlled so that they become available in blood only in quantities that can be used rapidly. If the fuels are mobilized from stores too quickly, their blood levels will increase and directly stimulate pancreatic insulin release, which then will slow this recruitment process.

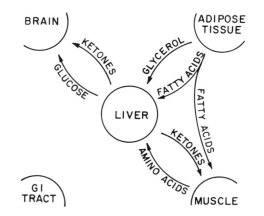

Figure 15.2 Mobilization and disposal of metabolic fuels in the postabsorptive state. Compared to the flood of nutrients right after a meal, the postabsorptive mobilization of metabolic fuels from reserves is conservative. Stores are used only in response to tissue needs, maintaining the body for as long as possible during food deprivation. The lipid depot in adipose tissue normally contains 80% to 90% of all stored calories. Triglycerides in adipose tissue cells are hydrolyzed to form glycerol and free fatty acids, which are then released into the blood. The liver transforms the glycerol into glucose and either uses the free fatty acids for energy or converts them to ketone bodies. Also in the liver, glucose is synthesized from amino acids and mobilized from stored glycogen. Glucose is released into the blood, and the major portion of it is used by the brain. The ketone bodies, in contrast, are used as metabolic fuels by muscle as well as brain. Free fatty acids not taken up by the liver provide a major fuel for muscle but cannot be used by the brain. (Adapted from Friedman and Stricker, 1976.[384])

The control of food ingestion seems to be linked to these two phases of caloric homeostasis: satiety (the feeling of not being hungry) occurs when the stomach is full and the intestinal supply of caloric nutrients to the circulation is ample (figure 15.3), whereas hunger occurs in the postabsorptive period when the stomach has emptied, the intestinal supply of nutrients has slowed to a trickle or stopped altogether, and metabolic fuels are being recruited from body stores. Satiety is signaled both by gastric chemoreceptors or stretch receptors that respond to the presence of food in the stomach, and by postgastric receptors that respond to the storage and utilization of metabolic fuels in the liver.[1000] Hunger occurs when these signals are absent.

Note that hunger is never associated with an *absolute* need for metabolic fuels unless the animal has exhausted all depots of stored caloric nutrients and is literally starving. Thus, despite the obvious discomfort of hunger and the sense of urgency to eat that it creates, there are no prominent physiological dysfunctions that result when individuals skip single meals or even a series of meals. Survival certainly is not threatened, and there is more than adequate time for animals to find and consume food. Rather than reflecting true need, hunger emerges when there is a change in the predominant source of metabolic fuels from exogenous sources (food in the gastrointestinal tract) to endogenous body stores.[384] Thus, hunger provides a very early warning that ensures the continued maintenance of adequate fuel supplies.

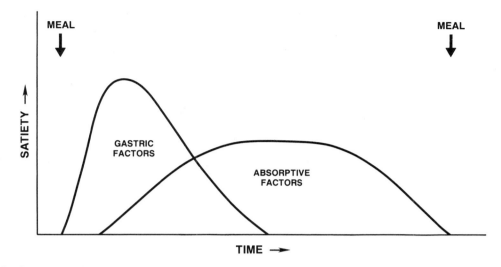

Figure 15.3 Sequence of factors that promote satiety after ingestion of a meal. Each meal generates both gastric and absorptive inhibitory signals that have to fade before the animal will seek another meal. According to this perspective, food intake occurs when inhibitory satiety signals are absent, rather than when a direct excitatory stimulus is present. (From Stricker and Verbalis, 1990.[1008])

Also note that there are other important influences on food consumption that have little or nothing to do with caloric homeostasis.[1008] For example, the familiar inclination to eat a palatable dessert at the end of a meal usually occurs after hunger has disappeared and satiety signals are present. Conversely, dehydration and nausea are much more potent inhibitors of eating than is satiety, and they will prevent feeding even when the stomach is empty and a favorite food item is available. These mechanisms for controlling eating appear to be quite different from those that maintain caloric homeostasis (figure 15.4), and they will be discussed later in this chapter.

Fluid Homeostasis

Fluid homeostasis requires balancing the intake and excretion of both water and sodium. Although these matters can be described separately, they are closely related and should be considered together. There are two dimensions to this consideration of fluid balance: the regulation of fluid volume itself, and the regulation of fluid osmolality, i.e., the concentration of dissolved particles or solutes (e.g., ions and protein molecules) in body fluids.

For osmoregulation, the ratio of dissolved particles to blood plasma volume is monitored closely and maintained within 1% to 2% of normal levels by a combination of physiological and behavioral responses. For example, when the ratio *decreases* because of excessive water consumption, AVP secretion is inhibited. Consequently, water reabsorption from urine diminishes in the kidneys, and the excess water is excreted. Moreover, as we will discuss below, thirst disappears. Conversely, when the ratio *increases* after water deprivation or due

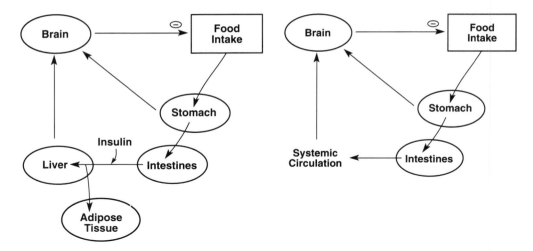

Figure 15.4 Schematic representation of some of the physiological factors that appear to be involved in the control of food intake. *Left*, Controls associated with caloric homeostasis. During a meal, afferent neural signals from gastric chemoreceptors tell the brain that abundant food is present, thereby inhibiting further food intake. Inhibition continues in the absorptive state, when ingested caloric nutrients plus insulin stimulate afferent neural signals from the liver.

Right, Controls associated with nonhomeostatic factors. During a meal, afferent neural signals from gastric stretch receptors inform the brain when the stomach is "full" and thereby inhibit further food intake. Food may contain toxic substances, which are detected in the circulation by chemoreceptors in the brain stem; food also contains solutes such as sodium, which are detected in the circulation by osmoreceptors in the forebrain. In either case, a central system is stimulated that inhibits food intake independent of caloric supplies and needs. (Adapted from Stricker, 1984.[1000])

to a solute load (say a very salty meal), AVP secretion is stimulated, and consequently water reabsorption from urine increases, causing excretion of urine that is much more concentrated than plasma.[861] The resultant water conservation slows the rise in plasma osmolality, but water is still needed for complete osmoregulation to occur. That need underlies thirst. It is interesting that AVP secretion appears slightly sooner than thirst, and relatively little AVP is needed to produce very concentrated urine. Consequently, water conservation in the kidneys begins with incipient dehydration, and the distraction of thirst and stimulated drinking behavior is thereby delayed until dehydration has progressed somewhat.[860]

When we consider the regulation of fluid volume per se, it should be noted that the volume in question is that of blood, not total body fluid. A moderate *decrease* in blood volume (hypovolemia) affects primarily the venous side of the circulation because veins are much more distensible than the thicker-walled arteries. Stretch receptors in the walls of the great veins leading to the right side of the heart can therefore detect blood volume loss. These receptors send afferent neural signals to the brainstem, and in response the central nervous system initiates a number of important reflex responses. One of these responses is AVP secretion. AVP not only promotes water conservation in urine, but when secreted in large amounts it also becomes a potent pressor

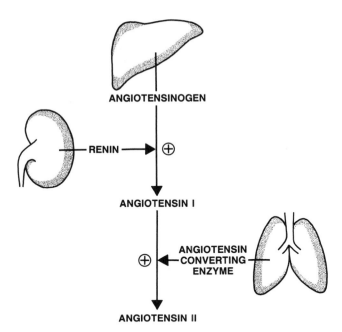

Figure 15.5 Cascade of biosynthetic steps in the renin-angiotensin system. Renin is an enzyme secreted from the kidneys when blood volume is low (hypovolemia). Renin cleaves four amino acid fragments from a plasma protein made in the liver (angiotensinogen), to produce angiotensin I, which itself has little biological activity. However, two additional amino acid fragments are cleaved by a converting enzyme found in the lungs and other tissues (including brain), thus producing angiotensin II. Angiotensin II is a potent pressor agent (i.e., it causes blood vessels to constrict) and additionally may stimulate aldosterone secretion, thirst, and sodium appetite, depending on the presence of other factors (see text).

agent (i.e., it causes blood vessels to constrict and thereby increases blood pressure). This action reduces blood flow to the periphery and intestines, thereby restricting blood to the central circulation that supplies the critical organs such as the liver, kidneys, and brain.[225]

Another reflex response to hypovolemia involves the neural outflow from the sympathetic nerves exiting the thoracic and lumbar spinal cord. Some of these sympathetic nerves innervate the adrenal medulla and stimulate the release of norepinephrine and epinephrine. These responses all act to increase heart rate and peripheral vasoconstriction.[225] In addition, sympathetic nerves to the kidneys stimulate the secretion of renin. Renin is an enzyme that acts on a plasma protein to form the hormone angiotensin I, which is soon cleaved by other enzymes (in the lungs) to form angiotensin II (AII) (figure 15.5). AII acts on blood vessels as a pressor agent, stimulating the adrenal cortex to secrete aldosterone. Aldosterone in turn acts upon the kidneys to promote sodium conservation, as mentioned previously.

More severe degrees of blood loss activate stretch receptors on both the venous and the arterial sides of the circulation, augmenting the above volume-regulating responses. They also provide a direct stimulus of renin release from

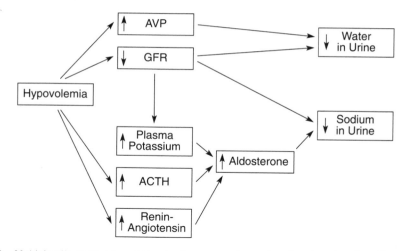

Figure 15.6 Multiple effects of reduced blood volume on water and sodium loss in urine. Hypovolemia is detected by cardiovascular stretch receptors, which provide afferent neural signals that activate secretion of arginine vasopressin (AVP, also known as antidiuretic hormone), from the posterior pituitary and secretion of pressor agents from the sympathoadrenal and renin-angiotensin systems. When blood loss is severe and blood pressure is low sufficient AVP is secreted to serve as an additional pressor agent. Also, renal baroreceptors can stimulate renin release independently of the sympathoadrenal system. Angiotensin II (AII) also stimulates aldosterone secretion, promoting urinary sodium conservation. Adrenocorticotropic hormone (ACTH) secreted from the anterior pituitary also stimulates aldosterone secretion, as does potassium accumulated in the blood when renal blood flow and glomerular filtration rate (GFR) are reduced. Decreased GFR of the kidneys also promotes water and sodium conservation in urine independently of AVP and aldosterone.

the kidneys, elevating blood AII to very high levels. Marked hypovolemia additionally decreases filtration of blood in the kidneys, which reduces urine formation independently of AVP and also increases blood levels of potassium, stimulating aldosterone secretion from the adrenals. Moreover, such severe volume depletion elicits pituitary secretion of adrenocorticotropic hormone (ACTH), which acts in the adrenal cortex to further promote secretion of aldosterone (figure 15.6).

In short, there are many compensatory physiological responses after an extensive loss of blood or a reduction of blood pressure, including activation of the sympathoadrenal and renin-angiotensin systems, secretion of AVP and aldosterone, peripheral vasoconstriction, and conservation of water and sodium in urine. It should not be surprising that multiple complex physiological mechanisms such as these have evolved to preserve cardiovascular function. Collectively, these varied responses stabilize fluid volume and pressure in the cardiovascular system and minimize further fluid loss. As discussed later, they are accompanied by increases in the specific appetites for water and sodium chloride (NaCl), which are needed to replace the deficits.

Direct Effects of Hormones on Ingestive Behavior

We will now discuss whether the hormones we have mentioned so far, insulin, AVP, aldosterone, and AII, also have direct effects on ingestive behavior. We

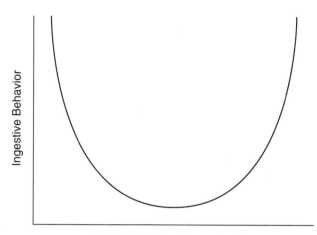

Figure 15.7 Stylized U-shaped function relating blood hormone concentration to ingestive behavior. This function appears to be appropriate when discussing changes in food and NaCl intake that result in the absence of insulin and aldosterone, respectively, and when the two hormones are present in excessive amounts. However, this function is not useful when considering the asymmetrical effects on ingestive behavior of vasopressin (whose absence increases water intake but whose presence does not) and angiotensin II (whose presence stimulates water and NaCl intake but whose absence does not).

will also review the evidence that two other hormones, cholecystokinin (CCK) and oxytocin, may influence ingestive behaviors as well.

Insulin

A direct stimulatory effect of insulin on food intake was first considered 50 years ago on the basis of observations that injections of insulin elicited hunger in humans and other animals. Taken together with the increased eating associated with untreated diabetes mellitus, it appears that a U-shaped function relates blood insulin levels to food intake (figure 15.7). Nevertheless, considerable evidence now indicates that insulin itself is neither a "hunger hormone" nor a "satiety hormone."

With regard to the right-hand side of this U-shaped function, hyperinsulinism stimulates food intake by accelerating glucose storage in peripheral tissue and thereby decreasing available glucose for the brain. The brain detects the falling glucose supply and triggers the sensation of being hungry. This point is most clearly demonstrated by experiments showing that the cerebral chemoreceptors respond only when blood glucose levels fall below a threshold value of approximately 70 mg/dl, which is the amount of glucose needed to provide maximal transport of glucose into the brain. Similarly, food intake is stimulated when cerebral glucose deprivation is produced by a drug that specifically inhibits glucose metabolism without raising blood insulin levels or lowering blood glucose levels.

Three prominent responses are initiated when cerebral glucose utilization is compromised: (1) a massive sympathetic discharge, which stimulates glucose mobilization from body stores while inhibiting pancreatic insulin secretion; (2) increased gastric emptying, which speeds the absorption of ingested nutrients from the intestines; and (3) increased hunger and food intake, which provides caloric nutrients from outside the body. These adaptive responses elevate blood glucose levels and thereby restore cerebral nourishment.[327,1003] Note that such severe hypoglycemia constitutes an unnatural emergency condition, and because cerebral glucose deprivation might never occur in the lifetime of an animal, it would provide an unsuitable explanation for the regular appearance of hunger.

On the left-hand side of the curve in figure 15.7 we see a marked increase in food intake associated with diabetes mellitus. Because insulin is required for both the storage and utilization of carbohydrates, rats with diabetes mellitus eat very large amounts of food when provided with a high-carbohydrate diet, but, without insulin, they receive little nourishment. However, such diabetic rats consume normal amounts when given a high-fat diet,[383] which can be stored and utilized even in the absence of insulin. So it is possible to reach satiety without insulin. These and other findings suggest that insulin permits ingested carbohydrates to be satiating but in itself probably has no direct effect on food intake. There is some other evidence suggesting that insulin may also have a direct effect on the brain to reduce food intake,[1115] but the issue is unsettled, and it would be premature to consider insulin a satiety hormone.

Vasopressin (AVP)

The two most prominent responses to dehydration are AVP secretion and thirst. That coincidence suggests that AVP itself may stimulate thirst during dehydration. However, that does not seem to be the case. The great thirst that accompanies urinary water loss during diabetes insipidus proves that AVP is not *necessary* for the development of thirst. Nor is AVP alone *sufficient* to stimulate thirst because when injected systemically it does not elicit water intake. In fact, as mentioned, AVP treatment has the opposite effect— indirectly limiting thirst by increasing water conservation in urine and thereby postponing the need for drinking.

On the other hand, there is some evidence suggesting that AVP can lower the set point of cerebral osmoreceptors, thereby sensitizing the animal to the effects of dehydration.[1018] Moreover, hypothalamic AVP is also secreted from centrally projecting neurons into the cerebrospinal fluid during dehydration. It is possible that AVP, acting as a neurotransmitter in the brain (rather than as a hormone in the circulation), may have an important role in mediating thirst during dehydration. However, that attractive possibility requires further examination, and in any case a direct and substantial effect of pituitary AVP on water intake appears unlikely.

Aldosterone

In most animals the lack of aldosterone stimulates an increase in NaCl (salt) intake because sodium is lost through urine, just as the lack of AVP causes water loss and therefore drinking. Moreover, similar to the effects of insulin (but not AVP), substantial NaCl intake is stimulated when large amounts of aldosterone or its biosynthetic precursor, desoxycorticosterone (DOC), are injected in rats. Thus, there is also apparently a U-shaped curve relating plasma aldosterone levels to NaCl intake in rats (see figure 15.7).

This stimulating effect of mineralocorticoids such as aldosterone on salt intake is a curious phenomenon because these hormones cause pronounced sodium *retention* in urine. Thus, in this situation sodium appetite occurs in the absence of sodium need; indeed, it occurs despite surplus body sodium. For this reason, it has been assumed that these steroid hormones must have direct effects on the brain to stimulate sodium appetite. However, recent findings indicate that intracranial administration of an aldosterone receptor blocking agent does not reduce sodium appetite in aldosterone-treated rats. It therefore appears that the effects of these hormones on sodium appetite are indirect, i.e., they somehow affect the body, which in turn affects the brain.[1009] This issue is considered further when we consider the role of AII in the control of water and NaCl intake.

Cholecystokinin (CCK)

Cholecystokinin (CCK) is a peptide hormone secreted from the intestines after ingestion of dietary fat and protein. CCK influences pancreatic exocrine secretion and gallbladder contraction and is also known to stimulate insulin secretion. In the early 1970s reports indicated that CCK also produced a dose-related inhibition of food intake in rats without disrupting other ingestive behavior, for example, water intake. Indeed, CCK elicited a pattern of behaviors that closely resembled the activities of rats that had just finished a meal. During this so-called satiety sequence, rats groomed themselves, explored the cage, and then rested. These observations led to the proposal that CCK may be an endogenous satiety hormone that was secreted during a meal and thereby served to limit further food intake.[399]

However, later observations indicated that CCK was more effective in inhibiting food intake when food was present in the stomach than when the stomach was empty. Moreover, cutting nerve afferents from the stomach to the brainstem eliminated the inhibitory effects of CCK on food intake. It was as though CCK magnified the signal of a full stomach, thereby mimicking the effect of a very large meal. On the other hand, high doses of CCK could inhibit eating even when rats were "sham- feeding"—that is, when ingested food was drained through a chronic gastric fistula and rats neither experienced gastric distension nor absorbed nutrients from their meal.[399]

While there is no doubt that exogenous CCK inhibits food intake in several species, there remains considerable controversy about how this happens. The initial presumption that CCK reduces food intake by stimulating the sensation of satiety still is uncertain. An alternative possibility is that CCK reduces food intake by causing nausea. Consistent with this possibility are recent findings that treatment of rats with lithium chloride (LiCl), a toxic substance that when given in low doses causes nausea and vomiting in humans, inhibits sham-feeding in hungry rats rather like CCK. Moreover, like CCK, LiCl has little effect on water intake in thirsty rats and also produces the satiety sequence of behaviors seen after a meal. In fact, even when the experimenter abruptly removes food in the middle of a meal, rats groom, explore, and then rest.[359] So this sequence of behaviors may appear whenever rats stop eating and may not necessarily indicate that they are satiated.

The question posed by these studies—how do the rats feel after CCK treatment?—is, of course, very difficult to answer. Extreme nausea can be inferred when animals display emesis (vomiting), but rats do not vomit, even when they are sick. But when rats become sick (or are made sick with LiCl treatment) after ingesting a particular substance (say a novel sweet-tasting saccharin solution), they act as though the food made them sick and avoid that food in the future.[389] In contrast, the sensation of satiety is a positive experience and should not lead to such conditioned taste aversions. It appears that CCK treatment can be substituted for LiCl to produce conditioned taste aversions in rats. Moreover, injection of a drug that reduces nausea in humans also blunts the inhibitory effects of CCK on food intake in rats. These findings suggest that exogenous CCK decreases food intake in rats at least in part by causing nausea rather than by inducing satiety.[277]

More compelling evidence regarding the sensations caused by CCK can be obtained only through human subjects, and the results of such experiments are consistent with the idea that CCK causes nausea in rats.[716] Specifically, CCK given in doses comparable to those that inhibit food intake in rats causes vomiting in humans. Smaller doses of CCK produced nausea but not emesis, whereas still smaller doses did not cause nausea but still produced abdominal cramps. In other words, the administration of CCK in doses that affect food intake appears to produce a variety of effects ranging from mild gastric malaise to frank emesis in human subjects, and, by implication, CCK probably does so in animal subjects as well. It is possible that very small doses of CCK stimulate satiety without having any adverse effects, but such doses of CCK also would have very small effects on food intake. Taken together, these experiments suggest that administered CCK does not elicit satiety but instead induces the unpleasant sensations of sickness, which interrupts food intake even more effectively than does satiety.

When considering how chemical agents reduce food intake, it would be best actually to measure some biological variable that is always associated with nausea rather than drawing inferences about induced sensations from behavioral studies of animals. In humans, nausea usually is associated with pituitary secretion of AVP in even greater amounts than after blood loss.[860] This response presumably occurs because AVP constricts the blood vessels in the intestines, and such diversion of blood away from the intestines after consuming toxin-containing food helps limit further absorption of poison.

Curiously, this same endocrine response does not occur in rats. Although different drugs (LiCl, copper sulfate, and apomorphine) each cause nausea and vomiting in humans, and each can be used to produce learned taste aversions in rats, none of these agents increase plasma AVP levels in rats except at very high doses. However, each of these drugs did increase plasma levels of the very similar pituitary hormone oxytocin in a dose-related manner.[1076] Perhaps oxytocin has the same special ability to reduce intestinal blood flow in rats that AVP has in humans. Regardless of its function, however, pituitary oxytocin secretion can be used as a biological marker of gastric malaise in rats as long as other stimuli known to affect oxytocin secretion are absent.

This oxytocinergic response was used in the following studies of rats. One group of experiments revealed a dose-related increase in plasma oxytocin levels when rats were given CCK in the same doses that inhibit food intake.[1075] The regression line relating plasma oxytocin levels to inhibition of food intake after injection of CCK was very similar to that produced by LiCl treatment. Other experiments showed that pituitary oxytocin secretion was increased when CCK was given to rats after a gastric preload, in parallel with the enhanced inhibitory effect of CCK on food intake. Furthermore, oxytocin secretion was abolished when the gastric afferent nerves were destroyed.[1077] Remember that this surgery also abolishes the effect of CCK on feeding.

The effects of CCK and LiCl on pituitary peptide secretion are relatively short lasting compared to their effects on food intake, as if these hormones signaled the onset of nausea rather than its duration. But we can consider a second biological marker of nausea, the inhibition of gastric motility and emptying. This response effectively slows absorption of toxin-containing material that has been eaten. The adaptive value of this effect may result from the relatively slow entry of the toxin into the circulation, which might be better tolerated than if it were absorbed rapidly. Slow gastric emptying also would allow time for vomiting to rid the body of toxin in animals that vomit. In any case, rats show pronounced inhibition of gastric motility and gastric emptying after LiCl treatment, and the duration of these effects is comparable to the LiCl-induced inhibition of food intake. Moreover, inhibition of gastric function was also observed after systemic injection of CCK in rats, and the same regression line relating inhibition of gastric emptying to inhibition of food intake was obtained for both LiCl and CCK.[679]

To summarize, it appears from this series of studies that CCK treatment potently reduces food intake, not by acting centrally to cause satiety but in large part by acting peripherally to cause nausea or gastric malaise. However, this conclusion does not preclude the possibility that endogenous CCK acts elsewhere to promote satiety, and that issue is another subject of lively debate. One approach has been to inject a CCK receptor blocking agent prior to a meal and then determine its effect on food intake. If CCK is a satiety signal, this treatment should lead to increased eating. Several such studies in rats have shown that there is indeed an increase in food intake under these circumstances, but it seems possible that the drug might have facilitated gastric emptying or otherwise blocked the signal of pronounced gastric distention resulting when food-deprived rats ate a large meal. Furthermore, there is no evidence as yet that a similar effect occurs in rats when smaller, more normal-sized meals are consumed, and thus it is unclear whether endogenous CCK contributes to the cessation of eating. In human subjects, CCK blockers do not appear to affect gastric emptying of normal meals, but their effect on food intake remains to be determined.

It is interesting that in rats dehydration stimulates not only AVP but also oxytocin secretion[1005] and decreases gastric function and food intake in a manner analogous to the effects produced by CCK and toxins.[360] Of course, it is clear in the case of dehydration that the animals are experiencing thirst rather than nausea. But these findings emphasize the point that an increase in plasma oxytocin level is accompanied by an inhibition of food intake and gastric function in rats when widely different types of stimuli for pituitary oxytocin secretion are used.

Brain mechanisms that mediate the pituitary secretion of AVP and oxytocin, the inhibition of gastric motility and emptying, and the anorexia (lack of appetite) seen in response to toxins and dehydration can be conceptualized as follows. Pituitary AVP and oxytocin are synthesized in the magnocellular neurons of the supraoptic and paraventricular nuclei of the hypothalamus. Smaller parvocellular oxytocinergic neurons, projecting from the paraventricular nucleus to the dorsomotor nucleus of the vagus in the brainstem (figure 15.8), have been shown to be involved in the inhibition of gastric motility in rats.[865] Still other parvocellular projections from the hypothalamus, some of which may also be oxytocinergic, appear to inhibit food intake.[787] Hence, when the hypothalamus is stimulated, as might occur after consumption of toxins, after treatment with large doses of CCK, or during dehydration, there is simultaneous activation of magnocellular neurons controlling pituitary hormone secretion and parvocellular neurons controlling the inhibition of gastric motility and food intake. In this way, the hypothalamus may provide integrated control of neuroendocrine secretion, autonomic function, and ingestive behavior.[1016]

Angiotensin II (AII)

As mentioned earlier, angiotensin II (AII) is a peptide hormone formed in blood as the final step of a cascade that begins with secretion of renin from the kidneys (see figure 15.5). In the late 1960s, reports appeared indicating that infusion of AII produced a dose-related increase in drinking. Because plasma AII levels are known to increase during hypovolemia and hypotension (low blood pressure), it seemed reasonable to suggest that AII may contribute to the thirst

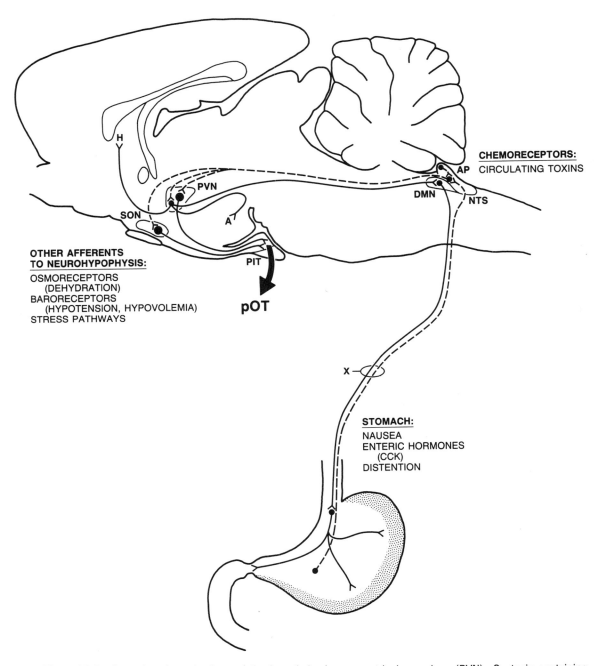

Figure 15.8 Oxytocinergic projections of the hypothalamic paraventricular nucleus (PVN). Oxytocin-containing neurons from magnocellular cells project to the posterior pituitary (PIT), from which oxytocin is secreted and raises plasma levels (pOT). Neurons from parvocellular cells in PVN project throughout the brain, including the amygdala (A), hippocampus (H), and the dorsal motor nucleus of the vagus nerve (DMN) and nucleus tractus solitarius (NTS) in the brain stem. Oxytocin acting as a neurotransmitter appears to be involved in the central control of gastric function and ingestive behavior. In contrast, oxytocin-containing neurons from the hypothalamic supraoptic nucleus (SON) project only to the posterior pituitary. Stimuli for oxytocin secretion from both magnocellular and parvocellular PVN neurons are conducted through vagal afferent nerves (X) from the stomach, and also arise from the area postrema (AP) and other afferents. (Adapted from Verbalis and Stricker, 1991.[1077])

caused by a decrease in blood volume or pressure. That hypothesis was consistent with subsequent findings that nephrectomy (removing the kidneys, which eliminates the source of renin) abolished the increase in water intake normally seen in rats after drug-induced hypotension.[357]

On the other hand, there are alternative explanations of these observations. For example, AII is an important pressor agent, and therefore removal of the kidneys should compromise blood pressure maintenance and thereby debilitate an animal made hypotensive. In fact, these drugs severely lowered arterial blood pressure in nephrectomized rats to an extent that might cause loss of consciousness in humans. As might be expected, when rats were also deprived of water before nephrectomy and hypotensive drug treatment, they drank little despite the presumed presence of thirst, probably because blood pressure was too low for them to manage to drink. Thus, the conclusion reached from these studies is that AII is vital for increased water intake during hypotension, not as a direct stimulus of thirst but as an indirect stimulus of drinking by maintaining blood pressure.[998]

The contribution of AII to water intake has been examined further in studies of thirst after a more gradual loss of blood volume, in which case arterial blood pressure is stable even in nephrectomized animals. One way to cause a gradual loss of plasma volume in rats is by injecting a colloidal solution subcutaneously, which leeches plasma fluid into the interstitial space. Colloid-treated rats are not debilitated by volume depletions of up to 30% to 35%, and they both secrete renin and drink readily in proportion to the induced hypovolemia. However, nephrectomized rats cannot produce renin, and yet they drink water after colloid treatment too, in the same amounts as intact control rats. Thus, despite the significant positive correlation between activation of the renin-angiotensin system and water intake in colloid-treated rats, neither renin nor AII appears to be necessary for thirst to appear. Instead, the drinking that occurs when blood loss is moderate and hypotension is not present seems to be mediated primarily by neural signals from vascular stretch receptors.[998]

Nevertheless, it seems clear that AII can directly stimulate the brain to produce thirst under pathophysiological or pharmacological circumstances when plasma AII levels are very high. AII appears to act upon the subfornical organ (SFO), a small diencephalic tissue mass protruding into the dorsal portion of the third cerebral ventricle.[960] Injection of AII directly into the SFO produces dose-related increases in water intake, whereas destruction of the SFO eliminates the drinking response to systemically infused AII. Similarly, injection of an AII receptor blocker into the SFO prevents the drinking elicited by systemic AII. Although AII does not penetrate into most of the brain, the SFO, like a number of tissues surrounding the cerebral ventricles, lacks a tight blood–brain barrier, so it can detect and respond to circulating AII much like peripheral tissue.

AII is also synthesized within brain neurons, like many other peptides found in the periphery.[837] This fact helps to explain the otherwise paradoxical finding that systemic injection of drugs that block conversion of AI to AII in the periphery produces a marked increase in drinking during colloid-induced hypovolemia in rats. In explanation, the peripherally acting enzyme-inhibitor enhances renin secretion from the kidney, which causes AI to be produced in unusually large amounts, and the excess AI is converted to AII in the brain, where it stimulates drinking.

AII in large doses raises blood pressure and thereby increases the excretion of sodium in urine. These effects are seen readily when AII is injected into the cerebral ventricles. Thus, prolonged infusion of AII into the brain has been found to increase sodium loss in urine and ultimately to stimulate salt intake in rats. In other words, AII can indirectly affect sodium appetite in rats. However, when the sodium-excreting effect of AII is blunted by pretreating rats with mineralocorticoids, the sodium appetite still is enhanced and, in fact, appears more rapidly.[365] Those observations led to the hypothesis that AII also has a direct role in mediating sodium appetite in rats, acting synergistically in the brain with mineralocorticoids. Thus, it was suggested that the two hormones that are critically important in maintaining blood pressure and limiting sodium loss in urine during hypovolemia or sodium deficiency also stimulate an adaptive increase in NaCl intake.

Recent studies of rats after colloid treatment have added new insights to this phenomenon, including the possibility that central oxytocin secretion also plays a role in the control of sodium appetite.[1007] These experiments initially focused on the observations that subcutaneous colloid treatment elicits thirst in rats and about 5 hours later also stimulates intake of NaCl solution. It seems paradoxical that thirst appears soon after colloid treatment while sodium appetite is delayed because ingested water is distributed largely into cells, and extracellular sodium is required to keep water outside the cells and thereby repair the volume depletion. Later studies indicated that the 5-hour delay resulted from the time required for the consumed water to dilute plasma osmolality.[999] Evidently osmotic dilution facilitates sodium appetite when it is present together with hypovolemia.

Osmotic dilution also inhibits thirst and the pituitary secretion of AVP and oxytocin, even in the presence of continued hypovolemia.[997,1005] To determine whether the inhibition of AVP or oxytocin was always correlated with sodium appetite, neurohypophyseal hormone secretion also was examined in rats with elevated NaCl intake caused by adrenalectomy or DOC treatment. These treatments had no effect on plasma AVP levels, but caused plasma oxytocin levels to fall.[1006] Moreover, when plasma oxytocin levels were measured following various other manipulations to increase sodium appetite in rats, an inverse correlation always was found. For example, maintenance of rats on a sodium-deficient diet for 2 days increased sodium appetite after colloid treatment and reduced the pituitary secretion of oxytocin that usually follows colloid treatment.[1002] Indeed, 8 days of a sodium-deficient diet alone produced a marked sodium appetite in rats, and under those circumstances oxytocin secretion seemed to be eliminated altogether.

Complementing these studies are experimental findings that LiCl treatment, which produced very high plasma levels of oxytocin, always inhibited sodium appetite in rats that were sodium-deficient and hypovolemic. Similarly, systemic injections of hypertonic NaCl solution caused the release of oxytocin and inhibited sodium appetite in adrenalectomized rats (while potentiating thirst), and the inhibition of salt intake lasted as long as the oxytocin secretion.[1002] However, when the stimulating effects of hypertonic NaCl solution on pituitary oxytocin secretion and thirst were prevented by destroying the osmoreceptors located in the forebrain,[391] rats showed a spontaneous sodium appetite that was not associated with hypovolemia, sodium deficiency, or stimulation of the renin-angiotensin-aldosterone system.[390]

These experiments collectively led to the hypothesis that pituitary oxytocin secretion somehow was associated with inhibition of sodium appetite in rats. Inhibition did not result from circulating oxytocin itself because infusion of oxytocin did not reduce sodium appetite in colloid-treated rats, and blocking peripheral oxytocin receptors did not enhance sodium appetite.[1002] Rather, evidence suggests that sodium appetite is inhibited by some central neuronal system whose activity is *correlated* with the activity of magnocellular neurons in the supraoptic and paraventricular nuclei projecting to the posterior pituitary gland. We noted earlier that some oxytocinergic cells in the paraventricular nucleus project centrally (figure 15.8). In fact, neurons in the parvocellular portion of the paraventricular nucleus appear to be activated by the same treatments that inhibit sodium appetite and provoke pituitary oxytocin secretion in rats (i.e., hypotension, LiCl, and osmotic dehydration).[1009] The important role of those neurons in the central control of sodium appetite was demonstrated in recent experiments showing that their stimulation inhibited NaCl consumption in colloid-treated rats, whereas that inhibitory effect was abolished by injecting an oxytocin receptor blocker into the cerebral ventricles.[1074]

To summarize, during hypovolemia rats need both water and NaCl to repair their plasma volume deficits. The best source of these substances would be isotonic saline (i.e., water with a concentration of salt approximating plasma). When given access to both pure water and hypertonic NaCl solution, neural signals from vascular stretch receptors appeared to stimulate water intake at first, but they also stimulate some central system that inhibits sodium appetite and is accompanied by oxytocin release. Because of this induced water intake, there is osmotic dilution of body fluids, which inhibits further water intake and oxytocin secretion and apparently inhibits the central system suppressing sodium appetite as well. This latter effect is seen when the animals start drinking NaCl solution. But as they do, plasma osmolality again becomes elevated, thereby disinhibiting thirst and oxytocin secretion. Animals then drink water, reestablishing osmotic dilution and permitting sodium appetite to emerge again. This explanation, summarized schematically in figure 15.9, accounts for the observed alternation between water and NaCl intakes by rats during hypovolemia. Hypovolemia and AII provide the excitatory stimuli for sodium appetite, which is revealed only when osmotic dilution eliminates their inhibitory effects on sodium appetite.

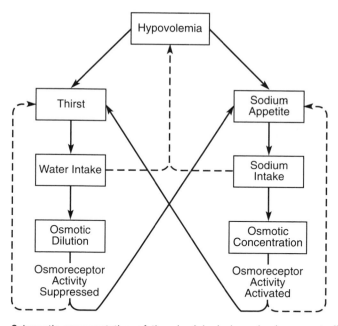

Figure 15.9 Schematic representation of the physiological mechanisms controlling thirst and sodium appetite during hypovolemia (low blood volume) in rats. Solid arrows indicate stimulation; broken arrows indicate inhibition. Hypovolemic rats alternately drink water and concentrated NaCl solution, depending on the current plasma osmolality, and in the long run consume sufficient water and salt to repair the volume deficit. However, drinking is limited when animals have access to only one of the drinking fluids because an inhibitory osmoregulatory pathway is activated. Conversely, neither inhibitory pathway is activated when hypovolemic rats drink isotonic NaCl solution, and drinking proceeds unabated. (Adapted from Stricker and Verbalis, 1990.[1009])

Because pituitary oxytocin secretion appears to be a marker of the central inhibition of both food and NaCl intake in rats, it is interesting to consider whether this coincidence indicates the presence of an integrative mechanism common to both of these ingestive behaviors. At present, it seems likely that the central inhibitory system limiting NaCl intake is the same system that inhibits food intake after injection of CCK, LiCl, or hypertonic NaCl solution. When active, this system could decrease the general inclination of animals to consume any substance that would increase body fluid osmolality. Since food provides salts as well as caloric nutrients, this motivation could be expressed as a loss of appetite both for food and for NaCl solution. Such a central integrative system presumably is also present in mammals other than rats, although pituitary oxytocin secretion may not be a marker of its activation in other species (particularly primates) because AVP rather than oxytocin is secreted in response to hyperosmolality, hypovolemia, CCK, and LiCl.

Summary

1. Insulin has a critical role in the control of food intake; it is required to make carbohydrates utilizable in the liver, which thereby generates a signal of

satiety. Insulin's absence allows metabolic fuels to be mobilized from stores, thereby generating a signal of hunger. But in these instances, insulin seems to act in the periphery, and the nervous system generates satiety and hunger when it detects these changes.

2. Pituitary oxytocin is secreted in rats (and AVP is secreted in primates) when conditions other than satiety inhibit food intake, such as nausea or dehydration. Again, the plasma levels of these hormones appear to be associated with activity in some central hunger-suppressing system, and the systemically released hormones themselves do not directly inhibit food intake. Exogenous CCK also provokes neurohypophyseal hormone secretion while suppressing the urge to eat, but there is no definite evidence that circulating levels of either oxytocin, AVP, or CCK have a direct and significant influence on food intake.

3. At present, no definite role for hormones in the control of osmoregulatory thirst is known. However, AVP clearly limits dehydration indirectly by promoting water conservation in urine. Aldosterone similarly limits sodium deficiency by promoting sodium conservation in urine, and thereby affects sodium appetite indirectly. In contrast, AII definitely contributes to the stimulation of sodium appetite during hypovolemia by acting directly on the brain to increase NaCl intake.

4. Pituitary oxytocin secretion can be used as a marker of a central system inhibiting sodium appetite, but the circulating oxytocin itself seems to have no direct effect on salt intake. Rather, the systemic release of oxytocin may simply be correlated with activation of oxytocinergic synapses within the nervous system.

5. In short, several hormones have important but indirect effects on ingestive behavior. In contrast, AII has a direct stimulating effect on sodium appetite and, under certain circumstances, on thirst as well. However, the data at present do not support such a direct role for insulin or CCK in the inhibition of food intake, nor for aldosterone in the excitation of sodium appetite. These considerations are based on research conducted during the past 20 years, especially the last decade. Future research may reveal new hormones with comparable effects on ingestive behavior as well as new roles for familiar hormones in the control of ingestive behavior. In this regard, there have been recent proposals that food intake is inhibited by systemic administration of glucagon and bombesin, hormones secreted by the pancreas and intestines, respectively. Similarly, tachykinins found in the brain and a peptide hormone secreted by the heart, atrial natriuretic peptide, have been found to inhibit salt intake when injected into the brains of rats. Full evaluation of the physiological significance of these recent findings remains a project for future research.

16 Hormones and Biological Rhythms

Lawrence P. Morin and John Dark

In physiology, as in humor, timing is everything. We will find that hormones are almost always secreted in pulses and patterns across time. The timing of these pulses, both in terms of their duration and the time of day at which they occur, can have a significant impact on their effects. Animals have evolved a quite sophisticated neural clock that keeps track of the time of day, the season of the year, and their own reproductive status to help them anticipate future conditions and breed successfully. You will not be surprised to learn that hormones respond to this clock to help animals prepare for the future.

Why must animals keep track of the time of day and season of the year, and what neural structures provide this information? What are the various temporal patterns of hormone release and which environmental stimuli regulate the patterns? Can hormones affect the time-keeping mechanism itself?

Introduction and Definitions

The word rhythm indicates a movement or function with regular recurrence. Thus, in music the rhythm is the uniform recurrence of the beat or accent in the music. In physiological systems a biological event that recurs at regular intervals is said to be rhythmic. A heartbeat is an example of a simple biological rhythm. In many ways, rhythmicity is a property of all biological systems. Indeed, some scientists believe that rhythmicity is a major organizing principle in biology. In this chapter we will present the view that an understanding of biological rhythms is critical to a clear understanding of the capabilities of any physiological system.

A number of examples demonstrating that a wide variety of neuroendocrine and behavioral systems depend upon an integrated rhythm will be developed to illustrate the importance of these concepts to the study of hormones and behavior. An astute reader will of course realize that many, if not all, other physiological systems are also rhythmic. There have been several recent reviews of the properties of rhythmicity and the significance of oscillatory systems in biology. Interested readers are referred to reviews by Moore-Ede,[745] Morin,[751] and Rapp.[839,840]

The appreciation of biological rhythms has an ancient history. For example, there is evidence from ancient writings that humans noted very early that most species of vertebrates are seasonal breeders. Modern study of seasonality has emerged from the study of daily rhythms. In 1936, Bunning[170] proposed that reproductive seasonality is the consequence of an interaction between an **endogenous clock** timing daily rhythms and **seasonal changes** in the time of day at which light is perceived by the animals. The endogenous clock is the heart of circadian rhythm biology. The ability to respond to seasonal changes in the clock-light relations is known as photoperiodism. Bunning's hypothesis proposed that these two phenomena are functionally related.

Consider the remarkable consequence of Bunning's hypothesis: Animals can use a daily clock to generate a rhythm that lasts about a year. This same daily clock is also thought to generate estrous cycles that are 4 days long.[1023] Similarly, the ability of many other animals to undergo estrous or menstrual cycles is dependent on the interaction of several endocrine rhythms with *altogether different frequencies*. In other words, with his simple hypothesis about seasonal rhythms Bunning also provided a generic hypothesis for many interactive rhythmic events. Bunning's hypothesis is a "coincidence" hypothesis. It requires the coincidence of two rhythms (e.g., an endogenous daily clock and the light-dark cycle) to obtain a specific biological rhythm. Such coincidence hypotheses have provided the basis of understanding the relations among neuroendocrine events modulating reproduction. The discussion below is designed to elaborate on this basic regulatory organization.

Biological Rhythm Terminology

Every rhythm is characterized by its period (or frequency), phase, and amplitude (figure 16.1). **Period** is amount of time it takes to complete one cycle of the rhythm (e.g., 24 hours). **Frequency** refers to the number of recurrences or cycles during a given amount of time (e.g., 1 cycle/24 hours). Thus, frequency is the inverse of period, and the two words are used interchangeably to describe the rate of recurrence of a given cycle. For daily rhythms, there is one cycle per day (frequency), and the length of the cycle is 24 hours (period).

Rhythmic processes by definition change over time. Since the cycle is continuously changing, someone at some time has had to pick a time and say, "Let's start here." Time points during a cycle, therefore, are defined according to an arbitrary reference time. **Phase** refers to the location of a second point in time on a rhythm, relative to this arbitrary reference time.

Finally, during the period of a rhythm the variation from the mean can be determined. **Amplitude** describes the magnitude of the variation from the mean of the phases of the rhythm. Thus, the greater the variation, the larger the amplitude. These parameters are clear in a simple sine function but are much less so in the typical locomotor rhythm of a hamster (figure 16.1), for example.

A true biological rhythm is self-sustaining and endogenous to the animal. For the most part, this chapter will present material pertaining to such self-sustained, endogenous rhythms. However, in several instances, rhythmicity emerges as a complex interaction (a "mixed mode") of endogenous processes

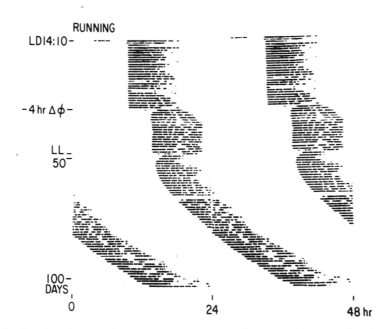

Figure 16.1 Running rhythm of a normal male hamster. The animal is housed under light-dark (LD) 14: 10 conditions with lights going off at 1400 hours. More than 100 days of activity records are stacked day below preceding day, with the figure photographically doubled to clarify the running pattern. Activity is shown on each day by the dark areas of the record. Therefore, under LD 14:10, the animal begins running shortly after the lights go off and runs intermittently throughout the night. The phase of the rhythm is here measured relative to the lighting schedule. On day 28, the onset of dark is delayed by 4 hours. The activity rhythm shifts quickly to reentrain to the shifted LD cycle. At day 48, the lights are left on permanently, and the activity rhythm assumes a free-running period that stabilizes at 24.7 hours in length. The amplitude of this rhythm would be indicated by the number of wheel revolutions per unit time (e.g., per 5-minute interval) but is not easily obtained from this type of data plot. (From Morin, 1985.[749])

and exogenous stimuli. These are inherently interesting and closely related in function and physiological basis to strictly endogenous biological rhythms. Therefore, this chapter also will include data of this type when useful. Purely exogenous rhythms such as might be forced upon an animal by a periodic stimulus (e.g., vitamin D synthesis in human skin in response to daily exposure to sunlight) are not considered here.

Biological rhythms are classified according to their *period length or domain*. Four groups are generally recognized: (1) circadian, (2) ultradian, (3) infradian, and (4) circannual. The suffix *dian* is derived from the Latin word *dies* meaning "day." The prefix *circa* is from the Latin word meaning "approximately." Therefore, **circadian** means "approximately a day." This definition is important because it implicitly contains the features necessary to demonstrate true biological rhythmicity.

For a 24-hour rhythm to be considered circadian, it must be self-sustained and endogenous and must have a period approximating 24 hours. To demonstrate that a rhythm is endogenous requires that the rhythm persist after all known time cues (**Zeitgebers**, literally, "time-givers") are removed from the environment. In the life of most organisms, the daily light-dark cycle constitutes the most potent Zeitgeber.

When the light-dark cycle cues are removed (by creating either constant light or constant dark conditions), an endogenous rhythm persists if it is a true circadian rhythm. Because the rhythm is no longer synchronized to the 24-hr day, however, it will normally have a period that deviates from 24 hours by a constant amount. It is similar to a wristwatch that gains or loses a few minutes every day. If you do not reset it each day, it will drift further and further from the true time. This rhythm is considered to be "**freerunning**" and demonstrates that there is an endogenous clock-like mechanism within the animal. In this instance, it is a freerunning circadian rhythm. It is endogenous, self-sustained, and has an approximately 24-hour period. The average freerunning circadian rhythm period ranges from about 20 to 30 hours. Freerunning periods vary between species. In the laboratory and under natural conditions, of course, the circadian rhythm is entrained to the light-dark cycle.

Ultradian rhythms are those with greater frequency than the range of circadian rhythms. Examples of ultradian rhythms are heartbeat, respiration, pulsatile hormone release, meal timing, and certain regular electroencephalogram (EEG) waves. The period range is very large, from milliseconds to hours in duration. There is seldom a Zeitgeber that is clearly associated with entrainment of each cycle of a rhythm. Sometimes, however, the light-dark cycle entrains some part of an ultradian cycle (e.g., the start or end time of the ultradian cycle).

Infradian rhythms are less frequent than circadian cycles but more frequent than circannual rhythms. Reproductive cycles are common examples of such rhythms. The hamster has the shortest known reproductive cycle—4 days. In contrast, mammals with a functional luteal phase in the reproductive cycle (as discussed in chapter 3) have cycles that are longer (e.g., guinea pig, 16 to 18 days; human, 24 to 33 days; baboon, 29 to 42 days).

At the long end of the rhythm spectrum are the **circannual** rhythms. In wild animals, these are typically synchronized with environmental events of the year, but will freerun under laboratory conditions. Freerunning circannual rhythms, such as those for body weight in golden-mantled ground squirrels, have an average period of about 345 days.

Synchronization of a Rhythm to a Periodic Stimulus

Entrainment is the process of synchronizing a rhythm to a periodic stimulus. The most complete example of entrainment comes from the circadian rhythm literature. For this type of rhythm, light is overwhelmingly the most potent timing event or Zeitgeber. The process of entrainment and the neural pathways and mechanisms regulating entrainment are under intense investigation. A detailed discussion of these mechanisms is beyond the scope of this chapter.

However, an appreciation of the entrainment process is necessary for an understanding of the interactions between rhythms.

In principle, any rhythm can become entrained by any periodic stimulus providing: (1) there is some form of physical interaction between the two rhythmic processes; (2) the amplitude of the periodic stimulus is sufficient to modify the period of the target rhythm; and (3) the two periodic processes have frequencies that are similar to each other.[242] If (2) and (3) are in effect, then entrainment occurs if the period of the target rhythm becomes equal to that of the periodic stimulus. This means that an exogenous periodic stimulus (e.g., the light-dark cycle) might act to modify the function of an endogenous clock. Although the following description is derived from work on rodent locomotor rhythm entrainment to the light-dark cycle, it is most important to recognize that the example can be applied to any rhythmic process and its Zeitgeber.

If a hamster living in a room where the light cycle is controlled so that there are 14 hours of light and 10 hours of darkness during each 24 hours (light-dark, 14:10 photoperiod) is then given free access to a running wheel, it will show a wheel running rhythm. Typically, it will enter the wheel 5 to 10 minutes after the lights go off and begin running (figure 16.1). More than 99% of running activity will occur at night for this species. If the lights fail to go back on some morning, the locomotor rhythm will continue to be expressed but with a period slightly different from 24 hours. This demonstrates two things: First, the locomotor rhythm is a circadian rhythm because it persists in a freerunning form in the absence of the light-dark cycle. Second, the behavior was entrained to the light-dark cycle prior to the constant darkness. Under the light-dark conditions, the locomotor rhythm maintains a constant phase relationship to the Zeitgeber (i.e., the animal's activity begins at the same time each day). Additionally, all animals will have circadian rhythms that average exactly 24 hours. Thus, one effect of light on a circadian clock is to control the rhythm's phase. Phase of the locomotor rhythm in a light-dark cycle is typically measured with respect to the time the lights go off. Under constant conditions, the circadian onset of locomotor activity for hamsters is used as a phase reference. It is described as circadian time 12, where circadian time 12 refers to the arbitrary midpoint of the approximately 24-hour (or circadian) day.

Light's effect on circadian rhythm phase is demonstrable by giving animals in constant darkness a single "pulse" of light at a variety of times during the circadian day. Examination of the running records (figure 16.2) reveals a systematic effect of light on the phase of running activity onset. When all the points are plotted, three quite different responses emerge on the graph (figure 16.2B): (1) There is a portion of the circadian day during which light has little or no effect on rhythm phase (the "dead zone"); (2) there is a portion during which light results in a delay of wheelrunning onset, and this "phase delay" persists indefinitely; and (3) there is a portion of the circadian day during which a light pulse will evoke an advance of wheelrunning onset, and this "phase advance" persists indefinitely. This plot of the effect of light on the

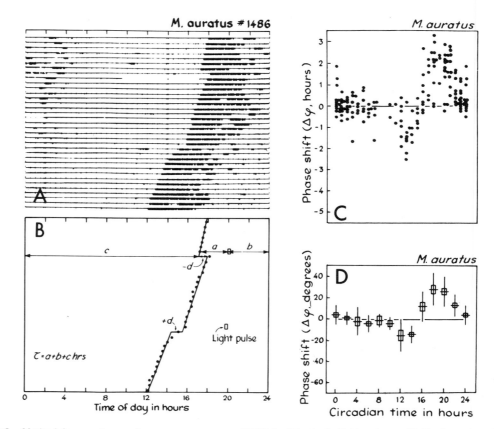

Figure 16.2 Method for creating a phase response curve (PRC) to 15-minute light pulses with the hamster. *A*, Free-running activity rhythm of an animal in constant dark. The phase changes in activity onset occur in response to light pulses given at the times indicated by the open boxes in *B*. The magnitudes of a large number of such phase changes from many animals, measured as delays in activity onset (−d, a negative phase change) or advances in activity onset (+d, a positive phase change), are plotted in *C*, and the smoothed curve with standard errors is shown in *D*. (Data from Daan and Pittendrigh, 1976[243]; figure reprinted from Morin, 1985.[749])

phase of the circadian rhythm is called the phase response curve. The dead zone corresponds to the "subjective day" of the animal. The phase delay and phase advance portions of the curve are considered the "subjective night" or that part of the phase response curve during which the Zeitgeber can modify the circadian rhythm's phase.

Entrainment can be demonstrated using a single daily light pulse.[325,821] The freerunning period usually deviates from 24 hours; for example, a circadian period may be measured at 24.2 hours. It is entrained to a Zeitgeber with a 24-hour period by the Zeitgeber inducing a daily phase advance of 0.2 hour. This is just enough to correct the difference between the biological clock and the 24-hour day. The same thing is occurring for an animal entrained to a light-dark cycle. At some time each day, light must be stimulating either the phase advance or the phase delay portion of the phase response curve such that it "corrects" the error caused by the circadian clock. In the same way a person with a faulty wristwatch must set his watch back or ahead each day.

As noted earlier, the principles of entrainment apply to all biological rhythms for whatever Zeitgeber. If the conditions of: (1) physical coupling of sufficient magnitude between the Zeitgeber and the target rhythm, and (2) sufficient similarity between the Zeitgeber frequency and that of the target rhythm are achieved, entrainment will occur.

The above list of rhythm domains and their definitions provides the basis for this chapter. There is an essentially infinite range of allowable periodicities. This enables enormous latitude in physiological regulation. Rhythmic regulation has been called **homeokinesis**.[1124] This term is used to indicate the dynamic interplay of physiological events configured to change in a rhythmic manner. For example, a house thermostat may have a built-in timer. House temperature is kept cool at night, but it is turned up shortly before the inhabitants rise in the morning. It is again turned down during the day while the people who live there are at work, then up again during the evening. The temperature is maintained at different set points at different times of day. Some of the advantages[839] conferred by rhythmic control systems are (1) prediction of repetitive events or "predictive homeostasis",[745] and (2) increased efficiency of biological systems. When rhythmicity is designed into physiological systems, the temporal characteristics of the signal can become an important aspect of physiological regulation. Thus, modulation of the frequency of a hormonal rhythm becomes a method for subtly controlling a physiological function. The magnitude of the response depends on the hormonal rhythm's frequency, not on the amount of hormone being received. Such is the case for the relationship between dihydrotestosterone and the regulation of pituitary luteinizing hormone (LH) release in rats (discussed later).

Rhythmic Expression of Hormone Secretion and Variation in Responsiveness to Hormones

Biological rhythms influence the expression of essentially every hormonal system. Table 16.1 shows numerous examples in humans. Much of the information in this table, especially that pertaining to daily and circadian rhythms, comes from a book on endocrine rhythms by Krieger.[602] This book is recommended as an excellent starting point for anyone wishing to pursue this topic in greater depth.

Any given hormone is not necessarily described by a single rhythm. A hormone may show ultradian and circadian as well as seasonal changes in its production and systemic release. An observed rhythm in the secretion of a hormone does not necessarily mean that the rhythm is driven directly by a biological clock. Release of a hormone may be driven by other factors, such as a specific behavior (e.g., sleep and growth hormone) or environmental conditions (e.g., low temperatures and thyroid hormone).

Table 16.1   The Rhythmic Expression of Several Major Human Endocrine Products

Hormone	Pulsatile	Daily	(Circadian)	Infradian	Annual	(Circannual)
				RHYTHM DOMAIN		
GH	Yes	Yes	No	?	?	—
ACTH	Yes	Yes	Yes	?	?	—
Cortisol	No	Yes	Yes	No	?	—
TSH	Yes	Yes	?	No	?	—
T4 (T3)	?	Yes	?	No	?	—
LH	Yes	No	—	Yes	Yes*	?
FSH	Yes	No	—	Yes	Yes*	?
Estradiol	Yes	Yes	?	Yes	?	—
Testosterone	Yes	Yes	?	—	Yes	?
Prolactin	Yes	Yes	No	Yes	?	—
Melatonin	No	Yes	Yes	?	Yes	?
Insulin	Yes	Yes	No	No	?	—
Epinephrine	No	Yes	No	?	?	—
Vasopressin	No	Yes	No	Yes†	?	—

Abbreviations: GH, growth hormone; ACTH, adrenocorticotropic hormone; TSH, thyroid-stimulating hormone; T4, thyroxine; T3, triiodothyronine; LH, luteinizing hormone; FSH, follicle-stimulating hormone.
? Indicates insufficient or conflicting data.
— Indicates not applicable.
* Indicates indirect evidence available; there are pronounced seasonal cycles in spermatogenesis.
† Indicates that there is no menstrual cycle in vasopressin release, but there is a cycle in sensitivity to vasopressin.

An important function of biological rhythms is the control of timing of the production and release of hormones, be it on a daily, monthly, or annual basis. Equally important is the change induced by biological clocks in the responsiveness of target tissues to hormones. In the absence of changes in hormone availability, altered sensitivity of tissues to hormones on a daily or annual basis will have a major impact on behavior. This is evident in the expression of annual rhythms, and numerous examples will be provided in the descriptions of photoperiodic and circannual rhythms given subsequently.

Biological Rhythms in Physiology and Behavior

The concepts and issues presented below have been selected for three basic reasons. One, they illustrate the breadth of rhythmicity in physiology and behavior. Two, they clearly demonstrate how strongly normal physiology depends on many rhythm frequencies. Three, each example is well documented in the scientific literature. It is our greatest hope that these examples will represent but a fraction of similar results and processes described by the end of this century.

The Circadian Corticosteroid Rhythm: Hierarchical Control of Rhythms

The general organization of the hypothalamo-hypophyseal system and its modulation of target endocrine organs has been described elsewhere in this book (see chapter 1). In this section, we will expand upon that organization to demonstrate the pervasiveness of biological rhythms within the neuroendo-crine system. In particular, we will illustrate the hierarchical organization of circadian rhythms evident in the control of adrenal steroid release in the rat.

In the context of clinical medicine, the adrenal corticosteroid rhythm is perhaps the most widely known and acknowledged circadian rhythm. Cortisol and its synthetic variants are extremely potent drugs used to control inflammation. The rhythm of cortisol is one of the very few rhythms regularly considered by physicians making therapeutic recommendations involving treatment with adrenal hormones. The cortisol rhythm of primates, including humans, reaches its daily peak within a few hours after waking.[392] In the rat, a nocturnal animal, the rhythm peak has a phase fitting that nocturnality, rising to a maximum shortly after the onset of darkness when the rat is maximally active.[245]

As discussed in previous chapters, the release of corticotropin-releasing hormone (CRH) from the hypothalamus stimulates adrenocorticotropin (ACTH) output from the pituitary and is under the inhibitory feedback control of the hippocampus. The ACTH stimulates the adrenal gland to produce a variety of steroid hormones. However, control of the adrenal is strongly rhythmic, involving large variations in the releasing hormone, the trophic hormone, and the steroid hormones from one time of day to another. How is this rhythmicity controlled? It could be that the pituitary and adrenal glands are themselves inherently rhythmic. Alternatively, there might be a circadian clock gating the release of ACTH or controlling the release of CRH. In fact, the master circadian clock controlling the adrenal rhythm lies in the suprachiasmatic nucleus of the hypothalamus. This nucleus receives photic stimulation enabling the clock to be synchronized to the environmental photoperiod.

The relationships between the circadian clock and the several elements of the neuroendocrine system have been studied in the rat and the rhesus monkey. As described earlier, the daily corticosteroid cycle is known to be a circadian rhythm. The rhythm of blood ACTH peaks with the same phase as that of the adrenal corticosteroid rhythm, and there is a daily rhythm of CRH.[10,392,550]

At least two mechanisms regulate rhythmicity of the adrenal system, one associated with circadian clocks and one controlling hormone synthesis and release. The corticosteroid rhythm is normally synchronized to the light-dark cycle but freeruns under constant conditions. Adrenal cortex incubated in vitro may have a freerunning corticosteroid rhythm,[28] and there is apparently a daily corticosteroid rhythm in hypophysectomized animals (given tonic ACTH and thyroid hormone replacement therapy.[704,792] In addition, there appears to be a daily rhythm of adrenal responsiveness to acute ACTH treatment in hypophysectomized animals.[793] These data suggest that there may be circadian oscillators located in the adrenal gland itself that control steroid synthesis.

In the absence of the adrenal, ACTH concentrations in serum are very high, and there is no rhythm.[10] Is the usual ACTH rhythm[326] imposed by the adrenal? Experiments in which a constant low dose of corticosteroid is infused have been conducted to address this question. The reduction in ACTH amplitude varied according to the time of day. As a consequence, a clear rhythm of ACTH release emerges despite a constant corticosteroid background.[10] This experiment suggests that the sensitivity of ACTH to corticosteroid feedback varies according to a rhythm in addition to any variation in the adrenal gland itself.

The concept of rhythmic sensitivity to stimulation is also found in the response of the adrenal to ACTH stimulation.[246,554] The adrenal corticosteroid response to acute ACTH injection is much larger in the early hours of darkness than during the early daytime hours. Under ordinary conditions, the rhythm in blood ACTH varies diurnally in phase with the corticosteroid rhythm (i.e., they peak at the same time). This temporal correlation may invoke the misleading inference that the amount of adrenal steroid released is directly related to the amount of ACTH available. Instead, experiments show that two separable events are occurring. First, more ACTH is released as the lights are about to go off. Second, corticosteroid output is maximized by the increasing sensitivity to ACTH that reaches a daily peak at that time, thereby further magnifying the adrenal steroid response. As Kaneko and associates[554] remark, the greater responsiveness of the evening adrenal to ACTH stimulation provides greatly enhanced sensitivity to small changes in trophic hormone levels.

The independence of rhythmic target sensitivity from rhythmic hormone secretion is a novel and important concept. Either type of rhythm can potentially alter the likelihood of some hormone-contingent physiological or behavioral response. The significance of this issue will be considered again in the context of rhythmic control of sexual behavior.

Rhythmic Control of Sexual Behavior

Figure 16.3 shows the patterns of the major ovarian steroids and pituitary trophic hormones during the 4-day hamster reproductive cycle. Under favorable environmental conditions, these patterns are repeated continuously during the entire reproductive life of the individual. Note also the peak of each hormone early in the afternoon of cycle day 4. It is not a chance phenomenon that the hormonal peaks happen at the same time of day. In the hamster, photoperiod affects reproductive functioning on a daily and seasonal basis. An unfavorable photoperiod for a golden hamster is one that has fewer than 12.5 hours of light per 24-hour day. Such a "short" photoperiod cannot maintain reproductive function. The ovary ceases to produce mature follicles, ovarian interstitial tissue hypertrophies, and ovulation stops. Three other environmental conditions can cause the ovary to become anovulatory. These conditions are chronic cold exposure, lactation, and food deprivation.

The hormonal events of the hamster estrous cycle are similar to those in the rat (discussed in detail in chapter 3). In both species, the circadian clock triggers the acute preovulatory release of gonadotropins (LH and follicle-stimulating hormone [FSH]. In the hamster, the ovaries release sufficient estradiol to act on the brain for 12 to 24 hours, the circadian clock will trigger the

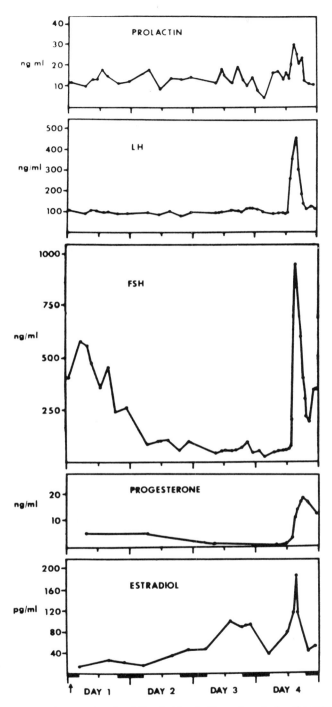

Figure 16.3   Levels of hormones circulating in blood of hamsters during the estrous cycle. The abscissa shows the approximate time of ovulation (arrow) for animals housed in LD 14:10 (lights off at 2100 hours). The intermittent black bars indicate the hours of darkness. Day 4 corresponds to "proestrus." (Data from Bast and Greenwald, 1974 [prolactin, LH, FSH][68]; Saidapur and Greenwald, 1978 [progesterone][897]; and Baranczuk and Greenwald, 1974 [estradiol].[52])

release of LH and FSH from the pituitary. The release of LH and FSH always occurs approximately 3.5 hours prior to the onset of the daily locomotor activity period.[734] Therefore, the hamster estrous cycle (and estrous cycles of similar animals, e.g., the rat) is the result of coincidence between two cyclic functions, the circadian clock and the cycle of endocrine events. If the circadian clock in the brain is destroyed, the estrous cycle is lost.[988]

The present summary of the pattern of ovarian and pituitary hormones demonstrates their rhythmic nature. Most important, normal hamster estrous cyclicity results from the coincidence between (1) a phase of the reproductive cycle characterized by high estradiol concentrations, and (2) a circadian rhythm of neural origin.[332,987] This coincidence leads to the release of a preovulatory surge of gonadotropins and preparation for pregnancy or the next estrous cycle. It is upon this neuroendocrine background that some environmental conditions can act to produce an anovulatory condition and the absence of reproductive behavior.

TIMING OF REPRODUCTIVE BEHAVIOR
The timing of the hamster estrous cycle can be measured very accurately using a simple method. Every 4 days the female hamster comes into estrus and will show lordosis behavior in response to tactile stimulation. An adequate stimulus can be as uncomplicated as a soft paintbrush stroked across the animal's hindquarters. When estrus is initiated, it reaches maximum responsiveness very rapidly. In the space of a few minutes, a female will go from unreceptive to fully sexually receptive. An understanding of the hamster's hormones and behavior and reference to figure 16.3 suggest why this happens.

As estradiol release from the maturing follicles increases, it activates neural structures in the hypothalamus. This priming action (see chapter 3) prepares the brain for the acute behavior-facilitating effect of progesterone. Timing of preovulatory progesterone is under the control of the circadian clock. It is released from the ovarian interstitium in direct response to the acute surge of LH.[332] Progesterone rises immediately and begins the process leading to the facilitation of sexual behavior. In the hamster, this process is so tightly controlled that sexual behavior can be elicited every 96 hours (4 × 24 hours) with only a few minutes deviation.[21,356]

Central to the organization of the hamster estrous cycle is the timing of sperm transmission from the male to the ova in the female, such that sperm arrive at a time that ensures fertilization. This is not a simple problem, and evolution has selected a large number of ways to solve it. In the case of the hamster, the process requires temporal coordination between the copulatory behavior necessary for sperm transmission and the ovulatory events that allow fertilization. This is the primary point of this discussion: the process of temporal reproductive coordination requires the presence of a circadian clock.

A second important function of the circadian clock is the synchronization of the social aspects of reproduction. Estrus normally lasts 14 to 18 hours if no copulation takes place.[639] Most of this time is during the night, which corresponds to the hours of greatest locomotor activity of male and female hamsters. Males show sexual behavior only during the nocturnal active phase despite the presence of ample testosterone at other times of day. The net result is clear. The nocturnal phases of sexual activity that occur daily in males and every 4 days in females must coincide or copulation will not be successful (see Morin and Zucker[757] for a discussion). These phases coincide when males and females are entrained to a common Zeitgeber.

Stimulus Conditions Inducing an Anovulatory State: Short Photoperiod   The above description of the hamster reproductive cycle is contingent upon the presence of a "long" photoperiod. A standard long photoperiod is 14 hours of light and 10 hours of darkness. In nature, such a constant photoperiod never occurs. The photoperiod varies seasonally. The daily amount of daylight ranges from a minimum of 9 hours 9 minutes on December 21 to a maximum of 14 hours 30 minutes on June 21 at 40 degrees north latitude (e.g., Pittsburgh, PA, Indianapolis, IN, and Denver, CO). A number of experiments have begun to elucidate the relationship between hamster reproductive seasonality and annual changes in photoperiod.

When hamsters are transferred from a 14:10 light-dark cycle to a 6:18 light-dark cycle, they become reproductively quiescent in 5 to 7 weeks. This means that the ovaries are no longer developing follicles. As a consequence no estradiol is secreted from the ovaries,[12] and neither sexual behavior or ovulation occurs. There persists, however, a small daily release of LH and FSH.[733,933] The precise neuroendocrine mechanism leading to the short photoperiod-induced anovulatory state is unknown. However, melatonin from the pineal gland appears to be important for transducing changes in day length into neuroendocrine information. This aspect has been well documented and is discussed later in this chapter.

Acute Food Deprivation   When female hamsters are food deprived for several days, they fail to ovulate.[750] The ovaries of these animals reveal the same histological picture that is found after exposure to a short photoperiod. The follicles are undeveloped, and there is interstitial tissue hypertrophy. An absence of adequate metabolizable fuels precipitates the loss of ovulatory capacity.[927] Furthermore, food deprivation is most damaging during a specific phase of the estrous cycle. The greatest sensitivity occurs in response to 48 hours of deprivation beginning on estrous cycle day 1.[750]

The major endocrine question concerns the nature of the events by which food deprivation prevents follicular development. Our best guess is that inadequate metabolizable fuel prevents the normal pulsatile release of LH on estrous cycle days 1 and 2. LH pulses are necessary for follicular development (also see the later section on puberty). The presence of undeveloped follicles leads to inadequate estradiol release, which has two consequences. First, if estradiol is insufficient, the circadian clock will not trigger a preovulatory gonadotropin surge. Second, there will be inadequate priming of the brain for the display of lordosis.

In summary, the relationship between food consumption and ovulation is highly dependent upon rhythms of several period lengths. (1) In the ultradian domain, LH pulses regulate follicular development; they are suppressed by food deprivation. (2) In the circadian domain, the low estradiol levels that follow food deprivation block the neural clock from triggering a preovulatory gonadotropin surge. (3) In the infradian domain, availability of adequate metabolic fuel is most crucial during the initial phase of the estrous cycle.

Lactation During pregnancy, the rhythmic hormonal environment is greatly modified to suit the maintenance of pregnancy and the development of the fetuses.[441] Estrous cycles also are suppressed during the subsequent lactation period. As with the other environmental conditions discussed, some facet of the lactational state results in a pattern of ovarian histology characterized by undeveloped follicles and interstitial tissue hypertrophy.[440] The anovulatory condition seen in hamsters during lactation is virtually identical to that seen after short photoperiod exposure.[149]

Chronic Cold Exposure Exposure to a cold environment for 6 to 12 weeks leads to an anovulatory state.[846] The ovary is histologically similar to its appearance following food deprivation or short photoperiod exposure. Changes in the rhythmic release of or in the response to hormones have not been documented for cold exposure.

The common ovarian condition found in response to each of the four environmental conditions described implies the existence of a common neuroendocrine mechanism causing that syndrome. This view is indicated in figure 16.4. The small daily release of LH and FSH from the undeveloped follicles of short photoperiod-exposed and lactating animals probably also occurs in animals that are exposed to chronic cold or to chronic food shortage.

PROLACTIN AND RAT PREGNANCY
Adler (see Adler and Allen, 1983) has performed a series of experiments defining how female rats become pregnant. The answer may seem simple but is in fact complicated. For pregnancy to occur, information from the internal and external environments must be integrated in a series of events resulting in development of a fetus. This series of events includes the use of a circadian clock to time the preovulatory gonadotropin surge. This surge stimulates progesterone release, which acts synergistically with estradiol to facilitate sexual behavior. Sensory information from cervical stimulation during copulation is neurally transmitted to the brain. If stimulation is sufficient,[6] rhythmic endocrine changes[1024] provide an environment for blastocyst implantation on the uterine wall.

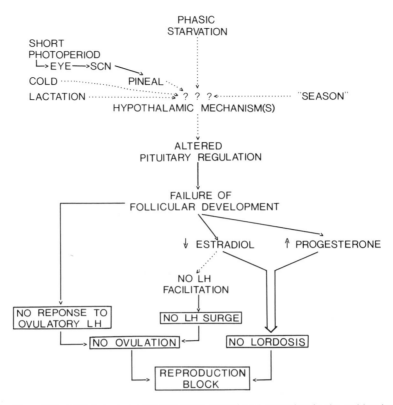

Figure 16.4 The relationship between environmental stimuli and ovulation in the golden hamster. Photoperiod, cold, lactation, and phasic starvation act through uncertain hypothalamic mechanisms to presumably modify the release of pituitary gonadotropins. This change prevents normal follicular development leading to reduced estradiol but elevated progesterone during the estrous cycle. This state blocks the display of lordosis behavior. The follicles remain immature, and ovulation cannot occur. In addition, either the hypothalamus or the pituitary is altered to prevent the acute ovulatory release of LH. The ultimate consequence of theses changes is full behavioral and endocrinological reproduction block.

An afternoon surge of prolactin is released at the same time as LH and FSH and is also elicited by the circadian clock.[1126] Copulatory stimulation, however, induces a second peak of prolactin late that night.[970,1024] Thus, copulatory behavior transforms the prolactin pattern from a single afternoon peak (near the time of lights off) to a bimodal pattern with a second peak at the time of lights on.[1970] The bimodal pattern persists during pregnancy.[377, 422, 971, 1127]opulation-induced prolactin release initiates and maintains the corpus luteum and, as a result, the secretion of progesterone.[969] Although the rhythmic events leading to sexual behavior are many, without the rhythmic endocrine changes that follow copulation, pregnancy fails despite the presence of normal fertilized eggs.

CONTROL OF PUBERTY

Bronson has developed a model accounting for the impact of many environmental variables on the timing of puberty (see Bronson[158] for an extensive

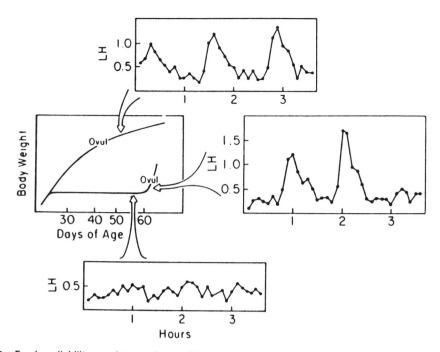

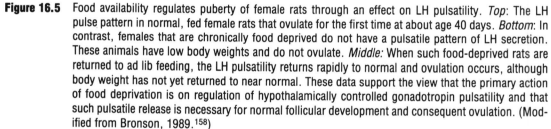

Figure 16.5 Food availability regulates puberty of female rats through an effect on LH pulsatility. *Top*: The LH pulse pattern in normal, fed female rats that ovulate for the first time at about age 40 days. *Bottom*: In contrast, females that are chronically food deprived do not have a pulsatile pattern of LH secretion. These animals have low body weights and do not ovulate. *Middle*: When such food-deprived rats are returned to ad lib feeding, the LH pulsatility returns rapidly to normal and ovulation occurs, although body weight has not yet returned to near normal. These data support the view that the primary action of food deprivation is on regulation of hypothalamically controlled gonadotropin pulsatility and that such pulsatile release is necessary for normal follicular development and consequent ovulation. (Modified from Bronson, 1989.[158])

presentation of these issues). One such variable is food availability. In a series of papers, Bronson has shown that prolonged food restriction will indefinitely block pubertal onset in female rats and that the block is dependent upon the loss of pulsatile gonadotropin-releasing hormones (GnRH).

If developing female rats are food deprived to prevent weight gain, first ovulation is restored only if ad lib food is made available. Ovulation occurs within 3 to 4 days[157] as the pattern of LH release returns to normal when food is made available. During food restriction, LH is consistently low (figure 16.5), and no animals show evidence of LH pulses. After 12 hours of ad lib food, half the animals average about 0.4 pulses of LH/hour; After 24 hours of ad lib food, pulses per hour increase to about 0.6, which is no different from normal.

The implication is that the loss of LH pulses may be due to food restriction blocking the GnRH pulse generator. If this is true, then pulsatile infusion of GnRH should restore LH pulses and ovulatory capacity in food-restricted animals. In fact, when 1 ng of GnRH is infused intravenously every hour into food-restricted rats, all individuals ovulate after 4 to 6 days. GnRH clearly has potent effects after as few as 3 days of pulsatile infusion. Estradiol from the newly developing follicles induces a fivefold increase in uterine weights by day 3.

The results from prepubertal female rats are consistent with the view that food deprivation, whether it occurs during the estrous cycle (see above)[750,927] or during puberty,[157] retards follicular development. The causative chain of events includes the absence of pulsatile LH trophic activity on the ovary; follicular development during the rat pubertal period is rendered static. Pulsatile LH is missing because the GnRH pulse generator is not functioning normally. Although Bronson has demonstrated that GnRH replacement can overcome most of the effects of food restriction, pulsatile GnRH therapy requires 1 to 2 days more than ad lib food to restore ovulation. The reason for this difference may be related to the fact that pulsatile prolactin and growth hormone are also suppressed by food restriction (see Bronson[157] for references). Many of these same issues are pertinent to the above discussion concerning the disruption of the hamster estrous cycle by acute food deprivation.

Neuroendocrine Bases of Annual Rhythms

Annual rhythms are widespread among living things and are exemplified by autumn color changes in the foliage of deciduous trees, winter dormancy of bears, and seasonal migration of species as diverse as Monarch butterflies, Canada geese, and Arctic caribou. The correlation between the changing seasons and the expression of annual rhythms of animal behavior has been appreciated by humans for a long time. Only during the last 75 years, however, have we begun to understand the mechanisms underlying the generation and expression of annual rhythms, and only in the past two decades have we come to recognize the vital role played by hormones in mediating seasonal changes in behavior.

Annual rhythms of animal behavior and physiology can be divided into those that are at least partially dependent upon the environment for their generation (type I) and others that are generated entirely by an endogenous biological clock (type II[1142]). Type I rhythms are generally referred to as "photoperiodic" because seasonal changes in day length are necessary for expression of at least some part of the annual cycle. For example, in late summer and autumn meadow voles reduce their food intake and lose body weight, their gonads involute, and reproductive behaviors cease. These responses are dependent upon decreasing day length and can be simulated in animals in the laboratory solely by decreasing the length of the photoperiod from summertime values (e.g., 14 hours of light/day) to those characteristic of winter (e.g., 10 hours of light/day).[256] Springtime increases in food intake, body weight, redevelopment of the reproductive system, and the return of reproductive behavior are mediated by an internal timing mechanism and occur spontaneously: environmental input is unnecessary. The onset of a second cycle, however, requires a return to long day lengths and a subsequent exposure to short days.

Type II annual rhythms are generated by an endogenous clock that does not require environmental input. These are referred to as circannual rhythms; to qualify as a circannual rhythm, a freerunning behavior or physiological measure must persist for at least one to two cycles under constant environmental conditions.[449] For example, the European starling is a migratory species in which individuals increase fat stores prior to spring migration and, upon completion of migration, a molt occurs. Annual changes in premigratory fattening, migratory restlessness (Zugenruhe), and molt persist in the laboratory under constant conditions of photoperiod, temperature, and food availability.[449] Each animal freeruns with an idiosyncratic period of approximately a year in much the same way as freerunning circadian rhythms are expressed. As is the case with circadian rhythms, freerunning animals eventually become desynchronized from each other as well as from the environment.

Photoperiodic Annual Rhythms

Animals living at more extreme latitudes face a marked seasonal cycle in environmental conditions. Summer is generally a period of bounty and moderate temperatures, but winters are challenging. Availability and nutritional content of food resources are reduced at a time when low temperatures increase the energetic costs of foraging. As a consequence, seasonal changes in energy balance and thermoregulation have evolved to maximize overwinter survival and restrict the birth of young to the time of the year that is optimal for successful development. It would be inefficient if animals waited until winter conditions were upon them before initiating adaptations to the cold; making changes prior to the onset of winter is advantageous. The most reliable environmental predictor of seasonal change is photoperiod. Many seasonal changes that have been studied in the laboratory are mediated by photoperiod. Note, however, that because photoperiod is a sufficient cue does not mean that other environmental factors, such as temperature, are not important signals as well.[158]

Photoperiodic rhythms have been studied in numerous mouse and hamster species. Meadow voles or Siberian hamsters, for example, born in long day lengths simulating those of summer rapidly reach reproductive maturity and adult size (within 1 to 1.5 months). As long as day lengths remain long, they continue to resemble animals in summer. Moving them to short day lengths characteristic of winter, however, induces numerous winter adaptations normally seen in winter-acclimatized animals.[256,493,1054] Most notably, the gonads involute (figure 16.6). In males, testicular weight decreases, spermatogenesis is arrested, and accessory organ size diminishes as a consequence of reduced androgen levels. Additionally, food intake decreases and body weight and fat stores are reduced (figure 16.6). Although various hormones such as insulin and glucagon are very important to the control of food intake and the maintenance of energy balance (see chapter 15), very little is known about their role in photoperiod-mediated changes in food intake and body weight.

After approximately 15 weeks of exposure to short day lengths in the laboratory, animals begin to return to their summer condition even though they

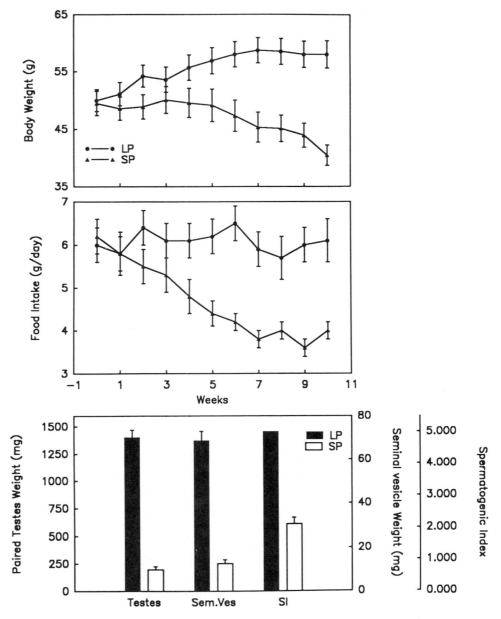

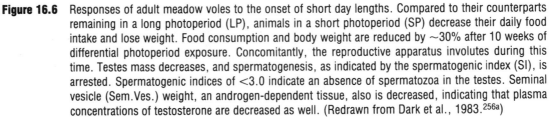

Figure 16.6 Responses of adult meadow voles to the onset of short day lengths. Compared to their counterparts remaining in a long photoperiod (LP), animals in a short photoperiod (SP) decrease their daily food intake and lose weight. Food consumption and body weight are reduced by ~30% after 10 weeks of differential photoperiod exposure. Concomitantly, the reproductive apparatus involutes during this time. Testes mass decreases, and spermatogenesis, as indicated by the spermatogenic index (SI), is arrested. Spermatogenic indices of <3.0 indicate an absence of spermatozoa in the testes. Seminal vesicle (Sem.Ves.) weight, an androgen-dependent tissue, also is decreased, indicating that plasma concentrations of testosterone are decreased as well. (Redrawn from Dark et al., 1983.[256a])

remain in short day lengths. By 26 weeks, this "spontaneous regrowth of the gonads" is complete.[1054,1141] The animals are said to become refractory to the effects of short day length. They remain insensitive to short day lengths until refractoriness is broken by exposure to long day length, which normally occurs during the ensuing summer.

THE SUPRACHIASMATIC NUCLEUS-PINEAL AXIS

How is photoperiodic time measurement mediated? The neuroendocrine pathway that transduces changes in day length into seasonal rhythms in physiology and behavior has received much attention; hormones play an important role in both generation and expression of seasonal rhythms. Photoperiodic time measurement is mediated by the suprachiasmatic nucleus-pineal axis.[1142]

The majority of projections from the retina of the eye terminate in the lateral geniculate nucleus of the thalamus and the superior colliculus as the classic visual pathway, but a significant number of direct retinal fibers project to the hypothalamus. The target of these retinohypothalamic fibers is the suprachiasmatic nucleus (SCN) of the hypothalamus. The SCN is a densely packed cell grouping nestled atop the optic chiasm (figure 16.7). Ablation of the SCN eliminates photoperiodic responsiveness in mammals. Efferent fibers from the SCN terminate in the paraventricular nucleus of the hypothalamus, which in turn projects to the thoracic spinal cord. Fibers from this nucleus proceed to the superior cervical ganglion, and postganglionic fibers innervate the pineal gland (figure 16.7). In most animals the pineal gland is located on the dorsal surface of the brain within a sinus situated between the cerebellum and the caudal aspects of the cerebral hemispheres.

Through this pathway the SCN generates a circadian rhythm in the pineal gland's output of the hormone melatonin and synchronizes this cycle with the light-dark cycle. Melatonin is produced and released solely during the dark phase, and thus duration of the daily melatonin pulse is dependent upon the duration of the dark phase. As a consequence, mammals in long day lengths have a short melatonin pulse, whereas melatonin release is extended in short days. Disruption of this pathway at any point, such as by pinealectomy, interferes with the animal's ability to respond to photoperiod. Pinealectomized Siberian hamsters and voles remain perpetually in reproductive condition even in short day lengths.[493,1142] Similarly, the effects of various photoperiods can be mimicked by manipulating the duration of the melatonin pulse.[414] If pinealectomized male hamsters receive daily infusions of exogenous melatonin of short duration (indicating long day lengths), they remain in summer condition and are reproductively competent. If, on the other hand, the daily melatonin pulse is lengthened beyond a critical value, the testes involute and body weight decreases regardless of the environmental photoperiod.

The eventual insensitivity to short day lengths is the result of the brain's refractoriness to the short-day melatonin signal.[121] Pinealectomized Syrian hamsters given daily melatonin injections simulating short day lengths undergo gonadal regression. Eventually, however, refractoriness to melatonin oc-

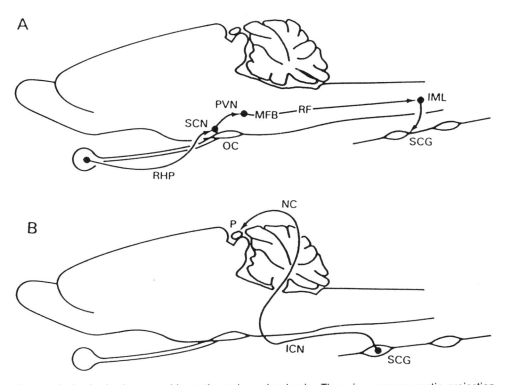

Figure 16.7 Proposed circuits in the suprachiasmatic nucleus-pineal axis. There is a monosynaptic projection from cells in the retina (retina-hypothalamic projection, RHP) to the suprachiasmatic nucleus (SCN). SCN cells project to the paraventricular nucleus (PVN) of the hypothalamus, which in turn then sends efferent fibers via the medial forebrain bundle (MFB) to the spinal cord. This projection terminates on cells of the intermediolateral cell column (IML); processes of these neurons then make synaptic connections in the superior cervical ganglion (SCG) of the sympathetic chain. Postganglionic noradrenergic fibers proceed in the inferior carotid nerve (ICN) and, later, in the nervii coronarii (NC) to innervate the pineal gland (P). (From Klein et al., 1983.[591])

curs, and the gonads redevelop even in the presence of melatonin. The short day melatonin profile remains, but melatonin target tissues have been rendered unresponsive by an endogenous timing mechanism. The specific brain sites upon which melatonin acts to effect photoperiodic responding are not yet clear but include depending upon the species studied, the anterior hypothalamus, the SCN, and the infundibular region of the pituitary.[1142] There is no reason to believe that a single site is crucial; perhaps numerous locations may be capable of mediating responses to melatonin.

THE HYPOTHALAMO-PITUITARY-GONADAL AXIS
The next question is, how does melatonin alter the hypothalamo-pituitary-gonadal axis to effect changes in gonadal activity and reproductive behavior? Again, melatonin alters tissue sensitivity to hormones. As described in earlier chapters, spermatogenesis and ovulation are controlled by gonadotropin levels. In turn, gonadotropin levels are in large part regulated by negative feedback of

gonadal androgen or estrogen. Photoperiod apparently readjusts hypothalamic sensitivity to gonadal steroid feedback. During reproductive quiescence, sensitivity to gonadal steroids is greatly increased; very low concentrations of circulating gonadal hormones are sufficient to all but shut down gonadotropin production. Decreased gonadotropin output results in gonadal inactivity, spermatogenesis and ovulation cease, and steroid output is reduced. During photorefractoriness, the hypothalamus spontaneously returns to its prior feedback sensitivity; existing low concentrations of steroids then are insufficient to inhibit gonadotropin secretion, high levels of gonadotropin result, and reproductive activity resumes.

The reduced concentrations of gonadal steroids in the photoperiod-inhibited hamster are insufficient to maintain normal reproductive behavior. This, however, is not the complete story. Steroid-sensitive target tissues that control reproductive behaviors also are modified by photoperiod. Unlike tissues controlling gonadotropin production, the sensitivity of the neural substrates mediating reproductive behaviors is decreased. As a result, even if gonadal hormones are increased through replacement therapy, normal reproductive behaviors are not restored. Responsiveness of the neural substrates for reproductive behavior to gonadal steroids has been suppressed by the inhibitory photoperiod. This is true for both male[757] and female hamsters.[43]

Photoperiodic species undergo seasonal adaptations in other regulatory systems, but less is known about the mechanism by which photoperiod and melatonin induce these changes. How are changes in food intake and fat deposition effected? Without being cold, why do animals build thicker, warmer nests? How is the heat-generating capacity of brown adipose tissue increased prior to exposure to cold temperatures? We know these changes occur, but how they are effected is not known. It is very likely that hormonal systems will be found to be involved.

PHOTOPERIOD-DELAYED PUBERTY

The discussion of photoperiodic seasonal rhythms up to this point has been concerned with the effects of photoperiod on adult animals. Photoperiodic effects in immature animals are even more striking.[412] Among many small mammals, multiple litters are born during the breeding season. Season of birth has quite pronounced effects on development of young (figure 16.8). Meadow voles have a breeding season lasting from April to September. Voles born in spring or early summer mature rapidly. Within 1 to $1\frac{1}{2}$ months they have reached reproductive maturity and have joined the breeding population in the season of their birth. Voles born in late summer or autumn, on the other hand, do not mature for 6 to 7 months, not until the following spring. This difference in the timing of puberty is mediated by photoperiod and can be mimicked in the laboratory by rearing newborn litters in long versus short day lengths. Short days delay onset of puberty, but the eventual occurrence of puberty is mediated by an endogenous timing mechanism. Voles born in short days under-

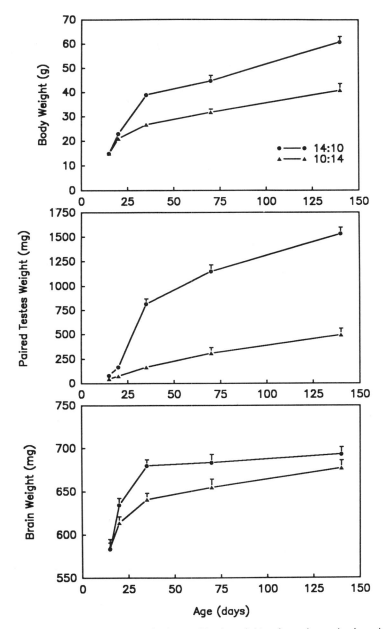

Figure 16.8 Growth curves for body, testicular, and brain weights of meadow voles born into short (10:14) versus long (14:10) photoperiods. Developing in short day lengths markedly retards body growth as well as the maturation of the reproductive system and postnatal myelination of the brain. Thus, puberty of voles born in the fall is delayed until the following spring. At this time, fall-born animals "catch-up" with their spring- or summer-born counterparts. (Adapted from Dark et al., 1990.[254])

go puberty about 6 months later despite being kept in short day lengths. Thus, many of the underlying mechanisms are similar to those in adults.[256,1142]

Reproductive development and fat deposition are not the only functions suppressed in meadow voles born into short photoperiods. Final skeletal growth is arrested until the time of puberty. Additionally, postnatal brain maturation is retarded (figure 16.8). Male voles born into short day lengths possess brains weighing less and containing fewer cells than their counterparts reared in long days.[254] Neurogenesis is essentially complete by birth, but brain myelination is retarded by short day lengths, and those areas of the brain containing the greatest density of myelinated fiber tracts (the midbrain and hindbrain) undergo the greatest weight reductions and decreases in myelin content.[979] Although photoperiod-induced reductions in brain weight are primarily the result of changes in myelination, this does not rule out the possibility of neural effects as well. Neuron size may differ between brains from animals born into long or short days[369]. In some species, there are even changes in neuron number, particularly in areas organized by gonadal steroids, such as the song system of the canary (see chapters 2 and 7).

Circannual Rhythms

Circannual rhythms are expressed by a wide range of mammals, including bats, ferrets, squirrels, marmots, sheep, deer, and nonhuman primates.[1142] The presence of numerous annual rhythms in humans and circannual clocks in nonhuman primates raises the interesting question of whether or not humans have a circannual clock. Although humans probably do possess the capability for expressing true circannual rhythms, it is even more likely that this will never be tested empirically. To do so would require isolating human subjects from all variations in environmental cues, including social ones, for a period of approximately 2 years.

The most intensively studied circannual mammals are ground squirrels and marmots. The hibernating ground squirrel's life history revolves around a strict annual cycle of weight change and reproduction. During the summer, they lay down large quantities of body fat. Body weight reaches a plateau in the fall, and the animals enter their underground burrows, or hibernaculae, where they spend the winter. Most species overwinter without eating by utilizing fat deposited during the summer months and by entering deep torpor. During deep torpor, their body temperature drops to just a few degrees above the ambient temperature of their hibernaculum, generally about 2° to 5°C. Ground squirrels do not remain in deep torpor throughout the entire hibernation season but arouse periodically, generally every 1 to 14 days. There is a final, or terminal, arousal in spring, and animals then resume activity above ground. Upon emergence, ground squirrels are in reproductive condition and soon mate; females bear a single litter each year. The cycle begins anew with the completion of the reproductive phase. All of these annual changes in physiology and behavior persist in the laboratory under constant conditions of temperature, photo-

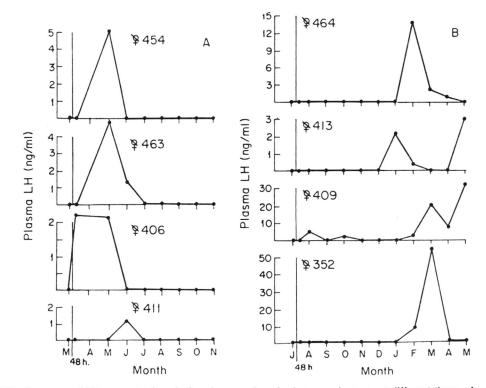

Figure 16.9 Response of LH concentrations in female ground squirrels to ovariectomy at different times of year. When animals are ovariectomized (vertical line) in March (*A*) just prior to the onset of the reproductive season, there is an immediate but temporary elevation of LH concentrations. On the other hand, if ovariectomies are performed in July (*B*) after the end of the reproductive season, there is no postsurgical elevation in plasma LH concentrations. LH levels remain depressed until the following reproductive season (~March). The circannual clock turns off feedback sensitivity to steroid feedback during all seasons of the year except the reproductive season. (From Zucker, 1988.[1138])

period, and food availability (Zucker et al., 1990). Although the various circannual rhythms may be generated by a single circannual oscillator, the expression of circannual reproductive, body fat, and hibernation rhythms will be discussed separately.

REPRODUCTION

Female golden-mantled ground squirrels are in reproductive condition at the time of spring emergence, and mating and fertilization occur within the first few days above ground. During the remainder of the year, the reproductive tract is unstimulated and small. Annual changes in the sensitivity of the hypothalamo-hypophyseal axis to steroid feedback could underlie this cycle, as occurred in type I rhythms, but this does not appear to be the case. Monthly blood samples taken from laboratory-housed intact female squirrels over the course of a year failed to discover measurable levels of LH (figure 16.9), even though the reproductive tract was stimulated in the spring as indicated by vaginal patency.[1138] LH may be elevated only very briefly, and the monthly blood sampling may have missed the transitory elevation of LH. This appears even more likely when data from ovariectomized females are examined. LH levels are elevated in ovariectomized squirrels only during the time of year when intact females are normally in reproductive condition (figure 16.9). At other times of year, LH levels are undetectable. The circannual timing system appears to turn on steroid feedback sensitivity during the reproductive season, and during the remainder of the year the hypothalamo-hypophyseal axis is not at all responsive to steroid feedback. Again, a biological clock alters the dependence of gonadotropin release on steroid hormone feedback.

As described previously, ground squirrels undergo a terminal arousal prior to emergence and mating. In female squirrels, terminal arousal is facultative, or flexible. The frequency of female arousals increases as the time for emergence approaches, but terminal arousal does not occur until the burrow entrance is free of snow and food is available above ground.[378] Although final arousal and subsequent mating occur when above ground food is available, female ground squirrels possess their lowest level of fat reserves at this time.[255,569] This is unlike other mammalian species, in which ovulation and conception are very dependent upon adequate fat reserves[158] (see discussion above).

The male's circannual reproductive rhythm is very different from that of females. Monthly blood sampling of intact, laboratory-housed male squirrels reveals a marked annual cycle in plasma LH titers that closely corresponds to the annual testosterone cycle.[1138] LH is undetectable most of the year except during the reproductive phase of the annual cycle, when it reaches maximal levels. Unlike females, orchidectomy during the nonreproductive period results in elevated levels of LH; LH rises after removal of gonadal steroids and remains elevated throughout the year.[1138] Male ground squirrels resemble species with type I rhythms in that reproductive quiescence depends upon an increased sensitivity to steroid feedback, and thus males are dissimilar to females of their own species, in whom reproductive quiescence is independent of steroid feedback.

The reproductive pattern of male ground squirrels differs from females in other ways as well. Females reproduce at emergence from their first hibernation phase (1 year of age); males do not become reproductively active until emergence from their second hibernation phase (2 years of age). Puberty is delayed an entire year in juvenile males. Females are facultative terminators of hibernation; males are facultative their first year, but in subsequent years they undergo an obligatory terminal arousal from hibernation. That is, they cease hibernating at a specific time of year, possibly dictated by the circannual oscillator, whether the burrow entrance is free of snow and food is available or not. Males cannot undergo testicular development and spermatogenesis at the low body temperatures of deep torpor (see later discussion); therefore, to be reproductively functional at the first appearance of receptive females, they must arouse from hibernation and remain warm prior to emergence. Early arousal is necessarily dependent upon the availability of significant energy reserves, so,

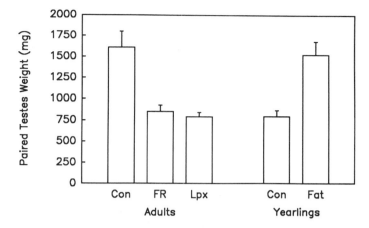

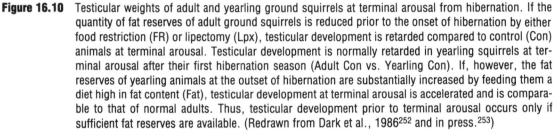

Figure 16.10 Testicular weights of adult and yearling ground squirrels at terminal arousal from hibernation. If the quantity of fat reserves of adult ground squirrels is reduced prior to the onset of hibernation by either food restriction (FR) or lipectomy (Lpx), testicular development is retarded compared to control (Con) animals at terminal arousal. Testicular development is normally retarded in yearling squirrels at terminal arousal after their first hibernation season (Adult Con vs. Yearling Con). If, however, the fat reserves of yearling animals at the outset of hibernation are substantially increased by feeding them a diet high in fat content (Fat), testicular development at terminal arousal is accelerated and is comparable to that of normal adults. Thus, testicular development prior to terminal arousal occurs only if sufficient fat reserves are available. (Redrawn from Dark et al., 1986[252] and in press.[253])

unlike females, reproductive development in males is very dependent upon body fat reserves. Indeed, if adult males are put on a diet to reduce fat stores or if body fat is surgically removed prior to the onset of hibernation, testicular development is suppressed in the spring[252] (figure 16.10). Ground squirrels become fatter at the end of their second summer than at the end of their first,[255] which may explain why juvenile squirrels do not become reproductively active their first year; they have inadequate fat reserves to undergo an obligatory early terminal arousal. If, however, body fat reserves are increased by means of a high-fat diet eaten prior to hibernation, juvenile squirrels spontaneously terminate hibernation in spring, and reproductive development is accelerated[253] (figure 16.10).

To summarize, there is a circannual cycle of gonadal steroid production in ground squirrels that underlies a corresponding cycle of reproductive behavior. This cycle is generated by altering gonadotropin production. In males, the circannual mechanism changes the sensitivity of the hypothalamo-hypophyseal axis to gonadal steroid feedback. In females, however, the circannual mechanism switches feedback sensitivity on and off. Additionally, this system is influenced by fat reserves in male squirrels but not in females.

FAT RESERVES
During the summer weight gain phase of the circannual cycle, ground squirrels increase fat stores[255] (figure 16.11). Appetite and food intake increase correspondingly, but these are secondary to changes in fat deposition. If ground

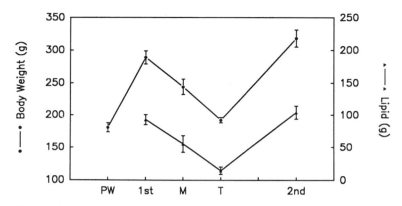

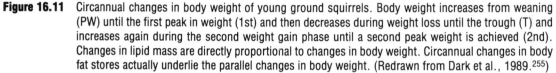

Figure 16.11 Circannual changes in body weight of young ground squirrels. Body weight increases from weaning (PW) until the first peak in weight (1st) and then decreases during weight loss until the trough (T) and increases again during the second weight gain phase until a second peak weight is achieved (2nd). Changes in lipid mass are directly proportional to changes in body weight. Circannual changes in body fat stores actually underlie the parallel changes in body weight. (Redrawn from Dark et al., 1989.[255])

squirrels are prevented from increasing their food intake during the weight gain phase by provision of a daily food ration comparable to their intake at the end of the loss phase, they still undergo weight gain and increased fat deposition.[252] Similarly, if they are food restricted during the weight gain phase so that no weight gain occurs, a persistent increase in fat stores occurs at the expense of other body components.[347] Thus, there are circannual changes in fat deposition and mobilization that in turn produce circannual rhythms in eating behavior.

Insulin is the primary regulator of fat deposition (see chapter 15), and changes in insulin levels have been measured during the circannual cycle of the marmot (Marmota flaviventris). There is a circannual rhythm of plasma insulin corresponding to annual changes in body fat (figure 16.11). Basal levels of insulin are increased threefold during the weight gain phase, but more importantly, glucose-stimulated insulin release is increased sixfold.[364] Thus, pancreatic β-cell glucose sensitivity varies on a circannual basis. In addition to circannual insulin release, there are circannual changes in fat cell sensitivity to insulin as well. In vitro insulin sensitivity of fat cells obtained during weight gain is elevated. Insulin sensitivity of fat cells is decreased during the weight loss phase.[364] How the circannual system effects changes in fat cell sensitivity is not known.

Weight loss during hibernation proceeds at a programmed pace. We know little about circannual regulation of fat mobilization and how it alters eating behavior. In addition to decreased insulin sensitivity and reduced plasma insulin titers during weight loss, fat cell sensitivity to the sympathetic nervous system neurotransmitter norepinephrine is also altered. Although various hormones (glucagon, epinephrine, and growth hormone) can promote lipolysis, sympathetic innervation of adipose tissue is the primary regulator of energy mobilization from fat. In vitro norepinephrine-stimulated lipolysis in adipose tissue taken during weight gain is reduced compared to adipose tissue taken from animals in weight loss.[364] Again, how circannual changes in sensitivity to norepinephrine are brought about remains unknown.

HIBERNATION

Hibernation is restricted to the weight loss phase of the circannual cycle. During weight gain, squirrels will not enter hibernation even if kept in the cold and deprived of food. Gonadotropin and gonadal steroid levels are low through most of the hibernation season in both male and female ground squirrels. In adult males, gonadotropin levels rise toward the end of the hibernation season, but testicular tissues are insensitive to the stimulating effects of gonadotropins at the low body temperatures ($\sim 2°$ to $5°C$) characteristic of deep torpor. Testes must be at least $\sim 20°C$ before gonadotropins are effective; as a result, testicular development and steroid production during the hibernation phase are restricted to the periods of spontaneous arousal when the animals are normothermic.[58]

Thus, in adult male ground squirrels, there is testicular development prior to terminal arousal. The presence of testosterone has been determined to prevent hibernation in several species that exhibit type I rhythms (e.g., Turkish hamsters[413]). Similarly, testosterone is also incompatible with the ability to enter deep torpor in most ground squirrels.[616] Terminal arousal may in part be due to increased plasma titers of testosterone. As the end of the hibernation season approaches, gonadotropin levels begin to increase. There is greater and greater testicular development during successive spontaneous arousals. Eventually, steroid production is sufficient during an arousal to prevent the animal from re-entering torpor. Elevated testosterone levels may play a role in the normal occurrence of terminal arousal, but terminal arousal is also controlled independently of gonadal steroids by the circannual mechanism. Hibernating males of several circannual species undergo a terminal arousal even if castrated.

WHERE IS THE CIRCANNUAL CLOCK?

At this point in time, we do not know the neural substrate for circannual rhythms. We do know that the suprachiasmatic-pineal axis, which is necessary for the generation of type I cycles, is not necessary for the generation of circannual (type II) cycles.[1142] Neither suprachiasmatic nuclear nor paraventricular nuclear lesions are sufficient to prevent expression of circannual rhythms. Additionally, circannual rhythms persist after pinealectomy. Although these structures do not prevent the generation of circannual rhythms, this pathway mediates their entrainment to annual changes in photoperiod. In the field, ground squirrels see a naturally changing photoperiod from approximately April to October; they are in constant darkness in their underground hibernaculae during the remainder of the year. A laboratory lighting regimen that imitates these annual changes in photoperiod also entrains the circannual rhythms of ground squirrels.[1142] Entrainment is disrupted, however, by suprachiasmatic nuclear lesions. Whether the suprachiasmatic nucleus mediates

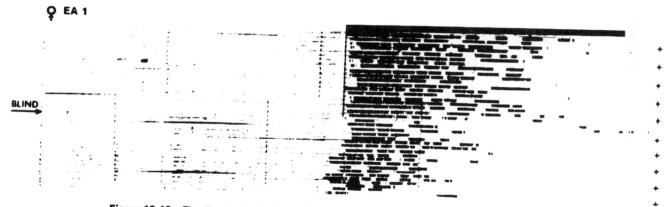

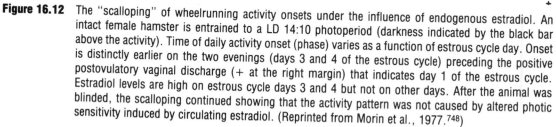

Figure 16.12 The "scalloping" of wheelrunning activity onsets under the influence of endogenous estradiol. An intact female hamster is entrained to a LD 14:10 photoperiod (darkness indicated by the black bar above the activity). Time of daily activity onset (phase) varies as a function of estrous cycle day. Onset is distinctly earlier on the two evenings (days 3 and 4 of the estrous cycle) preceding the positive postovulatory vaginal discharge (+ at the right margin) that indicates day 1 of the estrous cycle. Estradiol levels are high on estrous cycle days 3 and 4 but not on other days. After the animal was blinded, the scalloping continued showing that the activity pattern was not caused by altered photic sensitivity induced by circulating estradiol. (Reprinted from Morin et al., 1977.[748])

entrainment directly through neural connections or hormonally through the pineal gland is unknown; pineal involvement in entrainment has not been evaluated.

Hormones and the Control of Clock Frequency

Curt Richter was one of the pioneers in the field of biological rhythms. The goal of many of Richter's rhythm experiments was to find the site of the circadian clock. In pursuit of this goal, Richter ablated many areas of the brain and removed most of the endocrine organs. Although he never did definitely identify the suprachiasmatic nucleus of the hypothalamus as the site of the circadian clock, he came close.[851] Stephan and Zucker[986] and Moore and Eichler[744] published papers in 1972 identifying the SCN as the probable site of the clock.

Richter was looking for big effects, the loss of rhythmicity, in particular. With all of the brain and endocrine manipulations he made, the circadian locomotor rhythm remained essentially unperturbed and stable. The major exception to this was the observation that deuterium oxide (heavy water) could lengthen the circadian period. Richter, however, missed something in his own data (see figures II.9 and II.21 in Richter[851]) concerning the effect of estradiol on the timing of the circadian locomotor rhythm. Morin and colleagues[755] observed "scalloping" in the onset of daily locomotor activity of female hamsters across the estrous cycle. Scalloping is derived from the fact that on days of the estrous cycle during which estradiol is high, the animal starts its nocturnal activity phase earlier (figure 16.12). Further experimentation demonstrated that estradiol has a direct effect on the circadian clock. When estradiol is given to ovariectomized hamsters, the period of the locomotor rhythm shortens. Similar effects have been observed in rats.[11] Collectively, these results demonstrate that (1) endogenous substances have access to the circadian clock; (2) the circadian clock can be altered by the internal environment; and (3) there is hope for discovery of pharmacological or external environmental probes that will enable us to manipulate the clock. This would greatly facilitate the study of the clock and its circuitry. Indeed, this goal has become a major current thrust of biological rhythm research.

Other steroid hormones besides estradiol have been shown to alter the circadian period. These include progesterone, which lengthens the period in hamsters.[1020] Progesterone may act by antagonizing the actions of estradiol.[748] In hamsters, the response to estradiol is sexually differentiated.[1141] Males (or neonatally masculinized females) do not show a change in rhythm period with estradiol stimulation. The sexual differentiation process may affect a closely linked input pathway that can modulate clock frequency, or the circadian clock itself may be sexually dimorphic.

An essential feature of this work on circadian rhythms relates to the control of ovulation by circadian clock processes. A circadian rhythm is necessary for the timing of the gonadotropin surge that stimulates ovulation. The gonadotropin surge is not expressed in male hamsters or rats. In essence, the process of sexual differentiation has disconnected the circadian clock from hypothalamic control of gonadotropins. Thus, sexual differentiation in the hamster does two things: First, it prevents estradiol from altering clock frequency, and second, it prevents estradiol from eliciting an ovulatory gonadotropin surge. A parsimonious interpretation of these facts would be that the two events are functionally related. Because the gonadotropin surge depends on the circadian clock and on elevated levels of estradiol, it is reasonable to believe that masculinizing neonatal androgen interferes with the mechanism by which estradiol alters clock expression. Failure to ovulate would be a necessary consequence. Although the clock may not be affected by neonatal androgen, there are some suggestions that sex differences do affect circadian clock expression.[264,754]

Insight into the functional importance of steroid hormones altering circadian clock function has been gained. Experiments have evaluated the consequences of estradiol action on phasic release of LH. The effect of estradiol on phasic release of LH has been shown in intact and ovariectomized animals. After 3 weeks of exposure to short day lengths, ovariectomized hamsters show a daily LH surge occurring 1 hour after onset of darkness.[733] In contrast, intact animals still showing estrous cycles have a peak LH release 3 hours earlier. By 8 weeks, both ovariectomized animals and those with photoperiod-induced atrophic ovaries have a daily release of LH about 1 hour after the lights are turned off. The advanced phase of the LH surge at 3 weeks is most likely the consequence of persistent estradiol release from the still functioning ovary; estrous cycles do not cease until after 5 to 7 weeks of exposure to short photoperiods. Exogenous estradiol given to ovariectomized hamsters in short day lengths advances peak LH release by about 2 hours. These results support the observation that estradiol can alter circadian clock function to shorten the rhythm period and advance the phase of LH release.

Modulation of circadian clock frequency by other hormones has been suggested from studies of hypophysectomized animals and from animals that have had thyroid gland manipulations. Both male and female hamsters show marked lengthening of the circadian period if they are hypophysectomized. The specific endocrine cause of this phenomenon is unknown.[1141] However, it is unlikely to relate to the presence or absence of sex steroids because the rhythm period of males is unaffected by gonadal status.[753,1141] A more likely hormonal source of the altered rhythmicity in both sexes is the thyroid. Combined thyroidectomy and thyroid metabolic suppression by thiourea lengthen the circadian period. The circadian period of both male and female hamsters is lengthened by administration of the potent thyroid hormone blocking agent propylthiouracil.[756] It now appears more likely that propylthiouracil itself induces the rhythm changes than does the reduction of available thyroid hormones.[752] Although surgical thyroidectomy causes a decrease in the circadian period, this effect cannot rightfully be attributed to the thyroid until reversal of the extirpation effects are observed after hormone replacement. Such studies have not yet been completed.

Summary and Conclusions

From the examples given in this chapter, you should now have an appreciation of the importance of biological rhythms to the physiology and behavior of organisms. Other chapters have described the many ways in which hormones alter behavior. This chapter differs from the others in that it describes mechanisms that control the interaction between hormones and behavior.

Endogenous clocks control the timing of hormone release as well as rhythmically altering target tissue sensitivity to hormones. Thus, they provide appropriate temporal coordination between internal events—for example, the timing of estradiol and LH release, or the temporal coordination of receptive behavior and ovulatory events necessary for fertilization. Also, rhythmic control of endocrine events allows predictive changes to be made in advance of changes in the external world. Secretion of many hormones increases in the morning before you wake up, anticipating your onset of activity. Photoperiod-induced changes in pineal melatonin allow endocrine-mediated winter adaptations to be initiated prior to the actual onset of cold weather. In summary, biological rhythms temporally organize the substrates underlying behavioral endocrinology.

Glossary

A priori   Before the fact. Here, the prediction or construction of hypotheses before the conduct of the experiment. Contrast with a posteriori (post hoc, after the fact), or the construction of a hypothesis after the experiment is completed.

Accessory sex structures   Tissues and organs that are part of the reproductive tract and important in the transport of gametes. In males these consist of the epididymis, vas deferens, prostate, seminal vesicles, and, in reptiles, the renal sex segment. In females these consist of the uterus and fallopian tubes.

Action potential   An all-or-none change in the membrane potential of an axon that results in synaptic transmission for communication between neurons.

Activational effects of hormones   Transient actions of hormones, usually in adulthood. Activational effects may be defined by the occurrence of a given behavioral response only in the presence of a given hormone.

Active space   Here, the distance one electric fish can be from another and still have its electric organ discharges detected.

Adenohypophysis   Anterior pituitary.

Adrenal gland   Located just above the kidneys. Among the hormones secreted are epinephrine (=adrenaline) from the medulla, and glucocorticoids from the cortex.

Adrenalectomy   Surgical removal of the adrenal glands.

Adrenaline   See Epinephrine.

Adrenocorticotropic hormone (ACTH)   Hormone released by the pituitary that stimulates the adrenal to secrete corticosteroids.

Age-limited song learning   Song learning that is confined to the first year of life; a characteristic of certain song birds such as zebra finches.

Aggression   Behavioral sequences that could result in one animal injuring or killing another animal. In humans, the behavior must be accompanied by the intent to do harm.

Agonist   A substance that binds to receptors, mimicking the effects of the natural hormone or neurotransmitter.

α-Fetoprotein (AFP)   A protein found in plasma that, in rodents, can bind to estrogens but not androgens.

α-Flupenthixol   A dopamine receptor antagonist.

Alternative life-history strategies   The presence, in the same sex of a species, of different phenotypes and different behavioral characteristics; these traits may be either inherited or environmentally induced.

Altricial Refers to young birds or mammals born in an immature condition, with poorly developed vision, learning, and locomotion, and dependent upon the parent for nutrition.

Amnesia Partial or total loss of memory. See also anterograde and retrograde amnesia.

Amphetamine Drug that acts by stimulating catecholamine release and blocking catecholamine reuptake into synaptic terminals.

Amphibian and basilar papillae The auditory organs of frogs; the hair cells are located within these structures.

Amygdala Brain structure (nucleus). Portion of the limbic system located in the anterior forebrain and involved in the control of aggressive and sexual behaviors. Receives input from the vomeronasal system among others.

Anabolism A term in physiology referring to the building up of the body. Contrast with catabolism.

Androgen A class of steroid hormones secreted primarily from the testes, including testosterone, dihydrotestosterone, and androstenedione.

Angiogenesis The growth of new capillaries. This is a process that occurs often when tumors begin to grow; such tumors release "angiogenesis factors" that stimulate capillary ingrowth to the tumor as a means of supplying blood.

Annual rhythms (type I) Annual rhythms that are dependent to some degree upon the environment for their expression; Type I rhythms do not persist in constant environmental condition.

Annual rhythms (type II) Annual rhythms that are generated independently of the environment by an endogenous clock but rely upon the environment for entrainment to a period of 365 days; Type II rhythms freerun in constant environment conditions.

Anorexia Loss of appetite.

Antagonists Substances that bind to receptors and thereby block the natural hormones or neurotransmitters from acting at the receptor.

Anterograde amnesia Inability to form new memories.

Anurans Frogs and toads.

Aphasia An impairment in the production and comprehension of speech or written language following brain damage.

Apomorphine A dopamine receptor agonist.

Apraxia An impairment in the production of manual or oral movements following brain damage, which may reflect an underlying motor programming disorder; occurs in the absence of paralysis or paresis.

Aromatase An enzyme that catalyzes the conversion of testosterone into estradiol.

Assay A method for determining the quantity of a substance present in a sample.

Associated reproductive pattern Close temporal relationship between the maturation of the gametes, increase in circulating concentrations of sex hormones, and the display of mating behaviors.

Ataxia Loss or lack of motor coordination.

Attractivity The value of a given individual as a stimulus capable of eliciting sexual responses from another individual.

Axon A single, small extension of a neuron that (usually) branches many times and serves to transmit information from that neuron to target cells through propagation of action potentials. Bundles of axons form nerves.

Bag cells Two clusters of about 400 neurons each that are located on the anterior connectives of the abdominal ganglion in the sea slug, *Aplysia*. The cells in a cluster are electrically coupled and secrete egg-laying hormone and associated peptides.

Basal ganglia Functional group of brain nuclei, consisting of the caudate nucleus, putamen, and the globus pallidus.

Behavioral facilitation of reproduction The stimulation of reproductive processes in one sex by the behavior of a member of the other sex.

Bioassay An assay that uses a biological response to detect the presence and quantity of a substance in a sample.

Biogenic amines Small aromatic amines that include epinephrine, norepinephrine, dopamine, octopamine, and serotonin. They may act locally as neurotransmitters or neuromodulators or systemically as neurohormones.

Biphasic effects of progesterone The ability of progesterone to at first facilitate and later inhibit sexual behavior in female vertebrates.

Blood–brain barrier A cellular barrier consisting of brain blood vessels and surrounding glial cells that prevent free passage of components of the blood into the brain.

Bradykinesia A neurological symptom characterized by a reduction of the speed of movements.

Brain nucleus Aggregation of neuron cell bodies within the central nervous system (pl. brain nuclei).

Bruce effect The blocking of pregnancy in a female rodent by the odor of a strange male.

Bunning's hypothesis That seasonality is the consequence of an interaction between an endogenous clock timing daily rhythms and the circadian time of day at which an animal is stimulated by light. The circadian clock regulates a "sensitive" phase during which light stimulates reproductive maturity.

Cannula Small-diameter tube used to deliver drug or hormone to a specific site, usually the brain (pl. cannulae).

Castration Removal of gonads, usually referring to testes.

Catabolism A term in physiology referring to the breaking down of the body. Contrast with anabolism.

Catecholamines Collective term for the neurotransmitters epinephrine (= adrenaline), norepinephrine (= noradrenaline), and dopamine.

Caudate nucleus Brain structure (nucleus), which, together with the putamen and globus pallidus, forms the basal ganglia.

Central gray Area in the midbrain important for lordosis behavior in the female rat.

Central pattern generator A functional group of central neurons that produces a sequence of temporally and spatially coordinated motor activity. The patterned activity can occur in the absence of sensory feedback and provides the basis for many rhythmic behaviors.

Cerebellum Portion of the brain involved in the control of balance and coordinated movement.

Cerebral lateralization Specialization of one or the other cerebral hemisphere for a particular function.

Chemoreceptor Receptor cells that detect changes in the chemical environment. This can refer to either the external environment, such as chemoreceptors in the vomeronasal organ detecting pheromones, or the internal environment, such as chemoreceptors in the hypothalamus that respond to a decrease in glucose utilization.

Chirps Electrical signals used in male courtship in the glass knife gymnotid fish *Eigenmania virescens.*

Chorea graviderum A rare complication of pregnancy in which the woman spontaneously exhibits rapid, dance-like contorted movements.

Chorea Refers to rapid, dance-like, movements of the limbs or facial features and resulting from neurological disorder.

Chromosome Long, filament-like structure found in cell nuclei, consisting of twisted coils of DNA.

Circadian clock Mechanism(s) generating a master circadian rhythm; located in the suprachiasmatic nucleus in mammals.

Circadian rhythm An endogenous, self-sustained oscillation having a freerunning period of approximately 24 hours.

Circadian time 12 Arbitrary designation of the time (phase) of locomotor activity onset of a freerunning, nocturnal animal. The time is relative to a circadian "day" consisting of 24 circadian hours, each of which may be longer or shorter than 60 minutes depending upon whether the freerunning "day" is longer or shorter than 24 hours.

Circannual rhythm A rhythm generated by a self-sustained, endogenous clock having a period approximating 365 days.

Coincidence hypothesis An hypothesis concerning the regulation of a seasonal event in which occurrence of the event depends upon the "coincidence" (simultaneous occurrence) of specific elements or phases of two or more rhythms, e.g., Bunning's hypothesis.

Complement Here, a series of bloodborne proteins produced by the immune system that can be triggered to attack and destroy bacteria or other cells.

Complementarity The combination of parts required for completion. Here the requirement of stimulus and response, signal and receiver, hormone and receptor, mounting and receptivity.

Congenital adrenal hyperplasia (CAH) An inherited adrenal enzyme deficiency that results in overproduction of androgens, beginning in the prenatal period and continuing until controlled with appropriate medications.

Congenital Present at birth; contrast with hereditary.

Conspecific Member of the same species.

Constraints Here, factors that restrict or limit the development of new adaptations.

Copulation The act of individuals exchanging gametes.

Corpora allata Endocrine glands, situated behind the brain of insects, which secrete juvenile hormone.

Corpus callosum Brain structure (fiber pathway). Fiber pathway connecting the two cerebral hemispheres.

Cortex An external layer, as in the brain or adrenal gland.

Corticosteroid binding globulin A protein that binds and transports most glucocorticoids in the bloodstream. Because of the hydrophobic nature of steroid molecules, such protein transporters act to keep the steroids in solution in the circulation.

Corticotropin-releasing factor (CRF) Hormone released by the hypothalamus that stimulates the pituitary to secrete adrenocorticotropic hormone (ACTH).

Cortisol The primary adrenal steroid hormone in primates.

Courtship Actions of a member of one sex that induce a member of the opposite sex to mate with the individual performing the behavior.

Crystallized song The final stage in song development in which birds produce songs with a well-defined structure and a stereotyped manner in successive renditions.

Cytoplasm Interior of cell body surrounding and separate from the nucleus.

Dead zone The portion of a phase response curve to light in which a light pulse will not induce either rhythm phase delays or advances. The dead zone is equivalent to the "subjective day."

Dendrite Branch-like extensions of a neuron that receive information from (usually) many cells.

Dentate gyrus Brain structure (nucleus). Region of the hippocampus.

Deoxyribonucleic acid (DNA) The chemical repository of genetic information. The sequence of nucleotides in DNA specifies a specific sequence of nucleotides in RNA for the production of a protein.

Diabetes insipidus A disorder caused by the absence (or ineffectiveness) of vasopressin, and consequent loss of its antidiuretic actions in the kidneys. The disorder is characterized by excessive excretion of water in urine and compensatory large increases in water intake.

Diabetes mellitus A disorder caused by the absence (or relative ineffectiveness) of insulin, and consequent loss of its actions in the storage of ingested calories as glycogen in the liver and triglycerides in adipose tissue. The disorder is characterized by elevated levels of blood glucose (hyperglycemia) and the appearance of glucose in urine (glycosuria).

Dichotic listening A type of perceptual test in which different auditory stimuli are presented simultaneously to the two ears.

Dihydrotestosterone (DHT) Metabolite of testosterone formed from testosterone by the action of the 5α-reductase enzyme. DHT has androgenic effects on the brain, accessory sex structures, and peripheral secondary sex characteristics.

Diethylstilbestrol (DES) A synthetic estrogen agonist. DES was formerly administered clinically to prevent miscarriage, which may have had masculinizing or defeminizing effects on the brain of female children born to these mothers.

Dioecious The characteristic of having two structurally distinct sexes (= gonochorism). The opposite of monoecious.

Dissociated reproductive pattern Maturation of gametes and the display of mating behaviors occurring at different times of the year.

DNA fingerprinting A method for describing individual differences in patterns of DNA.

Dopamine A neurotransmitter, member of the catecholamine family.

Dyadic Involving two individuals.

Dynorphin An opioid compound produced by the brain.

Ecdysis The event in arthropods of shedding the old exoskeleton at the end of each molt.

Ecdysteroids A family of steroid hormones that trigger molting in insects.

Eclosion The term applied to the final ecdysis to the adult stage in insects that undergo complete metamorphosis.

Eclosion hormone A 62-amino acid neuropeptide found in insects. Its principal target is the CNS, on which it acts to trigger the ecdysis behavior programs.

Egg-laying hormone A 36-amino acid neuropeptide first found in the sea slug, *Aplysia californica.* It triggers the stereotyped sequence of behaviors seen during egg-laying.

Ejaculation   The pulsatile expulsion of semen during copulation.

Electric organ discharge (EOD)   A general name for the electrical signals made by mormyrid and gymnotid fish.

Electrocytes   Modified muscle cells of some fish that are capable of producing electrical discharges.

Electroreceptors   Modified hair cells that can respond to electrical signals. In some fish species electroreceptor organs are called knollenorgen because they look like knobs ("knolle" in German).

Endocrinology   The study of endocrine glands, their functions, and their products; in particular, the release of hormones in response to hormonal, neural, and other signals.

Endogenous   Originating from within. Here, referring to hormones or neurotransmitters actually produced by an individual itself. Opposite of exogenous.

Endogenous clock   Any of a variety of possible mechanisms in an organism that may generate a self-sustained rhythm, regardless of period length.

Endorphin   A 31-amino acid protein that serves as an endogenous morphine or opioid by acting as a neurotransmitter in the brain and a hormone in the pituitary and gut.

Enkephalin   A 5-amino acid peptide neurotransmitter with opioid properties.

Entrainment   The process by which a rhythm is synchronized to a periodic time-giving stimulus or Zeitgeber.

Epigamic or intersexual selection   The evolutionary result of organisms choosing a mate nonrandomly from many different available individuals. In many species, epigamic selection has led to the evolution of male courtship signals, and females choose among many potential mates on the basis of these traits.

Epinephrine   Hormone released by adrenal medulla, critical for adapting to stress. Along with the related hormone norepinephrine, these hormones are known as catecholamines, and their secretion is under the regulation of the sympathetic nervous system (= adrenaline).

Estrogen   A class of steroid hormones secreted primarily from the ovaries, including estradiol, estrone, and estriol.

Estrous cycle   Cyclic events associated with the maturation of ovarian follicles and characterized by a distinct period of female sexual receptivity (estrus). Estrus is usually coordinated with ovulation, either through patterns of ovarian hormone secretion or through induced ovulation.

Estrus   The period of sexual receptivity in females.

Eukaryotic   Cells that have a distinct nucleus containing genetic information.

Exocytosis   Process by which internal vesicles first fuse with external membrane of a cell and then open to release chemicals outside the cell or into the intercellular space.

Exogenous   Originating from outside. Here, referring to hormones introduced by an experimenter into an individual.

External fertilization   Eggs fertilized by sperm after being released into the environment.

Extrapyramidal motor system   Brain areas involved in the control of movement that are not part of the pyramidal system. This includes the basal ganglia and cerebellum.

Facultative   The occurrence of a response that is flexible and contingent upon suitable environmental conditions; e.g., female ground squirrels terminate hibernation facultatively when food becomes available above ground. Does not imply causation.

Fallopian tube   Structure through which the ovum travels to reach the uterus, where in mammals fertilization usually occurs.

Fat deposition   The storage of excess metabolic fuel as triglyceride in adipose tissue; opposite of fat mobilization.

Fat mobilization   The release of stored metabolic energy from adipose tissue as glycerol and fatty acids; opposite of fat deposition.

Feedback   Here, the nature of control over a physiological system. Negative feedback involves maintenance of a steady state or homeostasis as occurs in the regulation of body temperature. Positive feedback refers to the movement away from a set point as occurs in ovulation or spermiation.

Fistula   An opening that allows material to flow from one passage to another. An abnormal condition, usually the result of congenital defect or surgery.

Follicle   Ovarian compartment housing an individual ovum. In the process of development and maturation the follicle produces the hormonal changes necessary for ovulation and sexual behavior.

Follicle-stimulating hormone (FSH)   A glycoprotein hormone released by the pituitary. FSH stimulates follicular development in the ovary and sperm formation in the testis and is therefore referred to as a gonadotropin.

Follicular development   Process by which a follicle evolves from a primordial state through growth, ovulation, and subsequent change into a corpus luteum.

Freerunning   A rhythm that is not entrained by (synchronized to) a time-giving stimulus (Zeitgeber).

Frequency   Number of rhythm cycles per unit time, e.g., a circadian rhythm with a freerunning period of $24\frac{1}{2}$ hours has a frequency of 1.02 cycles/day.

Gamete   Specialized cells for contributing genetic material from parents for sexual reproduction, i.e., sperm or eggs.

Gametogenesis   Egg or sperm production by the gonad.

Ganglion (invertebrate)   A discrete collection of neurons that may make up part of the CNS or may be found in the periphery.

Gender identity   The sex role a person assumes in private thoughts.

Gender role   The sex role a person assumes in social interactions.

Gene   A particular stretch of DNA that codes for a specific string of RNA nucleotides that code for a particular protein. Such a protein may be cleaved into several different active proteins.

Genotype   The sum of all the genetic information possessed by an individual. See phenotype.

Gestation   The period from fertilization of the ovum until delivery of the young in viviparous animals.

Globus pallidus   Brain structure (nucleus). Together with the putamen and the caudate nucleus it forms the basal ganglia.

Glucagon   A pancreatic hormone released during stress that contributes to the mobilization of energy from storage sites during stress.

Glucocorticoids   Steroid hormones secreted by the adrenal gland that are critical to adapting to stress. The primary glucocorticoid in primates and humans is cortisol, whereas in other animals it is corticosterone.

Gluconeogenesis   The ability of the liver to generate "new" glucose, typically by conversion of amino acids to sugars. The process is stimulated by glucocorticoids and catecholamines and is part of the metabolic stress-response.

Glucoprivation   A decrease in the metabolic utilization of glucose in cells.

Gonad   Organ that produces gametes (i.e., ovary and testis).

Gonadectomy   Removal of the gonads; i.e., ovariectomy or castration (= orchidectomy).

Gonadotropin-releasing hormone (GnRH)   A peptide produced in the hypothalamus that modulates secretion of pituitary hormones (= LHRH).

GnRH pulse generator   A mechanism in the brain, presumably the hypothalamus, that generates an ultradian clock-like output controlling the pulsatile release of GnRH (gonadotropin-releasing hormone).

Gonadotropins   Pituitary hormones that stimulate the gonad, i.e., the glycoprotein hormones luteinizing hormone (LH) and follicle-stimulating hormone (FSH).

Gonochorism   The species characteristic of having separate sexes in separate individuals (= dioecious).

Gravid   Full of ripe ova or, in egg-laying animals, shelled eggs.

Growth hormone (GH)   A pituitary hormone whose actions promote normal growth in developing organisms, tissue repair, and energy metabolism in adults. See also Somatomedin and Somatostatin.

Hair cell   A sensory receptor found in the vestibular (balance) organ, the ear, and, in modified form, in the lateral line system and electroreceptor organs of aquatic organisms.

Haloperidol   A dopamine receptor antagonist; a neuroleptic drug used in the treatment of schizophrenia.

Heritable   The relative amount of variance in a trait that is due to genetic factors and therefore can be passed on to the offspring.

Hermaphrodite   The species characteristic whereby individuals possess both male and female reproductive structures. This can occur either simultaneously or sequentially at different stages of the life cycle.

Heterogametic   Property of having different sex chromosomes; e.g., XY or ZW.

Hibernaculum   The underground burrow or den in which hibernating animals spend the winter.

Hierarchical control of rhythms   The concept that a master clock acts as a pacemaker generating a primary output rhythm. This primary rhythm then generates one or more secondary rhythms that can, in turn, generate tertiary rhythms, and so forth.

Hippocampus   An area of the brain involved in learning and memory.

Homeokinesis   The concept of dynamic regulation (regulation of change), as opposed to static regulation (regulation around a constant set-point).

Homeostasis   The coordinated physiological and behavioral mechanisms by which animals maintain a relatively constant internal state despite living in an environment that fluctuates widely. Among the many variables that are homeostatically regulated are body temperature, blood glucose, blood pressure, and extracellular fluid osmolality.

Homogametic   Property of having similar sex chromosomes, e.g., XX or ZZ.

Hormone   A chemical, released from cells, that travels to and affects other cells.

Hormone replacement therapy   Administration of exogenous hormones to supplement deficient levels of endogenous hormones, such as estrogen therapy in postmenopausal women.

Hormone-sensitive genes   Genes whose expression is regulated by hormones, often by binding of the activated hormone receptor complex to a particular DNA sequence in the gene's regulatory region.

Huntington's disease   Hereditary disease of the basal ganglia characterized by progressive cell loss in the striatum and other brain regions, chorea, and progressive dementia.

Hybrid   The offspring of parents of different species.

6-Hydroxydopamine (6-OHDA)   A substance that is selectively toxic to catecholamine neurons.

Hyperprolactinemia   Increased or excessive release of prolactin.

Hypogonadism   Lack of gonads or gonadal secretions.

Hypoglycemia   Low blood sugar.

Hypophysectomy   Removal of the pituitary gland.

Hypophysis   The pituitary.

Hypothalamus   Brain structure (group of nuclei). A neural center, at the base of the diencephalic region of the brain, involved in the control of rhythmic and regulatory functions, including pituitary hormone release.

Hypotonia   Loss of muscle tone.

Hypoxia-ischemia   Lack of oxygen combined with lack of blood flow.

Hysterectomy   Surgical removal of the uterus in mammals.

Ibotenic acid   A neurotoxin used in the brain to produce lesions of cell bodies while sparing fibers of passage.

Implantation   Attachment of fertilized egg to the wall of the uterus by the formation of a placenta in mammals.

Incubation   Period of development, usually referring to shelled eggs.

Indifferent gonad   An early stage in gonadal development when the gonad appears structurally intermediate between a testis and an ovary.

Induced estrus   Estrus that occurs only following exposure to stimuli from a male.

Induced ovulation   Ovulation in response to stimulation by a male.

Infradian rhythm   A self-sustained, endogenous oscillation with a freerunning period greater than circadian but less than circannual (e.g., 28-day menstrual cycle).

Insulin   A pancreatic hormone released in response to increases in circulating glucose concentrations, or in response to stimulation of the parasympathetic nervous system. Insulin promotes uptake and storage of glucose and other energy substrates and thus is classically an anabolic hormone.

Internal fertilization   Eggs fertilized by male sperm while still inside the female's body.

Interneurons   Neurons whose axons do not leave the brain nucleus where the cell body is found.

Intrasexual selection   Competition among members of the same sex for access to mates. Fights usually involve ritualized aggressive displays.

Intromission   Insertion of a penis into the vagina.

Involution   Reduction in size. Here, the functional inactivity and, frequently, the reduced size of the gonads during the nonreproductive portion of the annual cycle.

Ion channels   Pores formed by proteins that cross the cell membrane. These channels permit ions (typically sodium, potassium, and calcium) to travel into or out of the cell.

Juvenile hormones   A family of sesquiterpenoid hormones that act in the larval stages of insects to prevent metamorphosis.

Kallman's syndrome   A pathologic condition in humans that is characterized by an inability to smell and lack of gonadal development.

Klinefelter's syndrome   Externally masculine individuals who possess two X chromosomes and a Y chromosome (XXY).

Lactation   Milk production and its release during suckling of young.

Larynx   A sound-producing organ in vertebrates. In the clawed frog, contraction of the laryngeal muscles causes sound-producing discs to pop apart, resulting in a click.

Lateral line organs   Organs located on the body surface of aquatic organisms that detect water movements; the sensory receptor is a hair cell.

Lee-Boot effect   A suppression of estrous cycles in females due to overcrowding.

Leydig cell   Specialized cells located in the testes between the seminferous tubules; source of androgens.

Light-dark cycle   The natural or experimental environmental photoperiod.

Limbic system   Brain structure (functional group of structures). Term refers to a constellation of interconnected brain areas that regulate social and sexual behaviors. Includes the hypothalamus, amygdala, septum, hippocampus, bed nucleus of the stria terminalis (= emotional brain).

Lipolysis   The physiological process that breaks down stored triglycerides from adipose tissue into glycerol and fatty acids in adipose tissue; opposite of lipogenesis.

Locomotor activity   Unit of measure of activity, usually in open-field tests or in running wheels.

Lordosis   A sexual posture characterized by immobility with a species-typical posture that facilitates vaginal penetration by the penis of the male. In rodents, this usually consists of an arching of the back by extending the hindlegs and lateral deflection of the tail.

Luteinizing hormone (LH)   A glycoprotein hormone released by the pituitary. LH stimulates estrogen and progesterone secretion by the ovary, and testosterone secretion by the testes and is referred to as a gonadotropin.

Mate call   A vocalization displayed during courtship.

Maternal aggression   The high level of aggression displayed by females soon after delivering young or laying eggs.

Maternal imprinting   A process characterized by the young following the mother. Usually seen in precocial birds and mammals during the first few hours or days after hatching or birth.

Melatonin   Primary hormone of the pineal gland, thought to be important in biological rhythms.

Menstrual cycle   Cyclic changes in the output of reproductive hormones in women, revolving around the maturation of egg follicles in the ovaries.

Menstrual phase   The portion of the menstrual cycle characterized overtly by menstruation, i.e., shedding of the uterine lining.

Metabolic fuel   Any chemical substance, derived from food, that can be oxidized by cells to produce energy. Glucose and lipids are the main such fuels when animals are well nourished, but ketone bodies and free fatty acids derived from energy stores (fat) also become important fuels during fasting.

Metamorphosis   The process by which a transition is made between life stages—e.g., tadpole turning into a frog or caterpillar into a moth.

Microdialysis   Method by which small amounts of neurotransmitters in the extracellular fluid are collected for later analysis; involves diffusion across a semipermeable membrane at the base of a cannula.

Midluteal phase   A portion of the menstrual cycle characterized by high concentrations of estradiol and progesterone, occurring about midway between ovulation and onset of menstruation.

Migratory restlessness   Enhanced locomotor activity by birds, particularly at night, that occurs at the time of migration (= Zugenruhe).

Modality   The sensory domain of a particular stimulus (e.g., the visual modality, the auditory modality, etc.).

Molting   The series of events in arthropods that are involved in the production of a new exoskeleton and the shedding (ecdysis) of the old one.

Mormyrids and gymnotids   Two orders of weakly electric fish.

Motoneuron   Neuron whose cell body is located in the nervous system and whose axonal terminal synapses on a muscle fiber.

Motor pattern generator   A nucleus or set of nuclei in the central nervous system that produces a patterned discharge that affects the activity of motoneurons.

Motor tape   The representation of a stereotyped sequence of behaviors that is stored in the CNS.

Müllerian ducts   A duct system connecting the gonad to the external body wall; present in both sexes early in development but differentiates in females into the fallopian tubes, uterus, and inner vagina.

Müllerian regression factor (MRF)   A protein hormone secreted by the developing testes that inhibits development of the müllerian ducts into patent ducts (= müllerian inhibiting substance [MIS]).

N-methyl-D-aspartate (NMDA)   An excitatory amino acid that can be used as a neurotoxin to destroy cell bodies of neurons.

Naloxone   An opioid receptor antagonist.

Natural selection   Evolutionary process whereby traits that provide adaptational responses to the social, ecological, or physical environment are retained.

Neonatal   Occurring soon after birth.

Nephrectomy   Surgical removal of the kidneys.

Neuroeffectors   Motoneurons and the muscles they innervate.

Neurohormone   Chemical released by a neuron into general circulation or into the hypothalamic-pituitary-portal system.

Neurohypophysis   The posterior portion of the pituitary gland where axon terminals from neurons in the hypothalamus secrete of oxytocin and vasopressin into the blood (= posterior pituitary).

Neuroleptic drug   Dopamine receptor antagonists with antipsychotic, therapeutic value; used for treatment of schizophrenia.

Neuromodulation   A rather loose classification of the action of many neuropeptides and biogenic amines. These actions are characterized by a slower time-course and actions that occur over a broader area than that seen for classical neurotransmission.

Neuron   A nerve cell, capable of receiving and transmitting information.

Neuropeptides   Small chains of amino acids produced in the brain and used in neurotransmission or neuromodulation.

Neuropsychological test   Sensory, perceptual, cognitive, or motor tests that have been shown experimentally to depend on particular regions of the brain.

Neurosecretory cell   Specialized neuron that releases its neurotransmitter into the bloodstream rather than into a synapse.

Neurotransmitter Chemical released by a neuron to relay information to other cells, usually other neurons.

Nonspatial maze learning Learning to navigate in space using cues in the immediate or proximate environment (e.g., turn left at the corner with a stop sign; turn right after the large oak tree). Contrast with Spatial maze learning.

Norepinephrine A catecholaminergic neurotransmitter (= noradrenaline).

Normothermic Maintaining a body temperature within normal limits—e.g., 37°C in humans. Contrast with Torpor.

Nucleotide One of several chemicals that make up DNA and RNA. The different nucleotides provide the specificity of information in such molecules. For DNA the nucleotides are thymine, guanine, cytosine, and adenine; RNA uses the same nucleotides except that uridine replaces thymine.

Nucleus Either the spherical receptacle of genetic information in a eukaryotic cell, or a cluster of neuronal cell bodies found within the nervous system (pl. nuclei).

Open-ended song learning The ability of certain bird species to learn new songs even as adults (i.e., beyond the first year of life).

Open-field activity Standard measure for activity; refers to locomotor behavior shown by organism when placed in a large open arena.

Opiates Compounds derived from opium, such as heroin and morphine.

Opioids Compounds made in the body or synthesized exogenously that have opiate-like effects.

Orchidectomy Surgical removal of the gonads (= gonadectomy).

Organizational effects of hormones Actions during development, usually perinatally, that alter subsequent adult neural structures and functions.

Organizational hypothesis The proposal that androgens secreted by the developing testes permanently masculinize the developing nervous system, resulting in an adult that will more readily display male-typical behaviors.

Osmoreceptor Cerebral cells that detect changes in extracellular fluid osmolality (concentration of solute particles) that result from the induced movement of water by osmosis across the cell membrane.

Oviparity Egg-laying mode of reproduction with either internal or external fertilization.

Ovoviviparity Retention of fertilized egg with reduced nutrient and waste exchange between embryo and mother and usually some kind of shell barrier.

Ovulation The physical release of a mature egg from the ovary. See Spontaneous ovulation; Reflex ovulation.

Pain pathways Neural pathways carrying pain information, beginning with peripheral pain receptors, afferent projections to the spinal cord, ascending spinal pathways, and parts of the brain including the raphe complex and the periaqueductal gray.

Parkinson's disease A neurological disease in which the dopamine neurons of the substantia nigra degenerate; characterized by motor and cognitive deficits.

Parthenogenesis Reproductive mode whereby fertilization is not required for a female to give birth; in parthenogenesis only daughter(s) are produced, and they contain only the mother's genes.

Peptide A molecule consisting of about 50 or fewer amino acids.

Perceptual speed The ability to perceive quickly and accurately the details of a visual configuration or stimulus.

Periaqueductal gray See Pain pathways.

Perinatal   Occurring around the time of birth, including both the prenatal and neonatal periods. During this period many vertebrates, particularly rodents, are susceptible to the organizational effects of hormones.

Perineum   The pelvic floor, i.e., the region including the genitalia and underlying structures adjacent to, but separate from, the abdomen.

Period   The duration of a rhythm measured as the time between the appearance of an arbitrary phase point until the reappearance of that phase point; the inverse of frequency.

Phase advance   A shift of a rhythm caused by a Zeitgeber stimulus such that all subsequent phases of the rhythm occur *relatively earlier* than expected prior to application of the stimulus.

Phase   Any temporal location of a rhythm, e.g., each of the 360-degrees of a sine wave is a phase of that rhythm.

Phase delay   A shift of a rhythm caused by a Zeitgeber stimulus such that all subsequent phases of the rhythm occur *relatively later* than expected prior to application of the stimulus.

Phase response curve (PRC)   A curve showing the amount and direction of phase shift as a function of the circadian time of stimulus application. The PRC to light consists of a subjective day and a subjective night.

Phenotype   The sum of all physical characteristics of an individual that are expressed at a particular time. These traits are the result of the interplay of the genotype and environment up to that point.

Pheromone   Chemical signal produced by one organism that is capable of altering the reproductive behavior or physiology of another member of the same species. Pheromones may act slowly (priming effects), may act quickly (releasing effects), or communicate specific information (signaling effects).

Photoperiodic annual rhythms   Annual rhythms that are dependent to some degree upon seasonal changes in day length; photoperiodic annual rhythms, unlike circannual annual rhythms, do not persist or freerun when animals are kept in constant environmental conditions (= photoperiodic time measurement or photoperiodism).

Pineal   A gland lying outside of, but attached to, the brain. The pineal secretes melatonin under the rhythmic control of the circadian clock to regulate environmentally sensitive reproductive activity.

Pituitary   An endocrine gland found beneath the brain and controlled by the hypothalamus.

Plastic song   The intermediate stage of song development in which birds produce song syllables that have a well-defined structure but vary in order and number in successive renditions.

Postpartum estrus   The phenomenon in which a female ovulates and becomes sexually receptive immediately after parturition, shown by a large number of mammals.

Preadaptation   Anatomical structure or behavior that appears in evolution or in development to serve one function but then serves another at a future time (= exaptation).

Precocial   Refers to young birds or mammals born in a more mature condition with well-developed vision, hearing, and locomotion, and a relatively short period of dependence upon the parent for nutrition.

Predictive homeostasis   An advantage of a rhythm control system consisting of the ability to predict the timing of repetitive events.

Preovulatory gonadotropin surge   Sudden large increase of luteinizing hormone (LH) that acts as the final hormonal stimulus for the next ovulation.

Preovulatory phase   The portion of the menstrual cycle just prior to ovulation in which estradiol levels reach peak concentrations.

Presynaptic terminal   Portion of the axon usually characterized by concentration of synaptic vesicles containing neurotransmitters that are released by exocytosis in response to the arrival of an action potential.

Primates   The order of mammals including monkeys, apes, and humans.

Proceptive behaviors   Behaviors used to indicate the willingness of an organism to approach or solicit a member of the opposite sex.

Proceptivity   Extent to which an individual engages in behaviors likely to initiate mating from another individual. In female rats, ear wiggling and hopping and darting appear to be proceptive behaviors.

Prolactin   A pituitary hormone that is secreted during nursing to promote lactation, during mating to promote progesterone release and successful implantation, or during stress to inhibit reproduction.

Propylthiouracil   A potent blocker of thyroid hormone metabolism.

Prostaglandins   A class of fatty acid-derived compounds that have a vast array of biological actions throughout the body.

Prostate gland   Accessory sex organ in male vertebrates that contributes fluid to semen, necessary for insemination to occur. The prostate has an absolute requirement for dihydrotestosterone for normal function.

Protein   A molecule consisting of a long string of amino acids. A short string of amino acids is referred to as a peptide.

Protein kinase   A diverse class of enzymes that transfer a phosphate group from ATP to proteins. Most second messengers alter cellular function through the activation of specific protein kinases.

Prothoracic glands   Insect endocrine glands that secrete the molting hormones, the ecdysteroids.

Proximate causation   Here, those stimuli used by an organism to initiate, maintain, and terminate breeding.

Proximate mechanism   The genetic and physiological processes that contribute to behavioral expression.

Puberty   Time at which an individual first becomes capable of reproduction.

Pulsatile release   Acute bursts of hormones released as "pulses," usually one to three times per hour, e.g., release of GnRH under the control of the GnRH pulse generator.

Pulse EOD   Type of electric organ discharge (EOD) in the weakly electric fish in which the interval between EOD pulses is long compared to the duration of the pulse itself.

Purkinje cells   Large cells in the cerebellum.

Putamen   Brain structure (nucleus). Forms the basal ganglia together with the caudate nucleus and the globus pallidus.

Pyramidal system   Brain structure (fiber pathway). Output system connecting neurons in the motor cortex with spinal cord motoneurons for the activation of motor output (muscle movement).

Radioimmunoassay (RIA)   Method of using antibodies and radiolabeled hormone to measure hormonal levels in a biological sample.

Radiolabeled   Describing a molecule in which one or more atoms are made up of radioactive isotopes, making it relatively easy to detect said molecule by detecting the radioactivity.

Receptivity Extent to which an animal will mate, often measured in female rodents by quantification of the frequency or duration of the lordosis reflex.

Reductase 5α-reductase catalyzes the conversion of testosterone into 5α-dihydro-testosterone (DHT).

Reflex ovulation Ovulation of mature eggs in response to tactile (usually cervical) stimuli associated with copulation. A characteristic of cats, rabbits, and ferrets.

Releasing factor One of many chemicals released by the hypothalamus into the hypothalamic-pituitary portal system that increase or decrease the release of specific hormones from the pituitary.

Reliability Here, the extent to which a biological phenomenon is repeatedly observed.

Reproductive isolation The prevention of interbreeding between species either by behaviors characteristic of the species (premating mechanisms) or by infertility following mating (postmating mechanisms).

Reproductive success The extent to which a given individual's genes are present in succeeding generations. In practice, this quality is usually measured by determining the number of offspring that themselves survive to reproduce.

Reproductive synergism Coordination and synchronization of hormonal, gonadal, and sexual events by behavioral interaction.

Resting potential The electrical charge across a cell membrane. In neurons this refers to the charge seen in the absence of synaptic input.

Resting tremor Regular, involuntary oscillating movement of a body part when it is at rest.

Retrograde amnesia Loss of memory of events prior to some event such as trauma.

Ribonucleic acid (RNA) The chemical messenger, similar in structure to DNA, which is itself transcribed from DNA and serves as the template for the translation of genetic directions into a specific string of amino acids to form a protein or peptide.

Ritualization The evolutionary process whereby full-scale behavioral interchanges, such as fights, are replaced by highly stereotyped representations of the behavior such as aggressive displays. The result is exaggerated displays that are effective in social communication.

Rotational behavior Persistent 360-degree circles or turns made in one predominant direction.

Runningwheel activity Standard measure of activity in which the animal, usually small rodents, turns a wheel while running.

Scalloping The pattern of daily locomotor activity onset characterized by earlier onsets on days of high estradiol availability.

Scrotum The pouch of skin containing the testes.

Seasonality (seasonal breeding) The occurrence of various physiological and behavioral responses during a specific season (or seasons) of the year.

Secondary sex characteristics Anatomical structures that may or may not contribute to reproduction and are usually sexually dimorphic. Examples include mammary glands and male pattern baldness.

Secretagogs Term for a collection of hormones, usually released together.

Semialtricial Refers to young birds or mammals born with vision and hearing but with poor locomotion and therefore dependent upon the parent for nutrition.

Seminal vesicles Accessory sex organ in male vertebrates.

Seminiferous tubules Site of sperm production in the testes.

Sensory neurons   Neurons that respond directly to sensory stimuli or are excited by sensory receptors.

Sensory receptors   Cells that respond to external stimuli and alter the activity of adjacent sensory neurons.

Sex chromosome   A chromosome that contributes to sex determination; e.g., X and Y chromosomes for mammals, W and Z chromosomes for birds.

Sex determination   The point at which an individual begins developing as either a male or a female. In mammals this takes place at fertilization, depending on whether the sperm has contributed an X or a Y chromosome.

Sexual cycle   Cycle of ovarian follicular development, ovulation, and corpora lutea formation including hormone secretion.

Sexual differentiation   The process by which a developing individual assumes the characteristics of either a male or a female. In vertebrates, gonadal hormones released following sex determination implement this decision by guiding developing somatic structures, including the brain.

Sexual dimorphism   The species characteristic of having males and females that are structurally different.

Sexual motivation   Interest in and attempts to engage in copulatory activity. A conceptual term referring to the inclination of an individual to seek out and approach another individual for the purpose of mating.

Sexual receptivity   The willingness to engage in copulatory behaviors. Receptivity in mammals is usually indexed by the probability that a female will show lordosis in response to flank stimulation or by the frequency or duration of female lordosis within a given time period.

Sexual selection   A counterpart to natural selection. Sexual selection arises when individuals of a species differ in their ability to compete with members of the same sex for access to mates (intrasexual) or to attract members of the opposite sex (epigamic or intersexual selection).

Sexually dimorphic   Characters or behaviors that occur in different forms in the sexes.

Sexually dimorphic nucleus of the preoptic area (SDN-POA)   A densely staining region of the preoptic area that is larger in males than females for both rodents and humans.

Silastic   A silicon rubber compound through which steroid hormones readily dissolve. Surgically implanted steroid-filled Silastic capsules slowly release the steroid into the circulation.

Sodium appetite   A strong motivation to seek, obtain, and consume salty foods and fluids, typically as a consequence of sodium deficiency. Analogous to hunger and thirst as a drive.

Somatic   Refers to nonreproductive cells or tissues.

Somatomedin   A class of compounds released by the liver in response to growth hormone; somatomedins mediate some of the stimulatory effects caused by growth hormone.

Somatostatin   Hypothalamic hormone that inhibits the pituitary release of growth hormone.

Song learning, age-limited.   *See* Age-limited song learing

Song learning, open-ended.   *See* Open-ended song learning.

Song repertoire   The number of different versions of species-specific song that an individual produces.

Spatial maze learning   The ability to navigate in space. For example, navigation achieved by imagining or visualizing the location or orientation of objects, or features of objects, in three-dimensional space. Contrast with non-spatial maze learning.

Spinal nucleus of the bulbocavernosus (SNB)   Group of motoneurons in spinal cord that innervate several muscles attached to the base of the penis.

Spontaneous ovulation   Endogenous timing of ovulation occurring in the absence of stimulation from the male; often regulated by photoperiod.

Sprouting   Here, the formation of new neuronal connections following neuronal injury.

Stereotyped behaviors   Any seemingly mechanical repetitive movements. Here, repetitive movements of the head, mouth, facial features, or forelimbs.

Steroid hormone receptors   A family of proteins that act as transcription factors when bound to hormones. Members include receptors for sex steroids (androgens, estrogens, progestins), thyroid hormones, and retinoic acid. These proteins have several domains, one of which binds the hormone and another that binds to DNA.

Steroidogenesis   The production and secretion of steroid hormones.

Steroids   Biologically active compounds that share a particular molecular structure resembling cholesterol, consisting of four linked rings of carbon atoms.

Stomatogastric ganglion   A small ganglion composed of about 30 neurons and found in decapod crustaceans such as crabs and lobsters. It controls the movements of the various regions of the stomach.

Stress dwarfism   A pediatric disorder in which children, exposed to considerable amounts of stress, occasionally cease growing. If the child is moved to a less stressful environment rapidly enough, growth may resume and catch up with normal levels (= Psychogenic dwarfism).

Stress-induced analgesia   The phenomenon in which, following exposure to certain types of stressors, organisms become less sensitive to pain.

Stretch receptor   Receptor cells, located on the outside of an elastic vessel, that detect changes in tension of the vessel's walls. For example, such receptors signal the brain when the stomach is empty, the bladder is full, and the venous blood vessels are contracted.

Striatum   Brain structure (nucleus). One of a group of nuclei that, with the globus pallidus, composes the basal ganglia. The putamen and caudate nucleus are referred to collectively as the striatum.

Sub-song   The first stage of song development in which birds produce crude sounds that are highly variable in structure in successive renditions and bear little similarity to adult song.

Subjective day   The portion of the circadian day in which a light stimulus produces neither phase advances nor delays. Corresponds to the time of low locomotor activity for nocturnal animals.

Subjective night   The portion of the circadian day in which a light stimulus produces a phase shift. During the early subjective night, these are phase delays that give way to phase advances during the late subjective night.

Substantia nigra   Brain structure (nucleus). Brain nucleus containing neurons that produce and deliver dopamine to the striatum.

Suprachiasmatic nucleus   Brain structure (nucleus). Brain site of the mechanisms generating "clock" activity controlling circadian rhythmicity in mammals.

Sympathoadrenal system   A division of the autonomic nervous system consisting of the sympathetic nerves and the adrenal medulla, which responds to conditions of stress by secreting catecholamine hormones (e.g., epinephrine, norepinephrine) that prepare the animal physiologically for attack, defense, or escape.

Synapse Site of "connection" between two neurons. The site where presynaptic terminals connect with a postsynaptic cell.

Synaptic transmission The passage of information between two cells across a synapse.

Synthetic Manufactured at the conscious direction of humans.

Systemic Overall. Here referring to hormones available throughout the body through the circulatory system. Opposite of local.

Teats Nipples of mammary glands.

Testicular feminization mutation (TFM) A genetic mutation that renders androgen receptors nonfunctional.

Testis determination factor (TDF) The protein, a product of a gene on the Y chromosome, that instructs the indifferent gonad to develop as a testis.

Testosterone A steroid hormone that is the principal secretion of the testes.

Thermoregulation Ability of animals to regulate their body temperature at an optimal temperature for physiological functioning.

Thiourea A chemical inhibitor of thyroid hormone function.

Thymidine A chemical precursor to thymine, the nucleotide found in DNA but not RNA. Radioactively labeled thymidine will be incorporated into newly duplicated DNA of cells about to divide, marking the "birthdate" of those cells.

Ticking A vocalization given by sexually unreceptive female or by male clawed frogs when mounted by a male clawed frog that results in release from the male's clasp.

Torpedo The electric ray, a fish that can stun prey with shocks produced by the electric organ.

Torpor A state of reduced metabolic functioning characterized by decreases in body temperature beyond the normal range of variability; e.g., mammals exhibiting shallow daily torpor (Siberian hamster, deer mice, etc.) reduce their body temperatures from 37°C to 15° to 20°C, for up to several weeks.

Transcription The creation of a specific string of RNA encoded by a gene.

Translation The creation of a specific protein encoded by RNA.

Trophic relationships A dependent relation between a neuron and the cell(s) it innervates. When one of these cells is removed, the remaining cell may die.

Turner's syndrome Externally feminine individuals that possess a single X chromosome but no Y chromosome (XO).

Ultimate causation Evolutionary factors that result in individuals within populations responding in particular ways to changing environmental conditions.

Ultradian rhythm A class of rhythms with a range of periods shorter than the circadian range.

Urethra Duct from the bladder that releases urine outside the body.

Uterus Structure connecting the fallopian tubes to the vagina; usual site of embryo implantation and fetal development.

Vaginal code Refers to the number and patterning of intromissions characteristic of a species mating behavior. This "code" is essential for the induction of the progestational state (pregnancy). It is possible to mimic the necessary tactile cues by mechanical means.

Validity Here, the extent to which laboratory findings apply to situations outside of the laboratory.

Vandenbergh effect Acceleration of puberty in a young female rodent due to odorant from an adult male.

Vasopressin A hormone that has a variety of effects throughout the body. Vasopressin can be released from the posterior pituitary, where it affects water balance. It also can be released from the hypothalamus, where it acts as a secretagogue at the pituitary, stimulating secretion of adrenocorticotropic hormone (ACTH). Thus, hypothalamic vasopressin is typically released during stress.

Verbal fluency Facility in generating words, phrases, or sentences that fulfill specific semantic or phonetic criteria.

Vesicle Small, spherical-shaped structure for transporting protein(s).

Viviparity Mode of reproduction whereby embryos are retained in the mother's body and nutrients and waste are exchanged.

Voltammetry Method by which the pattern of electrical current at the membrane is measured.

Vomeronasal organ Receptor organ for detecting chemical signals and, in particular, pheromones.

Wandering behavior Here, behavior shown by some caterpillars in preparation for metamorphosis. It involves the cessation of feeding and the display of sustained locomotion and other behaviors associated with the construction of a chamber for metamorphosis.

Wave EOD Type of electric organ discharge (EOD) in which the interval between EOD pulses is short compared to the pulse duration itself.

Whitten effect The induction of estrus in a female rodent by the odor of a strange male.

Wolffian ducts A duct system connecting the gonad to the external body wall. Present in both sexes early in development but differentiating in males into the epididymis, vas deferens, and seminal vesicles and regressing in females.

Zeitgeber Stimulus used to impart information about time. Literally, "time-giver."

Zugenruhe Migratory restlessness.

Zygote A fertilized egg, i.e., the single celled beginning of an individual.

References

1. Abplanalp, J. M., Rose, R. M., Donnelly, A. F., and Livingston-Vaughan, L. (1979) Psychoendocrinology of the menstrual cycle: II. The relationship between enjoyment of activities, moods, and reproductive hormones. Psychosom. Med. 41:605–615.

2. Adams, D. B. (1983) Hormone-brain interactions and their influence on agonistic behavior. In B. B. Svare (Ed.), Hormones and Aggressive Behavior. Plenum, New York, pp. 223–245.

3. Adams, D. B., Gold, A. R., and Burt, A. D. (1978) Rise in female initiated sexual activity at ovulation and its suppression by oral contraceptives. N. Engl. J. Med. 229:1145–1150.

4. Adkins-Regan, E. (1989) Sex hormones and sexual orientation in animals. Psychobiology 16:335–347.

5. Adkins-Regan, E. and Ascenci, M. (1987) Social and sexual behaviour of male and female zebra finches treated with oestradiol during the nestling period. Anim. Behav. 35:1100–1112.

6. Adler, N. T. (1969) The effect of male's copulatory behavior on successful pregnancy of the female rat. J. Comp. Physiol. Psychol. 69:613–622.

7. Adler, N. T. and Allen, T. O. (1983) The origin of sexual behavior: A functional analysis. In E. Satinoff and P. Teitelbaum (Eds.), Motivation. Plenum, New York, pp. 475–509.

8. Ahdieh, H. B., Mayer, A. D., and Rosenblatt, J. S. (1987) Effects of brain antiestrogen implants on maternal behavior and on postpartum estrus in pregnant rats. Neuroendocrinology 46:522–531.

9. Ahdieh, H. B., Mayer, A. D., and Rosenblatt, J. S. (1990) Estrogen-progesterone interaction in the stimulation of maternal behavior in the rat. 22nd Annual Conference on Reproductive Behavior, June 8–11, 1990, Emory University, Atlanta, Georgia, p. 40.

10. Akana, S., Cascio, C. S., Du, J.-Z., Levin, N. and Dallman, M. F. (1986) Reset of feedback in the adrenocortical system: An apparent shift in sensitivity of adrenocroticotropin to inhibition by corticosterone between morning and evening. Endocrinology 119:2325–2332.

11. Albers, H. E. (1981) Gonadal hormones organize and modulate the circadian system of the rat. Am. J. Physiol. 241:R62–R66.

12. Albers, H. E., Moline, M. L., and Moore-Ede, M. C. (1984) Sex differences in circadian control of LH secretion. J. Endocrinol. 100:101–105.

13. Albert, D. J., Walsh, M. L., Gorzalka, B. B., Siemens, Y., and Louie, H. (1986) Testosterone removal in rats results in a decrease in social aggression and a loss of social dominance. Physiol. Behav. 36:401–407.

14. Alberts, J. R. and Gubernick, D. J. (1983) Reciprocity and resource exchange: A symbiotic model of parent-offspring relations. In L. A. Rosenblum and H. Moltz (Eds.), Symbiosis in Parent-Offspring Interactions. Plenum, New York, pp. 7–44.

15. Alcock, J. (1989) Animal Behavior. An Evolutionary Approach. Sinauer Associates, Sunderland, Mass.

16. Alderson, L. M. and Baum, M. J. (1981) Differential effects of gonadal steroids on dopamine metabolism in mesolimbic and nigrostriatal pathways of male rat brain. Brain Res. 218:189–206.

17. Allen, L. S. and Gorski, R. A. (1986) Sexual dimorphism of the human anterior commissure. Anat. Rec. 214:3A.

18. Allen, L. S., Hines, M., Shryne, J. E., and Gorski, R. A. (1989) Two sexually dimorphic cell groups in the human brain. J. Neurosci. 9:497–506.

19. Allen, T. O. and Adler, N. T. (1985) Neuroendocrine consequences of sexual behavior. In N. Adler, D. Pfaff, and R. W. Goy (Eds.), Handbook of Behavioral Neurobiology, Vol. 7, Reproduction. Plenum, New York, pp. 725–766.

20. Allen, T. O. and Adler, N. T. (1989) Effects of sexual behavior on gonadal function in rodents. In R. Brush and S. Levine (Eds.), Psychoendocrinology. Academic Press, New York, pp. 227–269.

21. Alleva, J. J., Waleski, M. V., and Alleva, F. R. (1971) A biological clock controlling the estrous cycles of the hamster. Endocrinology 88:1368–1379.

22. Almeida, O. F. X., Nikolarakis, K. E. Sirinathsinghji, D. J. S., and Herz, A. (1989) Opioid-mediated inhibition of sexual behaviour and luteinizing hormone secretion by corticotrophin releasing hormone. In R. G. Dyer and R. J. Bicknell (Eds.), Brain Opioid Systems in Reproduction. Oxford University Press, Oxford, pp. 149–164.

23. Altemus, M., Wexler, B. E., and Boulis, N. (1989) Changes in perceptual asymmetry with the menstrual cycle. Neuropsychologia 27:233–240.

24. Altmann, S. A. (1962) A field study in the sociobiology of rhesus monkeys, *Macaca mulatta*. Ann. N.Y. Acad. Sci. 102:338–435.

25. Anderson, C. H. (1975) Localization of cells retaining ^{3}H-estradiol in the forebrain of rabbits. Anat. Rec. 69:287–291.

26. Anderson, C. O., Zarrow, M. X., Fuller, G. B., and Denenberg, V. H. (1971) Pituitary involvement in maternal nest-building in the rabbit. Horm. Behav. 2:183–189.

27. Anderson, E. I. (1972) Cognitive performance and mood change as they relate to menstrual cycle and estrogen level. Dissert. Abstr. Int. 33:1758-B.

28. Andrews, R. V. and Folk, G. E. (1964) Circadian metabolic patterns in cultured hamster adrenal glands. Comp. Biochem. Physiol. 11:393–409.

29. Anonymous (1970) Effects of sexual activity on beard growth in man. Nature 226:869–870.

30. Antoni, F. (1986) Hypothalamic control of adrenocorticotropic hormone secretion: Advances since the discovery of 41-residue corticotropin-releasing factor. Endocr. Rev. 7:351–373.

31. Ar, A. and Yom-Tov, Y. (1978) The evolution of parental care in birds. Evolution 32:655–669.

32. Archer, J. (1975) Rodent sex differences in emotional and related behavior. Behav. Biol. 14:451–479.

33. Arendash, G. W. and Gorski, R. A. (1983) Effects of discrete lesions of the sexually dimorphic nucleus of the preoptic area or other medial preoptic regions on the sexual behavior of male rats. Brain Res. Bull. 10:147.

34. Arletti, R. and Bertolini, A. (1985) Oxytocin stimulates lordosis behavior in female rats. Neuropeptides 6:247–253.

34a. Arnold, A. P. (1974) Behavioral effect of androgen in zebra finches and a search for its site of action. Ph.D. Dissertation, The Rockefeller University, New York.

35. Arnold, A. P. (1975) The effects of castration and androgen replacement on song, courtship, and aggression in zebra finches. J. Exp. Zool. 191:309–326.

36. Arnold, A. P., Bottjer, S. W., Brenowitz, E. A., Nordeen, E. J., and Nordeen, K. W. (1986) Sexual dimorphisms in the neural vocal control system in song birds: Ontogeny and phylogeny. Brain Behav. Evol. 28:22–31.

37. Arnold, A. P and Breedlove, S. M. (1985) Organizational and activational effects of sex steroid hormones on vertebrate behavior: A re-analysis. Horm. Behav. 19:469–498.

38. Arnold, A. P. and Gorski, R. A. (1984) Gonadal steroid induction of structural sex differences in the brain. Annu. Rev. Neurosci. 7:413–442.

39. Arnold, A. P., Nottebohm, F., and Pfaff, D. (1976) Hormone concentrating cells in vocal control and other areas of the brain of the zebra finch (*Poephilia guttata*). J. Comp. Neurol. 165:487–512.

40. Asso, D. (1985) Psychology degree examinations and the premenstrual phase of the menstrual cycle. Women & Health 10:91–104.

41. Attardi, B., Geller, L. N., and Ohno, S. (1976) Androgen and estrogen receptors in brain cytosol from male, female, and testicular feminized (tfm/y) mice. Endocrinology 98:864–874.

42. Axelson, J. F., Zoller, L. C., Tomassone, J. E., and Collins, D. C. (1986) Effects of silastic progesterone implants on activity cycles and steroid levels in ovariectomized and intact females rats. Physiol. Behav. 38:879–885.

43. Badura, L. L., Yant, W. R., and Nunez, A. A. (1987) Photoperiodic modulation of steroid-induced lordosis in golden hamsters. Physiol. Behav. 40:551–554.

44. Baker, M. (1990) Effects of ovariectomy on dyadic aggression and submission in a colony of peri-pubertal spotted hyenas. M. A. Thesis, University of California, Berkeley.

45. Baker, S. W. and Ehrhardt, A. A. (1974) Prenatal androgen, intelligence, and cognitive sex differences. In R. C. Friedman, R. M. Richart, and R. L. VandeWiele (Eds.), Sex Differences in Behavior. Wiley & Sons, New York, pp. 53–76.

46. Ball, G. F., Dufty, A. M., Goldsmith, A. R., and Buntin, J. D. (1988) Autoradiographic localization of brain prolactin receptors in a parental and non-parental songbird species. Soc. Neurosci. Abstr. 14:88.

47. Balthazart, J., Foidart, A., and Hendrick, J. C. (1990) The induction by testosterone of aromatase activity in the preoptic area and activation of copulatory behavior. Physiol. Behav. 47:83–94.

48. Bancroft, J. (1980) Endocrinology of sexual function. Clinics Obstet. Gynaecol. 7:253–281.
49. Bancroft, J., Tennent, T. G., Loucas, K., and Cass, J. (1974) Control of deviant sexual behaviour by drugs: Behavioural effects of oestrogens and anti-androgens. Br. J. Psychiat. 125:310–315.
50. Bancroft, J. and Wu, F. C. W. (1983) Changes in erectile responsiveness during androgen replacement therapy. Arch. Sex. Behav. 12:59–66.
51. Baptista, L. and Schuchmann, K. (1990) Song learning in the Anna's hummingbird (*Calypte anna*). Ethology 84:15–20.
52. Baranczuk, R. and Greenwald, G. S. (1973) Peripheral levels of estrogen in the cyclic hamster. Endocrinology 92:805–812.
53. Barber, P. V., Arnold, A. G., and Evans, G. (1973) Recurrent hormone dependent chorea: Effects of oestrogens and progestrogens. Clin. Endocrinol. 5:291–293.
54. Barberis, C. and Audigier, S. (1985) Des récepteurs à la vasopressine et à l'oxytocine dans la système nerveux central du rat. Ann. d'Endocrinol. (Paris) 46:35–39.
55. Barkley, M. S. and Goldman, B. D. (1977) Testosterone-induced aggression in adult female mice. Horm. Behav. 9:76–84.
56. Barkley, M. S. and Goldman, B. D. (1977) A quantitative study of serum testosterone, sex accessory organ growth, and the development of intermale aggression in the mouse. Horm. Behav. 8:208–218.
57. Barkley, M. S. and Goldman, B. D. (1978) Studies on opponent status and steroid mediation of aggression in female mice. Behav. Biol. 23:118–123.
58. Barnes, B. M., Licht, P., and Zucker, I. (1987) Temperature dependence of in vitro androgen production in testes from hibernating ground squirrels, Spermophilus lateralis. Can. J. Zool. 65:3020–3023.
59. Bartholomew, G. A. (1982) Scientific innovation and creativity: A zoologist's point of view. Am. Zool. 22:227–235.
60. Bartoshuk, L. M. (1977) Water taste in mammals. In J. A. W. Weijnen and J. Mendelson (Eds.), Drinking Behavior—Oral Stimulation, Reinforcement, and Preference. Plenum, New York, pp. 317–339.
61. Bass, A. H. (1986) A hormone-sensitive communication system in an electric fish. J. Neurobiol. 17:131–156.
62. Bass, A. H. (1986) Species differences in electric organs of mormyrids: Substates of species-typical electric organ discharge waveforms. J. Comp. Neurol. 244:313–330.
63. Bass, A. H. (1986) Electric organs revisited: Evolution of a vertebrate communication and orientation organ. In T. Bullock and W. Heiligenberg (Eds.), Electroreception. Wiley & Sons, New York, pp. 13–70.
64. Bass, A. H., Denziot, J.-P., and Marchaterre, M. A. (1986) Ultrastructural features and hormone dependent sex differences of mormyrid electric organs. J. Comp. Neurol. 254:511–528.
65. Bass, A. H. and Hopkins, C. (1984) Shifts in frequency tuning of electroreceptors in androgen-treated mormyrid fish. J. Comp. Physiol. [A] 155:713–724.
66. Bass, A., Segil, N., and Kelley, D. (1986) A steroid-sensitive electromotor pathway in mormyrid fish: Autoradiography and receptor biochemistry. J. Comp. Physiol. 159:535–544.
67. Bass, A. H. and Volman, S. (1987) From behavior to membranes: Testosterone-induced changes in action potential waveform duration in electric organs. Proc. Natl. Acad. Sci. U.S.A. 84:9295–9298.
68. Bast, J. D. and Greenwald, G. S. (1974) Serum profiles of follicle-stimulating hormone, luteinizing hormone and prolactin during the estrous cycle of the hamster. Endocrinology 94:1295–1299.
69. Bate, C. M. (1973) The mechanism of the pupal gin trap. II. The closure movement. J. Exp. Biol. 59:109–119.
70. Bate, C. M. (1973) The mechanism of the pupal gin trap. III. Interneurons and the origin of the closure mechanism. J. Exp. Biol. 59:121–135.
71. Baulieu, E. E., Lasnitzki, I., and Robel, P. (1968) Metabolism of testosterone and action of metabolites on prostate glands grown in organ culture. Nature 219:1155–1156.
72. Baum, M. J. (1976) Effects of testosterone propionate administered perinatally on sexual behavior of female ferrets. J. Comp. Physiol. Psychol. 90:300–310.
73. Baum, M. J. (1979) Differentiation of coital behavior in mammals: A comparative analysis. Neurosci. Biobehav. Rev. 3:265–284.
74. Baum, M. J., Canick, J. A., Erskine, M. S., Gallagher, C. A., and Shim, J. H. (1983) Normal differentiation of masculine sexual behavior in male ferrets despite neonatal inhibition of brain aromatase or 5α-reductase activity. Neuroendocrinology 36:277–284.
75. Baum, M. J., Carroll, R. S., Cherry, J. A., and Tobet, S. A. (1990) Steroidal control of behavioural, neuroendocrine and brain sexual differentiation: Studies in a carnivore, the ferret. J. Neuroendocrinol. 2:401–408.
76. Baum, M. J. and Erskine, M. S. (1984) Effect of neonatal gonadectomy and administration of testosterone on coital masculinization in the ferret. Endocrinology 115:2440–2444.

77. Baum, M. J., Erskine, M. S., Kornberg, E., and Weaver, C. E. (1990) Prenatal and neonatal testosterone exposure interact to affect differentiation of sexual behavior and partner preference in female ferrets. Behav. Neurosci. 104:183–198.

78. Baum, M. J., Everitt, B. J., Herbert, J., and Keverne, E. B. (1977) Hormonal basis of proceptivity and receptivity in female primates. Arch. Sex. Behav. 6:173–192.

79. Baum, M. J., Gallagher, C. A., Martin, J. T., and Damassa, D. A. (1982) Effect of testosterone, dihydrotestosterone and estradiol administered neonatally on sexual behavior of female ferrets. Endocrinology 111:773–780.

80. Baum, M. J., Gerlach, J. L., Drey, L. C., and McEwen, B. S. (1986) Biochemical and radioautographic analysis of estrogen-inducible progestin receptors in female ferret brain and pituitary: Correlations with effects of progesterone on sexual behavior and gonadotropin-releasing hormone-stimulated secretion of luteinizing hormone. Brain Res. 368:296–309.

81. Baum, M. J., Kingsbury, P. A., and Erskine, M. S. (1987) Failure of the synthetic androgen, methyltrienolone, R1881, to duplicate the activational effect of testosterone on mating in castrated male rats. J. Endocrinol. 113:15–20.

82. Baum, M. J., Melamed, E., and Globus, M. (1986) Dissociation of the effects of castration and testosterone replacement on sexual behavior and neural metabolism of dopamine in the male rat. Brain Res. Bull. 16:145–148.

83. Baum, M. J. and Schretlen, P. (1975) Neuroendocrine effects of perinatal androgenization in the male ferret. Prog. Brain Res. 42:343–355.

84. Baum, M. J., and Tobet, S. A. (1988) Endocrine control of coital sexual differentiation in the ferret: A model for higher mammals. In J. M. A. Sitsen and J. Money (Eds.), Handbook of Sexology. Vol. 6, The Pharmacology and Endocrinology of Sexual Function. Elsevier, Amsterdam, pp. 193–208.

85. Baum, M. J., Tobet, S. A., Starr, M. S., and Bradshaw, W. G. (1982) Implantation of dihydrotestosterone propionate into the lateral septum or medial amygdala facilitates copulation in castrated male rats given estradiol systemically. Horm. Behav. 16:208–223.

86. Baum, M. J. and Vreeburg, J. T. M. (1973) Copulation in castrated male rats following combined treatment with estradiol and dihydrotestosterone. Science 182:283–285.

87. Bazer, F. W. and First, N. L. (1983) Pregnancy and parturition. J. Anim. Sci. (Suppl.) 57:425–460.

88. Beach, F. A. (1942) Importance of progesterone to the induction of sexual receptivity in spayed female rats. Proc. Soc. Exp. Biol. Med. 51:369–371.

89. Beach, F. A. (1968) Coital behavior in dogs. III. Effects of early isolation of mating in males. Behaviour 30:218–238.

90. Beach, F. A. (1971) Hormonal factors controlling the differentiation, development and display of copulatory behavior in the ramstergig and related species. In E. Tobach, L. R. Aronson, and E. Shaw (Eds.), Biopsychology of Development. Academic Press, New York, pp. 249–296.

91. Beach, F. A. (1976) Sexual attractivity, proceptivity, and receptivity in female mammals. Horm. Behav. 7:105–138.

92. Beach, F. A. (1979) Animal models for human sexuality. In R. Potter and J. Whelan (Eds.), Sex, Hormones and Behaviour. Ciba Foundation Symposium 62. Excerpta Medica, Amsterdam, pp. 113–143.

93. Beach, F. A. (1983) Hormones and psychological processes. Can. J. Psychol. 37:193–210.

94. Beatty, W. W. (1979) Gonadal hormones and sex differences in nonreproductive behaviors in rodents: Organizational and activational influences. Horm. Behav. 12:112–163.

95. Becker, D., Creutzfeldt, O. D., Schwibbe, M., and Wuttke, W. (1982) Changes in physiological, EEG and psychological parameters in women during the spontaneous menstrual cycle and following oral contraceptives. Psychoneuroendocrinology 7:75–90.

96. Becker, J. B. (1990) Direct effect of 17β-estradiol on striatum: Sex differences in dopamine release. Synapse 5:157–164.

97. Becker, J. B. and Beer, M. E. (1986) The influence of estrogen on nigrostriatal dopamine activity: Behavioral and neurochemical evidence for both pre- and postsynaptic components. Behav. Brain Res. 19:27–33.

98. Becker, J. B. and Cha, J. (1989) Estrous cycle-dependent variation in amphetamine-induced behaviors and striatal dopamine release assessed with microdialysis. Behav. Brain Res. 35:117–125.

99. Becker, J. B. and Ramirez, V. D. (1980) Sex differences in the amphetamine stimulated release of catecholamines from rat striatal tissue in vitro. Brain Res. 204:361–372.

100. Becker, J. B., Robinson, T. E., and Lorenz, K. A. (1982) Sex differences and estrous cycle variations in amphetamine-elicited rotational behavior. Eur. J. Pharmacol. 80:65–72.

101. Becker, J. B., Snyder, P. J., Miller, M. M., Westgate, S. A., and Jenuwine, M. J. (1987) The influence of estrous cycle and intrastriatal estradiol on sensorimotor performance in the female rat. Pharmacol. Biochem. Behav. 27:53–59.

102. Bedard, P. J., P. Langelier, and A. Villeneuve (1977) Estrogens and the extrapyramidal system. Lancet 2:1367–1368.

103. Beeman, E. A. (1947) The effect of male hormone on aggressive behavior in mice. Physiol. Zool. 20:373–405.

104. Beletsky, L. D. (1983) Aggressive and pair-bond maintenance songs of female red-winged blackbirds. Z. Tierpsychol. 62:47–54.

105. Bell, A. D. and Variend, S. (1985) Failure to demonstrate sexual dimorphism of the corpus callosum in childhood. J. Anat. 143:143–147.

106. Bell, C. and Szabo, T. (1986) Electroreception in mormyrid fish: Central anatomy. In T. Bullock and W. Heiligenberg (Eds.), Electroreception. Wiley & Sons, New York, pp. 375–422.

107. Bengelloum, W. A., Nelson, D. J., Zent, H. M., and Beatty, W. W. (1976) Behavior of male and female rats with septal lesions: Influence of prior gonadectomy. Physiol. Behav. 14:201–206.

108. Bennett, M. and Grundfest, H. (1961) Studies on morphology and electrophysiology of electric organs III. Electrophysiology of electric organs in mormyrids. In C. Chagas and A. Paes de Carvalho (Eds.), Biogenesis. Elsevier, Amsterdam, pp. 113–115.

109. Ben Shaul, D. M. (1962) The composition of the milk of wild animals. International Zoo Yearbook 4:333–342.

110. Benton, A. L. (1972) The "minor" hemisphere. J. Hist. Med. All. Sci. 27:5–14.

111. Berenbaum, S. A. and Hines, M. (1989) Hormonal influences on sex-typed toy preferences. Presented at the Biennial Meeting of the Society for Research in Child Development, March 7–10, 1989, Kansas City, Missouri.

112. Beresford, O. D. and Graham, A. M. (1950) Chorea graviderum. J. Obstet. Gynecol. Br. Emp. 57:616–625.

113. Bern, H. A. (1972) Comparative endocrinology—The state of the field and the art. Gen. Comp. Endocrinol. Suppl. 3:7551–7561.

114. Bernstein, B. E. (1977) Effect of menstruation on academic performance among college women. Arch. Sex. Behav. 6:289–296.

115. Bernstein, I. S. (1981) Dominance: The baby and the bathwater. Behav. Brain Sci. 4:419–4567.

116. Bernstein, I. S., Gordon, T. P., and Rose, R. M. (1983) The interaction of hormones, behavior, and social context in nonhuman primates. In B. B. Svare (Ed.), Hormones and Aggressive Behavior. Plenum, New York, pp. 197–222.

117. Berta, P., Hawkins, J. R., Sinclair, A. H., Taylor, A., Griffiths, B. L., and Goodfellow, P. N. (1990) Genetic evidence equating SRY and the testis-determining factor. Nature 348:448–450.

118. Berthold, A. A. (1849) Transplantation der Hoden. Arch. Anat. Physiol. Wissensch. Med. pp. 42–46.

119. Bicker, G. and Menzel, R. (1989) Chemical codes for the control of behaviour in arthropods. Nature 337:33–39.

120. Bitran, D. and Hull, E. M. (1987) Pharmacological analysis of male rat sexual behavior. Neurosci. Biobehav. Rev. 11:365–389.

121. Bittman, E. L. (1978) Hamster refractoriness: The role of insensitivity of pineal target tissues. Science 202:648–650.

122. Blackburn, D. G. and Evans, H. E. (1986) "Why are there no viviparous birds?" Am. Nat. 128:165.

123. Blackwelder, R. E. and Shepard, B. A. (1981) The Diversity of Animal Reproduction. CRC Press, Boca Raton, Fla.

124. Blanchard, R. J. and Blanchard, D. C. (1977) Aggressive behavior in the rat. Behav. Biol. 21:197–224.

125. Blanchard, R. J., Blanchard, D. C., and Takahashi, L. K. (1977) Reflexive fighting in the albino rat: Aggressive or defensive behavior? Aggress. Behav. 3:145–155.

126. Bluhm, C. K. (1985) Social factors regulating avian endocrinology and reproduction. In B. K. Follett, S. Ishii, and A. Chandola (Eds.), The Endocrine System and the Environment. Japanese Scientific Society Press, Tokyo, pp. 247–264.

127. Bluhm, C. K., Phillips, R. E., Burke, W. H., and Gupta, G. N. (1984) Effects of male courtship and gonadal steroids on pair formation, egg-laying, and serum LH in canvasback ducks (Aythya valisineria). J. Zool. (Lond.) 204:185–200.

128. Bodnar, R. J., Romero, M.-T., and Kramer, E. (1988) Organismic variables and pain inhibition: Roles of gender and aging. Brain Res. Bull. 21:947–953.

129. Boice, R. (1981) Captivity and feralization. Psychol. Bull. 89:407–421.

130. Bojlen, K. and Bentzon, M. W. (1974) Seasonal variation in the occurrence of menarche. Dan. Med. Bull. 21:161–168.

131. Bollenbacher, W. E., Smith, S. L., Goodman, W., and Gilbert, L. I. (1981) Ecdysteroid titer during the larval-pupal-adult development of the tobacco hornworm, Manduca sexta. Gen. Comp. Endocrinol. 44:302–306.

132. Booth, A., Shelley, G., Mazur, A., Tharp, G., and Kittok, R. (1989) Testosterone, and winning and losing in human competition. Horm. Behav. 23:556–571.

133. Booth, J. E. (1977) Sexual behavior of neonatally castrated rats injected during infancy with oestrogen and dihydrotestosterone. J. Endocrinol. 72:135–142.

134. Booth-Kewley, S. and Friedman, H. (1987) Psychological predictors of heart disease: A quantitative review. Psychol. Bull. 101:343–362.

135. Bottjer, S. W. (1987) Ontogenetic changes in the pattern of androgen accumulation in song-control nuclei of male zebra finches. J. Neurobiol. 18:125–139.

136. Bowden, N. J. and Brain, P. F. (1978) Blockade of testosterone-maintained intermale fighting in albino laboratory mice by an aromatization inhibitor. Physiol. Behav. 20:543–546.

137. Bowen, W. D., Oftedal, O. T., and Boness, J. (1985) Birth weaning in 4 days: Remarkable growth in the hooded seal, Cystophora cristata. Can. J. Zool. 63:2841–2846.

138. Bradford, J. M. W. (1988) Treatment of sexual offenders with cyproterone acetate. In J. M. A. Sitse (Ed.), Handbook of Sexology. Vol. 6, The Pharmacology and Endocrinology of Sexual Function. Elsevier, Amsterdam.

139. Bradshaw, W. G., Baum, M. J., and Awh, C. C. (1981) Attenuation by a 5α-reductase inhibitor of the activational effect of testosterone propionate on penile erections in castrated male rats. Endocrinology 109:1047–1051.

140. Brain, P. F. (1983) Pituitary-gonadal influences on social aggression. In B. B. Svare (Ed.), Hormones and Aggressive Behavior. Plenum, New York, pp. 3–25.

141. Brain, P. F. and Evans, C. M. (1975) Attempts to influence fighting and threat behaviors in adult isolated female CFW mice in standard opponent aggression tests using injected and subcutaneously implanted androgens. Physiol. Behav. 14:551–556.

142. Brain, P. F., Simon, V., Hasan, S., Martinez, M., and Castano, D. (1988) The potential of anti-estrogen as centrally acting anti-hostility agent: Recent animal data. Int. J. Neurosci. 41:169–177.

142a. Breedlove, S. M. (1984) Steroid influences on the development and function of a neuromuscular system. Prog. Brain Res. 61:147–170.

143. Breedlove, S. M. and Arnold, A. A. (1980) Hormone accumulation in a sexually dimorphic motor nucleus of the rat spinal cord. Science 210:564–566.

144. Breedlove, S. M. and Arnold, A. P. (1983) Hormonal control of a developing neuromuscular system. I. Complete demasculinization of the spinal nucleus of the bulbocavernosus in male rats using the anti-androgen flutamide. J. Neurosci. 3:417–423.

145. Breedlove, S. M. and Arnold, A. P. (1983) Hormonal control of a developing neuromuscular system. II. Sensitive periods for the androgen induced masculinization of the rat spinal nucleus of the bulbocavernosus. J. Neurosci. 3:424–432.

146. Brenowitz, E. A. and Arnold, A. P. (1985) Lack of sexual dimorphism in steroid accumulation in vocal control brain regions of duetting song birds. Brain Res. 344:172–175.

147. Brenowitz, E. A., Arnold, A. P., and Levin, R. N. (1985) Neural correlates of female song in tropical duetting birds. Brain Res. 343:104–112.

148. Bridges, R. S. (1990) Endocrine regulation of parental behavior in rodents. In N. A. Krasnegor and R. S. Bridges (Eds.), Mammalian Parenting. Oxford University Press, New York, pp. 93–132.

149. Bridges, R. S. and Goldman, B. D. (1975) Diurnal rhythms in gonadotropins and progesterone in lactating and photoperiod-induced acyclic hamsters. Biol. Reprod. 13:617–622.

150. Bridges, R. S., Numan, M., Ronsheim, P. M., Mann, P. E., and Lupini, C. E. (1990) Central prolactin infusions stimulate maternal behavior in steroid-treated, nulliparous female rats. Proc. Natl. Acad. Sci. U.S.A. 87:8003–8007.

151. Bridges, R. S. and Ronsheim, P. M. (1990) Prolactin (PRL) regulation of maternal behavior in rats: Bromocriptine treatment delays and PRL promotes the rapid onset of behavior. Endocrinology 126:837–848.

151a. Brink, E., Modianos, D., and Pfaff, D. W. (1979) Ablations of epaxial deep back muscles. Effects on lordosis behavior in the female rat. Brain Behav. Evol. 17:67–88.

152. Brockway, B. F. (1965) Stimulation of ovarian development and egg laying by male courtship vocalization in budgerigars (Melopsittacus undulatus). Anim. Behav. 13:575–578.

153. Brockway, B. F. (1967) The influence of vocal behavior on the performer's testicular activity in budgerigar (Melopsittacus undulatus). Wilson Bull. 79:328–334.

154. Brodal, A. (1981) Neurological Anatomy in Relation to Clinical Medicine (3rd ed.). Oxford University Press, New York.

155. Broida, J. and Svare, B. (1984) Sex differences in the activity of mice: Modulation by postnatal gonadal hormones. Horm. Behav. 18:65–78.

156. Bronson, F. H. (1968) Pheromonal influence on mammalian reproduction. In M. Diamond (Ed.), Perspectives in Reproduction and Sexual Behavior. Indiana University Press, Bloomington, pp. 341–361.

157. Bronson, F. H. (1986) Food-restricted, prepubertal, female rats: Rapid recovery of luteinizing hormone pulsing with excess food, and full recovery of pubertal development with gonadotropin-releasing hormone. Endocrinology 118:2483–2487.

158. Bronson, F. H. (1989) Mammalian Reproductive Biology. University of Chicago Press, Chicago.

159. Bronson, F. H. and Desjardins, C. (1968) Aggression in adult mice: Modification by neonatal injections of gonadal hormones. Science 161:705–706.

160. Bronson, F. H. and Desjardins, C. (1970) Neonatal androgen administration and adult aggressiveness in female mice. Gen. Comp. Endocrinol. 15:320–325.

161. Broverman, D. M., Klaiber, E. L., Kobayashi, Y., and Vogel, W. (1968) Roles of activation and inhibition in sex differences in cognitive abilities. Psychol. Rev. 75:23–50.

162. Broverman, D. M., Vogel, W., Klaiber, E. L., Majcher, D., Shea, D., and Paul, V. (1981) Changes in cognitive task performance across the menstrual cycle. J. Comp. Physiol. Psychol. 95:646–654.

163. Brown, R. O., Pulst, S. M., and Mayeri, E. (1989) Neuroendocrine bag cells of Aplysia are activated by bag cell peptide-containing neurons in the pleural ganglion. J. Neurophysiol. 61:1142–1152.

164. Bruce, H. M. (1959) An exteroceptive block to pregnancy in the mouse. Nature 184:105.

165. Brush, F. and Nagase Shain, C. (1989) Endogenous opioids and behavior. In F. Brush and S. Levine (Eds.), Psychoendocrinology. Academic Press, New York, pp. 379–435.

166. Bryden, M. P. (1979) Evidence for sex-related differences in cerebral organization. In M. Wittig and A. C. Petersen (Eds.), Sex-Related Differences in Cognitive Functioning. Academic Press, New York, pp. 121–143.

167. Bull, J. J. and Vogt, R. C. (1979) Temperature dependent sex determination in turtles. Science 206:1186–1188.

168. Bullock, T. H. (1984) Comparative neuroscience holds promise for quiet revolutions. Science 225:473–478.

169. Bullock, T. H. and Horridge, G. A. (1965) Structure and Function in the Nervous Systems of Invertebrates, Vols. I and II. W. H. Freeman, San Francisco, p. 1719.

170. Bunning, E. (1973) The Physiological Clock (3rd ed.), Springer-Verlag, New York, pp. 1–258.

171. Buntin, J. D. (1986) Role of prolactin in avian incubation behavior and care of young: Is there a causal relationship? In B. R. Komisaruk, H. I. Siegel, M.-F. Cheng, and H. H. Feder (Eds.), Reproduction: A Behavioral and Neuroendocrine Perspective. New York Academy of Sciences, New York, pp. 252–267, 474.

172. Buntin, J. D., Cheng, M.-F., and Hansen, E. W. (1977) Effect of parental feeding activity on squab-induced crop sac growth in ring doves (Streptopelia risoria). Horm. Behav. 8:297–308.

173. Buntin, J. D. and Ruzycki, E. M. (1989) Prolactin-induced parental behavior in doves: Characteristics and sites of action. International Conference on Hormones, Brain and Behavior, Liège, Belgium, August 18–23, 1989, pp. 31–32.

174. Buntin, J. D. and Walsh, R. J. (1988) In vivo autoradiographic analysis of prolactin binding in brain and choroid plexus of the domestic ring dove. Cell Tissue Res. 251:105–109.

175. Burghardt, G. M. (1970) Chemical perception in reptiles. In J. W. Johnston, D. G. Moulton, and A. Turk (Eds.), Communication by Chemical Signals. Appleton-Century-Crofts, New York, pp. 241–308.

176. Burris, A. S., Gracely, R. H., Carter, C. S., Sherins, R. J., and Davidson, J. M. (1991) Testosterone therapy is associated with reduced tactile sensitivity in human males. Horm. Behav. 25:195–205.

177. Cahill, G. F., Jr. (1970) Starvation in man. N. Engl. J. Med. 282:668–675.

.77a. Caldwell, G. S. and Glickman, S. E. Unpublished observations.

178. Caldwell, G. S., Glickman, S. E., and Smith, E. R. (1984) Seasonal aggression independent of seasonal testosterone in wood rats. Proc. Natl. Acad. Sci. U.S.A. 81:5255–5257.

179. Caldwell, J. D., Prange, A. J. Jr., and Pedersen, C. A. (1986) Oxytocin facilitates the sexual receptivity of estrogen-treated female rats. Neuropeptides 7:175–189.

180. Camp, D. M., Becker, J. B., and Robinson, T. E. (1986) Sex differences in the effects of gonadectomy on amphetamine-induced rotational behavior in rats. Behav. Neural Biol. 46:491–495.

181. Cardwell, J. R. and Liley, N. R. (1991) Androgen control of social status in males of a wild population of stoplight parrot fish, Sparisoma viride. Horm. Behav. 25:1–18.

182. Cardwell, J. R. and Liley, N. R. (1991) Hormonal control of sex and color change in the stoplight parrot fish, Sparisoma viride (Scaridae). Gen. Comp. Endocrinol. 81:7–20.

183. Carlson, J. R. (1977) The imaginal ecdysis of the cricket (Teleogryllus oceanicus). I. Organization of motor programs and roles of central and sensory control. J. Comp. Physiol. 115:299–317.

184. Carmichael, M. S., Humbert, R., Dixen J., Palmisano, G., Greenleaf, W., and Davidson, J. M. (1987) Plasma oxytocin increases in the human sexual response. J. Clin. Endocrinol. Metabol. 64:27–31.

185. Carr, G. D., Fibiger, M. C., and Phillips, A. G. (1989) Conditioned place preference as a measure of drug reward. In J. M. Liebman and S. J. Cooper (Eds.), The Neuropharmacological Basis of Reward. Oxford Science Publications, Oxford, pp. 264–319.

186. Carson, H. L. (1987) The contribution of sexual behavior to Darwinian fitness. Behav. Genet. 17:597–611.

187. Carter, C. S. (1985) Female sexual behavior. In H. I. Siegel (Ed.), The Hamster: Reproduction and Behavior. Plenum, New York, pp. 173–189.

188. Carter, C. S. (1992) Oxytocin and sexual behavior. Neurosci. Biobehav. Rev., in press.

189. Carter, C. S., Bahr, J. M., and Ramirez, V. D. (1978) Monoamines, estrogen and female sexual behavior in the golden hamster. Brain Res. 144:109–121.

190. Carter, C. S., Getz, L. L., and Cohen-Parsons, M. (1986) Relationships between social organization and behavioral endocrinology in a monogamous mammal. Adv. Study Behav. 16:109–145.

191. Carter, C. S., Williams, J. R., and Witt, D. M. (1990) The biology of social bonding in a monogamous mammal. In J. Balthazart (Ed.), Hormones, Brain and Behaviour in Vertebrates. Karger, Basel, pp. 154–164.

192. Carter, C. S., Witt, D. M., Kolb, B., and Whishaw, I. Q. (1982) Neonatal decortication and adult female sexual behavior. Physiol. Behav. 29:763–766.

193. Casey, M., MacDonald, P., and Simpson, E. (1985) Endocrinological changes of pregnancy. In J. Wilson and D. Foster (Eds.), Textbook of Endocrinology (7th ed.). W. B. Saunders, Philadelphia, pp. 422–437.

194. Chadwick, A. (1977) Comparison of milk-like secretions found in non-mammals. Symp. Zool. Soc. (Lond.) 41:341–358.

195. Chambers, K. C. (1976) Hormonal influences on sexual dimorphism in rate of extinction of a conditioned taste aversion in rats. J. Comp. Physiol. Psychol. 90:851–856.

196. Chambers, K. C. (1985) Sexual dimorphisms as an index of hormonal influences on conditioned food aversion. Ann. N.Y. Acad. Sci. 443:126–144.

197. Chamley, W. A., Buckmaster, J. M., Cerini E., Cummings, I. A., Goding, J. R., Obst, J. M., Williams, A., and Winfield, C. (1973) Changes in levels of progesterone, corticosteroids, estrone, estradiol-17 beta and prolactin in the peripheral plasma of the ewe during late pregnancy and at parturition. Biol. Reprod. 9:30–35.

198. Chang, K. S. F., Chan, S. T., Low, W. D., and Ng, C. K. (1963) Climate and conception rates in Hong Kong. Hum. Biol. 35:366–376.

199. Cheng, M.-F. (1979) Progress and prospect in ring dove research: A personal view. In J. S. Rosenblatt, R. A. Hinde, C. G. Beer, and M.-C. Busnel (Eds.), Advances in the Study of Behavior. Academic Press, New York, pp. 97–129.

200. Cheng, M.-F., Desiderio, C., Havens, M., and Johnson, A. (1988) Behavioral stimulation of ovarian growth. Horm. Behav. 22:388–401.

201. Cheng, M.-F., and Silver, R. (1975) Estrogen-progesterone regulation of nest-building and incubation behavior in ovariectomized ring doves (Streptopelia risoria). J. Comp. Physiol. Psychol. 88:256–263.

202. Cherry, J. A., and Baum, M. J. (1990) Effects of lesions of a sexually dimorphic nucleus in the preoptic/anterior hypothalamic area on the expression of androgen- and estrogen-dependent sexual behaviors in male ferrets. Brain Res. 552:191–203.

203. Chiarello, C., McMahon, M. A., and Schaefer, K. (1989) Visual cerebral lateralization over phases of the menstrual cycle: A preliminary investigation. Brain Cogn. 11:18–36.

204. Chiu, A. Y., Hunkapiller, M. W., Heller, E., Stuart, D. K., Hood, L. E. and Strumwasser, F. (1979) Purification and primary structure of the neuropeptide egg-laying hormone of Aplysia californica. Proc. Natl. Acad. Sci. U.S.A. 76:6656–6660.

205. Chiu, A. Y. and Strumwasser, F. (1984) Two neuronal populations in the head ganglia of Aplysia californica with egg-laying hormone-like immunoreactivity. Brain Res. 294:83–93.

206. Christensen, L. W. and Clemens, L. G. (1975) Blockade of testosterone-induced mounting behavior in the male rat with intracranial application of the aromatase inhibitor, androst-1, 4, 6-triene-3, 17-dione. Endocrinology 97:1545–1551.

207. Christiansen, K. and Knussmann, R. (1987) Sex hormones and cognitive functioning in men. Neuropsychobiology 18:27–36.

208. Chrousos, G., Loriaux, D., and Gold, P. (1988) The concept of stress and its historical development. In G. Chrousos, D. Loriaux, and P. Gold (Eds.), Mechanisms of Physical and Emotional Stress. Plenum, New York, pp. 3–10.

209. Cihak, R., Gutmann, E., and Hanzlikova, V. (1970) Involution and hormone-induced persistance of the muscle sphincter (levator) ani in female rats. J. Anat. 106:93–110.

210. Clark, A. S. and Roy, E. J. (1983) Behavioral and cellular responses to pulses of low doses of estradiol-17β. Physiol. Behav. 30:561–565.

211. Clemens, J. A., Gallo, R. V., Whitmoyer, D. I., and Sawyer, C. H. (1971) Prolactin responsive neurons in the rabbit hypothalamus. Brain Res. 25:371–379.

212. Clemens, L. G., Dohanich, G. and Barr, P. (1983) Cholinergic regulation of feminine sexual behavior in laboratory rats. In J. Balthazart, E. Prove, and R. Gilles (Eds.), Hormones and Behavior in Higher Vertebrates. Springer-Verlag, Berlin, pp. 56–68.

213. Clemens, L. G., Gladue, B. A., and Coniglio, L. P. (1978) Prenatal endogenous androgenic influences on masculine sexual behavior and genital morphology in male and female rats. Horm. Behav. 10:40–53.

214. Clemens, L. G. and Weaver, D. R. (1985) The role of gonadal hormones in the activation of feminine sexual behavior. In N. Adler, D. Pfaff, and R. W. Goy (Eds.), Handbook of Behavioral Neurobiology. Vol. 7, Reproduction. Plenum, New York, pp. 183–227.

215. Cloues, R., Ramos, C., and Silver, R. (1990) Vasoactive intestinal polypeptide-like immunoreactivity during reproduction in doves: Influence of experience and number of offspring. Horm. Behav. 24:215–231.

216. Cohen-Parsons, M. and Carter, C. S. (1988) Males increase progestin receptor binding in brain of female voles. Physiol. Behav. 42:191–197.

217. Cohen-Parsons, M. and Roy, E. J. (1989) Social stimuli augment estrogen receptor binding in preoptic area of female prairie voles. Brain Res. 476:363–366.

218. Coirini, H., Johnson, A. E., and McEwen, B. S. (1989) Estradiol modulation of oxytocin binding in the ventromedial hypothalamic nucleus of male and female rats. Neuroendocrinology 50:193–198.

219. Colby, D. R. and Vandenbergh, J. G. (1979) Regulatory effects of urinary pheromones on puberty in the mouse. Biol. Reprod. 11:268–279.

220. Conaway, C. H. (1971) Ecological adaptation and mammalian reproduction. Biol. Reprod. 4:239–247.

221. Conner, R. L., Constantino, A. P., and Scheuch, G. C. (1983) Hormonal influences on shock-induced fighting. In B. B. Svare (Ed.), Hormones and Aggressive Behavior. Plenum, New York, pp. 119–144.

222. Coulson, J. C. (1966) The influence of the pair bond and age on the breeding biology of the kittywake gull, *Rissa tridactyla*. Anim. Ecol. 35:269–279.

223. Courchesne, E. and Barlow, G. W. (1971) Effect of isolation on components of aggressive and other behavior in the hermit crab, *Pagurus samuelis*. Z. vergl. Physiologie 75:32–48.

224. Cowie, A. T. (1984) Lactation. In C. R. Austin and R. V. Short (Eds.), Reproduction in Mammals. 3. Hormonal Control of Reproduction, Cambridge University Press, New York, pp. 195–231.

225. Cowley, A. W., Jr. (1982) Vasopressin and cardiovascular regulation. In A. C. Guyton and J. E. Hall (Eds.), Cardiovascular Physiology, IV (International Review of Physiology, Vol. 26). University Park Press, Baltimore, pp. 189–242.

226. Crespi, B. J. (1989) Facultative viviparity in a thrips. Nature 337:357–358.

227. Creutzfeldt, O. D., Arnold, P. M., Becker, D., Langenstein, S., Tirsch, W., Wilhelm, H., and Wuttke, W. (1976) EEG changes during spontaneous and controlled menstrual cycles and their correlation with psychological performance. Electroencephalogr. Clin. Neurophysiol. 40:113–131.

228. Crews, D. (1975) Effects of different components of male courtship behaviour on environmentally induced ovarian recrudescence and mating preferences in the lizard, *Anolis carolinensis*. Anim. Behav. 23:349–356.

229. Crews, D. (1975) Psychobiology of reptilian reproduction. Science 189:1059–1065.

230. Crews, D. (1982) On the origin of sexual behavior. Psychoneuroendocrinology 7:259–270.

231. Crews D. (1984) Gamete production, sex hormone secretion, and mating behavior uncoupled. Horm. Behav. 18:22–28.

232. Crews, D. (Ed.) (1987) Psychobiology of Reproductive Behavior. Prentice Hall, Englewood Cliffs.

233. Crews, D. (1991) Trans-seasonal action of androgen in the control of spring courtship in male red-sided garter snakes. Proc. Natl. Acad. Sci. U.S.A. 88:3545–3548.

234. Crews, D., Grassman, M., and Lindzey, J. (1986) Behavioral facilitation of reproduction in sexual and parthenogentic whiptail (*Cnemidophorus*) lizards. Proc. Natl. Acad. Sci. U.S.A. 83:9547–9550.

235. Crews, D. and Moore, M. C. (1986) Evolution of mechanisms controlling mating behavior. Science 231:121–125.

236. Crews, D. and Morgentaler, A. (1979) Effects of intracranial implantation of oestradiol and dihydrotestosterone on the sexual behaviour of the lizard. J. Endocrinol. 82:373–381.

237. Crews, D. and Silver, R. (1985) Reproductive physiology and behavior interactions in nonmammalian vertebrates. In N. Adler, D. Pfaff, and R. W. Goy (Eds.), Handbook of Behavioral Neurobiology, Vol. 7, Reproduction. Plenum, New York, pp. 101–182.
238. Crews, D. and Young, R. (1991) Pseudocopulation in nature in a unisexual whiptail lizard. Anim. Behav. 42:512–514.
238a. Crichton-Browne, J. (1880) On the weight of the brain and its component parts in the insane. Brain 2:42–67.
239. Cunningham, S. T., Rosenblatt, J. S., and Komisaruk, B. R. (1990) Evidence that Caesarian-section-induced ovulation in the rat is mediated by the pelvic and hypogastric nerves. Soc. Neurosci. Abstr. 16:396.
240. Cushman, P. (1972) Sexual behavior in heroin addiction and methadone maintenance. N.Y. State J. Med. 72:1261–1265.
241. Czaja, J. A. (1984) Sex differences in the activational effects of gonadal hormones on food intake and body weight. Physiol. Behav. 33:553–558.
242. Daan, S. and Berde, C. (1978) Two coupled oscillators: Simulations of the circadian pacemaker in mammalian activity rhythms. J. Theor. Biol. 70:297–313.
243. Daan, S. and Pittendrigh, C. S. (1976) A functional analysis of circadian pacemakers in nocturnal rodents. II. The variability of phase response curves. J. Comp. Physiol. 106:253–266.
244. Dacanay, R. J., Mastropaolo, J. P., Olin, D. A., and Riley, A. L. (1984) Sex differences in taste aversion learning: An analysis of the minimal effective dose. Neurobehav. Toxicol. Teratol. 6:9–11.
245. Dallman, M. F. (1984) Viewing the ventromedial hypothalamus from the adrenal gland. Am. J. Physiol. 246:R1–R12.
246. Dallman, M. F., Engeland, W. C., Rose, J. C., Wilkinson, C. W., Shinsako, J. and Siedenburg, F. (1978) Nycthemeral rhythm in adrenal responsiveness to ACTH. Am. J. Physiol. 235:R210–R218.
247. Dalton, K. (1960) Menstruation and accidents. Br. Med. J. 2:1425–1426.
248. Dalton, K. (1968) Ante-natal progesterone and intelligence. Br. J. Psychiat. 114:1377–1382.
249. Dalton, K. (1968) Menstruation and examinations. Lancet 2:1386–1388.
250. Dalton, K. (1976) Prenatal progesterone and educational attainments. Br. J. Psychiat. 129:438–442.
251. Damassa, D. A., Smith, E. R., Tennent, B., and Davidson, J. M. (1977) The relationship between circulating testosterone levels and male sexual behavior in rats. Horm. Behav. 8:275–286.
252. Dark, J., Forger, N. G. and Zucker, I. (1986) Regulation and function of lipid mass during the annual cycle of the golden-mantled ground squirrel. In H. C. Heller, X. J. Musacchia, and L. C. H. Wang (Eds.), Living in the Cold: Physiological and Biochemical Adaptations. Elsevier, New York, pp. 445–451.
253. Dark, J., Ruby, N. F. and Zucker, I. (in press) Increased body fat influences reproduction in juvenile but not adult ground squirrels.
254. Dark, J., Spears, N., Whaling, C. S., Meyer, J. S., Wade, G. N., and Zucker, I. (1990) Long day lengths promote brain growth of meadow voles. Dev. Brain Res. 53:264–269.
255. Dark, J., Stern, J., and Zucker, I. (1989) Adipose tissue dynamics during cyclic weight loss and weight gain of ground squirrels. Am. J. Physiol. 256:R1286–R1292.
256. Dark, J. and Zucker, I. (1985) Seasonal cycles in energy balance: Regulation by light. Ann. N.Y. Acad. Sci. 453:170–181.
256a. Dark, J., Zucker, I., and Wade, G. N. (1983) Photoperiodic regulation of body mass, food intake, and reproduction in meadow voles. Am. J. Physiol. 245:R334–R338.
257. Davidson, J. M. (1966) Activation of male rat's sexual behavior by intracerebral implanatation of androgen. Endocrinology 79:783–794.
258. Davidson, J. M. (1969) Effects of estrogen on the sexual behavior of male rats. Endocrinology 84:1365–1372.
259. Davidson, J. M. (1980) The psychobiology of sexual experience. In J. M. Davidson and R. J. Davidson (Eds.), The Psychobiology of Consciousness. Plenum, New York, pp. 271–332.
260. Davidson, J. M., Camargo, C., and Smith, E. R. (1979) Effects of androgen on sexual behavior in hypogonadal men. J. Clin. Endocrinol. Metab. 48:955–958.
261. Davidson, J. M., Chen, J. J., Crapo, L., Gray, G. D., Greenleaf, W. J., and Catania, J. A. (1983) Hormonal changes and sexual function in aging men. J. Clin. Endocrinol. Metab. 57:71–77.
262. Davidson, J. M., Kwan, M., and Greenleaf, W. (1982) Hormonal replacement and sexuality in men. In J. Bancroft (Ed.), Clinics in Endocrinology and Metabolism. Vol. II, Saunders, London, pp. 599–624.
262a. Davie, J. C. and Baldwin, M. (1967) Radiographic-anatomical study of the massa intermedia. J. Neurosurg. 28:483–487.
263. Davies, I. J. and Ryan, K. J. (1972) Comparative endocrinology of gestation, Vit. Horm. 30:223–279.

264. Davis, F. C., Darrow, J. M., and Menaker, M. (1983) Sex differences in the circadian control of hamster wheel-running activity. Am. J. Physiol. 244:R93–R105.

265. Davis, P. G. and Barfield, R. J. (1979) Activation of masculine sexual behavior by intracranial estradiol benzoate implants in male rats. Neuroendocrinology 28:217–227.

266. DeBold, J. F. and Clemens, L. G. (1978) Aromatization and the induction of male sexual behavior in male, female, and androgenized female hamsters. Horm. Behav. 11:401–413.

267. DeBold, J. F. and Miczek, K. A. (1981) Sexual dimorphism in the hormonal control of aggressive behavior of rats. Pharmacol. Biochem. Behav. 14:89.

268. De Jonge, F. H., Louwerse, A. L., Ooms, M. P. Evers, P., Endert, E., and van de Poll, N. E. (1989) Lesions of the SDN-POA inhibit sexual behavior of male Wistar rats. Brain Res. Bull. 23:483–492.

269. deLacoste, M. C., Holloway, R. L., and Woodward, D. J. (1986) Sex differences in the fetal human corpus callosum. Hum. Neurobiol. 5:93–96.

270. deLacoste, M. C. and Horvath, D. S. (1985) Sex differences in the development of morphological asymmetries in human fetuses. Am. J. Phys. Anthropol. 66:163.

271. deLacoste, M. C., Horvath, D. S., and Woodward, D. J. (in press). Sex differences in the developing human fetal brain. J. Clin. Exp. Neuropsychol.

272. deLacoste-Utamsing, C. and Holloway, R. L. (1982) Sexual dimorphism in the human corpus callosum. Science 216:1431–1432.

273. Demirgoren, S. and Pogun, S. (1990) Asymmetric distribution of estrogen and progesterone receptors in rat brain. Neuroendocrinol. Lett. 12:338.

274. Demski, L. S. (1987) Diversity in reproductive patterns and behavior in teleost fishes. In D. Crews (Ed.), Psychobiology of Reproductive Behavior. Prentice Hall, Englewood Cliffs, pp. 2–27.

275. Denenberg, V. H., Gaulin-Kremer, E., and Gandelman, R. (1973) The development of standard stimulus animals for mouse (Mus musculus) aggression testing by means of olfactory bulbectomy. Anim. Behav. 21:590–598.

276. Deslypere, J. P., Verdonck, L., Vermeulen, A. (1985) Fat tissue: A steroid reservoir and site of steroid metabolism. J. Clin. Endocrinol. Metab. 61:564–570.

277. Deutsch, J. A. (1990) Food intake: Gastric factors. In E. M. Stricker (Ed.), Handbook of Behavioral Neurobiology, Vol. 10. Plenum, New York, pp. 151–182.

278. DeVito, W. J. (1989) Immunoreactive prolactin in the hypothalamus and cerebrospinal fluid of male and female rats. Neuroendocrinology 50:182–186.

279. DeVoogd, T. J., Nixdorf, B., and Nottebohm, F. (1985) Synaptogenesis and changes in synaptic morphology related to acquisition of a new behavior. Brain Res. 329:304–308.

280. DeVoogd, T. J. and Nottebohm, F. (1981) Gonadal hormones induce dendritic growth in the adult avian brain. Science 214:202–204.

281. DeVries, G. J., DeBruin, G. J., Uylings, H. M. B., and Corner, M. A. (1984) Progress in Brain Research: Sex Differences in the Brain. Elsevier, Amsterdam.

282. Dewsbury, D. A. (1979) Description of sexual behavior in research on hormone-behavior interactions. In C. Beyer (Ed.), Endocrine Control of Sexual Behavior. Raven Press, New York, pp. 3–32.

283. Di Paolo, T., Dupont, A., and Daigle, M. (1982) Effect of chronic estradiol treatment on dopamine concentrations in discrete brain nuclei of hypophysectomized female rats. Neurosci. Lett. 32:295–300.

284. Di Paolo, T., Falardeau, P., and Morissette, M. (1988) Striatal D-2 dopamine agonist binding sites fluctuate during the rat estrous cycle. Life Sci. 43:665–672.

285. Di Paolo, T., Poyet, P., and Labrie, F. (1981) Effect of chronic estradiol and haloperidol treatment on striatal dopamine receptors. Eur. J. Pharmacol. 73:105–106.

286. Di Paolo, T., Rouillard, C., and Bedard, P. (1985) 17 beta-Estradiol at a physiological dose acutely increases dopamine turnover in rat brain. Eur. J. Pharmacol. 117:197–203.

287. Diamond, J. (1983) Laboratory, field, and natural experiments. Nature 304:586–587.

288. Diamond, M. (1970) Intromission pattern and species vaginal code in relation to the induction of pseudopregnancy. Science 169:995–997.

289. Diamond, M. (1972) Vaginal stimulation and progesterone in relation to pregnancy and parturition. Biol. Reprod. 6:281–287.

290. Diamond, M. (1982) Sexual identity, monozygotic twins reared in discordant sex roles and a BBC follow-up. Arch. Sex. Behav. 11:181–186.

291. Diamond, M., Diamond, L., and Mast, M. (1972) Visual sensitivity and sexual arousal levels during the menstrual cycle. J. Nerv. Ment. Dis. 155:170–176.

292. Diamond, M., Llacuna, A., and Wong, C. L. (1973) Sex behavior after neonatal progesterone, testosterone, estrogen or antiandrogens. Horm. Behav. 4:73–88.

293. Diamond, M. C., Dowling, G. A., and Johnson, R. E. (1981) Morphologic cerebral cortical asymmetry in male and female rats. Exp. Neurol. 71:261–268.

294. DiCarlo, R. and Muccioli, G. (1981) Presence of specific prolactin binding sites in the rabbit hypothalamus. Life Sci. 28:2299–2307.

295. Dickinson, P. S., Mecsas, C., and Marder, E. (1990) Neuropeptide fusion of two motor-pattern generating circuits. Nature 344:155–158.

296. Dittami, J. P. and Gwinner, E. (1985) Annual cycles in the African stonechat and their relationship to environmental factors. J. Zool. (Lond.) [A] 207:357–370.

297. Dluzen, D. E., Green, M. A., and Ramirez, V. D. (1986) The effect of hormonal condition on dose-dependent amphetamine-stimulated behaviors in the male rat. Horm. Behav. 20:1–6.

297a. Dluzen, D. E. and Ramirez, V. D. (1985) In vitro dopamine release from the rat striatum: diurnal rhythm and its modification by the estrous cycle. Neuroendocrinology 41:97–100.

298. Doherty, P. C., Baum, M. J., and Todd, R. B. (1986) Effects of chronic hyperprolactinemia on sexual arousal and erectile function in male rats. Neuroendocrinology 42:368–375.

299. Dohler, K. D., Hines, M., Coquelin, A., Davis, F., Shryne, J. E., and Gorski, R. A. (1982) Pre- and postnatal influence of diethylstilboestral on differentiation of the sexually dimorphic nucleus in the preoptic area of the female rat brain. Neuroendocrinol. Lett. 4:361.

300. Dominick, O. S. and Truman, J. W. (1984) The physiology of wandering behaviour in Manduca sexta. I. Temporal organization and the influence of the external and internal environments. J. Exp. Biol. 110:35–51.

301. Dominick, O. S. and Truman, J. W. (1985) The physiology of wandering behaviour in Manduca sexta. II. The endocrine control of wandering behaviour. J. Exp. Biol. 117:45–68.

302. Dominick, O. S. and Truman, J. W. (1986) The physiology of wandering behaviour in Manduca sexta. IV. Hormonal induction of wandering behaviour from the isolated nervous system. J. Exp. Biol. 121:133–152.

303. Dornan, W. A. and Malsbury, C. W. (1989) Neuropeptides and male sexual behavior. Neurosci. Biobehav. Rev. 13:1–15.

304. Dorner, G. (1976) Hormones and Brain Differentiation. Elsevier, Amsterdam.

305. Dorner, G., Rohde, W., Stahl, F., Krell, L., and Masius, W. G. (1975) A neuroendocrine predisposition for homosexuality in men. Arch. Sex. Behav. 4:1–8.

306. Doty, R., L., Snyder, P. J., Huggins, G. R., and Lowry, L. D. (1981) Endocrine, cardiovascular, and psychological correlates of olfactory sensitivity changes during the human menstrual cycle. J. Comp. Physiol. Psychol. 95:45–60.

307. Drago, F. and Scapagnini, U. (1986) Hormonal modulation of central dopaminergic transmission. J. Neural. Transm. Suppl. 22:47–54.

308. Drickamer, L. C. (1987) Behavioral aspects of rodent population biology. Am. Zool. 27:953–969.

309. Dryden, G. L. and Anderson, J. N. (1977) Ovarian hormones: Lack of effect on reproductive structures of female Asian musk shrews. Science 197:782–784.

309a. Dudai, Y. (1989) The Neurobiology of Memory. Oxford University Press, New York.

310. Duellman, W. E. and Maness, S. J. (1980) The reproductive behavior of some hylid marsupial frogs. J. Herpetol. 14:213–222.

311. Dunn, A. (1989) Psychoneuroimmunology for the psychoneuroendocrinologist: A review of animal studies of nervous system-immune system interactions. Psychoneuroendocrinology 14:251–274.

312. Dye, J. and Meyer, J. (1986) Control of the electric organ discharge. In T. Bullock and W. Heiligenberg (Eds.), Electroreception. Wiley & Sons, New York, pp. 71–102.

313. Edwards, D. A. (1970) Post-neonatal androgenization and adult aggressive behavior in female mice. Physiol. Behav. 5:465–467.

314. Edwards, D. A. and Herndon, J. (1970) Neonatal estrogen stimulation and aggressive behavior in female mice. Physiol. Behav. 5:993–995.

315. Ehrhardt, A. A. and Baker, S. W. (1974) Fetal androgens, human central nervous system differentiation, and behavior sex differences. In R. C. Friedman, R. M. Richart, and R. L. VandeWiele (Eds.), Sex Differences in Behavior. Wiley & Sons, New York, pp. 33–51.

316. Ehrhardt, A. A., Epstein, R., and Money, J. (1968) Fetal androgens and female gender identity in the early-treated adrenogenital syndrome. Johns Hopkins Med. J. 122:160–167.

317. Ehrhardt, A. A., Evers, K., and Money, J. (1968) Influence of androgen on some aspects of sexually dimorphic behavior in women with the late-treated adrenogenital syndrome. Johns Hopkins Med. J. 123:115–122.

318. Ehrhardt, A. A. and Meyer-Bahlburg, H. F. L. (1981) Effects of prenatal sex hormones on gender-related behavior. Science 211:1312–1318.

319. Ehrhardt, A. A., Meyer-Bahlburg, H. F. L., Rosen, L. R., Feldman, J. F., Veridiano, N. P., Zimmerman, I., and McEwen, B. S. (1985) Sexual orientation after prenatal exposure to exogenous estrogen. Arch. Sex. Behav. 14:57–78.

320. Ehrhardt, A. A. and Money, J. (1967) Progestin-induced hermaphroditism: IQ and psychosexual identity in a study of ten girls. J. Sex Res. 3:83–100.

321. Einon, D. (1980) Spatial memory and response strategies in rats: Age, sex and rearing differences in performance. Q. J. Exp. Psychol. 32:473–489.

322. Eisenberg, J. F., Muckenhirn, N. A., and Rudran, R. (1972) The relationship between ecology and social structure in primates. Science 176:863–874.

323. Ekstrom, R. B., French, J. W., and Harmon, H. H. (Eds.) (1976) Manual for Kit of Factor-Referenced Cognitive Tests. Educational Testing Service, Princeton, N. J.

324. Elkinton, J. R. (1961) Prerequisite of freedom: A hypertonic urine. Ann. Intern. Med. 54:827–831.

325. Elliott, J. A. (1976) Circadian rhythms and photoperiodic time measurement in mammals. Fed. Proc. 35:2339–2346.

326. Engeland, W. C., Shinsako, J., Winget, C. M., Vernikos-Danellis, J. and Dallman, M. F. (1977) Circadian patterns of stress-induced ACTH secretion are modified by corticosterone responses. Endocrinology 100:138–147.

327. Epstein, A. N., Nicolaidis, S., and Miselis, R. (1975) The glucoprivic control of food intake and the glucostatic theory of feeding behavior. In G. J. Mogenson and F. R. Calaresu (Eds.), Neural Integration of Physiological Regulations and Behaviour. University of Toronto Press, Toronto, pp. 148–168.

328. Erdelyi, G. J. (1962) Gynecological survey of female athletes. J. Sports Med. Phys. Fitness 2:174–179.

329. Erpino, M. J. and Chappelle, T. C. (1971) Interactions between androgens and progesterone in mediation of aggression in the mouse. Horm. Behav. 2:265–272.

330. Erskine, M. S. (1987) Serum 5α-androstane-3α, 17β-diol increases in response to paced coital stimulation in cycling female rats. Biol. Reprod. 37:1139–1148.

331. Erskine, M. S., Tobet, S. A., and Baum, M. J. (1988) Effect of birth on plasma testosterone, brain aromatase activity, and hypothalamic estradiol in male and female ferrets. Endocrinology 122:524–530.

332. Everett, J. W., Sawyer, C. H., and Markee, J. E. (1949) A neurogenic timing factor in control of the ovulatory discharge of luteinizing hormone in the cyclic rat. Endocrinology 44:234–250.

333. Everitt, B. J. (1990) Sexual motivation: A neural and behavioral anlaysis of the mechanisms underlying appetitive and copulatory responses of male rats. Neurosci. Biobehav. Rev. 14:217–232.

334. Everitt, B. J., Cador, M., and Robbins, T. W. (1989) Interactions between the amygdala and ventral striatum in stimulus-reward associations: Studies using a second-order schedule of sexual reinforcement. Neuroscience 30:63–75.

335. Everitt, B. J. and Stacey, P. (1987) Studies of instrumental behavior with sexual reinforcement in male rats: II. Effects of preoptic area lesions, castration and testosterone. J. Comp. Psychol. 101:407–419.

336. Ewer, R. F. (1968) Ethology of Mammals. Plenum, New York.

337. Fahrbach, S. E., Morrell, J. I., and Pfaff, D. W. (1984) Oxytocin induction of short-latency maternal behavior in nulliparous, estrogen-primed female rats. Horm. Behav. 18:267–286.

338. Fahrbach, S. E., Morrell, J. I., and Pfaff, D. W. (1985) Possible role for endogenous oxytocin in estrogen-facilitated maternal behavior in rats. Neuroendocrinology 40:526–532.

339. Fahrbach, S. E., Morrell, J. I., and Pfaff, D. W. (1985) Role of oxytocin in the onset of estrogen-facilitated maternal behavior. In J. A. Amico and A. G. Robinson (Eds.), Oxytocin: Clinical and Laboratory Studies. Excerpta Medica, New York, pp. 372–388.

340. Fahrbach, S. E., Morrell, J. I., and Pfaff, D. W. (1986) Effect of varying the duration of pre-test cage habituation on oxytocin induction of short-latency maternal behavior. Physiol. Behav. 37:135–139.

341. Fajans, S. S. and Floyd, J. C., Jr. (1972) Stimulation of islet cell secretion by nutrients and by gastrointestinal hormones released during digestion. In D. F. Steiner and N. Freinkel (Eds.), Handbook of Physiology. Section 7, Endocrinology. Vol. 1, Endocrine Pancreas. American Physiological Society, Washington, D.C., pp. 473–493.

342. Feder, H. H. (1981) Estrous cyclicity in mammals. In N. T. Adler (Ed.), Neuroendocrinology of Reproduction. Plenum, New York, pp. 279–348.

343. Feder, H. H. (1985) Peripheral plasma levels of gonadal steroids in adult male and adult, nonpregnant female mammals. In N. Adler, D. Pfaff, and R. W. Goy (Eds.), Handbook of Behavioral Neurobiology. Vol. 7, Reproduction. Plenum, New York, pp. 299–370.

344. Feder, H. H. and Whalen, R. E. (1965) Feminine behavior in neonatally castrated and estrogen-treated male rats. Science 147:306–307.

345. Federman, D. D. (1967) Abnormal Sexual Development. W. B. Saunders, Philadelphia.

346. Feingold, A. (1988) Cognitive gender differences are disappearing. Am. Pyschol. 43(2):95–103.
347. Feist, D., Florant, G., Greenwood, M. R. C., and Feist, C. (1986) Regulation of energy stores in Arctic ground squirrels: Brown fat thermogeneic capacity, lipoprotein lipase, and pancreatic hormones during fat deposition. In H. C. Heller, X. J. Musacchia, and L. C. H. Wang (Eds.), Living in the Cold: Physiological and Biochemical Adaptations. Elsevier, New York, pp. 281–285.
348. Fentress, J. C., Ryon, J., McCleod, P. J., and Havkin, G. Z. (1986) A multidimensional approach to agonistic behavior in wolves. In H. Frank (Ed.), Man and Wolf: Advances, Issues, and Problems in Captive Wolf Research. Dr. W. Junk Publishers, Dordrecht, The Netherlands.
349. Ferrari, M. and Zakon, H. (1989) The medullary pacemaker nucleus is unnecessary for electroreceptor tuning plasticity in Sternopygus. J. Neurosci. 9:1354–1361.
350. Findlay, A. L. R. and Roth, L. L. (1970) Long-term dissociation of nursing behavior and the condition of the mammary gland in the rabbit. J. Comp. Physiol. Psychol. 72:341–344.
351. Finegan, J., Bartleman, B., Zacher, J., and Mervyn, J. (1989) Prenatal testosterone and development at age 4 years. Presented at the Biennial Meeting of the Society for Research in Child Development, March 7–10, 1989, Kansas City, Missouri, April.
352. Fishman, R. B. and Breedlove, S. M. (1987) Androgen blockade of bulbocavernosus muscle inhibits testosterone-dependent masculinization of spinal motoneurons in newborn female rats. Soc. Neurosci. Abstr. 13:1520.
353. Fishman, R. B. and Breedlove, S. M. (1988) Neonatal androgen maintains sexually dimorphic perineal muscles in the absence of innervation. Muscle Nerve 11:553–560.
354. Fishman, R. B. and Breedlove, S. M. (1988) Sexual dimorphism in the developing nervous system. In E. Meisami and P. Timiras (Eds.), Handbook of Human Growth and Developmental Biology. CRC Press, Boca Raton, Fla.
355. Fishman, R. B., Chism, L., Firestone, G. L., and Breedlove, S. M. (1990) Evidence for androgen receptors in sexually dimorphic perineal muscles of neonatal male rats. Absence of androgen accumulation by the perineal motoneurons. J. Neurobiol. 21:694–705.
356. Fitzgerald, K. M. and Zucker, I. (1976) Circadian organization of the estrous cycle of the golden hamster. Proc. Natl. Acad. Sci. U.S.A. 73:2923–2927.
357. Fitzsimons, J. T. (1972) Thirst. Physiol. Rev. 52:468–571.
358. Flanagan, L. M., Verbalis, J. G., and Stricker, E. M. (1988) Unpublished observations.
359. Flanagan, L. M., Verbalis, J. G., and Stricker, E. M. (1989) Unpublished observations.
360. Flanagan, L. M., Verbalis, J. G., and Stricker, E. M. (1989) Effects of anorexigenic treatments on gastric motility in rats. Am. J. Physiol. 256:R955–R961.
361. Fleming, A. (1986) Psychobiology of rat maternal behavior: How and where hormones act to promote maternal behavior at parturition. Ann. N.Y. Acad. Sci. 474:234–251.
362. Floody, O. R. (1983) Hormones and aggression in female mammals. In B. B. Svare (Ed.), Hormones and Aggressive Behavior. Plenum, New York, pp. 39–89.
363. Florant, G. L., Lawrence, A. K., Williams, K. and Bauman, W. K. (1985) Seasonal changes in pancreatic B-cell function in euthermic yellow-bellied marmots. Am. J. Physiol. 249:R159–R165.
364. Florant, G. L., Tokuyama, K., and Rintoul, D. A. (1989) Carbohydrate and lipid utilization in hibernators. In A. Malan and B. Canguilhem (Eds.), Living in the Cold, II. John Libbey, London, pp. 137–145.
365. Fluharty, S. J. and Epstein, A. N. (1983) Sodium appetite elicited by intracerebroventricular infusion of angiotensin II in the rat. II. Synergistic interaction with systemic mineralocorticoids. Behav. Neurosci. 97:746–758.
366. Fogden, S. C. L. (1971) Mother-young behaviour at grey seal breeding beaches. J. Zool. (Lond.) 164:61–92.
367. Follett, B. K. and Sharp, P. J. (1969) Circadian rhythmicity in photoperiodically induced gonadotrophin release and gonadal growth in the quail. Nature 223:968–971.
368. Forger, N. G. and Breedlove, S. M. (1986) Sexual dimorphism in human and canine spinal cord: Role of early androgen. Proc. Natl. Acad. Sci. U.S.A. 83:7527–7531.
369. Forger, N. G. and Breedlove, S. M. (1987) Seasonal variation in mammalian striated muscle mass and motoneuron morphology. J. Neurobiol. 18:155–165.
370. Foster, R. G., Follett, B. K., and Lythgoe, J. N. (1985) Rhodopsin-like sensitivity of extra-retinal photoreceptors mediating the photoperiodic response in quail. Nature 313:50–52.
371. Fox, B. (1983) Current theory of psychogenic effects on cancer incidence and prognosis. J. Psychosoc. Oncol. 1:17–31.
372. Fox, C., Ismail, A., Love, D., Kirkham, K., and Loraine, J. (1972) Studies on the relation of plasma testosterone levels and human sexual activity. J. Endocrinol. 52:51–58.

373. Frank, L. G. (1986) Social organisation of the spotted hyaena: II. Dominance and reproduction. Anim. Behav. 35:1510–1527.

374. Frank, L. G., Glickman, S. E., and Licht, P. (1991) Fatal sibling aggression, precocial development and androgens in neonatal spotted hyaenas. Science 252:702–704.

375. Frank, L. G., Glickman, S. E., and Zabel, C. J. (1989) Ontogeny of female dominance in the spotted hyaena: Perspectives from nature and captivity. Symp. Zool. Soc. Lond. 61:127–146.

376. Frankenhaeuser, M. (1980) Psychoneuroendocrine approaches to the study of stressful person-environment transactions. In H. Selye (Ed.), Selye's Guide to Stress Research. Van Nostrand, New York, pp. 46–70.

377. Freeman, M. E. (1979) A direct effect of the uterus on the surges of prolactin induced by cervical stimulation in the rat. Endocrinology 105:387–390.

378. French, A. R. (1989) The impact of variations in energy availability on the time spent torpid during the hibernation season. In A. Malan and B. Canguilhem (Eds.), Living in the Cold, II. John Libbey, London, pp. 129–136.

379. Freund-Mercier, M. J., Stoeckel, M. F., Palicios, J. M., Pazos, A., Reichart, J. M., Porte, A., and Richard, P. H. (1987) Pharmacological characteristics and anatomical distribution of (^{3}H)oxytocin-binding sites in the wistar rat brain studied by autoradiography. Neuroscience 20:615–627.

380. Friedman, H. and Booth-Kewley, S. (1987) The "disease-prone personality": A meta-analytic view of the construct. Am. Psychol. 42:539–555.

381. Friedman, J. and Meares, R. A. (1978) Comparison of spontaneous and contraceptive menstrual cycles on a visual discrimination task. Aust. N.Z. J. Psychiat. 12:233–239.

382. Friedman, M. B. (1977) Interactions between visual and vocal courtship stimuli in the neuroendocrine response of female doves. J. Comp. Physiol. Psychol. 91:1408–1416.

383. Friedman, M. I. (1978) Hyperphagia in rats with experimental diabetes mellitus: A response to a decreased supply of utilizable fuels. J. Comp. Physiol. Psychol. 92:109–117.

384. Friedman, M. I. and Stricker, E. M. (1976) The physiological psychology of hunger: A physiological perspective. Psychol. Rev. 83:409–431.

385. Fuchs, A.-R. (1973) Parturition in rabbits and rats. In A. Klopper and J. Gardner (Eds.), Endocrine Factors in Labour. Memoirs of the Society for Endocrinology, Cambridge University Press, Cambridge, pp. 163–183.

386. Galea, L. and Kimura, D. (1991) Sex differences in route learning. University of Western Ontario Department of Psychology Research Bulletin #700.

387. Gamberale, F. (1985) Effects of menstruation on work performance. Ergonomics 28:119–123.

388. Gandelman, R. (1980) Determinants of maternal aggression in mice. In R. W. Bell and W. P. Smotherman (Eds.), Maternal Influences and Early Behavior. Spectrum, New York, pp. 87–104.

389. Garcia, J., Hankins, W. G., and Rusiniak, K. W. (1974) Behavioral regulation of the milieu interne in man and rat. Science 185:824–831.

390. Gardiner, T. W., Jolley, J. R., Vagnucci, A. H., and Stricker, E. M. (1986) Enhanced sodium appetite in rats with lesions centered upon nucleus medianus. Behav. Neurosci. 100:531–535.

391. Gardiner, T. W., Verbalis, J. G., and Stricker, E. M. (1985) Impaired secretion of vasopressin and oxytocin in rats after lesions of nucleus medianus. Am. J. Physiol. 249:R681–R688.

392. Garrick, N. A., Hill, J. L., Szele, F. G., Tomai, T. P., Gold, P. W., and Murphy, D. L. (1987) Corticotropin-releasing factor: A marked circadian rhythm in primate cerebrospinal fluid peaks in the evening and is inversely related to the cortisol circadian rhythm. Endocrinology 121:1329–1334.

393. Gaulin, S. J. C. and Fitzgerald, R. W. (1986) Sex differences in spatial ability: An evolutionary hypothesis and test. Am. Naturalist 127:74–88.

394. Gaulin, S. J. C, FitzGerald, R. W., and Wartell, M. S. (1990) Sex differences in spatial ability and activity in two vole species (Microtus ochrogaster and M. pennsylvanicus). J. Comp. Psychology. 104:88–93.

395. Gentsch, C., Lichtesteiner, M., and Feer, H. (1988) Genetic and environmental influences on behavioral and neurochemical aspects of emotionality in rats. Experientia 44:482–499.

396. Gerendai, I., Rotsztejn, W., Marchett, B., Kordon, C., and Scapagnini, U. (1978) Unilateral ovariectomy-induced luteinizing hormone-releasing hormone content changes in the two halves of the mediobasal hypothalamus. Neurosci. Lett. 9:333–336.

397. Geschwind, N. and Galaburda, A. M. (1985) Cerebral Lateralization. Biological Mechanisms, Associations, and Pathology. MIT Press, Cambridge.

398. Ghiselin, M. T. (1974) The Economy of Nature and the Evolution of Sex. University of California Press, Berkeley.

399. Gibbs, J. and Smith, G. P. (1986) Satiety: The roles of peptides from the stomach and the intestine. Fed. Proc. 45:1391–1395.

400. Gibori, G., Richards, J. S., and Keyes, P. L. (1979) Synergistic effects of prolactin and estradiol in the luteotropic process in the pregnant rat: Regulation of estradiol receptor by prolactin. Biol. Reprod. 21:419–423.

401. Giebultowicz, J. M., Zdarek, J. and Chroscikowska, U. (1980) Cocoon spinning behavior in *Ephestia kuehniella*: Correlation with endocrine events. J. Insect Physiol. 26:459–464.

402. Ginsburg, B. and Allee, W. C. (1942) Some effects of conditioning on social dominance and subordination in inbred strains of mice. Physiol. Zool. 15:485–506.

403. Giordano, A. L., Ahdieh, H. B., Mayer, A. D., Siegel, H. I., and Rosenblatt, J. S. (1990) Cytosol and nuclear estrogen receptor binding in the preoptic area and hypothalamus of female rats during pregnancy and ovariectomized rats after steroid priming correlation with maternal behavior. Horm. Behav. 24:231–255.

404. Giordano, A. L., Siegel, H. I., and Rosenblatt, J. S. (1989) Nuclear estrogen receptor binding in the preoptic area and hypothalamus of pregnancy-terminated rats: Correlation with the onset of maternal behavior. Neuroendocrinology 50:248–258.

405. Giordano, A. L., Siegel, H. I., and Rosenblatt, J. S. (1991) Nuclear estrogen receptor binding in microdissected brain regions of female rats during pregnancy. Physiol. Behav. 50:1263–1267.

406. Gladue, B. A., Green, R., and Hellman, R. E. (1984) Neuroendocrine response to estrogen and sexual orientation. Scienc 225:1496–1499.

407. Glickman, S. E. and Caldwell, G. S. (in press) Studying natural behaviors in artificial environments: The problem of salient elements. In E. F. Gibbons, Jr., E. W. Menzel, and E. J. Wyers (Eds.), Naturalistic Environments for Animal Behavior Research. State University of New York Press, Albany.

408. Glickman, S. E., Frank, L. G., Davidson, J. M., Smith, E. R., and Siiteri, P. K. (1987) Androstenedione may organize or activate sex-reversed traits in female spotted hyenas. Proc. Natl. Acad. Sci. U.S.A. 84:3444–3447.

409. Goh, H. H., Ratnam, S. S., and London, D. R. (1984) The feminisation of gonadotrophin responses in intact male transsexuals. Clin. Endocrinol. 20:591–596.

410. Goh, H. H., Wong, P. C., and Ratnam, S. S. (1985) Effects of sex steroids on the positive estrogen feedback mechanism in intact women and castrate men. J. Clin. Endocrinol. Metab. 61:1158–1164.

411. Goldfoot, D. A., Kravetz, M. A., Goy, R. W., and Freeman, S. K. (1976) Lack of effect of vaginal lavages and aliphatic acids on ejaculatory responses in rhesus monkeys: Behavioral and chemical analyses. Horm. Behav. 7:1–27.

412. Goldman, B. D. (1989) Photoperiodic control of puberty in hamsters. In S. M. Reppert (Ed.), Development of Circadian Rhythmicity and Photoperiodism in Mammals. Perinatology Press, Ithaca, pp. 193–207.

413. Goldman, B. D. (1989) Effects of photoperiod on the hibernation cycle of the Turkish hamster. In A. Malan and B. Canguilhem (Eds.), Living in the Cold, II. John Libbey, London, pp. 5–15.

414. Goldman, B. D. and Darrow, J. M. (1983) The pineal gland and mammalian photoperiodism. Neuroendocrinology 37:386–396.

415. Goldsmith, A. R. (1982) Plasma concentrations of prolactin during incubation and parental feeding throughout repeated breeding cycles in canaries (*Serinus canarius*). J. Endocrinol. 94:51–59.

416. Goldsmith, A. R. (1983) Prolactin in avian reproductive cycles. In J. Balthazart, E. Prove, and R. Giles (Eds.), Hormones and Behaviour in Higher Vertebrates. Springer-Verlag, Berlin, pp. 375–387.

417. Goldsmith, A. R., Edwards, C., Koprucu, M., and Silver, R. (1981) Concentrations of prolactin and luteinizing hormone in plasma of doves in relation to incubation and development of the crop gland. J. Endocrinol. 90:437–443.

418. Goodman, H. (1980) The pancreas and regulation of metabolism. In V. Mountcastle (Ed.), Medical Physiology (14th ed.). C. V. Mosby, St. Louis, pp. 1638–1676.

419. Gooren, L. (1986) The neuroendocrine response of luteinizing hormone to estrogen administration in heterosexual, homosexual, and transsexual subjects. J. Clin. Endocrinol. Metab. 63:583–588.

420. Gooren, L. (1986) The neuroendocrine response of luteinizing hormone to estrogen administration in the human is not sex specific but dependent on the hormonal environment. J. Clin. Endocrinol. Metab. 63:589–593.

421. Gordon, H. W. and Lee, P. A. (1986) A relationship between gonadotropins and visuospatial function. Neuropsychologia 24:563–576.

422. Gorospe, W. C. and Freeman, M. E. (1981) An ovarian role in prolonging and terminating the two surges of prolactin in pseudopregnant rats. Endocrinology 108:1293–1298.

423. Gorski, R. A. (1984) Critical role for the medial preoptic area in the sexual differentiation of the brain. Prog. Brain Res. 61:129.

424. Gorski, R. A., Gordon, J. H., Shryne, J. E., and Southam, A. M. (1978) Evidence for a morphological sex difference within the medial preoptic area of the rat brain. Brain Res. 143:333–346.
425. Gouchie, C. T. (1990) The relation between testosterone concentrations and cognitive performance in humans. Unpublished M. A. Thesis, University of Western Ontario, August.
426. Gouchie, C. T. and Kimura, D. (1991) The relationship between testosterone levels and cognitive ability patterns. Psychoneuroendocrinology 16:323–334.
427. Gould, E., Westlind-Danielsson, E., Frankfurt, M., and McEwen, B. S. (1990) Sex differences and thyroid hormone sensitivity of hippocampal pyramidal cells. J. Neurosci. 10:996–1003.
428. Gould, E., Wooley, C. S., Frankfurt, M., and McEwen, B. S. (1990) Gonadal steroids regulate dendritic spine density in hippocampal pyramidal cells in adulthood. J. Neurosci. 10:1288–1291.
429. Gould, S. J. (1981) The Mismeasure of Man. Norton, New York.
430. Gould, S. J. and Vrba, E. S. (1982) Exaptation—a missing term in the science of form. Paleobiology 8:4–15.
431. Goy, R. W., Bercovitch, F. B., and McBrair, M. C. (1988) Behavioral masculinization is independent of genital masculinization in prenatally androgenized female rhesus macaques. Horm. Behav. 22:552–571.
432. Goy, R. W. and McEwen, B. S. (1980) Sexual Differentiation of the Brain. MIT Press, Cambridge.
433. Goy, R. W. and Phoenix, C. H. (1971) The effects of testosterone proprionate administered before birth on the development of behavior in genetic female rhesus monkeys. In C. H. Sawyer and R. A. Gorski (Eds.), Steroid Hormones and Brain Function. University of California Press, Berkeley.
434. Goy, R. W. and Resko, J. A. (1972) Gonadal hormones and behavior of normal and pseudohermaphroditic female primates. Recent Prog. Horm. Res. 28:707–733.
435. Graham, C. A. and McGrew, W. C. (1980) Menstrual synchrony in female undergraduates living on a coeducational campus. Psychoneuroendocrinology 5:245–252.
436. Graham, E. A. and Glasser, M. (1985) Relationship of pregnanediol level to cognitive behavior and mood. Psychosom. Med. 47:26–34.
437. Grant, E. C. and Mackintosh, J. H. (1963) A comparison of the social postures of some common laboratory rodents. Behaviour 21:246–259.
438. Gray, G. D., Smith, E. R., and Davidson, J. M. (1980) Hormonal regulation of penile erection in castrated male rats. Physiol. Behav. 24:463–468.
439. Greenough, W. T. (1986) What's special about development? Thoughts on the bases of experience-sensitive synaptic plasticity. In W. T. Greenough and J. M. Juraska (Eds.), Developmental Neuropsychobiology. Academic Press, New York, pp. 387–407.
440. Greenwald, G. S. (1965) Histologic transformation of the ovary of the lactating hamster. Endocrinology 77:641–650.
441. Greenwald, G. S. (1985) Endocrinology of the pregnant hamster. In H. I. Siegel (Ed.), The Hamster. Plenum, New York, pp. 53–72.
442. Gregory, E. and Pritchard, W. S. (1983) The effects of neonatal androgenization of female hamsters on adult preferences for female hamster vaginal discharge. Physiol. Behav. 31:861–864.
443. Grimmelikhuijzen, C. J. P. (1986) FMRFamide-like peptides in the primitive nervous systems of coelenterates and complex nervous systems of higher animals. In G. B. Stefano (Ed.), Handbook of Comparative Opioid and Related Neuropeptide Mechanisms. CRC Press, Boca Raton, pp. 103–115.
444. Gross, M. R. (1984) Sunfish, salmon, and the evolution of alternative reproductive strategies and tactics in fishes. In G. W. Potts and R. J. Wooten (Eds.), Fish Reproduction: Strategies and Tactics. Academic Press, New York, pp. 55–75.
445. Gruendel, A. D. and Arnold, W. J. (1969) Effects of early social deprivation on reproductive behavior of male rats. J. Comp. Physiol. Psychol. 67:123–128.
446. Grunt, J. A., and Young, W. C. (1952) Differential reactivity of individuals and the response of the male guinea pig to testosterone propionate. Endocrinology 51:237–248.
447. Gurney, M. E. (1981) Hormonal control of cell form and number in the zebra finch song system. J. Neurosci. 1:658–673.
448. Gustafson, J. E. and Crews, D. (1981) Effect of group size and physiological state of a cagemate on reproductive effort in the parthenogenetic lizard Chemidophorus uniparens (Teiidae). Behav. Ecol. Sociobiol. 8:267–272.
449. Gwinner, E. (1986) Circannual Rhythms: Endogenous Annual Clocks in the Organization of Seasonal Processes. Springer-Verlag, Berlin.
450. Gysling, K., and Wang, R. Y. (1983) Morphine-induced activation of A10 dopamine neurons in the rat. Brain Res. 277:119–127.

451. Hackman, B. W. and Galbraith, D. (1976) Replacement therapy with piperazine oestrone sulphate ("Harmogen") and its effect on memory. Curr. Med. Res. Opin. 4:303–306.

452. Hagedorn, M. (1986) The ecology, courtship and mating of gymnotiform electric fish. In T. Bullock and W. Heiligenberg (Eds.), Electroreception. Wiley & Sons, New York, pp. 497–527.

453. Halpern, D. F. (1986) Sex Differences in Cognitive Abilities. Lawrence Erlbaum Associates, Hillsdale, N.J.

454. Hamilton, W. J., Tilson, R. L., and Frank, L. G. (1986) Sexual monomorphism in spotted hyenas, Crocuta crocuta. Ethology 71:63–73.

455. Hampson, E. (1990) Variations in sex-related cognitive abilities across the menstrual cycle. Brain Cogn. 14:26–43.

456. Hampson, E. (1990) Estrogen-related variations in human spatial and articulatory-motor skills. Psychoneuroendocrinology 15:97–111.

457. Hampson, E. and Kimura, D. (1988) Reciprocal effects of hormonal fluctuations on human motor and preceptual-spatial skills. Behav. Neurosci. 102:456–459.

458. Hannigan, P. and Kelley, D. (1986) Androgen-induced alterations in vocalizations of female Xenopus laevis: Modifiability and constraints. J. Comp. Physiol. [A] 158:517–528.

459. Hansen, S. and Drake af Hagelsrum, L. J. K. (1984) Emergence of displacement activities in the male rat following the thwarting of sexual behavior. Behav. Neurosci. 98:868–883.

460. Hansen, S., Kohler, C., Goldstein, M., and Steinbusch, H. W. M. (1982) Effects of ibotenic acid-induced neuronal degeneration in the medial preoptic and lateral hypothalamic area on sexual behavior in the male rat. Brain Res. 239:213–232.

461. Harder, J. D. and Fleming, M. W. (1981) Estradiol and progesterone profiles indicate a lack of endocrine recognition of pregnancy in the opossum. Science 212:1400–1402.

462. Hardie, J. and Lees, A. D. (1985) Endocrine control of polymorphism and polyphenism. In G. A. Kerkut and L. I. Gilbert (Eds.), Comprehensive Insect Physiology, Biochemistry, and Pharmacology, Vol. 8. Pergamon Press, Oxford, pp. 441–490.

463. Harding, C. F. (1983) Hormonal specificity and activation of social behavior in the male zebra finch. In J. Balthazart, E. Prove, and R. Gilles (Eds.), Hormones and Behaviour in Higher Vertebrates. Springer-Verlag, Berlin, pp. 275–289.

464. Harlan, R. E., Shivers, B. D., Fox, S. R., Schachter, B. S., Kaplover, K. A., and Pfaff, D. W. (1989) Distribution and partial characterization of immunoreactive prolactin in the rat brain. Neuroendocrinology 49:7–22.

465. Harris, G. W. (1964) Sex hormones, brain development and brain function. Endocrinology 75:627–648.

466. Harris, G. W. and Jacobson, D. (1952) Functional grafts of the anterior pituitary gland. Proc. R. Soc. [Biol.] 139:263–276.

467. Harshman, R. A., Hampson, E., and Berenbaum, S. A. (1983) Individual differences in cognitive abilities and brain organization. Part I: Sex and handedness differences in ability. Can. J. Psychol. 37:144–192.

468. Harshman, R. A. and Remington, R. (1976) Sex, language, and the brain. Part I: A review of the literature on adult sex differences in lateralization. UCLA Working Papers in Phonetics 31:86–103.

469. Hart, B. L. (1967) Testosterone regulation of sexual reflexes in spinal male rats. Science 155:1283–1284.

470. Hart, B. L. (1967) Sexual reflexes and mating behavior in the male dog. J. Comp. Physiol. Psychol. 64:388–399.

471. Hasan, S. A., Brain, P. F., and Castano, D. (1988) Studies on effects of tamoxifen (ICI 46474) on agonistic encounters between pairs of intact mice. Horm. Behav. 22:178–185.

472. Haskell, P. T. and Moorhouse, J. E. (1963) A blood-borne factor influencing the activity of the central nervous system of the desert locust. Nature 197:56–58.

473. Hatton, G. I. (1988) Cellular reorganization in neuroendocrine secretion. In D. Ganten and D. Pfaff (Eds.), Current Topics in Neuroendocrinology, Vol. 9. Springer-Verlag, Berlin, pp. 1–27.

474. Haug, M., Brain, P. F., and Kamis, A. B. (1986) A brief review comparing the effects of sex steroids on two forms of aggression in laboratory mice. Neurosci. Biobehav. Rev. 10:463–468.

475. Heap, R. B. and Flint, A. P. F. (1986) Pregnancy. In C. R. Austin and R. V. Short (Eds.), Hormonal Control of Reproduction (2nd ed.). Cambridge University Press, Cambridge, pp. 153–194.

476. Heimer, L. and Larsson, K. (1966/67) Impairment of mating behavior in male rats following lesions in the preoptic-anterior hypothalamic continuum. Brain Res. 3:248–263.

477. Heinsbroek, R. P., Feenstra, M. G., Boon, P., Van Haaren, F., and van de Poll, N. E. (1988) Sex differences in passive avoidance depend on the integrity of the central serotonergic system. Pharmacol. Biochem. Behav. 31:499–503.

478. Heinsbroek, R. P., van Haaren, F., and van de Poll, N. E. (1988) Sex differences in passive avoidance behavior of rats: Sex-dependent susceptibility to shock-induced behavioral depression. Physiol. Behav. 43:201–206.

479. Heinsbroek, R. P., van Haaren, F., Zantvoord, F., and van de Poll, N. E. (1987) Sex differences in response rates during random ratio acquisition: Effects of gonadectomy. Physiol. Behav. 39:269–272.

480. Heinsbroek, R. P., van Oyen, H., and van de Poll, N. E. (1984) The pituitary-adrenocortical system is not involved in the sex difference in passive avoidance. Pharmacol. Biochem. Behav. 20:663–668.

481. Heinsbroek, R. P., van Oyen, H., van de Poll, N. E., and Boer, G. J. (1983) Failure of dexamethasone to influence sex differences in acquisition of discriminated lever press avoidance. Pharmacol. Biochem. Behav. 19:599–604.

482. Heister, G., Landis, T., Regard, M., and Schroeder-Heister, P. (1989) Shift of functional cerebral asymmetry during the menstrual cycle. Neuropsychologia 27:871–880.

483. Hendricks, S. E., Graber, B., and Rodriguez-Sierra, J. F. (1989) Neuroendocrine responses to exogenous estrogen: No differences between heterosexual and homosexual men. Psychoneuroendocrinology 14:177–185.

484. Herrenkohl, L. R., and Fixenmaier-Campbell, C. (1976) Mechanical stimulation of mammary gland development in virgin and pregnant rats. Horm. Behav. 7:183–198.

485. Herrmann, K. and Arnold, A. P. (1988) Effect of HVc lesions on estradiol-induced masculinization of zebra finch song system. Soc. Neurosci. Abstr. 14:289.

486. Hewes, R. S. and Truman, J. W. (1991) Role of central and peripheral peptide release in the control of ecdysis behavior in *Manduca sexta*. J. Comp. Physiol. [A]

487. Hier, D. B. and Crowley, W. F. (1982) Spatial ability in androgen-deficient men. N. Engl. J. Med. 306:1201–1205.

488. Hinde, R. A. (1965) The integration of internal and external factors in integration of canary reproduction. In F. A. Beach (Ed.), Sex and Behavior. Wiley & Sons, New York, pp. 381–415.

489. Hines, M. (1982) Prenatal gonadal hormones and sex differences in human behavior. Psychol. Bull. 92:56–80.

490. Hines, M. (1991) Gonadal hormones and human cognitive development. In J. Balthazart (Ed.), Hormones, Brain and Behavior in Vertebrates. Karger, Basel.

491. Hines, M. and Shipley, C. (1984) Prenatal exposure to diethylstilbestrol (DES) and the development of sexually dimorphic cognitive abilities and cerebral lateralization. Devel. Psychol. 20:81–94.

492. Hoffmann, J. A. and Hetru, C. (1983) Ecdysone. In R. G. H. Downer and H. Laufer (Eds.), Endocrinology of Insects. Alan R. Liss, New York, pp. 65–88.

493. Hoffmann, K. (1981) The role of the pineal gland in the photoperiodic control of seasonal cycles in hamsters. In B. K. Follett and D. K. Follett (Eds.), Biological Clocks in Reproductive Cycles. John Wright, Bristol, pp. 237–250.

494. Hohn, E. O. (1962) A possible endocrine basis of brood parasitism. Ibis 104:418–421.

495. Holekamp, K. and Smale, L. (1992) Dominance acquisition during mammalian social development: The "inheritance" of maternal rank. Am. Zool., in press.

496. Holloway, R. L. and deLacoste, M. C. (1986) Sexual dimorphism in the human corpus callosum: An extension and replication study. Hum. Neurobiol. 5:87–91.

497. Hood, K. E. (1984) Aggression among female rats during the estrous cycle. In K. J. Flannelly, R. J. Blanchard, and D. C. Blanchard (Eds.), Biological Perspectives on Aggression. Alan R. Liss, New York.

498. Hood, K. E. (1988) Female aggression in albino ICR mice: Development, social experience, and the effects of selective breeding (*Mus musculus*). Int. J. Comp. Psychol. 2(1):27–41.

499. Hood, K. E. and Cairns, R. B. (1988) A developmental-genetic analysis of aggressive behavior in mice. II. Cross-sex inheritance. Behav. Genet. 18:605–619.

500. Hopkins, C. (1972) Sex differences in signalling in an electric fish. Science 176:1035–1037.

501. Hopkins, C. (1974) Electric communication in the reproductive behavior of *Sternopygus macrurus*. Z. Tierpsychol. 35:518–535.

502. Hopkins, C. (1986) Behavior of mormyridae. In T. Bullock and W. Heiligenberg (Eds.), Electroreception. Wiley & Sons, New York, pp. 527–576.

503. Hopkins, C. (1988) Neuroethology of electric communication. Annu. Rev. Neurosci. 11:497–536.

504. House, J., Landis, K., and Umberson, D. (1988) Social relationships and health. Science 241:540–544.

505. Hoyle, G. (1970) Cellular mechanisms underlying behavior—neuroethology. Adv. Insect Physiol. 7:349–444.

506. Hruska, R. E., Ludmer, L. M., Pitman, K. T., De Ryck M., and Silbergeld, E. K. (1982) Effects of estrogen on striatal dopamine receptor function in male and female rats. Pharmacol. Biochem. Behav. 16:285–291.

507. Hruska, R. E. and Silbergeld, E. K. (1980) Estrogen treatment enhances dopamine receptor sensitivity in the rat striatum. Eur. J. Pharmacol. 61:397–400.

508. Hudson, R. and Distel, H. (1984) Nipple search pheromone in rabbits: Dependence on season and reproductive state. J. Comp. Physiol. 155:13–17.

509. Hughes, A. M., Everitt, B. J., and Herbert, J. (1988) The effects of simultaneous or separate infusions of some pro-opiomelanocortin-derived peptides (beta-endorphin, melanocyte stimulating hormone and corticotrophin-like intermediate polypeptide) and their acetylated derivatives upon sexual and ingestive behavior of male rats. Neuroscience 27:689–698.

510. Hughes, A. M., Everitt, B. J., Lightman, S. L, and Todd, K. (1987) Oxytocin in the CNS and sexual behavior in male rats. Brain Res. 414:133–137.

511. Hughes, A. M., Herbert, J., and Everitt, B. J. (1990) Comparative effects of preoptic area infusions of opioid peptides, lesions and castration on sexual behavior in male rats: Studies of instrumental behavior, conditioned place preference and partner preference. Psychopharmacology 102:243–256.

512. Hughes, R. N. (1983) Menstrual cycle influences on perceptual disembedding ability. Percept. Mot. Skills 57:107–110.

513. Hughes, T. D. (1980) The imaginal ecdysis of the desert locust, *Schistocerca gregaria*. I. Description of the behaviour. Physiol. Entomol. 5:47–54.

514. Hutchison, R. E. (1975) Effects of ovarian steroids and prolactin on the sequential development of nesting behavior in female budgerigars. J. Endocrinol. 67:29–39.

515. Hutt, S. J., Frank, G., Mychalkiw, W., and Hughes, M. (1980) Perceptual-motor performance during the menstrual cycle. Horm. Behav. 14:116–125.

516. Hyde, J. S., Fennema, E., and Lamon, S. J. (1990) Gender differences in mathematics performance: A meta-analysis. Psychol. Bull. 107:139–155.

517. Hyde, J. S. and Linn, M. C. (1988) Gender differences in verbal ability: A meta-analysis. Psychol. Bull. 104:53–69.

518. Hyde, J. S. and Sawyer, T. F. (1977) Estrous cycle fluctions in aggressiveness of house mice. Horm. Behav. 9:290–295.

519. Imperato-McGinley, J., Guerrero, L., Gautier, T., and Peterson, R. E. (1974) Steroid 5-alpha-reductase deficiency in man: An inherited form of male pseudohermaphroditism. Science 186:1213–1215.

520. Imperato-McGinley, J., Peterson, R. E., Gautier, T., and Sturla, E. (1979) Androgens and the evolution of male-gender identity among male pseudohermaphrodites with 5-alpha-reductase deficiency. N. Engl. J. Med. 300:1233–1237.

521. Ingles, L. G. (1965) Mammals of the Pacific States. Stanford University Press, Stanford.

522. Inglis, J. and Lawson, J. S. (1981) Sex differences in the effects of unilateral brain damage on intelligence. Science 212:693–695.

523. Inglis, J., Ruckman, M., Lawson, J. S., MacLean, A. W., Monga, T. N. (1982) Sex differences in the cognitive effects of unilateral brain damage. Cortex 18:257–276.

524. Insel, T. R. (1990) Oxytocin and maternal behavior. In N. E. Krasnegor and R. S. Bridges (Eds.), Mammalian Parenting. Oxford University Press, New York, pp. 260–280.

525. Ivey, M. E. and Bardwick, J. M. (1968) Patterns of affective fluctuation in the menstrual cycle. Psychosom. Med. 30:336–345.

526. Jacklin, C. N., Wilcox, K. T., Maccoby, E. E. (1988) Neonatal sex-steroid hormones and cognitive abilities at six years. Dev. Psychobiol. 21:567–574.

527. Jacobs, L. F., Gaulin, S. J. C., Sherry, D. F., and Hoffman, G. E. (1990) Evolution of spatial cognition: Sex-specific patterns of spatial behavior predict hippocampal size. Proc. Natl. Acad. Sci. U.S.A. 87:6349–6352.

528. Jacobson, C. D. and Gorski, R. A. (1981) Neurogenesis of the sexually dimorphic nucleus of the preoptic area in the rat. J. Comp. Neurol. 196:519–529.

529. Jacobson, C. D., Shryne, J. E., Shapiro, R., and Gorski, R. A. (1980) Ontogeny of the sexually dimorphic nucleus of the preoptic area. J. Comp. Neurol. 193:541.

530. Jarvik, L. F. (1975) Human intelligence: Sex differences. Acta Genet. Med. Gemellol. 24:189–211.

531. Jensen, A. R. (1988) Sex differences in arithmetic computation and reasoning in prepubertal boys and girls. Behav. Brain Sci. 11:198–199.

532. Jensen, B. K. (1982) Menstrual cycle effects on task performance examined in the context of stress research. Acta Psychologia 50:159–178.

533. Johns, J. E. and Pfeiffer, E. W. (1963) Testosterone-induced incubation patches of phalarope birds. Science 140:1225–1226.

534. Johnson, A. E., Coirini, H., McEwen, B. S., and Insel, T. R. (1989) Testosterone modulates oxytocin binding in the hypothalamus of castrated male rats. Neuroendocrinology 50:199–203.

535. Johnson, M. H. and Everitt, B. J. (1984) Essential Reproduction (2nd ed.). Blackwell Scientific Publications, Oxford.

536. Johnston, P. and Davidson, J. M. (1972) Intracerebral androgens and sexual behavior in the male rat. Horm. Behav. 3:345–357.

537. Johnston, R. E. (1990) Chemical communication in golden hamsters: From behavior to molecules and neural mechanisms. In D. A. Dewsbury (Ed.), Contemporary Issues in Comparative Psychology. Sinauer Associates, Sunderland, Mass., pp. 381–409.

538. Johnston, R. E., Zahorick, D. M., Immler, K., and Zakon, H. (1978) Attractions of male sexual behavior by learned aversions to hamster vaginal sections. J. Comp. Physiol. Psychol. 92:85–93.

539. Jones, H. E. (1947) Sex differences in physical abilities. Hum. Biol. 19:12–25.

540. Jones, R. E. (1971) The incubation patch of birds. Biol. Rev. 46:315–339.

541. Jonescu, C. N. (1909) Vergleichende Untersuchungen über das Gehirn der Honigbiene. Jena Z. Naturw. 45:111–180.

542. Jost, A. (1979) Basic sexual trends in the development of vertebrates. In Ciba Foundation Symposium, No. 62. Sex, Hormones and Behavior. Elsevier, Amsterdam.

543. Joyce, J. N. and Van Hartesveldt, C. (1984) Behaviors induced by intrastriatal dopamine vary independently across the estrous cycle. Pharmacol. Biochem. Behav. 20:551–557.

544. Joyce, J. N. and Van Hartesveldt, C. (1984) Estradiol application to one striatum produces postural deviation to systemic apomorphine. Pharmacol. Biochem. Behav. 20:575–581.

545. Juraska, J. M. (1984) Sex differences in dendritic response to differential experience in the rat visual cortex. Brain Res. 295:27–34.

546. Juraska, J. M. (1986) Sex differences in developmental plasticity of behavior and brain. In W. T. Greenough and J. M. Juraska (Eds.), Developmental Neuropsychobiology. Academic Press, New York.

547. Juraska, J. M. (1991) Sex differences in "cognitive" regions of the rat brain. Psychoneuroendocrinology (in press).

548. Juraska, J. M., Fitch, J., and Washburne, D. L. (1989) The dendritic morphology of pyramidal neurons in the rat hippocampal CA3 area. II. Effects of gender and the environment. Brain Res. 479:115–119.

549. Kafatos, F. C. and Williams, C. M. (1964) Enzymatic mechanism for the escape of certain moths from their cocoons. Science 146:538–540.

550. Kalin, N. H., Shelton, S. E., Barksdale, C. M. and Brownfield, M. S. (1987) A diurnal rhythm in cerebrospinal fluid corticotropin-releasing hormone different from the rhythm of pituitary-adrenal activity. Brain Res. 426:385–391.

551. Kamimura, K. (1976) Epidemiology of twin births from a climatic point of view. Br. J. Prev. Soc. Med. 30:175–179.

552. Kanatani, H. and Nagahama, Y. (1980) Mediators of oocyte maturation. Biomed. Res. 1:273–291.

553. Kandel, E. R. and Schwartz, J. H. (1985) Principles of Neural Science. Elsevier Science Publications, New York.

554. Kaneko, M., Kaneko, K., Shinsako, J. and Dallman, M. F. (1981) Adrenal sensitivity to adrenocorticotropin varies diurnally. Endocrinology 109:70–75.

555. Katchadourian, H. (1977) The Biology of Adolescence. W. H. Freeman, San Francisco.

556. Kato, J. (1985) Progesterone receptors in brain and hypophysis. In D. Ganten and D. Pfaff (Eds.), Actions of Progesterone on the Brain. Springer-Verlag, New York, pp. 31–82.

557. Katz, P. S. and Harris-Warrick, R. M. (1990) Actions of identified neuromodulatory neurons in a simple motor system. Trends Neurosci. 13:367–373.

558. Kazandijian, A., Spyraki, C., Papadopoulou, Z., Sfikakis, A., and Varanos, D. D. (1988) Behavioral and biochemical effects of haloperidol during the oestrous cycle of the rat. Neuropharmacology 27:73–78.

559. Kazandijian, A., Spyraki, C., Sfikakis, A., and Varanos, D. D. (1987) Apomorphine-induced behavior during the oestrus cycle of the rat. Neuropharmacology 26:1037–1045.

560. Keller, C., Zakon, H. and Sanchez, D. (1986) Evidence for a direct effect of androgens upon electroreceptor tuning. J. Comp. Physiol. [A] 158:301–310.

561. Kelley, D. (1980) Auditory and vocal nuclei of frog brain concentrate sex hormones. Science 207:553–555.

562. Kelley, D. (1988) Sexually dimorphic behaviors. Annu. Rev. Neurosci. 11:225–251.

563. Kelley, D. and Dennison, J. (1990) The vocal motor neurons of Xenopus laevis: Development of sex differences in axon number. J. Neurobiol. 21:869–882.

564. Kelley, D., Fenstemaker, S., Hannigan. P. and Shih, S. (1988) Sex differences in the motor nucleus of cranial nerve IX–X in *Xenopus laevis*: A quantitative study. J. Neurobiol. 19:413–429.

565. Kelley, D. and Gorlick, D. (1990) Sexual selection and the nervous system. Bioscience 40:275–283.

566. Kelley, D. and Tobias, M. (1989) The genesis of courtship song: Cellular and molecular control of a sexually differentiated behavior. In T. Carew and D. Kelley, (Eds.), Perspectives in Neural Systems and Behavior. Alan R. Liss, New York, pp. 175–194.

567. Kelly, M. J., Moss, R. L., and Dudley, C. A. (1977) The effects of microelectrophoretically applied estrogen, cortisol and acetylcholine on medial preoptic-septal unit activity throughout the estrous cycle of the female rat. Exp. Brain Res. 30:53–64.

568. Kelly, P. H. (1983) Inhibition of voluntary activity by growth hormone. Horm. Behav. 17:163–168.

569. Kenagy, G. J. (1989) Daily and seasonal uses of energy stores in torpor and hibernation. In A. Malan and B. Canguilhem (Eds.), Living in the Cold, II. John Libbey, London, pp. 17–24.

570. Kendeigh, S. C. (1962) Parental Care and Its Evolution in Birds. University of Illinois Press, Urbana.

571. Kendrick, K. M. and Keverne, E. B. (1989) Effects of intracerebroventricular infusions of naltrexone and phentolamine on central and peripheral oxytocin release and on maternal behaviour induced by vaginocervical stimulation in the ewe. Brain Res. 505:329–332.

572. Kendrick, K. M., Keverne, E. B., and Baldwin, B. A. (1987) Intracerebroventricular oxytocin stimulates maternal behavior in the sheep. Neuroendocrinology 46:56–61.

573. Keverne, E. B. (1988) Central mechanisms underlying the neural and neuroendocrine determinants in maternal behavior. Psychoneuroendocrinology 13:127–141.

574. Keverne, E. B., Lévy, F., Poindron, P., and Lindsay, D. (1983) Vaginal stimulation: An important determinant of maternal bonding in sheep. Science 219:81–83.

575. Kimura, D. (1982) Left-hemisphere control of oral and brachial movements and their relation to communication, Philos. Trans. R. Soc. Lond. [Biol.] 298:135–149.

576. Kimura, D. (1983) Sex differences in cerebral organization for speech and praxic functions. Can. J. Psychol. 37:19–35.

577. Kimura, D. (1989) The effect of exogenous estrogen on motor programming skills in post-menopausal women. University of Western Ontario Department of Psychology Research Bulletin #684.

578. Kimura, D. and Harshman, R. A. (1984) Sex differences in brain organization for verbal and non-verbal functions. Prog. Brain Res. 61:423–441.

579. Kindler, P. M., Philipp, D. P., Gross, M. R., and Bahr, J. M. (1989) Serum 11-ketotestosterone and testosterone concentrations associated with reproduction in male bluegill (*Lepomis macrochirus*: Centrachidae). Gen. Comp. Endocrinol. 75:446–453.

580. Kinsey, A. C., Pomeroy, W. B., and Martin, C. E. (1948) Sexual Behavior in the Human Male. W. B. Saunders, Philadelphia.

581. Kinsey, A. C., Pomeroy, W. B., Martin, C. E., and Gebhard, P. H. (1953) Sexual Behavior in the Human Female. W. B. Saunders, Philadelphia.

582. Kinsley, C., Miele, J., Konen, C., Ghiraldi, L., and Svare, B. (1986) Intrauterine contiguity influences regulatory activity in adult female and male mice. Horm. Behav. 20:7–12.

583. Kirkham, T. C. and Blundel, J. E. (1987) Effects of naloxone and naltrexone on meal patterns of freely-feeding rats. Pharmacol. Biochem. Behav. 26:515–520.

584. Kirkpatrick, M. (1987) Sexual selection by female choice and polygynous animals. Annu. Rev. Ecol. Syst. 18:43–70.

585. Klaiber, E. L., Broverman, D. M., Vogel, W., Kobayashi, Y., and Moriarty, D. (1972) Effects of estrogen therapy on plasma MAO activity and EEG driving responses of depressed women. Am. J. Psychiat. 128:42–48.

586. Klaiber, E. L., Broverman, D. M., Vogel, W., and Mackenberg, E. J. (1974) Rhythms in cognitive functioning and EEG indices in males. In M. Ferin, F. Halberg, R. M. Richart, and R. L. VandeWiele (Eds.), Biorhythms and Human Reproduction. Wiley & Sons, New York, pp. 481–493.

587. Klaiber, E. L., Kobayashi, Y., Broverman, D. M., and Hall, F. (1971) Plasma monoamine oxidase activity in regularly menstruating women and in amenorrheic women receiving cyclic treatment with estrogens and a progestin. J. Clin. Endocrinol. Metab. 33:630–638.

588. Kleiman, D. G. (1977) Monogamy in mammals. Q. Rev. Biol. 52:39–69.

589. Kleiman, D. G. and Malcolm, J. R. (1981) The evolution of male parental investment in mammals. In D. J. Gubernick and P. H. Klopfer (Eds.), Parental Care in Mammals. Plenum, New York, pp. 347–387.

590. Klein, D. C. (1979) Circadian rhythms in the pineal gland. In D. T. Krieger (Ed.), Endocrine Rhythms. Raven Press, New York, pp. 203–223.

591. Klein, D. C., Smoot, R., Weller, J. L., Higa, S., Markey, S. P., Creed, G. J. and Jacobowitz, D. M. (1983) Lesions of the paraventricular nucleus area of the hypothalamus disrupt the suprachiasmatic-spinal cord circuit in the melatonin rhythm generating system. Brain Res. Bull. 10:647–652.

592. Klopfer, P. H. (1971) Mother love: What turns it on? Am. Sci. 59:404–407.

593. Kluver, H. and Bucy, P. C. (1939) Preliminary analysis of functions of the temporal lobes in monkeys. Arch. Neurol. Psychiat. 42:979–1000.

594. Koch, M. (1990) Effects of treatment with estradiol and parental experience on the number and distribution of estrogen-binding neurons in the ovariectomized mouse brain. Neuroendocrinology 51:505–514.

595. Koeppe, J. K., Fuchs, M., Chen, T. T., Hunt, L.-M., Kovalick, G. E., and Briers, T. (1985) The role of juvenile hormone in reproduction. In G. A. Kerkut and L. I. Gilbert (Eds.), Comprehensive Insect Physiology, Biochemistry, and Pharmacology, Vol. 8. Pergamon Press, Oxford, pp. 165–203.

596. Kolb, B. and Stewart, J. (1991) Sex-related differences in dendritic branching of cells in the prefrontal cortex of rats. J. Neuroendocrinol. 3:95–99.

597. Komnenich, P., Lane, D. M., Dickey, R. P., and Stone, S. C. (1978) Gonadal hormones and cognitive performance. Physiol. Psychol. 6:115–120.

598. Konishi, M. (1985) Birdsong: From behavior to neuron. Annu. Rev. Neurosci. 8:125–170.

599. Konishi, M. and Akutagawa, E. (1985) Neuronal growth, atrophy and death in a sexually dimorphic song nucleus in the zebra finch brain. Nature 315:145–147.

600. Kow, L. M., Malsbury, C. W., and Pfaff, D. W. (1974) Effects of progesterone on female reproductive behavior in rats: Possible modes of action and role in behavioral sex differences. In W. Montagna and W. A. Sadler (Eds.), Reproductive Behavior. Plenum, New York, pp. 179–210.

601. Kravitz, E. A. (1988) Hormonal control of behavior: Amines and the biasing of behavioral output in lobsters. Science 241:1775–1781.

602. Krieger, D. T. (1979) Endocrine Rhythms. Raven Press, New York.

603. Krieger, D. T. (1982) Cushing's Syndrome. (Monographs in Endocrinology, Vol. 22). Springer-Verlag, Berlin.

604. Krohmer, R. W. and Baum, M. J. (1989) Effect of sex, intrauterine position and androgen manipulation on the development of brain aromatase activity in fetal ferrets. J. Neuroendocrinol. 1:265–271.

605. Kroodsma, D. E. (1976) Reproductive development in a female songbird: Differential stimulation by quality of male song. Science 192:574–575.

606. Kroodsma, D. E. (1977) Correlates of song organization among North American wrens. Am. Nat. 111:995–1008.

607. Kruuk, H. (1972) The Spotted Hyena: A Study of Predation and Social Behavior. University of Chicago Press, Chicago.

608. Kuhn, N. J. (1969) Progesterone withdrawal as the lactogenic trigger in the rat. J. Endocrinol. 44:39–54.

609. Kupfermann, I. (1967) Stimulation of egg laying: Possible neuroendocrine function of bag cells of abdominal ganglion of Aplysia californica. Nature 216:814–815.

610. Lagerspetz, K. (1964) Studies on the Aggressive Behavior of Mice. Suomalainen Tudeakatemia, Helsinki.

611. Landefeld, P., Baskin, R., and Tittler, P. (1984) Brain aging correlates: Retardation by hormonal/pharmacological treatments. Science 214:581–584.

612. Lansdell, H. (1961) The effect of neurosurgery on a test of proverbs. Am. Psychol. 16:448.

613. Lansdell, H. and Davie, J. C. (1972) Massa intermedia: Possible relation to intelligence. Neuropsychologia 10:207–210.

614. Lea, R. W., Vowles, D. M., and Dick, H. R. (1985) Factors affecting prolactin secretion during the breeding cycle in the ring dove and its possible role in incubation. J. Endocrinol. 110:447–458.

615. LeBoeuf, B. J. and Reiter, J. (1988) Lifetime reproductive success in northern elephant seals. In T. H. Clutton-brock (Ed.), Reproductive Success. University of Chicago Press, Chicago, pp. 344–362.

616. Lee, T. M., Pelz, K., Licht, P., and Zucker, I. (1990) Testosterone influences hibernation in golden-mantled ground squirrels. Am. J. Physiol. 259:R760–R767.

617. Lehne, G. K. (1988) Treatment of sex offenders with medroxyprogesterone acetate. In J. M. A. Sitsen (Ed.), Handbook of Sexology, Vol. 6. The Pharmacology and Endocrinology of Sexual Function. Elsevier Science Publishers, New York.

618. Lehrman, D. S. (1955) The physiological basis of parental feeding behavior in the ring dove (Streptopelia risoria). Behaviour 7:241–246.

619. Lehrman, D. S. (1958) Induction of broodiness by participation in courtship and nest building in the ring dove (Streptopelia risoria). J. Comp. Physiol. Psychol. 51:32–36.

620. Lehrman, D. S. (1965) Interaction between internal and external environments in the regulation of the reproductive cycle of the ring dove. In F. A. Beach (Ed.), Sex and Behavior. Wiley & Sons, New York, pp. 335–380.

621. Lemon, R. E. (1968) The relation between organization and function of song in cardinals. Behaviour 32:158–178.
622. Leshner, A. I. (1975) A model of hormones and agonistic behavior. Physiol. Behav. 15:225–235.
623. LeVay, S. (1991) A difference in hypothalamic structure between heterosexualand homosexual men. Science 253:1034–1037.
624. Levesque, D., Gagnon, S., and Di Paolo, T. (1989) Striatal D1 dopamine receptor density fluctuates during the rat estrous cycle. Neurosci. Lett. 98:345–350.
625. Levesque, D. and Di Paolo, T. (1988) Rapid conversion of high into low striatal D2-dopamine receptor agonist binding states after an acute physiological dose of 17 beta-estradiol. Neurosci. Lett. 88:113–118.
626. Levin, R. N. (1988) The adaptive significance of antiphonal song in the Bay wren, *Thryothorus nigricapillus*. Ph.D. dissertation, Cornell University, Ithaca, New York.
627. Levine, R. B. and Truman, J. W. (1983) Peptide activation of a simple neural circuit. Brain Res. 279:335–338.
628. Levine, S. (1957) Infantile experience and resistance to physiological stress. Science 126:405–406.
629. Levine, S., Wiener, S., and Coe, C. (1989) The psychoneuroendocrinology of stress: A psychobiological perspective. In F. R. Brush and S. E. Levine (Eds.), Psychoendocrinology. Academic Press, New York.
630. Lévy, F., Gervais, R., Kindermann, U., Orgeur, P., and Piketty, V. (1990) Importance of β-noradrenergic receptors in the olfactory bulb of sheep for recognition of lambs. Behav. Neurosci. 104:464–469.
631. Lévy, F., Poindron, P., and Le Neindre, P. (1983) Attraction and repulsion by amniotic fluids and their olfactory control in the ewe around parturition. Physiol. Behav. 31:687–692.
632. Lewis, R. S., Hodson, S. B., Lipcamon, J., Chiu, L., and Hines, M. (1988) A sex difference in the structural asymmetry of the caudate nucleus using MRI scans in humans. Soc. Neurosci. Abstr. 14:1137.
633. Lieblich, I., Baum, M. J., Diamond, P., Goldblum, N., Iser, C., and Pick, C. G. (1985) Inhibition of mating by naloxone or morphine in recently castrated, but not intact male rats. Pharmacol. Biochem. Behav. 22:361–364.
634. Lillie, F. R. (1916) The theory of the freemartin. Science 43:611–613.
635. Lincoln, G. A., Guinness, ?. ?., and Short, R. V. (1972) The way in which testosterone controls the social and sexual behavior of the red deer stag (*Cervus elaphus*). Horm. Behav. 3:375–396.
636. Lindburg, D. G. (1971) The rhesus monkey in North India: An ecological and behavioral study. Primate Behav. 2:1–106.
637. Linn, M. C. and Petersen, A. C. (1985) Emergence and characterization of sex differences in spatial ability: A meta-analysis. Child Devel. 56:1479–1498.
638. Linsdaile, J. M. and Tevis, L. P., Jr. (1951) The Dusky-Footed Wood Rat. University of California Press, Berkeley.
639. Lisk, R. D. (1985) The estrous cycle. In H. I. Siegel (Ed.), The Hamster. Plenum, New York, pp. 23–51.
640. Lott, D. F. and Comerford, S. (1968) Hormonal initiation of parental behavior in inexperienced ring doves. Z. Tierpsychol. 25:71–75.
641. Lounibos, L. P. (1976) Initiation and maintenance of cocoon spinning behaviour by saturniid silkmoths. Physiol. Entomol. 1:195–206.
642. Lovejoy, J. and Wallen, K. (1988) Sexually dimorphic behavior in group-housed rhesus monkeys (*Macaca mulatta*) at 1 year of age. Psychobiology 16:348–356.
643. Loy, R., Gerlach, J. L., and McEwen, B. S. (1988) Autoradiographic localization of estradiol-binding neurons in the rat hippocampal formation and entorhinal cortex. Dev. Brain Res. 39:245–251.
644. Luine, V. N. and McEwen, B. S. (1985) Steroid hormone receptors in brain and pituitary. In N. Adler, D. Pfaff, and R. W. Goy (Eds.), Handbook of Behavioral Neurobiology. Vol. 7, Reproduction. Plenum, New York, pp. 665–721.
645. Lynch, A., Mychalkiw, W., and Hutt, S. J. (1978) Prenatal progesterone I. Its effect on development and on intellectual and academic achievement. Early Hum. Devel. 2/4:305–322.
646. Lynch, W. C. and Libby, L. (1983) Naloxone suppresses intake of highly preferred sacharin solutions in food-deprived and sated rats. Life Sci. 33:1909–1914.
647. Maccoby, E. E. and Jacklin, C. N. (1974) The Psychology of Sex Differences. Stanford University Press, Stanford.
648. Mackenberg, E. J., Broverman, D. M., Vogel, W., and Klaiber, E. L. (1974) Morning-to-afternoon changes in cognitive performances and in the electroencephalogram. J. Educ. Psychol. 66:238–246.
649. MacLusky, N. J., Naftolin, F., and Goldman-Rakic, P. S. (1986) Estrogen formation and binding in the cerebral cortex of the developing rhesus monkey. Proc. Natl. Acad. Sci. U.S.A. 83:513–516.
650. Madlafousek, J., Hlinak, Z., and Beran, J. (1976) Decline of sexual behavior in castrated male rats: Effects of female precopulatory behavior. Horm. Behav. 7:245–252.

651. Maier, R. N. (1963) Maternal behavior in the domestic hen: The role of physical contact. J. Comp. Physiol. Psychol. 56:357–361.
652. Malsbury, C. W. (1971) Facilitation of male rat copulatory behavior by electrical stimulation of the medial preoptic area. Physiol. Behav. 7:797–805.
653. Malsbury, C. W. and McKay, K. (1987) A sex difference in the pattern of substance P-like immunoreactivity in the bed nucleus of the stria terminalis. Brain Res. 420:365–370.
654. Marchlewska-Koj, A. (1983) Pregnancy blocking by pheromones. In J. G. Vandenbergh (Ed.), Pheromones and Reproduction in Mammals. Academic Press, New York, pp. 151–173.
655. Marder, E. and Hooper, S. L. (1985) Neurotransmitter modulation of the stomatogastric ganglion of decapod crustaceans. In A. I. Selverston (Ed.), Model Neural Networks and Behavior. Plenum, New York, pp. 319–337.
656. Marin, M., Tobias, M., and Kelley, D. (1990) Hormone-sensitive stages in the sexual differentiation of laryngeal muscle fiber number in Xenopus laevis. Development 110:703–711.
657. Marler, P. (1970) A comparative approach to vocal learning: Song development in white-crowned sparrows. J. Comp. Physiol. Psychol. 71, Suppl., 1–25.
658. Marler, P. and Peters, S. (1982) Subsong and plastic song: Their role in the vocal learning process. In D. E. Kroodsma and E. H. Millers (Eds.), Acoustic Communication in Birds, Vol. 2. Academic Press, New York, pp. 25–50.
659. Marler, P., Peters, S., Ball, G. F., Dufty, A. M., and Wingfield, J. C. (1989) The role of sex steroids in the acquisition and production of birdsong. Nature 336:770–772.
660. Marler, P., Peters, S., and Wingfield, J. (1987) Correlations between song acquisition, song production, and plasma levels of testosterone and estradiol in sparrows. J. Neurobiol. 18:531–548.
661. Marsden, C. D. (1987) What do the basal ganglia tell premotor cortical areas? Ciba Foundation Symposium. 132:282–300.
662. Marshall, J. R. and Henkin, R. I. (1971) Olfactory acuity, menstrual abnormalities, and ooctye status. Ann. Intern. Med. 75:207–211.
663. Marti, T., Takio, K., Walsh, K. A., Terzi, G. and Truman, J. W. (1987) Microanalysis of the amino acid sequence of the eclosion hormone from the tobacco hornworm Manduca sexta. FEBS Lett. 219:415–418.
664. Martin, J. B. and Reichlin, S. (1987) Clinical Neuroendocrinology. F. A. Davis, Philadelphia.
665. Martin, R. D. (1966) Tree shrews: Unique reproductive mechanism of systematic importance. Science 152:1402–1404.
666. Martinez, J. L. (1986) Memory: Drugs and hormones. In J. L. Martinez and R. P. Kesner (Eds.), Learning and Memory. A Biological View. Academic Press, New York, pp. 127–163.
667. Masaoka, K., Kitazawa, M. and Kumasaka, T. (1988) Pulsatile secretion of prolactin and luteinizing hormone and their synchronous relationship during the human menstrual cycle. Gynecol. Endocrinol. 2:293–303.
668. Masica, D. N., Money, J., and Ehrhardt, A. A. (1971) Fetal feminization and female gender identity in testicular feminizing syndrome of androgen insensitivity. Arch. Sex. Behav. 1:131–142.
669. Mason, J. (1968) A review of psychoendocrine research on the pituitary adrenal cortical system. Psychosom. Med. 30:576–583.
670. Mason, J. (1975) A historical view of the stress field. J. Human Stress 1:6–21.
671. Mason, R. T., Fales, H. M., Jones, T. H., Pannell, L. K., Chinn, J. W., and Crews, D. (1989) Sex pheromones in garter snakes. Science 245:290–293.
672. Masters, W. and Johnson, V. (1966) Human Sexual Response. Little, Brown, Boston.
673. Mateer, C. A., Polen, S. B., and Ojemann, G. A. (1982) Sexual variation in cortical localization of naming as determined by stimulation mapping. Behav. Brain Sci. 5:310–311.
674. May, R. R. (1976) Mood shifts and the menstrual cycle. J. Psychosom. Res. 20:125–130.
675. Mayer, A. D., Monroy, M. A., and Rosenblatt, J. S. (1990) Prolonged estrogen-progesterone treatment of nonpregnant ovariectomized rats: Factors stimulating home-cage and maternal aggression and short-latency maternal behavior. Horm. Behav. 24:342–364.
676. Mayer, A. D., Reisbick, S., Siegel, H. I., and Rosenblatt, J. S. (1987) Maternal aggression in rats: Changes over pregnancy and lactation in a Sprague-Dawley strain. Aggress. Behav. 13:29–43.
677. Mayer, A. D. and Rosenblatt, J. S. (1984) Prepartum changes in maternal responsiveness and nest defense in Rattus norvegicus. J. Comp. Psychol. 98:177–188.
678. Mayeri, E. and Rothman, B. S. (1985) Neuropeptides and the control of egg-laying behavior in Aplysia. In A. I. Selverston (Ed.), Model Neural Networks and Behavior. Plenum, New York, pp. 285–301.
679. McCann, M. J., Verbalis, J. G., and Stricker, E. M. (1989) LiCl and CCK inhibit gastric emptying and feeding and stimulate OT secretion in rats. Am. J. Physiol. 256:R463–R468.

680. McCarthy, M. M., Bare, J. E., and vom Saal, F. S. (1986) Infanticide and parental behavior in wild female house mice: Effects of ovariectomy, adrenalectomy and administration of oxytocin and prostaglandin F2 alpha. Physiol. Behav. 36:17–23.

681. McCarthy, M. M. and vom Saal, F. S. (1986) Inhibition of infanticide after mating in wild male house mice. Physiol. Behav. 36:203–209.

682. McClintock, M. K. (1971) Menstrual synchrony and suppression. Nature 229:244–245.

683. McClintock, M. K. (1987) A functional approach to the behavioral endocrinology of rodents. In D. Crews (Ed.), Psychobiology of Reproductive Behavior. Prentice Hall, Englewood Cliffs, pp. 176–203.

684. McDonald, P. G., Beyer, C., Newton, F., Brien, B., Baker, R., Tan, H. S., Sampson, C., Kitching, P., Greenhill, R., and Pritchard, D. (1970) Failure of 5α-dihydrotestosterone to initiate sexual behavior in the castrated male rat. Nature 227:964–965.

685. McEwen, B. S. (1980) Gonadal steroids: Humoral modulators of nerve cell function. Mol. Cell. Endocrinol. 18:151–164.

686. McEwen, B. S. (1980) The brain as a target organ of endocrine hormones. In D. T. Krieger and J. C. Hughes (Eds.), Neuroendocrinology. Sinauer Associates, Sunderland, Mass., pp. 33–44.

687. McEwen, B. S., Biegon, A., Fischette, C. T., Luine, V. N., Parsons, B., and Rainbow, T. C. (1984) Toward a neurochemical basis of steroid hormone action. In L. Martini and W. F. Ganong (Eds.), Frontiers in Neuroendocrinology, Vol. 8. Raven Press, New York, pp. 153–176.

688. McEwen, B. S. and Brinton, R. E. (1987) Neuroendocrine aspects of adaptation. In E. R. de Kloet, V. M. Wiegant, and D. de Wied (Eds.), Progress in Brain Research. Elsevier, New York, pp. 11–27, 72.

689. McEwen, B. S., Davis, P. G., Parsons, B., and Pfaff, D. W. (1979) The brain as a target for steroid hormone action. Annu. Rev. Neurosci. 2:65–112.

690. McEwen, B. S. and Krey, L. C. (1984) Properties of estrogen sensitive neurons: Aromatization, progestin receptor induction and neuroendocrine effects. In F. Celotti et al. (Eds.), Metabolism of Hormonal Steroids in the Neuroendocrine Structures. Raven Press, New York.

691. McGaugh, J. L. (1989) Involvement of hormonal and neuromodulatory systems in the regulation of memory storage. Annu. Rev. Neurosci. 12:255–287.

692. McGinnis, M. Y. and Dreifuss, R. M. (1989) Evidence for a role of testosterone-androgen receptor interactions in mediating masculine sexual behavior in male rats. Endocrinology 124:618–626.

693. McGlone, J. (1977) Sex differences in the cerebral organization of verbal functions in patients with unilateral brain lesions. Brain 100:775–793.

694. McGlone, J. (1978) Sex differences in functional brain asymmetry. Cortex 14:122–128.

695. McGlone, J. (1980) Sex differences in human brain asymmetry: A critical survey. Behav. Brain Sci. 3:215–263.

696. McGuire, L. S. and Omenn, G. S. (1975) Congenital adrenal hyperplasia. I. Family studies of IQ. Behav. Genet. 5:165–173.

697. McGuire, L. S., Ryan, K. O., and Omenn, G. S. (1975) Congenital adrenal hyperplasia. II. Cognitive and behavioral studies. Behav. Genet. 5:175–188.

698. McIntosh, T. K. and Drickamer, L. C. (1977) Excreted urine, bladder urine, and the delay of sexual maturation in female house mice. Anim. Behav. 25:999–1004.

699. McKeever, W. F., Rich, D. A., Deyo, R. A., and Conner, R. L. (1987) Androgens and spatial ability: Failure to find a relationship between testosterone and ability measures. Bull. Psychosom. Soc. 25:438–440.

700. McMurtry, J. P. and Anderson, R. H. (1971) Prevention of self-licking on mammary gland development in pregnant rats. Proc. Soc. Exp. Biol. Med. 137:354–356.

701. Meaney, J., Mitchell, J., Aitken, D., Bhatnager, S., Bodnoff, S., Iny, L., and Sarrieau, A. (1991) The effects of neonatal handling on the development of the adrenocortical response to stress: Implications for neuropathology and cognitive deficits in later life. Psychoneuroendocrinology 16:85–103.

702. Meaney, M. J., Aitken, D. H., van Berkel, C., Bhatnagar, S., and Sapolsky, R. M. (1988) Effect of neonatal handling on age-related impairments associated with the hippocampus. Science 766–768.

703. Mehrara, B. J. and Baum, M. J. (1990) Naloxone disrupts the expression but not the acquisition by male rats of a conditioned place preference response for an oestrous female. Psychopharmacology 101:118–125.

704. Meier, A. H. (1976) Daily variation in concentration of plasma corticosteroid in hypophysectomized rats. Endocrinology 98:1475–1479.

705. Meisel, R. L., O'Hanlon, J. K., and Sachs, B. D. (1984) Differential maintenance of penile responses and copulatory behavior by gonadal hormones in castrated male rats. Horm. Behav. 18:56–64.

706. Menaker, M. (1972) Nonvisual light reception. Sci. Am. 226:22–29.

707. Mendonça, M. T. and Crews, D. (1989) Effect of fall mating on ovarian development in the red-sided garter snake. Am. J. Physiol. 257:R1548–1550.

708. Merkle, S. (1989) Sexual differences as adaptations to the different gender roles in the frog Xenopus laevis Daudin. J. Comp. Physiol. [B] 159:473–480.

709. Mesce, K. A. and Truman, J. W. (1988) Metamorphosis of the ecdysis motor pattern in the hawkmoth, *Manduca* sexta. J. Comp. Physiol. [A] 163:287–299.

710. Meyer, J. H. (1983) Steroid influences upon the discharge frequency of a weakly electric fish. J. Comp. Physiol. 153:29–38.

711. Meyer, J. H. and Zakon, H. (1982) Androgens alter the tuning of electroreceptors. Science 217:635–637.

712. Meyer-Bahlburg, H. F. L. (1984) Psychoendocrine research on sexual orientation. Current status and future options. Prog. Brain Res. 61:375–398.

713. Meyer-Bahlburg, H. F. L., Nat, R., Boon, D. A., Sharma, M., and Edwards, J. A. (1984) Aggression and testosterone measures in man. Psychosom. Med. 36:269–274.

714. Meyerson, B. J. (1981) Comparison of the effects of beta-endorphin and morphine on exploratory and socio-sexual behavior in the male rat. Eur. J. Pharmacol. 69:453–458.

715. Meyerson, B. J., Malmnas, C. O., and Everitt, B. J. (1985) Neuropharmacology, neurotransmitters, and sexual behavior in mammals. In N. Adler, D. Pfaff, and R. W. Goy (Eds.), Handbook of Behavioral Neurobiology, Vol. 7. Reproduction. Plenum, New York, pp. 495–536.

716. Miaskiewicz, S. L., Stricker, E. M., and Verbalis, J. G. (1989) Neurohypophyseal secretion in response to cholecystokinin but not meal-induced gastric distention in humans. J. Clin. Endocrinol. Metab. 68:837–843.

717. Michael, R. P. and Bonsall, R. W. (1979) Hormones and the sexual behavior of rhesus monkeys. In C. Beyer (Ed.), Endocrine Control of Sexual Behavior. Raven Press, New York, pp. 279–302.

718. Michael, R. P. and Keverne, E. B. (1968) Pheromones and the communication of sexual status in primates. Nature 218:746–749.

719. Michael, R. P., Zumpe, D., and Bonsall, R. W. (1986) Comparison of the effects of testosterone and dihydrotestosterone on the behavior of male cynomolgus monkeys. Physiol. Behav. 36:349–355.

720. Michel, G. F. (1977) Experience and progesterone in ring dove incubation. Anim. Behav. 25:281–285.

721. Michel, G. F. and Moore, C. L. (1986) Contributions of reproductive experience to observation-maintained crop growth and incubation in male and female ring doves. Anim. Behav. 34:790–796.

722. Miernicki, M., Pospchal, M. W., and Powers, J. B. (1990) Short photoperiods affect male hamster sociosexual behaviors in the presence and absence of testosterone. Physiol. Behav. 47:95–106.

723. Miller, J. P. and Selverston, A. I. (1985) Neural mechanisms for the production of the lobster pyloric motor pattern. In A. I. Selverston (Ed.), Model Neural Networks and Behavior. Plenum, New York, pp. 37–48.

723a. Miller, J. C. (1983) Sex differences in dopaminergic and cholinergic activity and function in the nigrostriatal system of the rat. Psychoneuroendocrinology 8:225–236.

724. Miller, N. (1980) Effects of learning on physical symptoms produced by psychological stress. In H. Selye (Ed.), The Stress of Life. McGraw-Hill, New York.

725. Miller, R. E. and Caul, W. F. (1973) Effect of adrenocorticotropic hormone on appetitive discrimination learning in the rat. Physiol. Behav. 10:141–143.

726. Miller, R. L. and Baum, M. J. (1987) Naloxone inhibits mating and conditioned place preference for an estrous female in male rats soon after castration. Pharmacol. Biochem. Behav. 26:781–789.

727. Mills, A. and Zakon, H. (1987) Coordination of EOD frequency and pulse duration in a weakly electric fish: The influence of androgens. J. Comp. Physiol. 161:417–430.

728. Mills, M. G. L. (1990) Kalahari Hyenas. Unwin Hyman, London.

729. Milner, B., Teuber, H.-L, and Corkin, S. (1968) Further analysis of the hippocampal amnesic syndrome: 14 year follow up study of H. M. Neuropsychologia 6:215–234.

730. Mitchell, J. A. and Yochim, J. M. (1970) Influence of environmental lighting on duration of pregnancy in the rat. Endocrinology 87:472–480.

731. Mitchell, J. B. and Stewart, J. (1989) Effects of castration, steroid replacement, and sexual experience on mesolimbic dopamine and sexual behaviors in the male rat. Brain Res. 491:116–127.

732. Mitchell, J. B. and Stewart, J. (1990) Facilitation of sexual behaviors in the male rat associated with intra-VTA injections of opiates. Pharmacol. Biochem. Behav. 35:643–650.

733. Moline, M. L., Albers, H. E., and Moore-Ede, M. C. (1986) Estrogen modifies the circadian timing and amplitude of the luteinizing hormone surge in female hamsters exposed to short photoperiods. Biol. Reprod. 35:516–523.

734. Moline, M. L., Albers, H. E., Todd, R. B., and Moore-Ede, M. C. (1981) Light-dark entrainment of proestrous LH surges and circadian locomotor activity in female hamsters. Horm. Behav. 15:451–458.

735. Money, J. (1987) Sin, sickness, or status? Homosexual gender identity and psychoneuroendocrinology. Am. Psychol. 42:384–399.

736. Money, J. and Ehrhardt, A. A. (1972) Man and Woman, Boy and Girl. Johns Hopkins University Press, Baltimore.

737. Money, J. and Lewis, V. (1966) IQ, genetics and accelerated growth: Adrenogenital syndrome. Bull. Johns Hopkins Hosp. 118:365–373.

738. Money, J., Lewis, V., Ehrhardt, A. A., and Drash, P. W. (1967) IQ impairment and elevation in endocrine and related cytogenetic disorders. In J. Zubin (Ed.), Psychopathology of Mental Development. Grune & Stratton, New York, pp. 22–27.

739. Money, J., Schwartz, M., and Lewis, V. G. (1984) Adult heterosexual status and fetal hormonal masculinization and demasculinization: 46XX congenital virilizing adrenal hyperplasia and 46XY androgen-insensitivity syndrome compared. Psychoneuroendocrinology 9:405–414.

740. Monti, P. M., Brown, W. A. and Corriveau, D. P. (1977) Testosterone and components of aggression and sexual behavior in man. Am. J. Psychiatry 134(6):692–694.

741. Moore, C. L. (1976) The transition from sitting on eggs to sitting on young in ring doves, *Streptopelia risoria*: Squab-egg preference during the normal cycle. Anim. Behav. 24:36–45.

742. Moore, C. L. (1976) Experiential and hormonal conditions affect squab-egg choice in ring doves (*Streptopelia risoria*). J. Comp. Physiol. Psychol. 90:583–589.

743. Moore, M. C. (1984) Changes in territorial defense produced by changes in circulating levels of testosterone: A possible hormonal basis for mate-guarding behavior in white-crowned sparrows. Behaviour 88:215–226.

744. Moore, R. Y. and Eichler, V. B. (1972) Loss of a circadian adrenal corticosterone rhythm following suprachiasmatic lesions in the rat. Brain Res. 42:201–206.

745. Moore-Ede, M. C. (1986) Physiology of the circadian timing system: Predictive versus reactive homeostasis. Am. J. Physiol. 250:R735–R752.

746. Morali, G. and Beyer, C. (1979) Neuroendocrine control of mammalian estrous behavior. In C. Beyer (Ed.), Endocrine Control of Sexual Behavior. Raven Press, New York, pp. 3–32.

747. Morel, F. (1948) La massa intermedia ou commissure grise. Acta Anat. 4:203–207.

748. Morin, L. P. (1977) Progesterone: Inhibition of rodent sexual behavior. Physiol. Behav. 18:701–715.

749. Morin, L. P. (1985) Biological Rhythms. In H. I. Siegel (Ed.), The Hamster. Plenum, New York, pp. 323–361.

750. Morin, L. P. (1986) Environment and hamster reproduction: Responses to phase-specific starvation during estrous cycle. Am. J. Physiol. 251:R663–R669.

751. Morin, L. P. (1987) A concept of physiological time: Rhythms in behavior and reproductive physiology. Ann. N.Y. Acad. Sci. 474:331–351.

752. Morin, L. P. (1988) Propylthiouracil, but not other antithyroid treatments, lengthens hamster circadian period. Am. J. Physiol. 255:R1–R5.

753. Morin, L. P. and Cummings, L. A. (1981) Effect of surgical or photoperiodic castration, testosterone replacement or pinealectomy on male hamster running rhythmicity. Physiol. Behav. 26:825–838.

754. Morin, L. P. and Cummings, L. A. (1982) Splitting of wheelrunning rhythms by castrated or steroid treated male and female hamsters. Physiol. Behav. 29:665–675.

755. Morin, L. P., Fitzgerald, K. M., and Zucker, I. (1977) Estradiol shortens the period of hamster circadian rhythms. Science 196:305–307.

756. Morin, L. P., Gavin, M. L., and Ottenweller, J. E. (1986) Propylthiouracil causes phase delays and circadian period lengthening in male and female hamsters. Am. J. Physiol. 250:R151–R160.

757. Morin, L. P. and Zucker, I. (1978) Photoperiodic regulation of copulatory behaviour in the male hamster. J. Endocrinol. 77:249–258.

758. Morris, D. (1965) The Mammals. A Guide to Living Species. Harper & Row, New York.

759. Morris, N. M. and Udry, J. R. (1970) Variations in pedometer activity during the menstrual cycle. Obstet. Gynecol. 35:199–201.

760. Morton, D. B. and Truman, J. W. (1985) Steroid regulation of the peptide-mediated increase in cyclic GMP in the nervous system of the hawkmoth, *Manduca sexta*. J. Comp. Physiol. [A] 157:423–432.

761. Morton, D. B. and Truman, J. W. (1988) The EGPs—the eclosion hormone and cyclic GMP regulated phosphoproteins. I. Appearance and partial characterization in the CNS of *Manduca sexta*. J. Neurosci. 8:1326–1337.

762. Morton, D. B. and Truman, J. W. (1988) The EGPs—the eclosion hormone and cyclic GMP regulated phosphoproteins. II. Regulation of appearance by the steroid hormone 20-hydroxyecdysone in *Manduca sexta.* J. Neurosci. 8:1338–1345.

763. Moss, R. L. and Dudley, C. A. (1984) Molecular aspects of the interaction between estrogen and the membrane excitability of hypothalamic nerve cells. In G. DeVries, J. De Bruin, H. Uylings, and M. Corner (Eds.), Sex Differences in the Brain: The Relation Between Structure and Function. Prog. Brain Res. 61:3–22.

764. Mount, R. H. (1963) The natural history of the red-tailed skink *Eumeces egregius* Baird. Am. Midl. Nat. 70:356–385.

765. Moyer, K. E. (1968) Kinds of aggression and their physiological basis. Communic. Behav. Biol. 2:65–87.

766. Mulaikal, R. M., Migeon, C. J., and Rock, J. A. (1987) Fertility rates in female patients with congenital adrenal hyperplasia due to 21-hydroxylase deficiency. N. Engl. J. Med. 316:178–182.

767. Muldoon, T. G. (1987) Prolactin mediation of estrogen-induced changes in mammary tissue estrogen and progesterone receptors. Endocrinology 121:141–149.

768. Munck, A., Guyre, P., and Holbrook, N. (1984) Physiological actions of glucocorticoids in stress and their relation to pharmacological actions. Endocr. Rev. 5:25–48.

769. Murphy, M. R. (1980) Sexual preferences of male hamsters: Importance of preweaning and adult experience, vaginal secretion and olfactory or vomeronasal sensation. Behav. Neural Biol. 30:323–340.

770. Murphy, M. R., Seckl, J. R., Burton, S., Checkley, S. A., and Lightman, S. L. (1987) Changes in oxytocin and vasopressin secretion during sexual activity in men. J. Clin. Endocrinol. Metab. 65:738–741.

771. Naftolin, F., Ryan, K. J., Davies, I. J., Reddy, V. V., Flores, F., Petro, Z., Kuhn, M., White, R. J., Takaoka, Y., and Wolin, L. (1975) The formation of estrogens by central neuroendocrine tissues. Recent Prog. Horm. Res. 31:295–319.

772. Nausieda, P. A., Koller, W. C., Weiner, W. J., and Klawans, H. L. (1979) Chorea induced by oral contraceptives. Neurology 29:1605–1609.

773. Nijhout, H. F. and Wheeler, D. E. (1982) Juvenile hormone and the physiological basis of insect polymorphism. Q. Rev. Biol. 57:109–133.

774. Nock, B., Blaustein, J. B., and Feder, H. H. (1981) Changes in noradrenergic transmission alter the concentration of cytoplasmic progestin receptors in hypothalamus. Brain Res. 201:371–396.

775. Nordeen, E. J. and Nordeen, K. W. (1989) Estrogen stimulates the incorporation of new neurons into avian song nuclei during adolescence. Dev. Brain Res. 49:27–32.

776. Nordeen, K. W., Nordeen, E. J., and Arnold, A. P. (1986) Estrogen establishes sex differences in androgen accumulation in zebra finch brain. J. Neurosci. 6:734–738.

777. Nordeen, K. W., Nordeen, E. J., and Arnold, A. P. (1987) Estrogen accumulation in zebra finch song control nuclei: Implications for sexual differentiation and adult activation of song behavior. J. Neurobiol. 18:569–582.

778. Nordeen, E. J. and Yahr, P. (1982) Hemispheric asymmetries in the behavioral and hormonal effects of sexually differentiating mammalian brain. Science 218:391–394.

778a. Norman, A. W. and Litwack, G. (1987) Hormones. Academic Press, San Diego.

779. Norman, R. L. and Spies, H. G. (1986) Cyclic function in a male macaque: Additional evidence for a lack of sexual differentiation in the physiological mechanisms that regulate the cyclic release of gonadotropins in primates. Endocrinology 118:2608–2610.

780. Nottebohm, F. (1980) Testosterone triggers growth of brain vocal control nuclei in adult female canaries. Brain Res. 189:429–436.

781. Nottebohm, F. (1987) Plasticity in adult avian central nervous system: Possible relation between hormones, learning, and brain repair. In F. Plum (Ed.), Higher Functions of the Nervous System. Section 1, Handbook of Physiology. Williams & Wilkins, Baltimore, pp. 85–108.

782. Nottebohm, F. (1989) Hormonal regulation of synapses and cell number in adult canary brain and its relevance to theories of long-term memory storage. In J. M. Lakoskin, J. R. Perez-Plo, and D. K. Rassin (Eds.), Neural Control of Reproductive Function. Alan R. Liss, New York, pp. 583–601.

783. Nottebohm, F. and Arnold, A. (1976) Sexual dimorphism in vocal control areas of the songbird brain. Science 194:211–213.

784. Numan, M. (1988) Neural basis of maternal behavior in the rat. Psychoneuroendocrinology 13:47–62.

785. O'Connell, M. E., Reboulleau, C., Feder, H. H., and Silver, R. (1981) Social interactions and androgen levels in birds. I. Female characteristics associated with increased plasma androgen levels in the male ring dove (*Streptopelia risoria*). Gen. Comp. Endocrinol. 44:454–463.

786. O'Connell, M. E., Silver, R., Feder, H. H., and Reboulleau, C. (1981) Social interactions and androgen levels in birds. II. Social factors associated with a decline in plasma androgen levels in male ring doves (*Streptopelia risoria*). Gen. Comp. Endocrinol. 44:464–469.

787. Olson, B. R., Drutarosky, M. D., Chow, M. S., Hruby, V. J., Stricker, E. M., and Verbalis, J. G. (1991) Oxytocin and an oxytocin agonist administered centrally decrease food intake in rats. Peptides 12:113–118.

788. Olweus, D., Mattsson, A., Schalling, D., and Low, H. (1988) Circulating testosterone levels and aggression in adolescent males: A causal analysis. Psychosom. Med. 50:261–272.

789. Onuf, B. (1899) Notes on the arrangement and function of the cell group in the sacral region of the spinal cord. J. Nerv. Ment. Dis. 26:498–504.

790. Orians, G. H. (1969) On the evolution of mating systems in birds and mammals. Am. Nat. 103:589–603.

791. Orpen, B. G., Furman, H., Wong, P. Y., and Fleming, A. S. (1987) Hormonal influences on the duration of postpartum maternal responsiveness in the rat. Physiol. Behav. 40:307–315.

792. Ottenweller, J. E. and Meier, A. H. (1982) Adrenal innervation may be an extrapituitary mechanism able to regulate adrenocortical rhythmicity in rats. Endocrinology 111:1334–1338.

793. Ottenweller, J. E., Meier, A. H., Ferrell, B. R., Horseman, N. D., and Proctor, A. (1978) Extrapituitary regulation of the circadian rhythm of plasma corticosteroid concentration in rats. Endocrinology 103:1875–1879.

794. Pakkenberg, H. and Voigt, J. (1964) Brain weight of the Danes. Acta Anat. 56(4):297–307.

794a. Palade, G. E. and Farquar, M. G. (1981) Cell biology. In L. H. Smith and S. O. Thier (Eds.), Pathophysiology: The Biological Principles of Disease. W. B. Saunders, Philadelphia, pp. 1–56.

795. Panzica, G. C., Viglietti-Panzica, C., Calcagni, M., Anselmetti, G. C., Schumacher, M., and Balthazart, J. (1987) Sexual differentiation and hormonal control of the sexually dimorphic medial preoptic nucleus in the quail. Brain Res. 416:59–68.

796. Parker, G. A. (1979) Sexual selection and sexual conflict. In M. S. Blum and N. A. Blum (Eds.), Sexual Selection and Reproductive Competition in Insects. Academic Press, New York, pp. 123–166.

797. Parlee, M. B. (1983) Menstrual rhythms in sensory processes: A review of fluctuations in vision, olfaction, audition, taste, and touch. Psychol. Bull. 93:539–548.

798. Paxinos, G. and Watson, C. (1982) The Rat Brain in Stereotaxic Coordinates. Academic Press, New York.

799. Payne, R. B. (1983) Bird songs, sexual selection, and female mating strategies. In S. K. Wasser (Ed.), Social Behavior of Female Vertebrates. Academic Press, New York, pp. 55–90.

800. Pedersen, C. A., Caldwell, J. D., Fort, S. A., and Prange, A. J., Jr. (1985) Oxytocin antiserum delays onset of ovarian steroid-induced maternal behavior. Neuropeptides 6:175–182.

801. Pedersen, C. A., Caldwell, J. D., and Jirikowski, G. R. (1988) Oxytocin and reproductive behaviors. In S. Yoshida and L. Share (Eds.), Recent Progress in Posterior Pituitary Hormones 1988. Excerpta Medica, Amsterdam, pp. 127–132.

802. Pedersen, C. A. and Prange, A. J., Jr. (1987) Evidence that central oxytocin plays a role in the activation of maternal behavior. In N. A. Krasnegor, E. M. Blass, M. A. Hofer, and W. P. Smotherman (Eds.), Perinatal Development. A Psychobiological Perspective. Academic Press, New York, pp. 299–320.

803. Perel, D., Daniilescu, D., Kindler, S., Kharlip, L., Killinger, D. W. (1986) The formation of 5 alpha-reduced androgens in stromal cells from human breast adipose tissue. J. Clin. Endocrinol. Metab. 62:314–318.

804. Perlman, S. M. (1973) Cognitive abilities of children with hormone abnormalities: Screening by psychoeducational tests. J. Learn. Disabil. 6:26–34.

805. Peters, M., Servos, P. and Day, R. (1990) Marked sex differences on a fine motor skill task disappear when finger size is used as a covariate. J. Appl. Psychol. 75:87–90.

806. Peters, P. J., Bronson, F. H., and Whitsett, J. M. (1972) Neonatal castration and intermale aggression in mice. Physiol. Behav. 8:265–268.

807. Pfaff, D. W. (1970) Mating behavior of hypophysectomied rats. J. Comp. Physiol. Psychol. 72:45–50.

808. Pfaff, D. W. (1980) Estrogens and Brain Function. Springer-Verlag, New York.

809. Pfaff, D. W. (1982) Motivational concepts: Definitions and distinctions. In D. W. Pfaff (Ed.), The Physiological Mechanisms of Motivation. Springer-Verlag, New York, pp. 3–24.

810. Pfaff, D. W. (1988) Multiplicative responses to hormones by hypothalamic neurons. In S. Yoshida and L. Share (Eds.), Recent Progress in Posterior Pituitary Hormones 1988. Excerpta Medica, Amsterdam, pp. 257–267.

811. Pfaff, D. W. and Pfaffmann, C. (1969) Olfactory and hormonal influences on the basal forebrain of the male rat. Brain Res. 15:137–156.

812. Pfaff, D. W. and Schwartz-Giblin, S. (1988) Cellular mechanisms of female reproductive behaviors. In E. Knobil and J. Neill (Eds.), The Physiology of Reproduction. Raven Press, New York, pp. 1487–1568.

813. Pfaus, J. G. and Gorzalka, B. B. (1987) Opioids and sexual behavior. Neurosci. Biobehav. Rev. 11:1–34.

814. Pfaus, J. G., Newton, T. N., Blaha, C. D., Fibiger, H. C., and Phillips, A. G. (1989) Electrochemical detection of central dopamine efflux during sexual activity in male rats. Soc. Neurosci. Abstr. 15:558.

815. Pfeiffer, C. A. (1936) Sexual differences of the hypophyses and their determination by the gonads. Am. J. Anat. 58:195.

816. Phoenix, C. H., Copenhaver, K. H., and Brenner, R. M. (1976) Scanning electron microscopy of penile papillae in intact and castrated rats. Horm. Behav. 7:217–227.

817. Phoenix, C. H., Goy, R. W., Gerall, A. A., and Young, W. C. (1959) Organizing action of prenatally administered testosterone propionate on the tissues mediating mating behavior in the female guinea pig. Endocrinology 65:369–382.

818. Pierson, W. R. and Lockhart, A. (1963) Effect of menstruation on simple reaction and movement time. Br. Med. J. 1:796–797.

819. Pinsker, H. M. and Dudek, F. E. (1977) Bag cell control of egg-laying in freely behaving *Aplysia.* Science 197:490–493.

820. Pissonier, D., Thiery, J. C., Fabre-Nys, C., Poindron, P., and Keverne, E. B. (1985) The importance of the olfactory bulbs and noradrenaline for maternal recognition in sheep. Physiol. Behav. 35:361–363.

821. Pittendrigh, C. S. and Daan, S. (1976) A functional analysis of circadian pacemakers in nocturnal rodents. IV. Entrainment: Pacemaker as clock. J. Comp. Physiol. 106:291–331.

822. Plomin, R., DeFries, J. C., and McClearn, G. E. (1990) Behavioral Genetics: A Primer. W. H. Freeman, New York.

823. Plooij, F. (1979) How wild chimpanzee babies trigger the onset of mother-infant play and what the mother makes of it. In M. Bullowa (Ed.), Before Speech. Cambridge University Press, New York.

824. Poindron, P. and LeNeindre, P. (1980) Endocrine and sensory regulation of maternal behavior in the ewe. In J. S. Rosenblatt, R. A. Hinde, C. G. Beer, and M.-C. Busnel (Eds.), Advances in the Study of Behavior, Vol. 11. Academic Press, New York, pp. 75–119.

825. Poindron, P. and Lévy, F. (1990) Physiological, sensory, and experiential determinants of maternal behavior in sheep. In N. E. Krasnegor and R. S. Bridges (Eds.), Mammalian Parenting. Oxford University Press, New York, pp. 133–156.

826. Poindron, P., Lévy, F., and Krehbiel, D. (1988) Genital, olfactory, and endocrine interactions in the development of maternal behaviour in the parturient ewe. Psychoneuroendocrinology 13:99–125.

827. Pomerantz, S. M., Goy, R. W., and Roy, M. M. (1986) Expression of male-typical behavior in adult female pseudohermaphroditic rhesus: Comparisons with normal males and neonatally gonadectomized males and females. Horm. Behav. 20:483–500.

828. Powers, J. B. and Winans, S. S. (1975) Vomeronasal organ: Critical role in mediating sexual behavior of the male hamster. Science 187:961–963.

829. Prosser, C. L. (1986) Adaptational Biology: Molecules to Organisms. Wiley & Sons, New York.

830. Prosser, C. L. (1989) Comparative physiology and biochemistry: Challenges for the future. Comp. Biochem. Physiol. 93A:309–312.

831. Prove, E. (1974) Der Einfluss von Kastration und Testosteronsubstitution auf das Sexualverhaltern mannlicher Zebrafinken. J. Ornithologie 115:338–347.

832. Purves, D. and Lichtman, J. W. (1985) Principles of Neural Development. Sinauer Associates, Sunderland, Mass.

833. Purves, D. and Lichtman, J. W. (1985) Geometrical differences among homologous neurons in mammals. Science 228:298–302.

834. Rabin, D., Gold, P., Margioris, A., and Chrousos, G. (1988) Stress and reproduction: Physiologic and pathophysiologic interactions between the stress and reproductive axes. In G. Chrousos, D. Loriaux, and P. Gold, (Eds.), Mechanisms of Physical and Emotional Stress. Plenum, New York.

834a. Rabl, R. (1958) Strukturstudien an der Massa Intermedia des Thalamus Opticus. J. Hirnforsch 4:78–112.

835. Raisman, G. and Field, P. M. (1973) Sexual dimorphism in the neuropil of the preoptic area of the rat and its dependence on neonatal androgen. Brain Res. 54:1–20.

836. Ralls, K. (1974) Mammals in which females are larger than males. Q. Rev. Biol. 51:245–276.

837. Ramsay, D. J. (1979) The brain renin angiotensin system: A re-evaluation. Neuroscience 4:313–321.

838. Rand, M. N. and Breedlove, S. M. (1987) Ontogeny of functional innervation of bulbocavernosus muscles in male and female rats. Dev. Brain Res. 33:150–152.

839. Rapp, P. E. (1985) Communication and control in reproduction: The ubiquity of periodic phenomena. Biol. Reprod. 32:70–72.

840. Rapp, P. E. (1987) Why are so many biological systems periodic? Prog. Neurobiol. 29:261–273.

841. Reddy, V. V. R., Naftolin, F., and Ryan, K. J. (1974) Conversion of androstenedione to estrone by neutral tissues from fetal and neonatal rat. Endocrinology 94:117.

842. Reid, I. (1989) Pathogenesis and treatment of steroid osteoporosis. Clin. Endocrinol. 30:83–103.

843. Reinisch, J. M. (1981) Prenatal exposure to synthetic progestins increases potential for aggression in humans. Science 211:1171–1173.
844. Reinisch, J. M. and Karow, W. G. (1977) Prenatal exposure to synthetic progestins and estrogens: Effects on human development. Arch. Sex. Behav. 6:257–288.
845. Reinisch, J. M. and Sanders, S. A. (1984) Prenatal gonadal steroidal influences on gender-related behavior. Prog. Brain Res. 61:407–416.
846. Reiter, R. J. (1968) Changes in the reproductive organs of cold-exposed and light deprived female hamsters (*Mesocricetus auratus*). J. Reprod. Fertil. 16:217–222.
847. Resnick, S. M., Berenbaum, S. A., Gottesman, I. I., and Bouchard, T. J. (1986) Early hormonal influences on cognitive functioning in congenital adrenal hyperplasia. Dev. Psychol. 22:191–198.
848. Richard-Yris, M.-A. and Leboucher, G. (1986) Induction of maternal behaviour in the domestic hen: Influence of chick development on maternal responses. Biol. Behav. 11:157–166.
849. Richard-Yris, M.-A. and Leboucher, G. (1987) Initiation and maintenance of maternal behaviour in the domestic hen: Influence of testosterone and oestradiol treatments. Ethology 75:337–347.
850. Richter, C. P. (1942) Total self-regulatory functions in animals and human beings. Harvey Lectures 38:63–103.
851. Richter, C. P. (1967) Sleep and activity: Their relation to the 24-hour clock. Proc. Assoc. Res. Nerv. Ment. Dis. 45:8–27.
852. Riddiford, L. M. (1985) Hormone action at the cellular level. In G. A. Kerkut and L. I. Gilbert (Eds.), Comprehensive Insect Physiology, Biochemistry, and Pharmacology, Vol. 8. Pergamon Press, Oxford, pp. 37–84.
853. Riddiford, L. M. and Hiruma, K. (1990) Hormonal control of sequential gene expression in lepidopteran epidermis. In E. Ohnishi and H. Ishizaki (Eds.), Molting and Metamorphosis. Japan Scientific Society Press, Tokyo, pp. 207–222.
854. Riddoch, D., Jefferson, M., and Bickerstaff, E. R. (1971) Chorea and oral contraceptives. Br. Med. J. 4:217–218.
855. Ridewood, W. (1898) On the structure and development of the hyobranchial skeleton and larynx in *Xenopus* and *Pipa*; with remarks on the affinities of the aglossa. Linn. Soc. J. Zool. 26:53–128.
856. Rissman, E. (1987) Gonadal influences on sexual behavior in the male musk shrew (*Sucus murinus*). Horm. Behav. 21:132–136.
857. Rissman, E. F., Clendenon, A. L., and Krohmer, R. W. (1990) Role of androgens in the regulation of sexual behavior in the female musk shrew. Neuroendocrinology 51:468–473.
858. Robbins, S., Cotran, R., and Kumar, V. (1984) The gastrointestinal tract. In S. Robbins, R. Cotran, and V. Kumar (Eds.), The Pathological Basis of Disease (3rd ed.) W. B. Saunders, Philadelphia, pp. 797–883.
859. Roberts, W. W. and Keiss, H. O. (1964) Motivational properties of hypothalamic aggression in cats. J. Comp. Physiol. Psychol. 64:1–15.
860. Robertson, G. L. (1983) Thirst and vasopressin function in normal and disordered states of water balance. J. Lab. Clin. Med. 101:351–371.
861. Robertson, G. L. and Berl, T. (1986) Water metabolism. In B. M. Brenner, and F. C. Rector, Jr. (Eds.), The Kidney (3rd ed.). W. B. Saunders, Philadelphia, pp. 385–432.
862. Robinson, T. E., Camp, D. M., and Becker, J. B. (1981) Gonadectomy attenuates turning behavior produced by electrical stimulation of the nigrostriatal dopamine system in female but not male rats. Neurosci. Lett. 23:203–208.
863. Robinson, T. E., Camp, D. M., Jacknow, D. S., and Becker, J. B. (1982) Sex differences and estrous cycle dependent variation in rotational behavior elicited by electrical stimulation of the mesostriatal dopamine system. Behav. Brain Res. 6:273–287.
864. Roenneberg, T. and Aschoff, J. (1990) Annual rhythm of human reproduction: II. Environmental correlations. J. Biol. Rhythms 5:217–239.
865. Rogers, R. C. and Hermann, G. E. (1987) Oxytocin, oxytocin antagonist, TRH, and hypothalamic paraventricular nucleus stimulation: Effects on gastric motility. Peptides 8:505–513.
866. Rose, J. D. (1990) Forebrain influences on brainstem and spinal mechanisms of copulatory behavior: A current perspective on Frank Beach's contribution. Neurosci. Biobehav. Rev. 14:207–215.
867. Rose, R. (1985) Psychoendocrinology. In J. D. Wilson and D. Foster (Eds.), Williams Textbook of Endocrinology (7th ed.). W. B. Saunders, Philadelphia, pp. 653–681.
868. Rose, R. M., Berstein, I. S., and Holaday, J. W. (1971) Plasma testosterone, dominance rank and aggressive behavior in a group of male rhesus monkeys. Nature 231:366–368.
869. Rosedale, R. S. (1945) Nasogenital relationship. Arch. Otolaryngol. 42:235–238.
870. Rosenblatt, J. (1972) Learning in newborn kittens. Sci. Am. 227:18–29.

871. Rosenblatt, J. S. and Lehrman, D. S. (1963) Maternal behavior in the laboratory rat. In H. L. Rheingold (Ed.), Maternal Behavior in Mammals. Wiley & Sons, New York, pp. 8–57.

872. Rosenblatt, J. S. and Siegel, H. I. (1975) Hysterectomy-induced maternal behavior during pregnancy in the rat. J. Comp. Physiol. Psychol. 89:685–700.

873. Rosenblatt, J. S., and Siegel, H. I. (1981) Factors governing the onset and maintenance of maternal behavior among nonprimate mammals. In D. J. Gubernick and P. H. Klopfer (Eds.), Parental Care in Mammals. Plenum, New York, pp. 13–76.

874. Rosenblatt, J. S. and Siegel, H. I. (1981) Physiological and behavioural changes during pregnancy and parturition underlying the onset of maternal behavior in rodents. In R. W. Elwood (Ed.), Parental Behaviour of Rodents. Wiley & Sons, New York, pp. 23–66.

875. Rosenblatt, J. S., Siegel, H. I., and Mayer, A. D. (1979) Progress in the study of maternal behavior in the rat: Hormonal, nonhormonal, sensory, and developmental aspects. In J. S. Rosenblatt, R. A. Hinde, C. Beer, and M.-C. Busnel (Eds.), Advances in the Study of Behavior, Vol. 10. Academic Press, New York, pp. 225–311.

876. Rosenfeld, J. M., Daley, J. D., Ohno, S., and YoungLai, E. V. (1977) Central aromatization of testoterone in testicular feminized mice. Experientia 33:1392–1393.

877. Rossi, A. S. (1980) Mood cycles by menstrual month and social week. In A. J. Dan, E. A. Graham, and C. P. Beecher (Eds.), The Menstrual Cycle, Vol. 1. A Synthesis of Interdisciplinary Research. Springer-Verlag, New York, pp. 56–71.

878. Roth, L. L. and Rosenblatt, J. S. (1967) Changes in self-licking during pregnancy in the rat. J. Comp. Physiol. Psychol. 63:397–400.

879. Roth, L. L. and Rosenblatt, J. S. (1968) Self-licking and mammary development during pregnancy in the rat. J. Endocrinol. 42:363–378.

880. Rothman, B. S., Weir, G., and Dudek, F. E. (1983) Egg-laying hormone: Direct action on the ovotestis of Aplysia. Gen. Comp. Endocrinol. 52:134–141.

881. Rowan, W. (1925) Relation of light to bird migration and development changes. Nature 115:494–495.

882. Rowe, F. P. (1981) Wild house mouse biology and control. In R. J. Berry (Ed.), Biology of the House Mouse. Zoological Society of London Symposium 47. Academic Press, New York, pp. 575–590.

883. Rowell, T. (1972) Social Behaviour of Monkeys. Penguin, Middlesex, U.K.

884. Roy, E. J., Buyer, D. R., and Licari, V. A. (1990) Estradiol in the striatum: Effects on behavior and dopamine receptors but no evidence for membrane steroid receptors. Brain Res. Bull. 25:221–227.

885. Rozin, P. N. and Schulkin, J. (1990) Food selection. In E. M. Stricker (Ed.), Handbook of Behavioral Neurobiology, Vol. 10. Plenum, New York, pp. 297–328.

886. Rubin, B. S. and Barfield, R. J. (1983) Progesterone in the ventromedial hypothalamus facilitates estrous behavior in ovariectomized, estrogen-primed rats. Endocrinology 37:218–224.

887. Rubin, B. S. and Bridges, R. S. (1989) Immunoreactive prolactin in the CSF of estrogen-treated and lactating rats as determined by push-pull perfusion of the lateral ventricles. J. Neuroendocrinol. 1:345–349.

888. Rubin, R. T. (1982) Testosterone and aggression in men. In J. V. Beumont and G. D. Burrows (Eds.), Handbook of Psychiatry and Endocrinology. Elsevier Biomedical Press. Amsterdam.

889. Russell, M. J. S., G. M., and Thompson, K. (1980) Olfactory influences on the human menstrual cycle. Pharmacol. Biochem. Behav. 13:737–738.

890. Russert-Kraemer, L. (1989) "I'll see it when I believe it": Investigating nervous system/reproductive system interactions in animal organisms. Am. Zool. 29:1141–1155.

891. Ryan, M. J. (1985) The Tungara Frog. University of Chicago Press, Chicago.

892. Ryan, M. J. (1990) Sexual selection, sensory systems, and sensory exploitation. Oxford Surveys in Evolutionary Biology 7:157–196.

893. Ryan, M. J., Fox, J. H., Wilczynski, W., and Rand, A. S. (1990) Sexual selection for sensory exploitation in the frog Physalanaemus pustulosus. Nature 343:66–67.

894. Ryan, S. M. and Maier, S. F. (1988) The estrous cycle and estrogen modulate stress-induced analgesia. Behav. Neurosci. 102:371–380.

895. Sachs, B. D. (1982) Role of striated penile muscles in penile reflexes, copulation, and induction of pregnancy in the rat. J. Reprod. Fertil. 66:433–443.

896. Sachs, B. D. and Meisel, R. L. (1988) The physiology of male sexual behavior. In E. Knobil and J. Neill (Eds.), The Physiology of Reproduction, Vol. 2. Raven Press, New York, pp. 1393–1485.

897. Saidapur, S. K. and Greenwald, G. S. (1978) Peripheral blood and ovarian levels of sex steroids in the cyclic hamster. Biol. Reprod. 18:401–408.

898. Sanders, B., Soares, M. P., and D'Aquila, J. M. (1982) The sex difference on one test of spatial visualization: A nontrival difference. Child Devel. 53:1106–1110.

899. Sanders, D. and Bancroft, J. (1982) Hormones and the sexuality of women—The menstrual cycle. In J. Bancroft (Ed.), Clinics in Endocrinology and Metabolism, Vol. II. Saunders, London, pp. 639–660.

900. Sanders, D., Warner, P., Backstrom, T., and Bancroft, J. (1983) Mood, sexuality, hormones and the menstrual cycle. I. Changes in mood and physical state: Description of subjects and method. Psychosom. Med. 45:487–501.

901. Sandhu, S., Cooke, P., and Diamond, M. C. (1986) Rat cerebral cortical estrogen receptors: Male-female, right-left. Exp. Neurol. 92:186–196.

902. Sapolsky, R. M. (1985) Glucocorticoid toxicity in the hippocampus: Temporal aspects of neuronal vulnerability. Brain Res. 359:300–305.

903. Sapolsky, R. M. (1985) A mechanism for glucocorticoid toxicity in the hippocampus: Increased neuronal vulnerability to metabolic insults. J. Neurosci. 5:1228–1232.

904. Sapolsky, R. M. (1986) Glucocorticoid toxicity in the hippocampus: Reversal by supplementation with brain fuels. J. Neurosci. 6:2240–2244.

905. Sapolsky, R. M. (1987) Stress, social status and reproductive physiology in free-living baboons. In D. Crews (Ed.), Psychobiology of Reproductive Behavior: An Evolutionary Perspective. Prentice Hall, Englewood Cliffs, pp. 291–322.

906. Sapolsky, R. M. (1990) Stress in the wild. Sci. Am. 262:116–123.

907. Sapolsky, R. M. (1991) The effects of stress upon hippocampal function. In M. Brown, K. Rivier, and G. Koob (Eds.), The Neurobiology and Neuroendocrinology of Stress. Plenum, New York.

908. Sapolsky, R. M. (1991) Adrenocortical function, social status and personality among wild baboons. Biol. Psychiatry 28:862–878.

909. Sapolsky, R. M. (1991) Testicular function, social status and personality among wild baboons. Psychoneuroendocrinology 16:281–293.

910. Sapolsky, R. M., Armanini, M. P., Sutton, S. W., and Plotsky, P. M. (1989) Elevation of hypophysial portal concentrations of adrenocorticotropin secretagogues after fornix transection. Endocrinology 125:2881–2887.

911. Sapolsky, R. M., Krey, L. C., and McEwen, B. S. (1985) Prolonged glucocorticoid exposure reduces hippocampal neuron number: Implications for aging. J. Neurosci. 5:1222–1227.

912. Sapolsky, R. M., Krey, L. C., and McEwen, B. S. (1986) The adrenocortical axis in the aged rat: Impaired sensitivity to both fast and delayed feedback inhibition. Neurobiol. Aging 7:331–335.

913. Sapolsky, R. M. and Meaney, M. J. (1986) Maturation of the adrenocortical stress response: Neuroendocrine control mechanisms and the stress hyporesponsive period. Brain Res. 396:64–76.

914. Sapolsky, R. M., Packan, D. R., and Vale, W. W. (1988) Glucocorticoid toxicity in the hippocampus: In vitro demonstration. Brain Res. 453:367–371.

915. Sapolsky, R. M. and Plotsky, P. (1989) Hypercortisolism and its possible neural bases. Biol. Psychiatry 27:937–952.

916. Sapolsky, R. M., Uno, H., Rebert, C., and Finch, C. E. (1990) Hippocampal damage associated with prolonged glucocorticoid exposure in primates. J. Nurosci. 10:2897–2902.

917. Sarrieau, A., Mitchell, J., and Meaney, M. J. (1988) Androgen receptors in human temporal cortex. Soc. Neurosci. Abstr. 14:511.

918. Sassoon, D., Gray, G., and Kelley, D. (1987) Androgen regulation of muscle fiber type in the sexually dimorphic larynx of Xenopus laevis. J. Neurosci. 7:3198–3206.

919. Schaffer, C. E., Davidson, R. J., and Saron, C. (1983) Frontal and parietal electroencephalogram asymmetry in depressed and nondepressed subjects. Biol. Psychiatry 18:753–762.

920. Scheff, S. W. and Dekosky, S. T. (1989) Glucocorticoid suppression of lesion-induced synaptogenesis: Effect of temporal manipulation of steroid treatment. Exp. Neurol. 105:260–264.

921. Scheff, S. W., Hoff, S. F., and Anderson, K. J. (1986) Altered regulation of lesion-induced synaptogenesis by adrenalectomy and corticosterone in young adult rats. Exp. Neurol. 93:456–470.

922. Scheff, S. W., Morse, J. K., and DeKosky, S. T. (1988) Hydrocortisone differentially alters lesion-induced axon sprouting in male and female rats. Exp. Neurol. 100:237–241.

923. Scheff, S. W., Morse, J. K., and DeKosky, S. T. (1988) Neurotrophic effects of steroids on lesion-induced growth in the hippocampus. I. The asteroidal condition. Brain Res. 457:246–250.

924. Scheller, R. H., Jackson, J. F., McAllister, L. B., Rothman, B. S., Mayeri, E., and Axel, R. (1983) A single gene encodes multiple neuropeptides mediating a stereotyped behavior. Cell 32:7–22.

925. Schmidt, R. (1974) Neural correlates of frog calling: Trigeminal tegmentum. J. Comp. Physiol. 92:229–254.

926. Schmidt, R. (1976) Neural correlates of frog calling: Isolated brain stem. J. Comp. Physiol. 108:99–113.

927. Schneider, J. E. and Wade, G. N. (1989) Availability of metabolic fuels controls estrous cyclicity of Syrian hamsters. Science 244:1326–1328.

928. Schumacher, M. (1990) Rapid membrane effects of steroid hormones: An emerging concept in neuroendocrinology. Trends Neurosci. 13:359–362.

929. Schwanzel-Fukuda, M., Bick, D., and Pfaff, D. W. (1989) Luteinizing hormone-releasing hormone (LHRH)-expressing cells do not migrate normally in an inherited hypogonadal (Kallman) syndrome. Mol. Br. Res. 6:311–326.

930. Schwanzel-Fukuda, M. and Pfaff, D. W. (1989) Origin of luteinizing hormone-releasing hormone neurons. Nature 138:161–164.

931. Schwartz-Giblin, S., McEwen, B. S., and Pfaff, D. W. (1989) Mechanisms of female reproductive behavior. In R. Brush and S. Levine (Eds.), Psychoendocrinology. Academic Press, New York, pp. 41–104.

932. Scott, J. P. and Fredericson, E. (1951) The causes of fighting in mice and rats. Physiol. Zool. 24:273–309.

933. Seegal, R. F. and Goldman, B. D. (1975) Effects of photoperiod on cyclicity and serum gonadotropins in the Syrian hamster. Biol. Reprod. 12:223–231.

934. Seger, J. (1989) Diversity of little things. Nature 337:305–306.

935. Segraves, R. T., Madsen, R., Carter, C. S., and Davis, J. M. (1985) Erectile dysfunction associated with pharmacological agents. In R. T. Segraves and H. W. Schoenberg (Eds.), Diagnosis and Treatment of Erectile Disturbances. Plenum, New York, pp. 23–63.

936. Selander, R. K. (1960) Failure of estrogen and prolactin to induce brood patch formation in brown-headed cowbirds. Condor 62:65.

937. Selye, H. (1976) The Stress of Life. McGraw-Hill, New York.

938. Sharman, G. B. (1963) Delayed implantation in marsupials. In A. D. Enders (Ed.), Delayed Implantation. University of Chicago Press, Chicago, pp. 3–14.

939. Shekelle, R., Raynor, W., Ostfeld, A., Garron, D., Bieliauskas, L., Liu, S., Maliza, C., and Paul, O. (1981) Psychological depression and 17-year risk of death from cancer. Psychosom. Med. 43:117–125.

939a. Shepherd, G. M. (1988) Neurobiology. Oxford University Press, New York.

940. Sherman, P. W., Jarvis, J. U. M., and Alexander, R. D. (Eds.) (1991) The Biology of the Naked Mole-Rat. Princeton University Press, Lawrenceville, N.J.

941. Sherwin, B. B. (1988) A comparative analysis of the role of androgen in human male and female sexual behavior: Behavioral specificity, critical thresholds, and sensitivity. Psychobiology 16:416–425.

942. Sherwin, B. B. (1988) Estrogen and/or androgen replacement therapy and cognitive functioning in surgically menopausal women. Psychoneuroendocrinology 13:345–357.

943. Sherwin, B. B. and Gelfand, M. M. (1985) Sex steroids and affect in the surgical menopause: A double-blind, crossover study. Psychoneuroendocrinology 10:325–335.

944. Sherwin, B. B. and Phillips, S. (1990) Estrogen and cognitive functioning in surgically menopausal women. Ann. N.Y. Acad. Sci. 592:474–475.

945. Shivers, B. D., Harlan, R. E., and Pfaff, D. W. (1989) A subset of neurons containing immunoreactive prolactin is a target for estrogen regulation of gene expression in rat hypothalamus. Neuroendocrinology 49:23–27.

946. Shughrue, P. J., Stumpf, W. E., MacLusky, N. J., Zielinski, J. E., and Hochberg, R. B. (1990) Developmental changes in estrogen receptors in mouse cerebral cortex between birth and postweaning: Studied by autoradiography with 11 beta-methoxy-16 alpha-[^{125}I]iodoestradiol. Endocrinology 126:1112–1124.

947. Shute, V. J., Pellegrino, J. W., Hubert, L., and Reynolds, R. W. (1983) The relationship between androgen levels and human spatial abilities. Bull. Psychonom. Soc. 21:465–468.

948. Signoret, J. P. (1976) Chemical communication and reproduction in domestic mammals. In R. L. Doty (Ed.), Mammalian Olfaction, Reproductive Processes, and Behavior. Academic Press, New York, pp. 243–256.

949. Silver, R. (1984) Prolactin and parenting in the pigeon family. J. Exp. Zool. 232:617–625.

950. Silver, R. (1990) Avian behavioral endocrinology: Status and prospects. In M. Wada, S. Ishii, and C. G. Scanes (Eds.), Endocrinology of Birds, Molecular to Behavioral. Springer-Verlag, Berlin, pp. 261–272.

951. Silver, R. (1990) Biological timing mechanisms with special emphasis on the parental behavior of doves. In D. A. Dewsbury (Ed.), Contemporary Issues in Comparative Psychology. Sinauer Associates, Sunderland, Mass., pp. 252–277.

952. Silver, R. and Barbiere, C. (1977) Display of courtship and incubation behavior during the reproductive cycle of the male ring dove (Streptopelia risoria). Horm. Behav. 8:8–21.

953. Silver, R. and Feder, H. H. (1973) Role of gonadal hormones in incubation behavior of male ring doves (Streptopelia risoria). J. Comp. Physiol. Psychol. 84:464–471.

954. Silverin, B. and Goldsmith, A. R. (1983) Reproductive endocrinology of free living Pied flycatchers (*Ficedula hypoleuca*): Prolactin and FSH secretion in relation to incubation and clutch size. J. Zool. (Lond.) 200:119–130.

955. Silverman, E. M. and Zimmer, C. H. (1975) Speech fluency fluctuations during the menstrual cycle. J. Speech Hear. Res. 18:202–206.

956. Silverman, E. M., Zimmer, C. H., and Silverman, F. H. (1974) Variability of stutterers' speech disfluency: The menstrual cycle. Percept. Mot. Skills 38:1037–1038.

957. Simerly, R. B. (1990) Hormonal control of neuropeptide gene expression in sexually dimorphic olfactory pathways. Trends Neurosci. 13:104–109.

958. Simon, N. G. and Whalen, R. E. (1987) Sexual differentiation of androgen-sensitive and estrogen-sensitive regulatory systems for aggressive behavior. Horm. Behav. 21:493–500.

959. Simpkins, J. W., Kalra, S. P., and Kalra, P. S. (1980) Inhibitory effects of androgens on the preoptic area dopaminergic neurons in castrate rats. Neuroendocrinology 31:177–181.

960. Simpson, J. B., Mangiapane, M. L., and Dellman, H. D. (1978) Central receptor sites for angiotensin-induced drinking: A critical review. Fed. Proc. 37:2676–2682.

961. Sirinathsinghji, D. J. S., Whittington, P. E., Audsley, A., and Frazer, H. M. (1983) Beta-endorphin regulates lordosis in female rats by modulating LH-RH release. Nature 301:62–64.

962. Skutch, A. F. (1976) Parent Birds and Their Young. University of Texas Press, Austin.

963. Slimp, J. C., Hart, B. L., and Goy, R. W. (1975) Heterosexual, autosexual and social behavior of adult male rhesus monkeys with medial preoptic-anterior hypothalamic lesions. Brain Res. 142:105–122.

964. Slob, A. K., Bogers, H., and van Stolk, M. (1981) Effects of gonadectomy and exogenous gonadal steroids on sex differences in open field behaviour of adult rats. Behav. Brain Res. 2:347–362.

965. Sloviter, R. S., Valiquette, G., Abrams, G. M., Ronk, E. C., Sollas, A. I., Paul, L. A., and Neubort, S. L. (1989) Selective loss of hippocampal granule cells in the mature rat brain after adrenalectomy. Science 243:535–538.

966. Smith, A. J. (1950) Menstruation and industrial efficiency. I. Absenteeism and activity level. J. Appl. Psychol. 34:1–5.

967. Smith, A. J. (1950) Menstruation and industrial efficiency. II. Quality and quantity of production. J. Appl. Psychol. 34:148–152.

968. Smith, J. C. (1981) Senses and communication. In R. J. Berry (Ed.), Biology of the Mouse. Zoological Society of London Symposium 47. Academic Press, New York, pp. 367–394.

969. Smith, M. S., McLean, B. K., and Neill, J. D. (1976) Prolactin: The initial luteotropic stimulus of pseudo-pregnancy in the rat. Endocrinology 98:1370–1377.

970. Smith, M. S. and Neill, J. D. (1976) A "critical period" for cervically-stimulated prolactin release. Endocrinology 98:324–328.

971. Smith, M. S. and Neill, J. D. (1976) Termination at midpregnancy of the two daily surges of plasma prolactin initiated by mating in the rat. Endocrinology 98:696–701.

972. Smith, S. S. (1989) Estrogen administration increases neuronal responses to excitatory amino acids as a long-term effect. Brain Res. 503:354–357.

973. Smith, S. S., Woodward, D. J., and Chapin, J. K. (1989) Sex steroids modulate motor-correlated increases in cerebellar discharge. Brain Res. 476:307–316.

974. Snyder, D. A. B. (1978) The relationship of the menstrual cycle to certain aspects of perceptual cognitive functioning. Dissert. Abstr. Int. 39:962B–963B.

975. Soares, M. J. and Diamond, M. (1982) Pregnancy and chin marking in the rabbit, *Oryctolagus cuniculas*. Anim. Behav. 30:941–943.

976. Sodersten, P., Forsberg, G., Bednar, I., Eneroth, P., and Wiesenfeld-Hallin, Z. (1989) Opioid peptide inhibition of sexual behaviour in female rats. In R. G. Dyer and R. J. Bicknell (Eds.), Brain Opioid Systems in Reproduction. Oxford University Press, Oxford, pp. 203–215.

977. Sommer, B. (1972) Menstrual cycle changes and intellectual performance. Psychosom. Med. 34:263–269.

978. Sorensen, P. W. and Stacey, N. E. (1991) Identified hormonal pheromones in the goldfish: The basis for a model of sex pheromone function in teleost fish. In D. W. MacDonald, D. Muller-Schwarze, and S. E. Natynezuk (Eds.), Chemical Signals in Vertebrates. V. Oxford University Press, Oxford, pp. 302–311.

979. Spears, N., Meyer, J. S., Whaling, C. S., Wade, G. N., Zucker, I., and Dark, J. (1990) Long day lengths enhance myelination of midbrain and hindbrain regions of developing meadow voles. Dev. Brain Res. 55:103–108.

980. Spies, H. G., Forbes, Y. M., and Clegg, M. T. (1971) The influence of coitus, suckling and prolactin injections on pregnancy in pelvic neurectomized rats. Proc. Soc. Exp. Biol. Med. 138:470–474.

981. Spies, H. G. and Niswender, G. D. (1971) Levels of prolactin, LH and FSH in the serum of intact and pelvic-neurectomized rats. Endocrinology 88:937–943.

982. Springer, S. P. and Deutch, G. (1985) Left Brain, Right Brain (2nd ed.). W. H. Freeman, New York.

983. Squire, A. and Moller, P. (1982) Effects of water conductivity on electrocommunication in the weak-electric fish *Brienomyrus niger* (mormyriformes). Anim. Behav. 30:375–382.

984. Stanley, A. J., Gumbreck, L. G., Allison, J. E. (1973) Male pseudohermaphroditism in the laboratory rat. Recent Prog. Horm. Res. 29:43–64.

984a. Steiner, M., Katz, R. J., and Carroll, B. J. (1980) Behavioral effects of dopamine agonists across the estrous cycle in rats. Psychopharmacology 71:147–151.

985. Stenn, P. G. and Klinge, V. (1972) Relationship between the menstrual cycle and bodily activity in humans. Horm. Behav. 3:297–305.

986. Stephan, F. K. and Zucker, I. (1972) Circadian rhythms in drinking behavior and locomotor activity of rats are eliminated by hypothalamic lesions. Proc. Natl. Acad. Sci. U.S.A. 69:1583–1586.

987. Stetson, M. H. and Anderson, P. J. (1980) Circadian pacemaker times gonadotropin release in free-running female hamsters. Am. J. Physiol. 238:1223–1227.

988. Stetson, M. H. and Watson-Whitmyre, M. (1976) Nucleus suprachiasmaticus: The biological clock in the hamster? Science 191:197–199.

989. Stevens, R. and Goldstein, R. (1981) Effects of neonatal testosterone and estrogen on open-field behaviour in rats. Physiol. Behav. 26:551–553.

990. Stewart, J. and Cygan, D. (1980) Ovarian hormones act early in development to feminize adult open-field behavior in the rat. Horm. Behav. 14:20–32.

991. Stewart, J. and Kolb, B. (1988) The effects of neonatal gonadectomy and prenatal stress on cortical thickness and asymmetry in rats. Behav. Neural. Biol. 49:344–360.

992. Stocker, J. M. (1973) Motor performance and state anxiety at selected stages of the menstrual cycle. Dissert. Abstr. Int. 34:3971-A.

993. Stockman, E. R., Callaghan, R. S., and Baum, M. J. (1985) Effect of neonatal castration and testosterone treatment on sexual partner preference in the ferret. Physiol. Behav. 34:409–414.

994. Stone, C. P. (1939) Copulatory activity in adult male rats following castration and injections of testosterone propionate. Endocrinology 24:165–174.

995. Stoneham, M. D., Everitt, B. J., Hansen, S., Lightman, S. L., and Todd, K. (1985) Oxytocin and sexual behaviour in the male rat and rabbit. J. Endocrinol. 107:97–106.

996. Stout, J., Walikonis, R., and Atkins, G. (1989) The influence of age and JHIII levels on the phonotactic response of female crickets (*Acheta domestica*) to the male's calling song. In J. Erber, R. Menzel, H.-J. Pfluger, and D. Todt (Eds.), Neural Mechanisms of Behavior. G. Thieme Verlag, Stuttgart, p. 75.

997. Stricker, E. M. (1969) Osmoregulation and volume regulation in rats: Inhibition of hypovolemic thirst by water. Am. J. Physiol. 217:98–105.

998. Stricker, E. M. (1978) The renin-angiotensin system and thirst: Some unanswered questions. Fed. Proc. 37:2704–2710.

999. Stricker, E. M. (1981) Thirst and sodium appetite after colloid treatment in rats. J. Comp. Physiol. Psychol. 95:1–25.

1000. Stricker, E. M. (1984) Biological bases of hunger and satiety: Therapeutic implications. Nutr. Rev. 42:333–340.

1001. Stricker, E. M. (1990) Homeostatic origins of motivated behavior. In E. M. Stricker (Ed.), Handbook of Behavioral Neurobiology, Vol. 10. Plenum, New York, pp. 45–60.

1002. Stricker, E. M., Hosutt, J. A., and Verbalis, J. G. (1987) Neurohypophyseal secretion in hypovolemic rats: Inverse relation to sodium appetite. Am. J. Physiol. 252:R889–R896.

1003. Stricker, E. M. and McCann, M. J. (1985) Visceral factors in the control of food intake. Brain Res. Bull. 14:687–692.

1004. Stricker, E. M., McCann, M. J., Flanagan, L. M., and Verbalis, J. G. (1988) Neurohypophyseal secretion and gastric function: Biological correlates of nausea. In H. Takagi, Y. Oomura, M. Ito, and M. Otsuka (Eds.), Biowarning System in the Brain. University of Tokyo Press, Tokyo, pp. 295–307.

1005. Stricker, E. M. and Verbalis, J. G. (1986) Interaction of osmotic and volume stimuli in regulation of neurohypophyseal secretion in rats. Am. J. Physiol. 250:R267–R275.

1006. Stricker, E. M. and Verbalis, J. G. (1987) Central inhibitory control of sodium appetite in rats: Correlation with pituitary oxytocin secretion. Behav. Neurosci. 101:560–567.

1007. Stricker, E. M. and Verbalis, J. G. (1988) Hormones and behavior: The biological bases of thirst and sodium appetite. Am. Sci. 76:261–267.

1008. Stricker, E. M. and Verbalis, J. G. (1990) Control of appetite and satiety: Insights from biologic and behavioral studies. Nutr. Rev. 48:49–56.

1009. Stricker, E. M. and Verbalis, J. G. (1990) Sodium appetite. In E. M. Stricker (Ed.), Handbook of Behavioral Neurobiology, Vol. 10. Plenum, New York, pp. 387–419.

1010. Suomi, S. (1987) Genetic and maternal contributions to individual differences in rhesus monkey biobehavioral development. In N. Krasnegor, E. Blass, M. Hofer, and W. Smotherman (Eds.), Perinatal Development: A Psychobiological Perspective. Academic Press, New York.

1011. Susman, E. J., Inoff-Germain, G., Nottelmann, E. D., Loriaux, D. L., Cutler, G. B., and Chrousos, G. P. (1987) Hormones, emotional dispositions, and aggressive attributes in young adolescents. Child Dev. 58:1114–1134.

1012. Svare, B., Davis, P. G., and Gandelman, R. (1974) Fighting behavior in female mice following chronic androgen treatment during adulthood. Physiol. Behav. 12:399–403.

1013. Svare, B. B. and Mann, M. A. (1983) Hormonal influences on maternal aggression. In B. B. Svare (Ed.), Hormones and Aggressive Behavior. Plenum, New York, pp. 91–104.

1014. Swaab, D. F. and Fliers, E. (1985) A sexually dimorphic nucleus in the human brain. Science 228:1112–1115.

1015. Swaab, D. F. and Hofman, M. A. (1984) Sexual differentiation of the human brain. A historical perspective. Prog. Brain Res. 61:361.

1016. Swanson, L. W. and Sawchenko, P. E. (1983) Hypothalamic integration: Organization of the paraventricular and supraoptic nuclei. Annu. Rev. Neurosci. 6:269–324.

1017. Szabo, T. (1974) Anatomy of the specialized lateral line organs of electroreception. In A. Fessard (Ed.), Handbook of Sensory Physiology, Vol. III. Springer-Verlag, Berlin, pp. 13–18.

1018. Szczepanska-Sadowska, E., Kozlowski, S., and Sobocinska, J. (1974) Blood antidiuretic hormone level and osmotic reactivity of thirst mechanisms in dogs. Am. J. Physiol. 227:766–770.

1019. Taigen, T. and Wells, K. (1984) Energetics of vocalization by an anuran amphibian, *Hyla versicolor*. J. Comp. Physiol. [B] 155:163–170.

1020. Takahashi, J. S. and Menaker, M. (1980) Interaction of estradiol and progesterone: Effects on circadian locomotor rhythms in female golden hamsters. Am. J. Physiol. 239:R497–R504.

1021. Tanner, J. M. (1968) Earlier maturation in man. Sci. Am. 218:21–27.

1022. Tellegen, A., Horn, J. M., and Legrand, R. G. (1969) Opportunity for aggression as a reinforcer in mice. Psychonom. Sci. 14:104–105.

1023. Ter Haar, M. B. (1972) Circadian and estrual rhythms in food intake in rat. Horm. Behav. 3:213–219.

1024. Terkel, J. and Sawyer, C. H. (1978) Male copulatory behavior triggers nightly prolactin surges resulting in successful pregnancy in rats. Horm. Behav. 11:304–309.

1025. Therrien, B. A. (1982) Sex differences in the effects of hippocampal lesions on place navigation. Ph.D. dissertation, University of Michigan, Ann Arbor.

1026. Therrien, B. A., Camp, D. M., and Robinson, T. E. (1982) Sex differences in the effects of unilateral hippocampal lesions on spatial navigation. Soc. Neurosci. Abstr. 8:312.

1027. Thomas, C. S. and Coulson, J. C. (1988) Reproductive success of kittiwake gulls, *Rissa tridactyla*. In T. H. Clutton-Brock (Ed.), Reproductive Success. University of Chicago Press, Chicago, pp. 251–262.

1028. Thorpe, W. H. (1958) The learning of song patterns by birds, with especial reference to the song of the chaffinch, *Fringilla coelebs*. Ibis 100:535–570.

1029. Tindal, J. S., Beyer, C., and Sawyer, C. H. (1963) Milk ejection reflex and maintenance of lactation in the rabbit. Endocrinology 72:720–724.

1030. Tobet, S. A. and Baum, M. J. (1987) Role for prenatal estrogen in the development of masculine sexual behavior in the male ferret. Horm. Behav. 21:419–429.

1031. Tobet, S. A., Shim, J. H., Osiecki, S. T., Baum, M. J., and Canick, J. A. (1985) Androgen aromatization and 5α-reduction in ferret brain during perinatal development: Effects of sex and testosterone manipulation. Endocrinology 116:1869–1877.

1032. Tobias, M. L. and Kelley, D. B. (1987) Vocalizations by a sexually dimorphic isolated larynx: Peripheral constraints on behavioral expression. J. Neurosci. 7:3191–3197.

1033. Tobias, M. L. and Kelley, D. B. (1988) Electrophysiology and dye-coupling are sexually dimorphic characteristics of individual laryngeal muscle fibers in *Xenopus laevis*. J. Neurosci. 8:2422–2429.

1034. Tobias, M. L., Marin, M. L., and Kelley, D. B. (1991) Development of functional sex differences in the larynx of *Xenopus laevis*. Dev. Biol. 147:251–259.

1035. Tobias, M. L., Marin, M. L., and Kelley, D. B. (1991) Temporal constraints on androgen directed laryngeal masculinization in *Xenopus laevis*. Dev. Biol. 147:260–270.

1036. Todt, D., Hultsch, H., and Duvall, F. P., III (1981) Behavioral significance and social function of vocal and non-vocal displays in monogamous duet-singer *Cossypha heuglini* H. Zool. Beitr. 27:421–448.

1037. Tolman, J. and King, J. A. (1956) The effects of testosterone propionate on aggression in male and female C 57 B1/10 mice. Br. J. Anim. Behav. 6:147–149.

1038. Toran-Allerand, C. D. (1986) Sexual differentiation of the brain. In W. T. Greenough and J. M. Juraska (Eds.), Developmental Neuropsychobiology. Academic Press, New York, pp. 175–211.

1039. Toran-Allerand, C. D., MacLusky, N. J., Miranda, R. C., and Hochberg, R. B. (1990) Co-localization of estrogen receptor mRNA and protein in developing rat brain. Abstr. Soc. Neurosci. 16:327.

1040. Trivers, R. L. (1985) Social Evolution, Benjamin/Cummings Publishing, Menlo Park, Calif.

1041. Truman, J. W. (1971) Physiology of insect ecdysis. I. The eclosion behaviour of saturniid moths and its hormonal release. J. Exp. Biol. 54:805–814.

1042. Truman, J. W. (1978) Hormonal release of stereotyped motor programmes from the isolated nervous system of the Cecropia silkmoth. J. Exp. Biol. 74:151–174.

1043. Truman, J. W. (1980) Organization and hormonal release of stereotyped motor programs from the CNS of an insect. Front. Horm. Res. 6:1–15.

1044. Truman, J. W. (1984) The preparatory behavior rhythm of the moth Manduca sexta: An ecdysteroid-triggered circadian rhythm that is independent of the brain. J. Comp. Physiol. 155:521–528.

1045. Truman, J. W. (1985) Hormonal control of ecdysis. In G. A. Kerkut and L. I. Gilbert (Eds.), Comprehensive Insect Physiology, Biochemistry, and Pharmacology, Vol. 8. Pergamon Press, Oxford, pp. 413–440.

1046. Truman, J. W. (1988) Hormonal approaches for studying nervous system development in insects. Adv. Insect Physiol. 21:1–34.

1047. Truman, J. W. (1989) Interaction of steroid and peptide hormones in the regulation of insect behavior. In J. Erber, R. Menzel, H.-J. Pfluger, and D. Todt (Eds.), Neural Mechanisms of Behavior. G. Thieme Verlag, Stuttgart, pp. 67–72.

1048. Truman, J. W. and Copenhaver, P. F. (1989) The larval eclosion hormone neurones in Manduca sexta: Identification of the brain-proctodeal neurosecretory system. J. Exp. Biol. 147:457–470.

1049. Truman, J. W. and Endo, P. T. (1974) Physiology of insect ecdysis: Neural and hormonal factors involved in wing-spreading behaviour of moths. J. Exp. Biol. 61:47–55.

1050. Truman, J. W., Mumby, S. M., and Welch, S. K. (1980) Involvement of cyclic GMP in the release of stereotyped behaviour patterns in moths by a peptide hormone. J. Exp. Biol. 84:201–212.

1051. Truman, J. W. and Riddiford, L. M. (1970) Neuroendocrine control of ecdysis. Science 167:1624–1626.

1052. Truman, J. W., Rountree, D. B., Reiss, S. E., and Schwartz, L. M. (1983) Ecdysteroids regulate the release and action of eclosion hormone in the tobacco hornworm, Manduca sexta (L). J. Insect Physiol. 29:895–900.

1053. Tucker, D. M., Stenslie, C. E., Roth, R. S., and Shearer, S. L. (1981) Right frontal lobe activation and right hemisphere performance. Arch. Gen. Psychiat. 38:169–174.

1054. Turek, F. W. and Campbell, C. S. (1979) Photoperiodic regulation of neuroendocrine-gonadal activity. Biol. Reprod. 20:32–50.

1055. Turner, B. B. and Weaver, D. A. (1985) Sexual dimorphism of glucocorticoid binding in rat brain. Brain Res. 343:16–23.

1056. Tyler, L. E. (1965) The Psychology of Human Differences (3rd ed.). Appleton-Century-Crofts, New York.

1057. Tyler, M. J. and Carter, D. B. (1981) Oral birth of the young of the gastric brooding frog Rheobatrachus silus. Anim. Behav. 29:280–282.

1058. Ucker, D. (1987) Cytotoxic T lymphocytes and glucocorticoids activate an endogenous suicide process in target cells. Nature 327:62–64.

1059. Udry, J. R. and Morris, N. M. (1968) Distribution of coitus in the menstrual cycle. Nature 220:593–596.

1060. Uno, H., R. Tarara, R., Else, J. G., Suleman, M. A., and Sapolsky, R. M. (1989) Hippocampal damage associated with prolonged and fatal stress in primates. J. Neurosci. 9:1705–1711.

1061. Vandenberg, S. G. (1976) Mental Rotations Test. In R. B. Ekstrom, J. W. French, and H. H. Harmon (Eds.), Manual for Kit of Factor-Referenced Cognitive Tests. Educational Testing Service, Princeton, N.J. pp 21, 177.

1062. Vandenbergh, J. G. (1987) Regulation of puberty and its consequences on population dynamics of mice. Am. Zool. 27:891–898.

1063. Vandenbergh, J. G. (1988) Pheromones and mammalian reproduction. In E. Knobil et al. (Eds.), The Physiology of Reproduction. Raven Press, New York.

1064. Vandenbergh, J. G., Finlayson, J. S., Dobrogosz, W. J., Dills, S. S., and Kost, T. A. (1976) Chromatographic separation of puberty accelerating pheromone from male mouse urine. Biol. Reprod. 15:260–265.

1065. Van der Kloot, W. G. and Williams, C. M. (1953) Cocoon construction by the Cecropia silkworm. I. The role of the external environment. Behaviour 5:141–156.

1066. van Haaren, F. and van de Poll, N. E.(1984) The effect of a choice alternative on sex differences in passive avoidance behavior. Physiol. Behav. 32:211–215.

1067. van Haaren, F., M. Wouters, M., and van de Poll, N. E. (1987) Absence of behavioral differences between male and female rats in different radial-maze procedures. Physiol. Behav. 39:409–412.

1068. Van Hartesveldt, C. J., Cottrell, G. A., and Meyer, M. E. (1989) The effects of intrastriatal hormones on the dorsal immobility response in gonadectomized male and female rats. Pharmacol. Biochem. Behav. 34:459–463.

1069. Van Hartesveldt, C. J., Cottrell, G. A., and Meyer, M. E. (1990) Effects of intrastriatal hormones on the dorsal immobility response in male rats. Pharmacol. Biochem. Behav. 35:307–310.

1070. van Hest, A., Haaren, F. van, and van de Poll, N. E. (1987) Behavioral differences between male and female Wistar rats on DRL schedules: Effect of stimuli promoting collateral activities. Physiol. Behav. 39:255–261.

1071. van Leengoed, E., Kerker, E., and Swanson, H. H. (1987) Inhibition of post-partum maternal behaviour in the rat by injecting an oxytocin antagonist into the cerebral ventricles. J. Endocrinol. 112:275–282.

1072. Van Oortmerssen, G. A., Benus, I. and Dijk, D. J. (1985) Studies in wild house mice: Genotype-environment interactions for attack latency. Neth. J. Zool. 35(1,2):155–169.

1073. van Oyen, H. G., van de Poll, N. E., and de Bruin, J. (1980) Effects of retention interval and gonadectomy on sex differences in passive avoidance behavior. Physiol. Behav. 25:859–862.

1074. Verbalis, J. G., Blackburn, R. E., and Sticker, E. M. (1991) Naloxone inhibits sodium appetite in the hypovolemic rat by a mechanism involving central oxytocin. Soc. Neurosci. Abstr. 17:1190.

1075. Verbalis, J. G., McCann, M. J., McHale, C. M., and Stricker, E. M. (1986) Oxytocin secretion in response to cholecystokinin and food intake: Differentiation of nausea from satiety. Science 232:1417–1419.

1076. Verbalis, J. G., McHale, C. M., Gardiner, T. W., and Stricker, E. M. (1986) Oxytocin and vasopressin secretion in response to stimuli producing learned taste aversions in rats. Behav. Neurosci. 100:466–475.

1077. Verbalis, J. G. and Stricker, E. M. (1991) Cholecystokinin and neuroendocrine secretion. In C. A. Johnston and C. D. Barnes (Eds.), Brain-Gut Peptides and Reproductive Function. CRC Press, Boca Raton, Fla., pp. 209–237.

1078. Vignolo, L. A., Boccardi, E., and Caverni, L. (1986) Unexpected CT-scan findings in global aphasia. Cortex 22:55–69.

1079. vom Saal, F. S. (1979) Prenatal exposure to androgen influences morphology and aggressive behavior of male and female mice. Horm. Behav. 12:1–11.

1080. vom Saal, F. S. (1983) Models of early hormonal effects on intrasex aggression in mice. In B. B. Svare (Ed.), Hormones and Aggressive Behavior. Plenum, New York, pp. 197–222.

1081. vom Saal F. S., Gandelman, R., and Svare, B. (1976) Aggression in male and female mice: Evidence for changed neural sensitivity in response to neonatal but not adult androgen exposure. Physiol. Behav. 17:53–57.

1082. Vreeburg, J. T. M., Schretlen, P. J. M., and Baum, M. J. (1975) Specific, high-affinity binding of estradiol in cytosols from several brain regions and pituitary of intact and castrated adult male rats. Endocrinology 97:969–977.

1082a. Wada, J. (1976) Sex differences in brain asymmetry. International Neuropsychological Society, June 21–24, Toronto, Canada.

1083. Wada, J. A., Clarke, R., and Hamm, A. (1975) Cerebral hemispheric asymmetry in humans. Arch. Neurol. 32:239–246.

1084. Wade, G. N. and Zucker, I. (1970) Modulation of food intake and locomotor activity in female rats by diencephalic hormone implants. J. Comp. Physiol. Psychol. 72:328–336.

1085. Wallen, K. (1982) Social organization in the dusky-footed woodrat (*Neotoma fuscipes*): A field and laboratory study. Anim. Behav. 30:1171–1182.

1086. Wallen, K. (1990) Desire and ability: Hormones and the regulation of female sexual behavior. Neurosci. Biobehav. Rev. 14:233–241.

1087. Walsh, R. J., Slaby, F. J., and Posner, B. I. (1987) A receptor-mediated mechanism for the transport of prolactin from blood to cerebrospinal fluid. Endocrinology 120:1846–1850.

1088. Ward, I. L. and Reed, J. (1985) Prenatal stress and prepubertal social rearing conditions interact to determine sexual behavior in male rats. Behav. Neurosci. 99:301–309.

1089. Warren, M. (1983) Effects of undernutrition on reproductive function in the huyman. Endocrinol. Rev. 4:363–377.

1090. Wasser, S. K. and Barash, D. P. (1983) Reproductive suppression among female mammals: Implications for biomedicine and sexual selection theory. Q. Rev. Biol. 58:513–538.

1091. Wearing, M. P., Yuhosz, M. D., Campbell, R., and Love, E. J. (1972) The effect of the menstrual cycle on tests of physical fitness. J. Sports Med. 12:38–41.

1092. Weeks, J. C. and Truman, J. W. (1984) Neural organization of peptide-activated ecdysis behaviors during metamorphosis in *Manduca sexta*. I. Conservation of the peristalsis motor pattern at the larval-pupal transformation. J. Comp. Physiol. [A] 155:407–422.

1093. Weeks, J. C. and Truman, J. W. (1984) Neural organization of peptide-activated ecdysis behaviors during metamorphosis in *Manduca sexta*. II. Retention of the proleg motor pattern despite loss of the prolegs at pupation. J. Comp. Physiol. A 155:423–435.

1094. Weeks, J. C. and Truman, J. W. (1985) Independent steroid control of the fates of motoneurons and their muscles during insect metamorphosis. J. Neurosci. 5:2290–2300.

1095. Weiss, J. (1970) Somatic effects of predictable and unpredictable shock. Psychosom. Med. 32:397–414.

1096. Wells, K. (1977) The social behavior of anuran amphibians. Anim. Behav. 25:666–693.

1097. Wetzel, D., Haerter, U., and Kelley, D. (1985) A proposed efferent pathway for mate calling of male South African clawed frogs, *Xenopus laevis*. J. Comp. Physiol. [A] 157:749–761.

1098. Wetzel, D. and Kelley, D. (1983) Androgen and gonadotropin control of the mate calls of male South African clawed frogs, *Xenopus laevis*. Horm. Behav. 17:388–404.

1099. Whalen, R. E. (1977) Current issues in the neurobiology of sexual differentiation. In A. Vernadski and P. S. Timiras (Eds.). Hormones in Development and Aging. Spectrum Publications, New York.

1099a. Whishaw, I. Q., Kolb, B., and Sutherland, R. J. (1983) The analysis of behavior in the laboratory rat. In T. E. Robinson (Ed.), Behavioral Approaches to Brain Research. Oxford University Press, New York, pp. 141–202.

1100. Wickham, M. (1958) The effects of the menstrual cycle on test performance. Br. J. Psychol. 49:34–41.

1101. Wiesner, J. B. and Moss, R. L. (1989) A psychopharmacological characterization of the opioid suppression of sexual behaviour in the female rat. In R. G. Dyer and R. J. Bicknell (Eds.), Brain Opioid Systems in Reproduction. Oxford University Press, Oxford, pp. 187–202.

1102. Williams, C. L., Barnett, A. M., and Meck, W. H. (1990) Organizational effects of early gonadal secretions on sexual differentiation in spatial memory. Behav. Neurosci. 104:84–97.

1103. Wilson, F. E. (1991) Neither retinal nor pineal photoreceptors mediate photoperiodic control of seasonal reproduction in American tree sparrows (*Spizella arborea*). J. Exp. Zool. 259:117–127.

1103a. Wilson, J. D., George, F. W., and Griffin, J. E. (1981) The hormonal control of sexual development. Science 211:1278–1284.

1104. Wilson, J. R. and Vandenberg, S. G. (1978) Sex differences in cognition: Evidence from the Hawaii family study. In T. E. McGill, D. A. Dewsbury, and B. D. Sachs (Eds.), Sex and Behavior: Status and Prospectus. Plenum, New York, pp. 317–335.

1105. Winans, S. S., Lehman, M. N., and Powers, J. B. (1982) Vomeronasal and olfactory CNS pathways that control male hamster mating behavior. In W. Breipohl (Ed.), Olfaction and Endocrine Regulation. IRL Press, Oxford.

1106. Wingfield, J. C., Hegner, R. E., Dufty, A. M., and Ball, G. F. (1990) The "challenge hypothesis": Theoretical implications for patterns of testosterone secretion, mating systems and breeding strategies of birds. Am. Nat. 136:829–846.

1107. Witelson, S. F. (1985) The brain connection: The corpus callosum is larger in left-handers. Science 229:665–668.

1108. Witkin, H. A. and Berry, J. W. (1975) Psychological differentiation in cross-cultural perspective. J. Cross-Cult. Psychol. 6:4–87.

1109. Witt, D. M., Carter, C. S., and Walton, D. M. (1990) Central and peripheral effects of oxytocin administration in prairie voles (*Microtus ochrogaster*). Pharmacol. Biochem. Behav. 36:63–69.

1110. Wolff, C., Friedman, S., hofeer, M., Mason, J. (1964) Relationship between psychologic defenses and mean urinary 17-hydroxycorticosteroid excretion rates. Psychosom. Med. 26:576–583.

1111. Wong, R. and Judd, M. (1973) Infantile handling and successive spatial reversal learning in rats. Behav. Biol. 8:391–398.

1112. Wong, S. and Tong, J. E. (1974) Menstrual cycle and contraceptive hormonal effects on temporal discrimination. Percept. Mot. Skills 39:103–108.

1113. Woodfield, R. L. (1984) Embedded figures test performance before and after childbirth. Br. J. Psychol. 75:81–88.

1114. Woods, S. C. and Porte, D., Jr. (1974) Neural control of the endocrine pancreas. Physiol. Rev. 54:596–619.

1115. Woods, S. C. and Porte, D., Jr. (1978) The central nervous system, pancreatic hormones, feeding, and obesity. In R. Levine and R. Luft (Eds.), Advances in Metabolic Disorders, Vol. 9. Academic Press, New York, pp. 283–312.

1116. Wray, S., Grant, P., and Gainer, H. (1989) Evidence that cells expressing luteinizing hormone-releasing hormone mRNA in the mouse are derived from progenitor cells in the olfactory placode. Proc. Natl. Acad. Sci. U.S.A. 86:8132–8136.

1117. Wuttke, W., Arnold, P., Becker, D., Creutzfeldt, O., Langenstein, S., and Tirsch, W. (1975) Circulating hormones, EEG, and performance in psychological tests of women with and without oral contraceptives. Psychoneuroendocrinology 1:141–151.

1118. Wuttke, W., Arnold, P., Becker, D., Creutzfeldt, O., Langenstein, S., and Tirsch, W. (1976) Hormonal profiles and variations of the EEG and of performances in psychological tests in women with spontaneous menstrual cycles and under oral contraceptives. In T. M. Itil, G. Laudahn, and W. M. Herrman (Eds.), Psychotropic Action of Hormones. Spectrum, New York, pp. 169–182.

1119. Yaeger, D. (1982) A novel mechanism for underwater sound production in *Xenopus borealis*. Am. Zool. 122:887.

1120. Yalcinkaya, T., Glickman, S. E., and Licht, P. Virilization of the female spotted hyena (SH) in utero. Endocr. Soc. Abstr. June 1991.

1121. Yalom, I. D., Green, R., and Fisk, N. (1973) Prenatal exposure to female hormones: Effect on psychosexual development in boys. Arch. Gen. Psychiat. 28:554–561.

1122. Yamada, Y. (1979) Effects of testosterone on unit activity in rat hypothalamus and septum. Brain Res. 172:165–168.

1123. Yamamoto, J. T., Shields, K. M., Millam, J. R., Roudybush, T. E., and Grau, C. R. (1989) Reproductive activity of force-paired cockatiels (*Nymphicus Hollandicus*). The Auk 106:86–93.

1124. Yates, F. E. (1982) Outline of a physical theory of physiological systems. Can. J. Physiol. Pharmacol. 60:217–248.

1125. Yeo, J. A. G. and Keverne, E. G. (1986) The importance of vaginal-cervical stimulation for maternal behaviour in the rat. Physiol. Behav. 37:23–26.

1126. Yogev, L. and Terkel, J. (1980) Effects of photoperiod, absence of photic cues, and suprachiasmatic nucleus lesions on nocturnal prolactin surges in pregnant and pseudopregnant rats. Neuroendocrinology 31:26–33.

1127. Yogev, L. and Terkel, J. (1980) Timing of termination of nocturnal prolactin surges in pregnant rats as determined by the number of fetuses. J. Endocrinol. 84:421–424.

1128. Yokoyama K. and Farner, D. S. (1976) Photoperiodic responses in bilaterally enucleated white-crowned sparrows, *Zonotrichia leucophrys* gambelii. Gen. Comp. Endocrinol. 30:528–533.

1129. Zabel, C. J., Glickman, S. E., Frank, L. G., Woodmansee, K., and Keppel, G. (in press) Coalition formation in a colony of prepubertal spotted hyenas. In A. Harcourt and F. W. DeWaal (Eds.), Cooperation in Competition in Animals and Humans. Oxford University Press, Oxford.

1130. Zacharias, L. and Wurtman, R. J. (1964) Blindness: Its relation to age of menarche. Science 144:1154–1155.

1131. Zaharieva, E. (1965) Survey of sportswomen at the Tokyo Olympics. J. Sports Med. Phys. Fitness 5:215–219.

1132. Zakon, H. (1986) The electroreceptive periphery. In T. Bullock and W. Heiligenberg (Eds.), Electroreception. Wiley & Sons, New York, pp. 103–156.

1133. Zakon, H. (1987) Hormone mediated plasticity in the electrosensory system of weakly electric fish. Trends Neurosci. 10:416–421.

1134. Zakon, H., Thomas, P., and Yan, H.-Y. (1991) Plasma steroids, reproductive state and electric organ discharge in a natural population of the weakly electric fish *Sternopygus macrurus*. J. Comp. Physiol. [A]

1135. Zarrow, M. X., Denenberg, V. H., and Anderson, C. O. (1965) Rabbit: Frequency of suckling in the pup. Science 150:1835–1836.

1136. Zarrow, M. X., Gandelman, R. T., and Denenberg, V. H. (1971) Prolactin: Is it an essential hormone for maternal behavior in mammals? Horm. Behav. 2:343–354.

1137. Zimmerman, E. and Parlee, M. B. (1973) Behavioral changes associated with the menstrual cycle: An experimental investigation. J. Appl. Soc. Psychol. 3:335–344.

1138. Zucker, I. (1988) Neuroendocrine substrates of circannual rhythms. In D. J. Kupfer, T. H. Monk, and J. D. Barchas (Eds.), Biological Rhythms and Mental Disorders. Guilford Press, New York, pp. 219–251.

1139. Zucker, I., Cramer, C. P., and Bittman, E. L. (1980) Regulation by the pituitary gland of circadian rhythms in the hamster. J. Endocrinol. 85:17–25.

1140. Zucker, I., Fitzgerald, K. M., and Morin, L. P. (1980) Sex differentiation of the circadian system in the golden hamster. Am. J. Physiol. 238:R97–R101.

1141. Zucker, I., Johnston, P. G., and Frost, D. (1980) Comparative, physiological, and biochronometric analyses of rodent seasonal reproductive cycles. Prog. Reprod. Biol. 5:102–133.

1142. Zucker, I., Lee, T. M., and Dark, J. (1991) The suprachiasmatic nucleus and annual rhythms in mammals. In D. C. Klein, S. M. Reppert, and R. Y. Moore (Eds.), The Suprachiasmatic Nucleus: The Mind's Clock. Elsevier, New York.

1143. Zupanc, G. and Heiligenberg, W. (1989) Sexual maturity-dependent changes in neuronal morphology in the prepacemaker nucleus of adult weakly electric knifefish, *Eigenmannia*. J. Neurosci 9:3816–3827.

Index